Coronary Atherosclerosis

Coronary Atherosclerosis
Current Management and Treatment

Edited by

Chourmouzios Arampatzis, MD, PhD, FESC
Interbalkan Medical Center, Thessaloniki, Greece

Eugène P. McFadden, MD, FESC, FACC
Department of Cardiology, Cork University Hospital, Cork, Ireland

Lampros K. Michalis, MD, PhD, MRCP (UK), FESC
Department of Cardiology, Medical School, University of Ioannina, Ioannina, Greece

Renu Virmani, MD
CVPath Institute, Inc., Gaithersburg, MD, USA

Patrick W. Serruys, MD
Interventional Department, Heartcenter Rotterdam, Rotterdam, The Netherlands
Thoraxcenter, Erasmus Medical Center, Rotterdam, The Netherlands

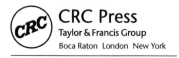

CRC Press
Taylor & Francis Group
Boca Raton London New York

CRC Press is an imprint of the
Taylor & Francis Group, an **informa** business

First published in 2012 by Informa Healthcare

Published 2020 by CRC Press
Taylor & Francis Group
6000 Broken Sound Parkway NW, Suite 300
Boca Raton, FL 33487-2742

First issued in paperback 2020

© 2012 by Taylor & Francis Group, LLC
CRC Press is an imprint of Taylor & Francis Group, an Informa business

No claim to original U.S. Government works

ISBN 13: 9780-3-675-7669-1 (pbk)
ISBN 13: 978-1-84184-853-2 (hbk)

Visit the Taylor & Francis Web site at
http://www.taylorandfrancis.com

and the CRC Press Web site at
http://www.crcpress.com

A CIP record for this book is available from the British Library.

Typeset by Exeter Premedia Services Private Ltd, Chennai, India

Dedication

To our friend and colleague Prof Wim van der Giessen 1954–2011.

Clinician and Scientist, Erasmus University, Rotterdam.

Contents

Recommended and key papers appear as shaded references at the end of each chapter.

Contents of online material

To access the extra online material for chapters 12, 13, 20, 32 and 34, you will need first to register at our website; https://informahealthcare.com/action/registration. Upon completion of the registration process, you will have the necessary login details. If you have previously registered, there is no need to register again.

After you have completed the registration procedure, please type the following link in your Web browser: http://informahealthcare.com/9781841848549/extras. The opening page will request your login details and, after signing in, the material listed below will be available for viewing.

Contributors

Takashi Akasaka
Department of Cardiovascular Medicine, Wakayama Medical University, Wakayama, Japan

Mario Albertucci
Interventional Cardiology, San Giovanni Hospital, Centro per la Lotta contro l'Infarto (CLI) Foundation, Rome, Italy

Dimitrios Alexopoulos
Cardiology Department, Patras University Hospital, Greece

Carlos L. Alviar
Zena and Michael A. Wiener Cardiovascular Institute, The Marie-Josee and Henry R. Kravis Cardiovascular Health Center, The Mount Sinai School of Medicine, NY, USA

John A. Ambrose
University of California San Francisco School of Medicine, Fresno, CA, USA

Dominick J. Angiolillo
University of Florida College of Medicine-Jacksonville, FL, USA

Antonios P. Antoniadis
Cardiovascular Division, Brigham and Women's Hospital, Harvard Medical School, Boston, MA, USA

Aris Bechlioulis
Department of Cardiology and Michaelidion Cardiac Center, University of Ioannina, Ioannina, Greece

Jan Bogaert
Radiology Department, Medical Imaging Research Center, University Hospitals Leuven, Herestraat Leuven, Belgium

Manolis Bountioukos
Thoraxcenter, Erasmus Medical Center, Rotterdam, The Netherlands

Emmanouil S. Brilakis
Dallas VA Medical Center, Dallas, TX, USA

Salvatore Brugaletta
Thoraxcenter, Erasmus Medical Center, Rotterdam, The Netherlands Thorax Institute, Department of Cardiology, Hospital Clinic, Barcelona, Spain

Andrew Cassar
Division of Cardiovascular Diseases, Mayo College of Medicine, Rochester, MN, USA

Kuang-Yuh Chyu
Oppenheimer Atherosclerosis Research Center, the Division of Cardiology and Cedars Sinai Heart Institute, Cedars Sinai Medical Center, Los Angeles, CA, USA

Antonio Colombo
EMO-GVM Centro Cuore Columbus, Milan, Italy

Filippo Crea
Institute of Cardiology, Catholic University, Rome, Italy

Pim J. de Feyter
Department of Radiology, Erasmus Medical Center, Rotterdam, The Netherlands Thoraxcenter, Erasmus Medical Center, Rotterdam, The Netherlands

Dominique de Kleijn
Laboratory of Experimental Cardiology, Utrecht, The Netherlands

Giuseppe De Luca
Division of Cardiology, 'Maggiore della Carità' Hospital, Università del Piemonte Orientale 'A. Avogadro', Novara, Italy

Ranil de Silva
National Heart and Lung Institute, Imperial College London, UK NIHR Biomedical Research Unit, Royal Brompton and Harefield NHS Foundation Trust, UK

Maria Drakopoulou
First Department of Cardiology, Hippokration Hospital, Athens Medical School, Athens, Greece

William F. Fearon
Division of Cardiovascular Medicine, Stanford University Medical Center, CA, USA

Charles L. Feldman
Cardiovascular Division, Brigham and Women's Hospital, Harvard Medical School, Boston, MA, USA

Eleonora Ficarra
Interventional Cardiology, San Giovanni Hospital, Centro per la Lotta contro l'Infarto (CLI) Foundation, Rome, Italy

Peter J. Fitzgerald
Division of Cardiovascular Medicine, Stanford University Medical Center, Stanford, CA, USA

Kim Fox
National Heart and Lung Institute,
Imperial College London, UK
NIHR Biomedical Research Unit,
Royal Brompton and Harefield NHS Foundation Trust, UK

Hector M. Garcia-Garcia
Thoraxcenter, Erasmus Medical Center, Rotterdam,
The Netherlands

Panagiota Georgiadou
2nd Division of Interventional Cardiology, Onassis Cardiac
Surgery Center, Athens, Greece

Bernard J. Gersh
Division of Cardiovascular Diseases,
Mayo College of Medicine, Rochester, MN, USA

Chrysafios Girasis
Interventional Cardiology, Thoraxcenter, Erasmus Medical
Center, Rotterdam, The Netherlands

Luca Golino
UOC Emodinamica/UTIC/Cardiologia – Belcolle Hospital,
Viterbo, Italy

Zhihua He
InfraReDx, Inc., Burlington, MA, USA

Imo Hoefer
Laboratory of Experimental Cardiology, Utrecht,
The Netherlands

Yasuhiro Honda
Division of Cardiovascular Medicine,
Stanford University Medical Center, Stanford, CA, USA

Krista Jansen
Thoraxcenter, Erasmus Medical Center, Rotterdam,
The Netherlands

Juan Carlos Kaski
Cardiovascular Sciences Research Centre,
Division of Clinical Sciences, St George's Hospital,
University of London, London, UK

Kazuhisa Kodama
Cardiovascular Division, Osaka Police Hospital,
Tennoji-ku, Osaka, Japan

Frank D. Kolodgie
CVPath Institute, Inc., Gaithersburg, MD, USA

Takashi Kubo
Department of Cardiovascular Medicine,
Wakayama Medical University, Wakayama, Japan

Gaetano Antonio Lanza
Institute of Cardiology, Catholic University, Rome, Italy

Joel A. Lardizabal
Cardiology Division, Department of Medicine,
University California San Francisco School of Medicine,
Fresno MEP, Fresno, CA, USA

Azeem Latib
EMO-GVM Centro Cuore Columbus, Milan, Italy

Pedro A. Lemos
Heart Institute (InCor), University of Sao Paulo Medical School,
Sao Paulo, Brazil Hospital Sirio Libanes, Sao Paulo, Brazil

Sean P. Madden
InfraReDx, Inc., Burlington, MA, USA

Pier Giorgio Masci
Fondazione C.N.R/Regione Toscana 'G.Monasterio'
Katholieke Universiteit Leuven
Leuven - Belgium

Lampros K. Michalis
Department of Cardiology and Michaelidion Cardiac Center,
University of Ioannina, Ioannina, Greece

Archontoula Michelongona
First Department of Cardiology, Hippokration Hospital,
Athens Medical School, Athens, Greece

Pedro R. Moreno
Zena and Michael A. Wiener Cardiovascular Institute, The
Marie-Josee and Henry R. Kravis Cardiovascular Health Center,
The Mount Sinai School of Medicine, New York, NY, USA

James E. Muller
InfraReDx, Inc., Burlington, MA, USA

Katerina K. Naka
Department of Cardiology and Michaelidion Cardiac Center,
University of Ioannina, Ioannina, Greece

Masataka Nakano
Cardiovascular Research Fellow
CVPath Institute, Inc.

Koen Nieman
Department of Radiology, Erasmus Medical Center, Rotterdam,
The Netherlands
Thoraxcenter, Erasmus Medical Center, Rotterdam,
The Netherlands

Peter Ong
Cardiovascular Sciences Research Centre, Division of Clinical
Sciences, St George's Hospital, University of London, London, UK

Michail I. Papafaklis
Cardiovascular Division, Brigham and Women's Hospital, Harvard Medical School, Boston, MA, USA

Gerard Pasterkamp
Laboratory of Experimental Cardiology, Utrecht, The Netherlands

Francesco Prati
Interventional Cardiology, San Giovanni Hospital, Centro per la Lotta contro l'Infarto (CLI) Foundation, Rome, Italy

Vito Ramazzotti
Interventional Cardiology, San Giovanni Hospital, Centro per la Lotta contro l'Infarto (CLI) Foundation, Rome, Italy

G. Russell Reiss
Center for Interventional Vascular Therapy and Department of Cardiothoracic Surgery, New York-Presbyterian Hospital, Columbia University, College of Physicians and Surgeons, New York, NY, USA

Francesco Saia
Institute of Cardiology, University of Bologna, Policlinico S. Orsola-Malpighi, Bologna, Italy

Kenji Sakamoto
Division of Cardiovascular Medicine, Stanford University Medical Center, Stanford, CA, USA

Arend F.L. Schinkel
Thoraxcenter, Department of Cardiology, Erasmus Medical Center, Rotterdam, The Netherlands

Gregory Angelo Sgueglia
UOC Emodinamica e Cardiologia Interventistica, Ospedale Santa Maria Goretti, Latina, Italy

Prediman K. Shah
Oppenheimer Atherosclerosis Research Center, the Division of Cardiology and Cedars Sinai Heart Institute, Cedars Sinai Medical Center, Los Angeles, CA, USA

Joanne Shannon
EMO-GVM Centro Cuore Columbus, Milan, Italy

Christodoulos Stefanadis
First Department of Cardiology, Hippokration Hospital, Athens Medical School, Athens, Greece

Peter H. Stone
Cardiovascular Division, Brigham and Women's Hospital, Harvard Medical School, Boston, MA, USA

Stephen T. Sum
InfraReDx, Inc., Burlington, MA, USA

Saeko Takahashi
Cardiovascular Division, Brigham and Women's Hospital, Harvard Medical School, Boston, MA, USA

Antonio Tello-Montoliu
University of Florida College of Medicine-Jacksonville, FL, USA

Gert-Jan R. ten Kate
Department of Radiology, Erasmus Medical Center, Rotterdam, The Netherlands
Thoraxcenter, Erasmus Medical Center, Rotterdam, The Netherlands
Interuniversity Cardiology Institute of the Netherlands, Utrecht, The Netherlands

Konstantinos Toutouzas
First Department of Cardiology, Hippokration Hospital, Athens Medical School, Athens, Greece

Eleftherios Tsiamis
First Department of Cardiology, Hippokration Hospital, Athens Medical School, Athens, Greece

Yasunori Ueda
Cardiovascular Division, Osaka Police Hospital, Tennoji-ku, Osaka, Japan

Ton van der Steen
Thoraxcenter, Erasmus Medical Center, Rotterdam, The Netherlands
Interuniversity Cardiology Institute of the Netherlands, Utrecht, The Netherlands

Gijs van Soest
Thoraxcenter, Erasmus Medical Center, Rotterdam, The Netherlands

Renu Virmani
President and Medical Director, CVPath Institute, Inc., Gaithersburg, MD, USA

Vassilis Voudris
2nd Division of Interventional Cardiology, Onassis Cardiac Surgery Center, Athens, Greece

Mathew R. Williams
Cardiovascular Transcatheter Therapies, Center for Interventional Vascular Therapy, New York-Presbyterian Hospital, Columbia University, New York, NY, USA
Department of Cardiothoracic Surgery, College of Physicians and Surgeons, New York, NY, USA

Ioanna Xanthopoulou
Cardiology Department, Patras University Hospital, Greece

Foreword

At a time when the number of cardiovascular journals is climbing exponentially, and the number of investigative and treatment options for patients with coronary artery disease (CAD) is growing at such a rapid pace, the launch of a comprehensive and definitive textbook in the burgeoning field of coronary atherosclerosis is timely indeed. It is my privilege to write this foreword and I can say, as someone who has worked for many years with CAD patients, that this text brings together all the relevant information in a superbly crafted manner. This book is a rich new resource for the cardiovascular community, and I commend the authors and editors for their efforts.

Allow me to explain the massive scope of the literature that now exists, and the need for a concise book that synthesizes this data. A quick search in PubMed using the term "coronary atherosclerosis" (taken directly from the title of this book), brings up some 121,000 references - a staggering number of papers. However, on breaking this down, the recent data explosion in coronary atherosclerosis becomes apparent. From 1900–1960 there were 694 publications; 1377 publications from 1960-70; 5927 from 1970 -80; 15797 from 1980–90; 30582 from 1990–2000; and 53186 from 2000–2010. In just the 2½ years from 2010–mid 2012, there were 16029 publications on coronary atherosclerosis, being more than the entire decade from 1980–1990! Clearly, there is no possibility that any researcher or clinician could hope to individually cover this literature. For some time the prevailing view was that guidelines and summary statements were the solution, but there are now so many of these documents in existence, emerging from numerous societies, and with new iterations and updates constantly appearing, even these are becoming overwhelming.

It is with this looming threat of information overload that Drs. Arampatzis, McFadden, Michalis, Virmani and Serruys saw a major unmet need, and set themselves the task of distilling this vast literature and producing a definitive text on the pathology, diagnosis and treatment of coronary atherosclerosis. These editors systematically sought out the current global thought leaders in this field and together they have laid out a book that logically steps through all the important elements. As it was my great pleasure to discover on reading this book, the sum of the individual parts here are far greater than the whole, and the writing team do a superb job in covering the full breadth and width of coronary atherosclerosis. The book begins exactly where it should – basic atherosclerotic pathobiology. The second section deals with imaging and diagnosis, first non-invasive and then invasive, covering topical modalities like fractional flow reserve and optical coherence tomography. Here, both interventional and non-interventional readers can take away many insights. The third section moves to treatment, starting with primary prevention and then sequentially covering relevant topics like risk stratification, pharmacotherapy,

NSTEMI, STEMI and microvascular angina. The book concludes with diverse perspectives on salient aspects such as the choice of bypass surgery versus percutaneous revascularization, long term outcomes and emerging therapies. In short, no stone is left unturned in this well balanced book.

The job description of a contemporary general physician, or even cardiologist, extends well beyond CAD. However, nobody would argue that coronary atherosclerosis remains the bread and butter of a great part of our daily clinical practice. Combined with the current intense research interest in this field and data explosion, "Coronary Atherosclerosis Current Management and Treatment" seems set to become an instant "go to" book. I'd advise all those just beginning with this book to clear ample space on your desk – this is not a text you will be filing away on a shelf. Bravo!

Valentin Fuster, MD, PhD
Physician-in-Chief, The Mount Sinai Medical Center, New York, USA
Director, Mount Sinai Heart, New York, USA
General Director, The Centro Nacional de Investigaciones Cardiovasculares (CNIC), Madrid, Spain
Past President, American Heart Association
Past President, World Heart Federation

Preface

In recent decades, new insights into the pathophysiology of coronary atherosclerosis, coupled with advances in imaging, the advent of appropriately powered randomized trials with relevant clinical endpoints, and the remarkable advances in the percutaneous and surgical techniques at our disposal, have resulted in dramatic changes in the management of patients with diverse presentations of coronary atherosclerosis.

For cardiologists training in the multiple sub-specialties that make up modern cardiology, it is difficult to imagine an era when the management of patients with heart disease was predominantly undertaken by physicians trained in general internal medicine, whose clinical acumen was supplemented by the meager diagnostic tools and limited therapeutic options available to them. Conversely, for those, with diverse backgrounds, who currently care for patients with coronary atherosclerosis, the pace of developments in the field has been so rapid that may prove difficult to determine which of the many novel risk factors, imaging techniques, and therapies are relevant to their daily practice.

Our aim is to provide established cardiologists and those in training with a comprehensive overview of the recent advances in the pathophysiology, diagnosis, and treatment of coronary atherosclerosis by key opinion leaders in the field.

The first section provides an overview of recent advances in the pathophysiology of atherosclerosis, of the role of conventional risk factors for coronary atherosclerosis, and looks at the potential of genomic and proteomic analysis to guide clinical management. It is completed by a clinical perspective on the current classification stratagems for patients who present with coronary disease and on the pivotal role of biomarkers in stratifying the risk of future clinical events.

The second section addresses the potential role of established and novel non-invasive and invasive techniques as aids to the diagnosis, risk stratification, and management of the patient with known or suspected coronary disease. It begins with an overview of the pivotal importance of the initial clinical assessment of the patient presenting with chest pain. It continues with a reassessment of basic non-invasive techniques in the initial evaluation of the patient with suspected coronary atherosclerosis and provides a critical evaluation of how newer non-invasive techniques might refine our approach to risk stratification by their ability to assess coronary anatomy and left ventricular function or to identify patients who will benefit from revascularization. Furthermore, it examines established and novel techniques that purport to evaluate the functional impact of atherosclerosis or the potential of atherosclerotic plaque to provide the substrate for future coronary events and looks at their putative role in guiding clinical decision making. Finally, it explores the relative strengths and weaknesses of currently available imaging tools for diagnosis and to guide treatment.

The third section provides a practical clinical approach to the treatment of patients with diverse clinical presentations of coronary disease. It highlights the pivotal role of primary and secondary prevention and reviews currently available pharmacologic agents. In addition it summarizes, in a clinically orientated fashion, the management of patients with different aspects of this multi-faceted disease.

The final section allows proponents of the different approaches to the treatment of coronary disease to present their perspective on current management strategies. It continues with an evidence-based assessment of the long-term results of percutaneous and surgical approaches and concludes with a perspective on future therapeutic options.

We hope that the contemporary knowledge, presented in this book by acknowledged leaders in the field, will provide the practicing clinician with a companion to optimize patient management.

Ch. Arampatzis, E.P. McFadden,
July 2012

Abbreviations

AACE	American Association of Clinical Endocrinologists
ABC	ATP-binding cassette
ACC	American College of Cardiology
ACE-I	angiotensin converting enzyme inhibitors
ACS	acute coronary syndrome
ADA	American Diabetes Association
AHA	American Heart Association
AMI	acute myocardial infarction
ARB	angiotensin receptor blocker
ARIC	Atherosclerosis Risk in Communities
ASA	acetyl salicylic acid
AVR	aortic valve replacement
BA	bifurcation angle
BIMA	bilateral internal mammary artery
BMI	body mass index
BMS	bare metal stent
CABG	coronary artery bypass grafting
CAC	coronary artery calcification
CAD	coronary artery disease
CKD	chronic kidney disease
CRP	high sensitivity C-reactive protein
CSA	chronic stable angina
CT	computed tomography
CT-CA	computed tomography coronary angiography
CTO	chronic total occlusion
CV	cardiovascular
CVD	cardiovascular disease
DASH	dietary approaches to stop hypertension
DBP	diastolic blood pressure
DCM	dilated cardiomyopathy
DES	drug-eluting stent
DM	diabetes mellitus
DMV	distal main vessel
DS	percent diameter stenosis
EAS	European Atherosclerosis Society
EASD	European Association for the Study of Diabetes
EBCT	electron beam CT
EPC	endothelial progenitor cells
ESC	European Society of Cardiology
ESH	European Society of Hypertension
FFR	fractional flow reserve
FH	familial hypercholesterolemia
FRS	Framingham Risk Score
GWAS	Genomewide association studies
HbA1c	glycated hemoglobin
HCR	hybrid coronary revascularization
HDL-c	high density lipoprotein cholesterol

HPR	healed plaque ruptures
HRT	hormone replacement therapy
HU	Houndsfield units
IB	integrated backscatter
ICA	invasive coronary angiography
IDF	International Diabetes Federation
IVOCT	intravascular optical coherence tomography
IVPA	intravascular photoacoustics
IVUS	intravascular ultrasound
LAD	left anterior descending
LCM	laser capture microdissection
LCP	lipid core plaque
LDL-c	low density lipoprotein cholesterol
LIMA	left internal mammary artery
LV	left ventricle
LVH	left ventricular hypertrophy
MACE	major adverse cardiac event
MI	myocardial infraction
MIDCAB	minimally invasive direct coronary artery bypass grafting
MLA/MLD	minimum lumen area/diameter
MMPs	matrix metalloproteinases
MPO	myeloperoxidase
MSCT	multi-slice computed tomography
NICE	National Institute of Health and Clinical Excellence
NIRS	near infrared reflection spectroscopy
OCT	optical coherence tomography
OMT	optimal medical therapy
OPCAB	off-pump coronary bypass
OR	operating room
PA	photoacoustics
PCI	percutaneous coronary intervention
PIT	pathologic intimal thickening
PMV	proximal main vessel
PROCAM	PROspective CArdiovascular Munster
PUFA	polyunsaturated fatty acids
QCA	quantitative coronary angiography
RVD	reference vessel diameter
SB	side-branch
SBP	systolic blood pressure
SCD	sudden coronary death; sudden cardiac death
SCORE	Systematic COronary Risk Evaluation
SMC	smooth muscle cell
SNP	single nucleotide polymorphism
STEMI	ST elevation myocardial infarction
SVG	saphenous vein graft
TAVR	transcatheter aortic valve replacement

TCFA	thin-cap fibroatheroma		2-D/3-D	two-dimensional/three-dimensional
TECAB	total endoscopic coronary bypass grafting		US	ultrasound
TIMI	thrombolysis in myocardial infarction		VH	virtual histology
TLR	target lesion revasularization			

1   Current concepts of plaque formation and the progression of atherosclerosis
Masataka Nakano, Renu Virmani, and Frank D. Kolodgie

OUTLINE

The 1994 American Heart Association classification incompletely described the variety of human atherosclerotic coronary lesions that lead to coronary thrombosis. In the modified classification, descriptive terminology was used to classify lesion diversity: adaptive intimal thickening, intimal xanthoma, pathologic intimal thickening, fibroatheroma, and thin-cap fibroatheroma as a precursor lesion to plaque rupture. Two other lesions that lead to thrombosis were also included and designated as plaque erosion and calcified nodule. This classification identified other forms of plaque events observed in sudden coronary death cases that represent asymptomatic events. These included healed plaque rupture lesions which were shown to cause luminal narrowing and are likely precursors of plaque progression and possible initiators of stable angina.

The process of atherosclerotic development involves a variety of factors including lipid accumulation at the initial stage, macrophage infiltration and apoptosis, intraplaque hemorrhage, oxidative stress, and matrix metalloproteases that lead to fibrous cap thinning with eventual rupture. Numerous studies have been conducted that focus on plaque rupture; however, the general understanding of disease progression, as described in this chapter, should be helpful in determining appropriate treatment for patients with various stages of plaque morphology that underlie the diverse clinical presentations of coronary atherosclerosis.

INTRODUCTION

Atheromatous coronary artery disease is the leading cause of death worldwide, constituting approximately 7,000,000 cases each year. To overcome the devastating effects of coronary artery disease, extensive clinical trials of pharmacotherapy and intervention have been conducted for decades in order to lower the high rates of mortality associated with this disease.

The initial knowledge on the progression of atherosclerosis was reported in the early 1980s by studying coronary lesions at autopsy (1,2). Despite these early reports, there remained an incomplete understanding of the relationship between lesion progression and acute coronary syndromes. The American Heart Association (AHA) perceived this gap in the mid-1990s and a committee was convened to summarize our understanding of plaque progression, also taking advantage of what had been learnt from animal models of atherosclerosis (3,4). Consensus reports demonstrated plaque rupture as the sole etiology of coronary thrombosis and proposed a classification scheme by which coronary atherosclerotic lesions were classified into six numerical categories staged in relation to plaque rupture. But no precursor lesion of plaque rupture was named, that is, no thin-cap fibroatheroma was described.

Our laboratory, which has one of the largest autopsy registries of sudden coronary death (SCD), recognized that the AHA nomenclature was incomplete since we had observed alternative substrates leading to acute coronary thrombosis, that is, plaque erosion (5) and nodular calcification (6). Moreover, the AHA nomenclature failed to describe healing processes, which also contribute to severe luminal narrowing with or without acute plaque rupture. Silent plaque ruptures may also lead to chronic total occlusion, which is observed at autopsy in approximately 30% of SCDs. These limitations led us to modify the AHA classification to one that does not use numeric categories but is more descriptive and easy to understand. It can easily be adopted and used by invasive and non-invasive imaging modalities that are constantly being introduced to improve the predictive ability in patients who are at high risk of developing acute coronary syndromes (6). Moreover, to improve the outcome of patients with ACS, it is essential to have a comprehensive understanding of the pathological processes involved in the progression of atherosclerosis, as discussed below.

DEFINITION

In the modified classification (Table 1.1, Fig. 1.1), the numeric AHA Types I–IV are replaced by descriptive terminology: adaptive intimal thickening, intimal xanthoma (fatty streak), pathologic intimal thickening, and fibroatheroma. Lesions alluded to in AHA Types V and VI were discarded because they failed to account for the three different causes of thrombotic morphologies (rupture, erosion, and calcified nodule) and because of their relationship with healed plaques, which is representative of stable angina. Since atherosclerosis is a dynamic process with multiple pathogenesis, it is useful to review the stages of development of atherosclerosis; however, as the mechanisms are better understood, the classification should be revised constantly and improved as new knowledge is gained.

Adaptive Intimal Thickening and Intimal Xanthoma (Fatty Streaks)

The earliest manifestation of vascular change is "adaptive intimal thickening" (AHA Type I), which consists of several layers of smooth muscle cells (SMCs) in an extracellular matrix with little or no inflammatory cell infiltration. Intimal thickening is observed in 35% of neonates, and the intima/media ratio at birth is 0.1, which increases progressively to reach 0.3 by the age of 2 years (7). This change is considered adaptive (non-atherosclerotic) since the SMC exhibits a very low proliferative activity and an anti-apoptotic phenotype (8). Although the adaptive intima becomes bigger with aging, very rarely does it grow to such an extent that it compromises blood flow. The change in the shear stress is a

Table 1.1 Modified AHA Consensus Classification Based on Morphologic Description

	Description	Thrombosis
Non-atherosclerotic intimal lesions		
Intimal thickening	Normal accumulation of smooth muscle cells (SMCs) in the intima in the absence of lipid or macrophage foam cells	Absent
Intimal xanthoma	Superficial accumulation of foam cells without a necrotic core or fibrous cap. Based on animal and human data, such lesions usually regress	Absent
Progressive atherosclerotic lesions		
Pathologic intimal thickening	SMC-rich plaque with a proteoglycan matrix and focal accumulation of extracellular lipids	Absent
Fibrous cap atheroma	Early necrosis: focal macrophage infiltration into areas of lipid pools with an overlying fibrous cap	Absent
	Late necrosis: loss of matrix and extensive cellular debris with an overlying fibrous cap	
Thin-cap fibroatheroma	A thin fibrous cap (<65 μm) infiltrated by macrophages and lymphocytes with rare or no SMCs and a relatively large underlying necrotic core. Intraplaque hemorrhage/fibrin may be present	Absent
Lesions with acute thrombi		
Plaque rupture	Fibroatheroma with cap disruption; the luminal thrombus communicates with the underlying necrotic core	Occlusive or non-occlusive
Plaque erosion	Plaque composition, as above; no communication of the thrombus with necrotic core. Can occur on a plaque substrate of pathologic intimal thickening or fibroatheroma	Usually non-occlusive
Calcified nodule	Eruptive (shedding) calcified nodule with an underlying fibrocalcific plaque with minimal or no necrosis	Usually non-occlusive
Lesions with healed thrombi		
Fibrotic (without calcification)	Collagen-rich plaque with significant luminal stenosis. Lesions may contain large areas of calcification with few inflammatory cells and absence of necrosis. These lesions may represent healed erosions or ruptures	Absent
Fibrocalcific (±necrotic core)		

Source: Adapted from Ref. 6.

trigger for abnormal responses in the endothelial lining (9) and for changes secondarily induced in the SMC phenotype (10); however, the detailed mechanism remains elusive.

"Fatty streak" or "intimal xanthoma" (AHA Type II) is a lesion that is not raised and is primarily composed of abundant foamy macrophages interspersed between SMCs. Although the AHA classification refers to this entity as the earliest lesion of atherosclerosis, our experience and reports of human and animal studies suggest that the lesion is reversible at least in some locations (11,12). Some reports suggest that the modification of extracellular matrix lays an important part in the progression of early atherosclerosis with an important role for biglycan and decorin proteoglycans (13), but the mechanism remains largely uncertain.

Pathologic Intimal Thickening

"Pathologic intimal thickening" (PIT) (AHA Type III) is recognized as the earliest progressive (irreversible) lesion by most research groups. The lesion is characterized by layers of proliferating SMCs near the lumen and an underlying lipid pool present at the intimal medial border. The origin of the lipid pool is not fully understood. The area of the lipid pool is rich in the proteoglycans versican and hyaluronan as well as extracellular lipid deposits but is devoid of SMCs and macrophages. It has been demonstrated that the lipid pool has an affinity for plasma

lipoproteins, which suggests that the accumulation of extracellular lipids is probably due to the influx of plasma lipoproteins (14). Williams and Tabas (15) proposed a "response-to-retention" hypothesis: namely that the retention of atherogenic lipoproteins associated with the extracellular matrix, such as the proteoglycans versican and hyaluronan, is an initiating event in early atherogenesis. Recent studies reinforce this hypothesis by demonstrating that structural changes in the glycosaminoglycan chain of proteoglycans are an initial proatherogenic step that promotes the binding and retention of lipoproteins (16). An alternative hypothesis proposed is that the membranes of apoptotic SMCs act as an alternative source for the lipids in PIT (17). Apoptotic SMCs within lipid pools are recognized by membrane remnants (cages of basal lamina) and the presence of microcalcification (18) representing calcified mitochondria. However, this mechanism remains speculative.

Another important feature of PIT is the presence of varying degrees of foamy macrophage accumulation near the luminal aspect of the plaque (apart from the lipid pool); however, this does not necessarily apply to all cases. Lesions demonstrating PIT with foamy macrophages are considered to be a more advanced stage of atherosclerosis, as reported by Nakashima et al. in their systematic study of early coronary plaques (19). We believe that macrophages invade the plaque from the luminal surface. Although the precise nature of focal macrophage accumulation in

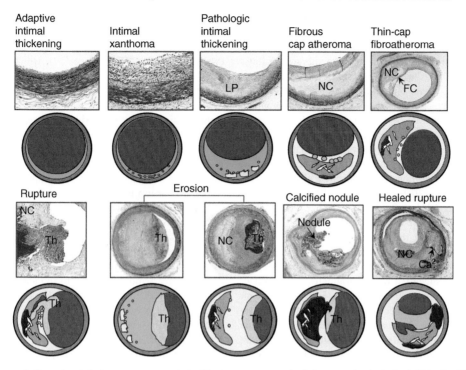

Figure 1.1 Spectrum of atherosclerosis in human coronary arteries. The two non-progressive lesions are adaptive intimal thickening (AHA Type I) and intimal xanthomas (foam cell collections known as fatty streaks, AHA Type II). Pathological intimal thickening (PIT, AHA Type III, transitional lesions) marks the first of the progressive plaques since they are considered to be precursors to more advanced fibroatheroma (FA). Thin-cap fibroatheromas are considered precursors to plaque rupture. Essentially missing from the AHA consensus classification are two alternative entities that give rise to coronary thrombosis, namely, erosion and calcified nodule. Erosions can occur on a substrate of PIT or FA, while calcified nodules (a minor but viable mechanisms of thrombosis) depict eruptive fragments of calcium that protrude into the lumen causing a thrombotic event. Lastly, healed plaque ruptures are lesions with generally smaller necrotic cores and focal areas of calcification where the surface generally shows areas of healing rich in proteoglycans. Multiple healed plaque ruptures are thought to be responsible for progressive luminal narrowing. *Abbreviations*: LP, lipid pool; NC, necrotic core; FC, fibrous cap; Th, thrombus. *Source*: Adapted from Ref. 6.

PIT is not fully elucidated, it is speculated that retention of modified lipoprotein and activation of vascular adhesion molecules such as VCAM-1 and ICAM-1 expressed by endothelial cells stimulate the recruitment of macrophages (20,21). In addition, lesions with PIT exhibit varying degrees of free cholesterol represented by empty fine crystalline structures in paraffin-embedded sections that accumulate within the lipid pools. Although it is assumed that free cholesterol originates from dead foam cells, it is not a likely source in PIT as the majority of macrophages when present are confined to the more luminal aspect of the plaque.

Fibroatheroma

Fibroatheroma (AHA Type IV) represents a further progressive stage of atherosclerotic disease and is histologically characterized by the presence of acellular necrotic cores that are distinct from the lipid pool of PIT as they lack the expression of hyaluronan and the proteoglycan versican. Recognition of early macrophage infiltration into the lipid pools and cell death along with a substantial increase in free cholesterol and breakdown of the extracellular matrix, which is presumably degraded by the matrix proteases released by macrophages, is classified as "early" necrotic core. In the early phase of necrotic core formation, there is an efficient system for the clearance of apoptotic bodies by macrophages; however, this system is soon overwhelmed and there is defective phagocytic clearance of apoptotic cells which is thought to further contribute to the vicious cycle of enlargement of the necrotic core and plaque progression (22). As the total plaque burden increases, compensatory enlargement of the vessel, that is, positive coronary arterial remodeling occurs to preserve the arterial lumen. According to Glagov et al., lumen compromise only occurs when luminal narrowing exceeds >40% of cross-sectional luminal narrowing (23). We have further classified fibroatheromas into "early" or "late" based on the type of the necrotic core observed. A necrotic core devoid of proteoglycans versican and hyaluronan or any collagen expression is termed "late" necrotic core; it has a thick fibrous cap that fully contains the necrotic core. On the other hand, "early" necrotic cores continue to focally express the proteoglycans versican and hyaluronan, especially toward the media, but there is an absence of matrix with macrophage infiltration toward the lumen.

Intraplaque Hemorrhage

In addition to the apoptotic macrophages that contribute to the accumulation of free cholesterol, other sources such as red blood cells (RBCs) may contribute to the expansion of the necrotic core. Studies from our SCD registry have shown that hemorrhage into a necrotic core is commonly observed in cases of plaque rupture and late necrotic core. The membranes of RBCs are enriched with lipids, which constitute 40% of their weight, and have a free cholesterol content that exceeds that of all other cell membranes (24). The excess cholesterol in the membranes of RBCs can phase-separate and form immiscible membrane domains consisting of pure cholesterol arranged in a tail-to-tail orientation that favors crystal formation (25). The extent of accumulated erythrocytes incorporated into the plaque and the abundant lipids, in addition to the impaired phagocytic efficiency of macrophages that makes them ineffective in cleaning up RBCs and other debris, influence both the biochemical composition and the size of the necrotic core (26,27).

There are contrasting theories about the origin of intraplaque hemorrhage. Some authors claim that it originates as a result of blood influx from the lumen via plaque fissuring, while others have suggested that it originates as a result of leakage from intraplaque microcapillaries. However, we favor the latter hypothesis since intraplaque erythrocyte extravasation is often seen in the absence of plaque fissuring but rather in association with a high intraplaque density of small vessels (Fig. 1.2). Further, some reports demonstrated the presence of incomplete mural cell coverage and dysfunctional endothelial cells of capillaries and arterioles with focal absence of

basement membranes and poorly formed endothelial junctions (28). It is possible that these immature or leaky vessels also allow diffusion of plasma proteins, diapedesis of leukocytes, and erythrocyte spillage (29), which may serve as a driving force for further centripetal angiogenesis from the adventitia (30).

Hemoglobin Toxicity and Oxidative Stress
Intraplaque hemorrhage could potentially also include inflammatory cells (31). The precise signaling pathways for the cellular response are not fully understood but it is postulated that the hemoglobin–haptoglobin (Hb–Hp) receptor CD163 on macrophages may be involved in the clearance of the complex and the release of anti-inflammatory cytokines may contribute to a decrease in inflammation (32). However, a recent study by our group has shown the significance of oxidative stress associated with extravasated erythrocytes, which results in a rapid increase of hemoglobin and continued inflammation in the intraplaque area (33). Free hemoglobin binds to and inactivates nitric oxide, a potent molecule that plays a critical role in the regulation of smooth muscle vasoreactivity and endothelial adhesion molecule expression—events that lead to inflammation within the vessel wall (34).

The function of haptoglobin (Hp) is primarily to handle hemoglobin released from RBCs following intravascular or extravascular hemolysis. There are two common alleles at the Hp

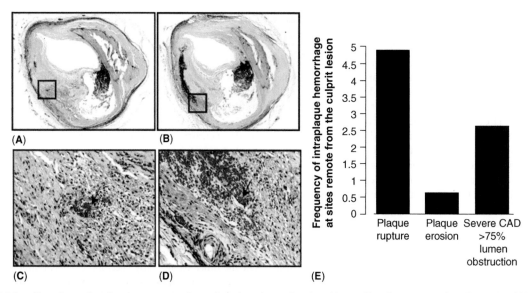

Figure 1.2 Intraplaque hemorrhage in a coronary artery. Recent intraplaque hemorrhage in a thin-cap fibroatheroma. Low- (**A** and **B**; ×20) and high-power views (**C** and **D**; ×200), represented by the black boxes, of a coronary artery with a thin-cap fibroatheroma ("vulnerable" plaque) and recent intraplaque hemorrhage. Parts **A** and **C** show the spillage of erythrocytes from the surrounding intraplaque vasa vasorum (arrow). Parts **B** and **D** depict serial sections of the lesion in A showing an expanded area of hemorrhage, with the higher power image demonstrating a large pool of extravasated erythrocytes surrounding proximate microvessels (arrow). Coronary sections were stained with Movat Pentachrome. (**E**) Bar graph representing the frequency of intraplaque hemorrhages at other coronary lesion sites in patients dying from plaque rupture, erosion, or severe coronary artery disease (CAD). Notably, patients dying from rupture had the highest number of remote sites with intraplaque hemorrhage. *Source*: From Ref. 64.

genetic locus denoted as 1 and 2, with two homozygous (1–1, and 2–2) and one heterozygous genotypes possible. There are clinically significant functional differences between the Hp 1 and Hp 2 protein products with respect to the degree of protection against hemoglobin-driven oxidative stress. Levy et al. (35) reported a three- to fivefold increased risk of cardiovascular disease in diabetic patients with the Hp 2–2 genotype when compared with those without the Hp 2–2 genotype. In particular, individuals with the Hp 2–2 genotype and diabetes mellitus appear to be at a significantly higher risk of microvascular and macrovascular complications.

In atherosclerotic plaques, the primary route for clearance of the Hb–Hp complex involves the CD163 receptor expressed on immunosuppressive macrophages with the M2 phenotype (36). Physiologically low concentrations of hemoglobin (heme) are cytoprotective as they induce the rapid upregulation of hemoxyenase-1 (HO-1), whereas excess pathological amounts of heme outstrip the ability of HO-1 to metabolize it such that the residual heme (liberated free iron) may destroy the tissue by pro-oxidative and pro-inflammatory effects (37). Also, when the capacity of the protective hemoglobin-scavenging mechanisms has been saturated, levels of cell-free hemoglobin increase, resulting in the consumption of nitric oxide and clinical sequelae. Nitric oxide plays a major role in vascular homeostasis and has been shown to be a critical regulator of basal and stress-mediated smooth muscle relaxation and vasomotor tone, endothelial adhesion molecule expression, and platelet activation and aggregation. Another product of excess heme is bilirubin, which has potential antioxidant activity. Free ferrous iron has potential pro-oxidant activity, although this may be limited because of its sequestration by ferritin.

Focus Box 1.1 Progression of Atherosclerotic Coronary Disease

The earliest vascular change is "intimal thickening", consisting of several layers of smooth muscle cell with a proteoglycan matrix

"Pathologic intimal thickening" (PIT) is the earliest progressive (irreversible) atherosclerotic change, which is characterized by the presence of a lipid pool. PIT contains varying degrees of foamy macrophages close to the lumen

Fibroatheroma is characterized by the presence of acellular necrotic cores that contain esterifiers and free cholesterol along with other lipoproteins. Many believe that macrophage apoptosis is a major contributor to the formation of the necrotic core

Intraplaque hemorrhage contributes to the expansion of the necrotic core by accumulation of excess free cholesterol from the RBC membrane

An increase in hemoglobin by extravasated erythrocytes induces oxidative stress leading to an increased presence of M2 macrophages (CD68+, CD163+) that have anti-inflammatory properties and contain smaller amounts of lipid droplets when compared with CD68+, CD163– macrophages

Thin-cap Fibroatheroma and Plaque Rupture

Thin-cap fibroatheroma (TCFA), traditionally designated as "vulnerable" plaque, has a morphological appearance that resembles a ruptured plaque (6). TCFAs generally contain a large necrotic core with overlying thin intact fibrous caps consisting mainly of type I collagen with varying degrees of macrophages and lymphocytes and very few, if any, α-actin-positive SMCs. The thickness of the fibrous cap is an indicator of plaque vulnerability; a TCFA is defined as having a cap thickness ≤65 μm, as the thinnest portion of the remnant cap in ruptured plaques was measured to be 23 ± 19 μm, whereas 95% of the ruptured caps measured <65 μm (38). When compared with ruptured plaques, TCFAs tend to have smaller necrotic cores and less macrophage infiltration. Cross-sectional luminal narrowing is also typically less in TCFAs than in ruptured plaques, and an occlusive thrombus generally shows greater underlying stenosis than lesions with a non-occlusive thrombus (39).

It has been shown that the rupture usually occurs at the weakest point, often the near shoulder regions. However, in our experience this is not always the case as we have observed an equivalent number of ruptures at the mid-portion of the fibrous cap, especially in individuals who died due to exertion (40). Therefore, it is reasonable to speculate that several processes may be involved in the mechanism of plaque rupture; for example, fibrous cap degradation by matrix metalloproteases (41), high shear stress (42), macrophage and SMC death (43), and microcalcification and iron accumulation within the fibrous cap (44) have all been implicated.

Once plaque rupture occurs and the necrotic contents are exposed to the flowing blood, it results in the triggering of the coagulation cascade in response to lipids, collagen, and tissue factors. The luminal thrombus at the site of the rupture is platelet-rich (white thrombus), while the sites that are proximal and distal to the rupture site (i.e., the sites of propagation of the thrombus) consist of a red thrombus, which is composed of layers of fibrin and erythrocytes. A study of aspirated thrombi from patients presenting with acute myocardial infarction (AMI), examined by scanning electron microscopy (SEM), confirmed a decrease in platelet content and an increase in fibrin content as the duration of ischemia increased (45).

Plaque Erosion

Plaque rupture of an atherosclerotic plaque is the primary cause of AMI and SCD, occurring in 60–75% of cases (46). In the mid-1990s, studies from our laboratory and that of van der Wal et al. reported an alternative mechanism of coronary thrombosis referred to as "plaque erosion" (5,47). In plaque erosion, the thrombus is confined to the luminal plaque surface that has an absence of fissures or communication with the underlying necrotic cores when it is present, which was validated by serial sectioning. In a study of 20 AMI patients, van der Wal et al. showed that the incidence of plaque ruptures (60%) was more frequent than that of "superficial erosion" (40%) (47). In our series of 50 consecutive cases of sudden death due to coronary artery thrombosis, plaque rupture was identified in 28 (56%) cases, while superficial erosion was observed in 22 (44%) cases, all of which had SMC-rich and proteoglycan-rich underlying plaques (5). In more recent studies of AMI and SCD cases, plaque erosion was identified as an important substrate of coronary thrombosis with its frequency being higher in women than in men (48).

The term "erosion" was used since the luminal surface beneath the thrombus was devoid of endothelium. Besides, there were clear morphologic differences between rupture and erosion with plaque erosions having fewer macrophages and T lymphocytes than plaque ruptures (5,49). In addition, eroded plaques tend to be more frequently eccentric with lesions rich in the proteoglycans versican and hyaluronan and type III collagen, unlike ruptured or stable plaques. Further, thrombi from sites of erosion express a greater number of myeloperoxidase positive cells and have a higher incidence of distal microemboli than thrombi from sites of ruptured plaques (50,51). Taken together, the above facts suggest that it is essential to better understand the mechanistic differences between erosion and rupture, as different strategies may be required for the diagnosis and treatment of erosions.

Calcified Nodule

A calcified nodule is the least frequent cause of coronary thrombosis. It is characterized by a lesion with underlying calcification that is fragmented into small amorphous nodules on the luminal surface with surrounding fibrin, while the deeper regions often show sheets of calcification. Morphologically it resembles an eruptive nodule (often multiple nodules with or without bone formation) protruding into the lumen, accompanied by a platelet-rich thrombus, which is usually non-occlusive. Little is known about the origin of nodular calcification. Histologically, fibrin is often present between the bony or calcified spicules, along with osteoblasts, osteoclasts, and inflammatory cells, indicating possible entrapment of circulating stem cells or cell transformation occurring from existing plaque cells (6). Lesions with nodular calcification are more common in older individuals, are more likely seen in men and chronic renal failure patients, and are preferentially found in tortuous middle-right coronary or left anterior descending coronary arteries. They also appear to be more prevalent in the carotid arteries than in the coronary arteries, which may be related to a greater frequency of calcification in carotid disease. The necrotic core, if present, is usually small in comparison with other atherothrombotic lesions.

Healed Plaque

The prevalence of silent plaque rupture or erosion in the clinical setting remains unknown as there are few studies that have demonstrated plaque progression following clinical events. It has been demonstrated in the National Heart, Lung, and Blood Institute Dynamic Registry, which includes consecutive patients undergoing percutaneous coronary interventions (PCIs) having a 6% rate of non-target lesion PCI by 1 year, that greater the coronary artery disease burden the higher is the risk. In another recent study in patients who presented with an acute coronary syndrome and underwent PCI, the rate of major cardiovascular

events in non-target lesions was 11.6% at 30 months and these lesions had angiographic mild disease, were most often TCFA, and were characterized by a large plaque burden and a small lumen area or a combination of these characteristics (52). Also, autopsy studies provide evidence that plaque progression, defined as cross-sectional luminal narrowing, occurs following repeated thrombotic events. Ruptured lesions with healed repair sites, referred to as healed plaque rupture (HPR), are discernible as breaks in the underlying old fibrous cap with a newly formed overlying tissue consisting of SMCs surrounded by proteoglycans and/or a collagen-rich matrix, depending on the phase of healing (53). Similar to plaque rupture, healing at the site of plaque erosion also leads to luminal narrowing. The early stage of healing is characterized by lesions that are rich in proteoglycans and type III collagen, with an underlying necrotic core and ruptured fibrous cap rich in type I collagen.

Davies showed that the mechanism of plaque progression was through HPRs (53). The frequency of HPR correlates with the degree of luminal narrowing such that HPR was identified in 8% of lesions with <20% diameter stenosis, 19% with 21–50% diameter stenosis, and 73% with >50% stenosis (53). We showed that, in patients who died due to SCD, the incidence of HPR was 61% and that the percentage of luminal narrowing was proportional to the increased number of healed rupture sites from previous ruptures. These data provide evidence that silent plaque rupture is a form of wound healing that results in plaque progression with luminal narrowing (54).

Calcified Stable Plaque

The extent of calcification has been shown to be a predictor of diffuse coronary disease by CT. Calcification of atherosclerotic plaques in SCD patients is observed in 80% of cases, but the degree of calcification varies significantly from patient to patient and does not necessarily correlate with disease severity or plaque vulnerability. Calcification is a likely consequence of multiple risk factors that include age/gender (55), renal function, diabetes (56), vitamin D levels and other aspects of bone metabolism (57), and genetic markers (58).

In humans, the initiation of calcification in atherosclerotic plaques is a marker of cell death, which is an essential component of all atherosclerotic plaques. Apoptotic SMCs are considered to be the earliest source of plaque calcification by an active or passive process involving calcification of cell organelles referred to as matrix vesicles, which are observed histologically as microcalcifications and were only identified following the use of special stains such as von Kossa (59). Macrophage cell death is thought to be another source of early calcium deposition. The calcified macrophages appear as small areas of calcification and are distinct from those of SMCs. We have observed that microcalcifications derived from apoptotic SMCs and macrophages generally begin within the lipid pool and in "early" necrotic cores close to the luminal surface. The mechanism by which the calcifications extend and lead to diffuse calcification involving other extracellular matrix proteins such as collagen and proteoglycans or through the expression of bone-forming proteins, at least *in vivo*, is poorly understood. An eventual transformation into plates of calcification that may appear as pipestem calcification, which involves the necrotic core, collagen, and inflammatory cells, and even bone formation in the late stages may be observed. Immunohistochemical and gene expression studies have demonstrated that bone morphogenic protein, osteopontin, bone sialoprotein, and the osteoblast-specific transcription factor for bone formation are highly expressed in calcified arteries when compared with non-calcified controls. In heavily calcified lesions that are regarded as burnt-out lesions, there is little if any macrophage infiltration and an absence of other inflammatory cells. Nevertheless, a fair proportion of the calcification is passive, purely degenerative without biological regulation, and consists of calcium phosphate crystals (60).

PLAQUE MORPHOLOGIES AND CLINICAL RELEVANCE
In histological studies of patients who died due to SCD, fresh thrombus has been reported in 50–75% of cases, while patients in the remaining cases have stable plaque with severe stenosis (>75% cross-sectional luminal narrowing) of the major coronary arteries. Of the various cases of fresh thrombus, the underlying pathologic lesions are mainly plaque rupture (60–75%), followed by erosion (30–40%) and calcified nodules (2–7%) (2,6,61–63). In cases where deaths are attributed to plaque rupture, 70% of cases have thin-cap fibroatheromas at sites remote from the ruptured lesion. On the other hand, the incidence of thin-cap fibroatheroma is markedly less (30% of cases) where death is associated with stable plaques with severe stenosis. Also, the incidence of thin-cap fibroatheroma is highest in patients dying of plaque rupture, less in those with stable plaques, and least in patients dying of plaque erosion (Fig. 1.2). The majority of thin-cap fibroatheromas occur predominantly in the proximal portion of the three major coronary arteries; the proximal portion of the left anterior descending artery is the most frequent location (43%), followed by the proximal right coronary artery (20%) and the left circumflex artery (18%) (39).

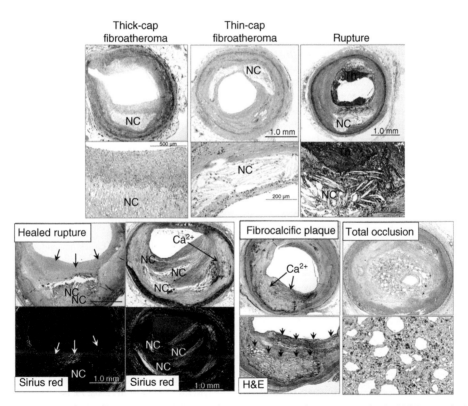

Figure 1.3 Fate of atherosclerotic plaques. Fibroatheromas are characterized by the presence of a necrotic core (NC) which is covered with a thick fibrous cap (upper left columns). As the plaque progresses, the fibrous cap becomes thin and the NC enlarges. Thin-cap fibroatheromas (upper middle columns) are considered to be precursors to lesions of plaque rupture (upper right columns). The lower left boxes demonstrate healed rupture lesions, where newly formed fibrous caps (arrows) rich in proteoglycans and type III collagen (greenish in Sirius red stain) with interspersed α-actin positive smooth muscle cells are observed overlying a necrotic core (NC) and ruptured type I collagen-rich thin fibrous caps (reddish on Sirius red stain). The lesion with repeated rupture episodes exhibits a multi-layered appearance with necrotic cores and overlying fibrous layers, resulting in severe luminal narrowing. Fibrocalcific plaques (lower middle box) are thought to be burnt-out lesions, which are associated with calcified sheets of plaque matrix (arrows). The lower right box shows a lesion of chronic total occlusion. The lumen is occupied by a recanalized organized thrombus that is rich in proteoglycan matrix showing the presence of iron deposition and macrophages.

In conclusion, although plaque rupture may lead to unstable angina, myocardial infarction, or sudden death, it may also occur without causing symptoms. Silent ruptures are know to heal, but their repeated occurrence at the same location leads to greater luminal area stenosis with each new rupture. The resulting lesions exhibit multiple necrotic cores separated by layers of collagen (Fig. 1.3). These repeated thrombotic events contribute to gradual luminal narrowing and plaque progression. The significant increase in plaque burden and luminal narrowing is due to previous repeated thrombosis that often occurs silently in the absence of cardiac symptoms. The prevalence of silent episodes of rupture in living patients is unknown. In our experience, 61% of SCD victims show at least one HPR lesion, where the incidence is greatest in deaths from stable plaques with severe stenosis (80%), followed by acute plaque rupture (75%), and the least in plaque erosions (9%) (54).

PERSONAL PERSPECTIVE

Although lipids along with other traditional risk factors play an essential role in the causation of coronary artery disease, the mechanistic link between lipids and diseases remains unknown. Similarly, plaque progression studies in humans have been derived mostly from autopsy studies and clinical studies in the last century have used investigative tools that concentrated on the study of luminograms and not the arterial wall, where most of the atherosclerotic diseases occur. Although animal models have failed to show events such as plaque rupture that occur commonly in human, without doubt, we have learned a lot about many disease mechanisms from genetically altered mice; however, the atherosclerotic lesions observed in the animal models do not in any way resemble those seen in humans. Similarly, animal models have not helped to predict the response, in humans, to novel treatments. Therefore, identification of various plaque characteristics by invasive or non-invasive means may be the only way we are likely to enhance our knowledge of plaque types and plaque progression in humans. We should continue to improve our imaging tools for the detection and characterization of coronary artery disease, by targeting detailed plaque morphology or specific metabolic processes, for example, local inflammation or biomarkers, which may permit strict monitoring of the activity of atherosclerotic disease. The development of a non-invasive imaging device for screening purposes in asymptomatic individuals may prove to be an indispensable predictive tool for the management of patients at high risk of clinical events.

Focus Box 1.2 Causes of Death Due To Atherosclerotic Coronary Disease

Fresh thrombosis accounts for 50–75% of cases of sudden coronary death

Of the cases with fresh thrombosis, the underlying pathologic lesions were mainly plaque rupture (60–75%), followed by erosion (30–40%) and calcified nodules (2–7%)

A thrombotic event may occur silently and contribute to gradual luminal narrowing and plaque progression which may finally result in acute coronary syndrome and sudden death

---

REFERENCES

1. Velican D, Velican C. Atherosclerotic involvement of the coronary arteries of adolescents and young adults. Atherosclerosis 1980; 36: 449–60.
2. Davies MJ, Thomas A. Thrombosis and acute coronary-artery lesions in sudden cardiac ischemic death. N Engl J Med 1984; 310: 1137–40.
3. Stary HC, Blankenhorn DH, Chandler AB, et al. A definition of the intima of human arteries and of its atherosclerosis-prone regions. A report from the Committee on Vascular Lesions of the Council on Arteriosclerosis, American Heart Association. Arterioscler Thromb 1992; 12: 120–34.
4. Stary HC, Chandler AB, Dinsmore RE, et al. A definition of advanced types of atherosclerotic lesions and a histological classification of atherosclerosis. A report from the Committee on Vascular Lesions of the Council on Arteriosclerosis, American Heart Association. Arterioscler Thromb Vasc Biol 1995; 15: 1512–31.
5. Farb A, Burke AP, Tang AL, et al. Coronary plaque erosion without rupture into a lipid core. A frequent cause of coronary thrombosis in sudden coronary death. Circulation 1996; 93: 1354–63.
6. Virmani R, Kolodgie FD, Burke AP, et al. Lessons from sudden coronary death: a comprehensive morphological classification scheme for atherosclerotic lesions. Arterioscler Thromb Vasc Biol 2000; 20: 1262–75.
7. Ikari Y, McManus BM, Kenyon J, et al. Neonatal intima formation in the human coronary artery. Arterioscler Thromb Vasc Biol 1999; 19: 2036–40.
8. Orekhov AN, Andreeva ER, Mikhailova IA, et al. Cell proliferation in normal and atherosclerotic human aorta: proliferative splash in lipid-rich lesions. Atherosclerosis 1998; 139: 41–8.
9. Davies PF, Civelek M, Fang Y, et al. Endothelial heterogeneity associated with regional athero-susceptibility and adaptation to disturbed blood flow in vivo. Semin Thromb Hemost 2010; 36: 265–75.
10. Wang L, Karlsson L, Moses S, et al. P2 receptor expression profiles in human vascular smooth muscle and endothelial cells. J Cardiovasc Pharmacol 2002; 40: 841–53.
11. Aikawa M, Rabkin E, Okada Y, et al. Lipid lowering by diet reduces matrix metalloproteinase activity and increases collagen content of rabbit atheroma: a potential mechanism of lesion stabilization. Circulation 1998; 97: 2433–44.
12. Velican C. A dissecting view on the role of the fatty streak in the pathogenesis of human atherosclerosis: culprit or bystander? Med Interne 1981; 19: 321–37.
13. Nakashima Y, Wight TN, Sueishi K. Early atherosclerosis in humans: role of diffuse intimal thickening and extracellular matrix proteoglycans. Cardiovasc Res 2008; 79: 14–23.
14. Hoff HF, Bradley WA, Heideman CL, et al. Characterization of low density lipoprotein-like particle in the human aorta from grossly normal and atherosclerotic regions. Biochim Biophys Acta 1979; 573: 361–74.
15. Williams KJ, Tabas I. The response-to-retention hypothesis of early atherogenesis. Arterioscler Thromb Vasc Biol 1995; 15: 551–61.
16. Merrilees MJ, Beaumont BW, Braun KR, et al. Neointima formed by arterial smooth muscle cells expressing versican variant v3 is

resistant to lipid and macrophage accumulation. Arterioscler Thromb Vasc Biol 2011; 31: 1309–16.

17. Preston Mason R, Tulenko TN, Jacob RF. Direct evidence for cholesterol crystalline domains in biological membranes: role in human pathobiology. Biochim Biophys Acta 2003; 1610: 198–207.

18. Kockx MM, De Meyer GR, Muhring J, et al. Apoptosis and related proteins in different stages of human atherosclerotic plaques. Circulation 1998; 97: 2307–15.

19. Nakashima Y, Fujii H, Sumiyoshi S, et al. Early human atherosclerosis: accumulation of lipid and proteoglycans in intimal thickenings followed by macrophage infiltration. Arterioscler Thromb Vasc Biol 2007; 27: 1159–65.

20. Cushing SD, Berliner JA, Valente AJ, et al. Minimally modified low density lipoprotein induces monocyte chemotactic protein 1 in human endothelial cells and smooth muscle cells. Proc Natl Acad Sci USA 1990; 87: 5134–8.

21. Klouche M, Gottschling S, Gerl V, et al. Atherogenic properties of enzymatically degraded LDL: selective induction of MCP-1 and cytotoxic effects on human macrophages. Arterioscler Thromb Vasc Biol 1998; 18: 1376–85.

22. Tabas I. Cholesterol and phospholipid metabolism in macrophages. Biochim Biophys Acta 2000; 1529: 164–74.

23. Glagov S, Weisenberg E, Zarins CK, et al. Compensatory enlargement of human atherosclerotic coronary arteries. N Engl J Med 1987; 316: 1371–5.

24. Yeagle PL. Cholesterol and the cell membrane. Biochim Biophys Acta 1985; 822: 267–87.

25. Tulenko TN, Chen M, Mason PE, et al. Physical effects of cholesterol on arterial smooth muscle membranes: evidence of immiscible cholesterol domains and alterations in bilayer width during atherogenesis. J Lipid Res 1998; 39: 947–56.

26. Kolodgie FD, Gold HK, Burke AP, et al. Intraplaque hemorrhage and progression of coronary atheroma. N Engl J Med 2003; 349: 2316–25.

27. Tabas I. Consequences and therapeutic implications of macrophage apoptosis in atherosclerosis: the importance of lesion stage and phagocytic efficiency. Arterioscler Thromb Vasc Biol 2005; 25: 2255–64.

28. Sluimer JC, Kolodgie FD, Bijnens AP, et al. Thin-walled microvessels in human coronary atherosclerotic plaques show incomplete endothelial junctions relevance of compromised structural integrity for intraplaque microvascular leakage. J Am Coll Cardiol 2009; 53: 1517–27.

29. Zhang Y, Cliff WJ, Schoefl GI, et al. Plasma protein insudation as an index of early coronary atherogenesis. Am J Pathol 1993; 143: 496–506.

30. Michel JB, Thaunat O, Houard X, et al. Topological determinants and consequences of adventitial responses to arterial wall injury. Arterioscler Thromb Vasc Biol 2007; 27: 1259–68.

31. Tavora F, Kutys R, Li L, et al. Adventitial lymphocytic inflammation in human coronary arteries with intimal atherosclerosis. Cardiovasc Pathol 2010; 19: e61–8.

32. Davis GE. The Mac-1 and p150,95 beta 2 integrins bind denatured proteins to mediate leukocyte cell-substrate adhesion. Exp Cell Res 1992; 200: 242–52.

33. Finn AV, Nakano M, Polavarapu R, et al. Hemoglobin directs macrophage differentiation and prevents foam cell formation in human atherosclerotic plaques. J Am Coll Cardiol 2012; 59: 166–77.

34. Rother RP, Bell L, Hillmen P, et al. The clinical sequelae of intravascular hemolysis and extracellular plasma hemoglobin: a novel mechanism of human disease. JAMA 2005; 293: 1653–62.

35. Levy AP, Hochberq I, Jablonski K, et al. Haptoglobin phenotype is an independent risk factor for cardiovascular disease in individuals with diabetes: The Strong Heart Study. J Am Coll Cardiol 2002; 40: 1984–90.

36. Boyle JJ, Harrington HA, Piper E, et al. Coronary intraplaque hemorrhage evokes a novel atheroprotective macrophage phenotype. Am J Pathol 2009; 174: 1097–108.

37. Wagener FA, van Beurden HE, von den Hoff JW, et al. The heme-heme oxygenase system: a molecular switch in wound healing. Blood 2003; 102: 521–8.

38. Burke AP, Farb A, Malcom GT, et al. Coronary risk factors and plaque morphology in men with coronary disease who died suddenly. N Engl J Med 1997; 336: 1276–82.

39. Kolodgie FD, Burke AP, Farb A, et al. The thin-cap fibroatheroma: a type of vulnerable plaque: the major precursor lesion to acute coronary syndromes. Curr Opin Cardiol 2001; 16: 285–92.

40. Burke AP, Farb A, Malcom GT, et al. Plaque rupture and sudden death related to exertion in men with coronary artery disease. JAMA 1999; 281: 921–6.

41. Sukhova GK, Schonbeck U, Rabkin E, et al. Evidence for increased collagenolysis by interstitial collagenases-1 and -3 in vulnerable human atheromatous plaques. Circulation 1999; 99: 2503–9.

42. Gijsen FJ, Wentzel JJ, Thury A, et al. Strain distribution over plaques in human coronary arteries relates to shear stress. Am J Physiol Heart Circ Physiol 2008; 295: H1608–14.

43. Kolodgie FD, Narula J, Burke AP, et al. Localization of apoptotic macrophages at the site of plaque rupture in sudden coronary death. Am J Pathol 2000; 157: 1259–68.

44. Vengrenyuk Y, Carlier S, Xanthos S, et al. A hypothesis for vulnerable plaque rupture due to stress-induced debonding around cellular microcalcifications in thin fibrous caps. Proc Natl Acad Sci USA 2006; 103: 14678–83.

45. Silvain J, Collet JP, Nagaswami C, et al. Composition of coronary thrombus in acute myocardial infarction. J Am Coll Cardiol 2011; 57: 1359–67.

46. Falk E, Shah PK, Fuster V. Coronary plaque disruption. Circulation 1995; 92: 657–71.

47. van der Wal AC, Becker AE, van der Loos CM, et al. Site of intimal rupture or erosion of thrombosed coronary atherosclerotic plaques is characterized by an inflammatory process irrespective of the dominant plaque morphology. Circulation 1994; 89: 36–44.

48. Kramer MC, van der Wal AC, Koch KT, et al. Histopathological features of aspirated thrombi after primary percutaneous coronary intervention in patients with ST-elevation myocardial infarction. PLoS One 2009; 4: e5817.

49. Kolodgie FD, Burke AP, Farb A, et al. Differential accumulation of proteoglycans and hyaluronan in culprit lesions: insights into plaque erosion. Arterioscler Thromb Vasc Biol 2002; 22: 1642–8.

50. Ferrante G, Nakano M, Prati F, et al. High levels of systemic myeloperoxidase are associated with coronary plaque erosion in patients with acute coronary syndromes: a clinicopathological study. Circulation 2010; 122: 2505–13.

51. Schwartz RS, Burke A, Farb A, et al. Microemboli and microvascular obstruction in acute coronary thrombosis and sudden coronary death: relation to epicardial plaque histopathology. J Am Coll Cardiol 2009; 54: 2167–73.

52. Stone GW, Maehara A, Lansky AJ, et al. A prospective natural history study of coronary atherosclerosis. N Engl J Med 2011; 364: 226–35.

53. Mann J, Davies MJ. Mechanisms of progression in native coronary artery disease: role of healed plaque disruption. Heart 1999; 82: 265–8.

54. Burke AP, Kolodgie FD, Farb A, et al. Healed plaque ruptures and sudden coronary death: evidence that subclinical rupture has a role in plaque progression. Circulation 2001; 103: 934–40.

55. Burke AP, Farb A, Malcom G, et al. Effect of menopause on plaque morphologic characteristics in coronary atherosclerosis. Am Heart J 2001; 141(2 Suppl): S58–62.

56. Burke AP, Taylor A, Farb A, et al. Coronary calcification: insights from sudden coronary death victims. Z Kardiol 2000; 89(Suppl 2): 49–53.

57. Watson KE, Abrolat ML, Malone LL, et al. Active serum vitamin D levels are inversely correlated with coronary calcification. Circulation 1997; 96: 1755–60.

58. Keso T, Perola M, Laippala P, et al. Polymorphisms within the tumor necrosis factor locus and prevalence of coronary artery disease in middle-aged men. Atherosclerosis 2001; 154: 691–7.

59. Proudfoot D, Shanahan CM. Biology of calcification in vascular cells: intima versus media. Herz 2001; 26: 245–51.

60. Sage AP, Tintut Y, Demer LL. Regulatory mechanisms in vascular calcification. Nat Rev Cardiol 2010; 7: 528–36.

61. el Fawal MA, Berg GA, Wheatley DJ, et al. Sudden coronary death in Glasgow: nature and frequency of acute coronary lesions. Br Heart J 1987; 57: 329–35.

62. Davies MJ, Bland JM, Hangartner JR, et al. Factors influencing the presence or absence of acute coronary artery thrombi in sudden ischaemic death. Eur Heart J 1989; 10: 203–8.

63. Burke AP, Farb A, Malcom GT, et al. Effect of risk factors on the mechanism of acute thrombosis and sudden coronary death in women. Circulation 1998; 97: 2110–16.

64. Virmani R, Kolodgie FD, Burke AP, et al. Atherosclerotic plaque progression and vulnerability to rupture: angiogenesis as a source of intraplaque hemorrhage. Arterioscler Thromb Vasc Biol 2005; 25: 2054–61.

2 Screening and identifying high-risk individuals in the general population by using traditional risk factors

Gregory Angelo Sgueglia, Gaetano Antonio Lanza, and Filippo Crea

OUTLINE

The traditional risk factors for cardiovascular (CV) disease, namely, cigarette smoking, hypertension, dyslipidemia, and diabetes mellitus, exhibit a dose-dependent and synergistic effect on CV risk. Thus, risk stratification has to be based on a global assessment of risk factors. Scoring algorithms and risk charts have been developed to this end and they are very efficient in risk stratification. Global risk assessment allows the identification of patients at low risk (10-year risk of CV events <10%), high risk (10-year risk of CV events >20%), and intermediate risk (10-year risk of CV events 10–20%). In patients at low risk it is important to achieve and maintain an optimal lifestyle. At the other extreme, in patients at high risk, who have a risk equivalent to that of patients with established CV disease, the pharmacological treatment of risk factors is needed in addition to the implementation of an optimal lifestyle. Patients at intermediate risk represent a heterogeneous population that needs to be re-stratified: further studies are warranted to establish which biomarkers or bio-imaging techniques are most efficient to this end.

INTRODUCTION

Cardiovascular diseases (CVDs) are the leading cause of death and disability across the world, in particular in developed countries. The lifetime risk of CVD for persons aged 50 years is estimated to be 52% for men and 39% for women (1).

Assessing CV risk is important for targeting lifestyle changes and implementing preventive medical treatments in individual patients who are asymptomatic but have a sufficiently high risk of developing CVD. The intensity of interventions that are shown to have an effect on CV risk factors should parallel the patient's level of absolute risk.

Although the definition of high risk is arbitrary, patients are usually considered to be in this risk category when the absolute risk of major CV events is comparable with that of patients with established disease such as those with a history of stable angina, acute coronary syndromes, or coronary revascularization procedures (2).

Clinical trials have shown that patients with a history of myocardial infarction have a 10-year risk for recurrent nonfatal or fatal myocardial infarction greater than 20% (3,4), and patients with stable angina pectoris have a 10-year risk of about 20% (5). Accordingly, asymptomatic patients who have a 10-year risk for non-fatal or fatal myocardial infarction greater than 20% are now considered to be at high risk, while those with risk from 10% to 20% are considered to be at intermediate risk.

The importance of stratifying patients relies on the fact that the benefit of CVD prevention strategies depends on the underlying level of CV risk. It is important to estimate the absolute reduction in risk to adequately assess the risk versus benefit of any prevention strategy. For a similar relative risk reduction across risk strata, the absolute reduction is indeed greater in a higher risk cohort than in a lower risk cohort.

Two different but complementary approaches are used for the prevention of CVD. Population-based strategies attempt to shift the burden of risk factors to lower levels by using public health measures. The impact of this approach on CVD death rates in the twentieth century has been remarkable. Most of the reduction in CV deaths observed in Western countries over the past decades is probably related to this strategy, and shifting the distribution of risk factors in the population should be the cornerstone of public health efforts for CVD prevention.

The population-based strategy, however, has some shortcomings. While preventive measures have a positive average impact on the entire population, the benefit is in fact limited to the subset of the population that would have had a CV event, resulting in overtreatment of the remaining individuals. This consideration is most relevant when pharmacologic therapies or other more aggressive measures are required to treat risk factors, which may result in unfavorable risk–benefit and cost–benefit ratios. Indeed, this approach is most rewarding when applied to lifestyle modifications (6).

A complementary strategy is the implementation of preventive measures in high-risk patients only. This approach involves setting a risk threshold and focusing treatment strategies on individuals who exceed this threshold. Traditional medical practice is based on this approach, which identifies patients with "illness" (or risk) requiring treatment. The advantage of this selective strategy is to deliver interventions characterized by a higher risk–benefit ratio than population-based strategies. Importantly, a selective strategy also improves the cost-effectiveness of implemented therapies. In addition, knowledge of CV risk enhances physician and patient motivation for the adoption of preventive measures.

The utility of the high-risk strategy in CVD prevention relies upon widely available, reliable measures of CV risk on which treatment algorithms can be based.

More than 100 independent CV risk factors have been identified during the past 50 years. However, only a small number have consistently been found to meet the accepted criteria of causation. Indeed, extensive epidemiologic studies and controlled randomized trials have consistently established that cigarette smoking, hypertension, dyslipidemia, and diabetes mellitus are independent modifiable risk factors for CVD and are also the causes of CVD. Because of the strength of evidence supporting their role in the pathogenesis of CVD, these four risk factors are often labeled as "traditional" risk factors.

CARDIOVASCULAR RISK FACTORS

A critically important feature of the traditional modifiable risk factors is that each of them has a continuous, dose-dependent relation to CV risk (7). Importantly, combinations of classical risk factors act synergistically in increasing the risk of CVD (8), and their global control results in a striking reduction of CV events (Fig. 2.1).

Cigarette Smoking

Cigarette smoking is the single most important modifiable CV risk factor and a potent predictor, in particular, of myocardial infarction, stroke, and peripheral artery disease.

Focus Box 2.1 Traditional Risk Factors for CVD
Cigarette smoking
Hypertension
Dyslipidemia
Diabetes mellitus

The negative effects of smoking concern both the development of atherosclerosis and the occurrence of acute thrombotic phenomena. Pathophysiologic studies have identified numerous mechanisms through which cigarette smoking may exert these adverse effects. Smokers have increased levels of oxidation products, including oxidized low-density lipoproteins (LDLs), and lower concentrations of the cardio-protective high-density lipoproteins (HDLs). These effects, along with the direct detrimental effects of carbon monoxide and nicotine, produce endothelial damage. Cigarette smoking has also been associated with increased levels of fibrinogen and enhanced platelet reactivity. Finally, the reduced capacity of the blood to carry oxygen contributes to the negative effects of smoking by lowering the threshold for myocardial ischemia.

The adverse effects of smoking are proportional to the number of cigarettes smoked daily and to the duration of smoking, and is similar in both sexes, in the young as in the elderly, and in all racial groups. Even smoking as few as four to five cigarettes per day results in a nearly twofold increase in the risk of acute myocardial infarction (Fig. 2.2) (9). There is no evidence that filters or other cigarette modifications reduce the risk. In contrast, pipe and cigar smoking, where the smoke is not inhaled, and oral tobacco use (either chewing tobacco or snuff) carry a somewhat smaller risk, which is, again, dose-dependent.

Importantly, passive smoking (i.e., exposure to environmental tobacco smoke) has increasingly been recognized as a modifiable

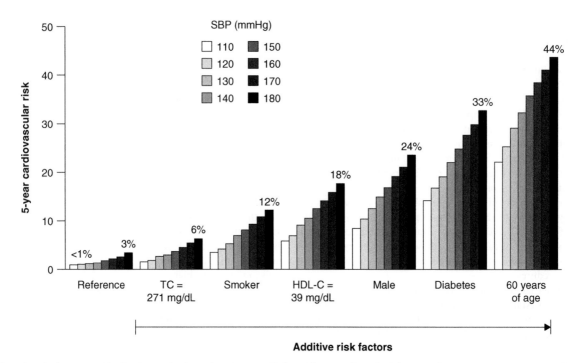

Figure 2.1 Absolute 5-year risk of cardiovascular disease in patients stratified according to traditional risk factors. Reference category refers to a non-diabetic, non-smoker female aged 50 years with total cholesterol of 155 mg/dL, HDL-cholesterol of 62 mg/dL, and systolic blood pressure <110 mmHg. The progressive addition of risk factors increases the 5-year risk of cardiovascular events from <1% to 44% (8). *Abbreviations*: HDL-C, high-density lipoprotein cholesterol; SBP, systolic blood pressure; TC, total cholesterol.

CV risk factor. In a meta-analysis of 18 epidemiologic studies, exposure to smoking was consistently associated with a 20–30% increase in the risk of CV events in non-smokers (10). Of note, smoking is the only CV risk factor that is significantly associated with vasospastic angina (11).

Because of the linear relationship between the number of cigarettes smoked per day, starting with as few as four to five cigarettes per day, and the risk of CV events, and because of the documented damage caused by passive smoking, the ultimate goal is to achieve total abstinence from smoking.

Hypertension

The potential mechanisms by which hypertension may promote atherosclerosis and favor acute CV events include impaired endothelial function, increased endothelial permeability to lipoproteins and adherence of leukocytes, increased oxidative stress, and increased hemodynamic stress, all of which may trigger acute plaque rupture. Furthermore, increased myocardial wall stress and oxygen demand favor myocardial ischemia and arrhythmias.

Systemic hypertension has been identified as a risk factor for CVD in both men and women, including the elderly, in a large number of prospective epidemiologic studies. Both systolic and diastolic values of blood pressure have a strong and graded relationship with the risk of CVD, without any evidence of a threshold value (12). In a meta-analysis of observational data in one million patients from 61 studies, death due to CVD increased progressively and linearly for blood pressure levels as low as 115 mmHg for systolic and 75 mmHg for diastolic values upward. The increased risk was present in all age groups, from 40 to 89 years, and there was a doubling of mortality due to CVD for every 20 mmHg increase for systolic or 10 mmHg increase for diastolic blood pressure (13). In addition, longitudinal data obtained from the Framingham Heart Study indicate that blood pressure values in the range 130–139/85–89 mmHg are associated with a more than twofold increase in the relative risk of CVD compared with blood pressure levels below 120/80 mmHg (12).

The large physiological variations in blood pressure impose that, to diagnose hypertension, blood pressure should be measured in each individual more than one time on separate occasions. In general, the diagnosis of hypertension should be confirmed during at least two or three visits, with a minimum of two blood pressure readings taken per visit. Blood pressure measurement should be carried out in the sitting position after the patient has rested for at least 5 minutes. At the initial visit, blood pressure values should be obtained from both arms to identify patients in whom atherosclerotic plaques in subclavian arteries result in substantial between-arm discrepancies. Under such circumstances, the highest reading should be selected. The use of a conventional sphygmomanometer with an appropriate bladder size has been considered the gold standard for clinical measurements of blood pressure. However, because the use of mercury has now been banned in some countries, non-mercury sphygmomanometers are being used more frequently. Accordingly, their accuracy should be properly tested and validated using standard protocols.

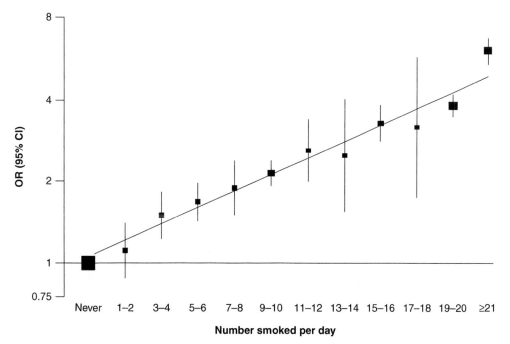

Figure 2.2 Risk of acute myocardial infarction with increasing numbers of cigarettes smoked per day. The risk almost doubles by smoking as few as three to four cigarettes per day (9).

The European Society of Hypertension (ESH) and the European Society of Cardiology (ESC) classify blood pressure levels as optimal (systolic <120 mmHg and diastolic <80 mmHg), normal (systolic 120–129 mmHg and diastolic 80–84 mmHg), high normal (systolic 130–139 mmHg and diastolic 85–89 mmHg), grade 1 hypertension (systolic 140–159 mmHg and diastolic 90–99 mmHg), grade 2 hypertension (systolic 160–179 mmHg and diastolic 100–109 mmHg), and grade 3 hypertension (systolic ≥180 mmHg and diastolic ≥110 mmHg) (14). A similar three-grade classification is also adopted by the WHO and the International Society of Hypertension (ISH) jointly (15) as well as the seventh report of the Joint National Committee on Prevention, Detection, Evaluation, and Treatment of High Blood Pressure that distinguishes three stages of hypertension and a pre-hypertension stage also called borderline hypertension, which refers to systolic values of 120–139 mmHg and diastolic values of 80–89 mmHg (16).

Compared with normotensive individuals, those with elevated blood pressure are more likely to have other risk factors for CVD. Indeed, hypertension is often associated with insulin resistance, hyperinsulinemia, glucose intolerance, dyslipidemia, and obesity, whereas it is found to be the sole risk factor in less than 20% of hypertensive individuals. Both the ESH/ESC and the WHO/ISH guidelines underscore that the diagnosis and treatment of hypertension has to be established based on the global CV risk (Fig. 2.3), focusing also on organ damage, in particular the presence of left ventricular hypertrophy and microalbuminuria (14,15).

The primary goal of treatment in hypertensive patients is to achieve a consistent reduction in the long-term risk of CVD. To this end, blood pressure should reach levels below 140/90 mmHg. Moreover, in diabetics and in subjects at high risk the goal is to achieve blood pressure levels below 130/80 mmHg. Yet this might be insufficient and the risk can remain high, or even very high, if the other risk factors, including smoking, dyslipidemia, and diabetes, are not appropriately treated (Fig. 2.3)

Dyslipidemia

In the second half of the previous century, several cross-sectional studies of cohorts living in different countries suggested that serum cholesterol levels were associated with death due to CVD. Prospective cohort studies bolstered this relationship whereas later investigations established that the association with CV mortality was attributable mainly to LDL-cholesterol. Indeed, in blood, lipids such as cholesterol and triglycerides, which are not water soluble travel in microspheres known as lipoproteins that contain a lipid core surrounded by a stratum of hydrophilic proteins (apoproteins). Apoproteins are not only important for lipid transportation but also have other functions including: (i) activation of key enzymes in lipid metabolism (lipoprotein lipase, hepatic lipase, lecithin cholesterol acyltransferase, and cholesteryl ester transfer protein) and (ii) binding to cell surface receptors.

The extent to which lipoproteins cause atherosclerosis depends on their type, size, and plasma concentration. Most of the cholesterol in blood is normally carried by LDLs; a strong and graded association has been consistently described between LDL-cholesterol and CV risk over a wide range of cholesterol concentrations, starting from levels as low as 50 mg/dL (17). This association applies to women and men, although the general level of risk is lower in women, at least until menopause. Furthermore, it applies to older as well as to younger people.

The relationship between elevated LDL-cholesterol and the development of coronary heart disease must be viewed as a multistep process beginning relatively early in life. The first stage of atherogenesis is the formation of the fatty streak, which consists largely of cholesterol-filled macrophages; most of the cholesterol

Blood pressure (mmHg)					
Other risk factors, OD or disease	Normal SBP 120–129 or DBP 80–84	High normal SBP 130–139 or DBP 85–89	Grade 1 HT SBP 140–159 or DBP 90–99	Grade 2 HT SBP 160–179 or DBP 100–109	Grade 3 HT SBP ≥ 180 or DBP ≥ 110
No other risk factors	Average risk	Average risk	Low added risk	Moderate added risk	High added risk
1–2 risk factors	Low added risk	Low added risk	Moderate added risk	Moderate added risk	Very high added risk
3 or more risk factors, MS, OD or diabetes	Moderate added risk	High added risk	High added risk	High added risk	Very high added risk
Established CV or renal disease	Very high added risk	Very high added risk	Very high added risk	Very high added risk	Very high added risk

Figure 2.3 Stratification of total cardiovascular risk in hypertensive patients according to cardiovascular risk factors and organ damage. The term "risk" refers to the probability of a cardiovascular event over 10 years; the term "added" indicates that in all categories the risk is greater than average. The dashed line indicates how the definition of hypertension varies according to total cardiovascular risk (14). *Abbreviations*: CV, cardiovascular; DBP, diastolic blood pressure; HT, hypertension; MS, metabolic syndrome; OD, organ damage; SBP, systolic blood pressure.

in fatty streaks is derived from LDL-cholesterol. The second stage consists of the formation of fibrous plaques in which a layer of scar tissue overlies a lipid-rich core. Other risk factors contribute to plaque growth in this phase. The third stage is represented by the development of unstable plaques that are prone to rupture and formation of luminal thrombosis. Plaque rupture (or erosion) is responsible for most acute coronary syndromes (myocardial infarction, unstable angina, and coronary death). Elevated LDL-cholesterol plays a role in the development of the mature coronary plaque, which is the substrate for the unstable plaque. Accordingly, lowering of LDL-cholesterol earlier in life slows atherosclerotic plaque development. This fact provides a rationale for long-term lowering of LDL-cholesterol in asymptomatic subjects with high levels of LDL-cholesterol or with moderate levels of LDL-cholesterol but high global risk. Recent evidence indicates that intensive LDL-cholesterol lowering in patients with an acute coronary syndrome reduces the short–medium-term risk of recurrence of coronary instability. This early effect of statins is more likely to be mediated by their anti-inflammatory effect rather than by their lipid-lowering effect. In contrast, the long-term beneficial effects of statins on CV events in asymptomatic subjects and in patients with established CVD are entirely mediated by LDL-cholesterol reduction.

Low concentrations of HDL-cholesterol are also clearly associated with early development of atherosclerosis. HDLs are antiatherogenic; it has been suggested that HDLs exert this effect through anti-inflammatory, antithrombotic, and anti-apoptotic mechanisms. The participation of HDL in cholesterol transportation to the liver from other organs and tissues, including the arterial wall, containing a surplus of cholesterol (termed reverse cholesterol transportation) is another mechanism by which HDL might protect the artery wall.

While total cholesterol and HDL-cholesterol are measured directly, LDL-cholesterol is usually calculated by the Friedewald formula:

$$\text{LDL-cholesterol} = \text{total cholesterol} - \text{HDL-cholesterol} - (0.2 \times \text{triglycerides})$$

However, this formula is valid only when the concentrations of triglycerides are less than approximately 400 mg/dL.

Hypertriglyceridemia is also associated with an increased risk of atherosclerotic disease, but it is still debated whether it is independent of the other risk factors, in particular diabetes mellitus.

With regard to the goals of treatment, an approach that is widely used and takes global risk assessment into account has been proposed by the National Cholesterol Education Program Adult Treatment Panel III (NCEP-ATP III) (18).

The ATP III identified three categories of risk that modify the goals and modalities of LDL-cholesterol lowering therapy having CVD as an end point. The category at the highest risk comprises asymptomatic subjects with a 10-year risk >20% and more than two risk factors and patients with established coronary heart disease or coronary heart disease equivalents, including diabetes, peripheral arterial disease, abdominal aortic aneurysm, carotid artery disease (symptomatic (e.g., transient

ischemic attack or stroke of carotid origin) or >50% stenosis on angiography or ultrasound). The LDL-cholesterol target in this category is <100 mg/dL. The second category consists of multiple (>2) risk factors and 10-year risk <20%. The LDL-cholesterol target in this category is <130 mg/dL. The third category consists of persons with zero to one risk factor. The LDL-cholesterol target in this category is <160 mg/dL. The major risk factors included in the NCEP-ATP III recommendations are cigarette smoking, blood pressure ≥140/90 mmHg or on antihypertensive medication, low HDL-cholesterol (<40 mg/dL), family history of premature coronary heart disease, and age ≥45 years in men or ≥55 years in women.

After the publication of the ATP III guidelines, several important trials on cholesterol lowering have been published. Therefore, updated management recommendations have been released (19) proposing the following LDL-cholesterol targets: (i) <100 mg/dL and optionally <70 mg/dL in subjects at high risk (as defined above); (ii) <130 mg/dL or optionally <100 mg/ dL in moderately high-risk subjects (>2 risk factors and a 10-year risk between 10% and 20%); (iii) <130 mg/dL in moderate-risk subjects (>2 risk factors and a 10-year risk <10%); (iv) <160 mg/dL in low-risk subjects (as defined above) (Fig. 2.4).

Diabetes Mellitus

Potential mechanisms by which diabetes may cause atherosclerosis include low HDL-cholesterol, high triglycerides, increased lipoprotein remnant particles, increased small, dense LDL-cholesterol, enhanced lipoprotein oxidation, glycation of LDL-cholesterol, increased fibrinogen, increased platelet aggregability, impaired fibrinolysis, increased von Willebrand factor, hyperinsulinemia, and impaired endothelial function.

Epidemiologic studies have demonstrated a linear association between increasing blood glucose levels and the risk of CVD. The relationship has been demonstrated using both the 2-hour value following an oral glucose tolerance test and the integrated measure of glycosilated hemoglobin.

Diabetes mellitus is an independent risk factor for CVD. Both type 1 and type 2 diabetes mellitus patients present a two to four times increased risk of CV events. CVD is responsible for three-fourths of deaths among people with diabetes. Some data have suggested that diabetic patients without a history of myocardial infarction have as high a risk of coronary mortality as non-diabetic patients with a history of myocardial infarction (20).

Diabetes abolishes the usual protection against CVD present in premenopausal women. Indeed, diabetic women have twice the risk of recurrent myocardial infarction compared with diabetic men. The greater risk of CVD in type II diabetic women than in diabetic men may, at least in part, be explained by the greater adverse effects that diabetes exerts on lipoproteins in women.

A joint document of the ESC and the European Association for the Study of Diabetes (EASD) (21) categorizes glucose metabolism, according to previous criteria issued by the WHO (22) and the American Diabetes Association (ADA) (23), into normal glucose regulation, impaired glucose metabolism, and diabetes. The WHO criteria are based on both fasting and

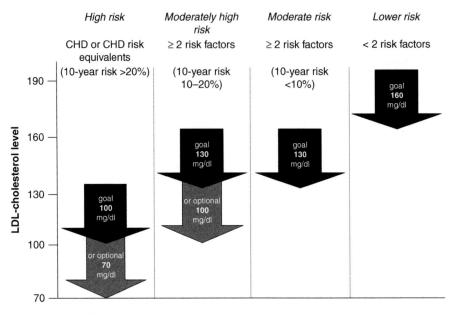

Figure 2.4 Target levels of LDL-cholesterol according to global risk as proposed by the guidelines of the Adult Treatment Panel III of the National Cholesterol Education Program (19). *Abbreviations*: CHD, coronary heart disease; LDL, low-density lipoprotein.

Focus Box 2.2

Combinations of traditional risk factors act synergistically in increasing the risk of cardiovascular events. Thus, global risk assessment plays a key role in primary prevention.

2-hour post-load plasma glucose whereas the ADA criteria strongly encourage the use of fasting glycemia only. Diabetes mellitus is defined as fasting plasma glucose ≥126 mg/dL or 2-hour post-load plasma glucose ≥200 mg/dL. These thresholds, also endorsed by the American Association of Clinical Endocrinologists (AACE) (24) and the International Diabetes Federation (IDF) (25), were primarily determined by the values at which the prevalence of diabetic retinopathy, which is a specific complication of hyperglycemia, starts to increase.

With regard to the treatment of diabetes it is becoming increasingly clear that the goal should be the control of hyperglycemia and of other risk factors frequently associated with diabetes. The Steno-2 Study (Fig. 2.5) has shown that the combined control of hyperglycemia, hypertension, and dyslipidemia results in a more than 50% reduction of CV events (26). With regard to diabetes in particular, the accepted goal is a value of glycated hemoglobin <7% for the ADA (23) and ≤6.5% for the ESC and EASD (21), AACE (24), and IDF (25). Recent trials suggest that a strict glycemic control may result in fatal episodes of hypoglycemia that might offset the potential benefits. Future guidelines will address this important issue probably by devising different target values based on clinical presentation.

OTHER CLINICAL RISK FACTORS

While the clinical importance of the traditional CV risk factors is well established, they are typically thought to only account for about half of the risk of developing CVD. Moreover, in recent years, many studies have suggested that other potentially modifiable risk factors, which are easily identifiable on clinical examination, might have clinical relevance and might constitute important targets to decrease the CV risk. The compelling INTERHEART study identified nine risk factors accounting for about 90% of the population-attributable risk of developing a myocardial infarction (Fig. 2.6) (27). These risk factors include abdominal obesity, psychosocial factors, sedentary lifestyle, lack of consumption of fruits and vegetables, and alcohol intake, in addition to the traditional risk factors (current smoking, dyslipidemia, hypertension, and diabetes mellitus).

However, their real independent association with CV risk remains under scrutiny and is still debated. Indeed, these risk factors frequently favor or cause the classical CV risk factors, including dyslipidemia, hypertension, and diabetes mellitus. Thus, it is plausible that most of their effects are mediated by the latter adverse conditions, and the benefit derived by their reduction might be due to the reduction of the traditional risk factors.

Although most studies, in recent years have underscored the importance of obesity as a pandemic issue, it is likely that most of the negative effects of obesity are, in fact, related to classical factors and that obesity by itself may not constitute an independent risk factor, as suggested by a recent study involving 221,934 individuals in 17 countries (28).

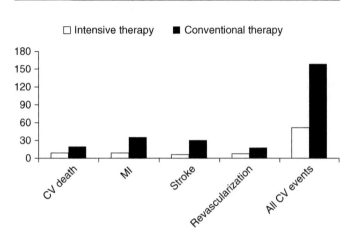

Steno-2 intensive treatment goals

Blood pressure < 130/80 mmHg

Cholesterol < 175 mg/dL

Triglycerides < 150 mg/dL

Glycosilated hemoglobin < 6.5%

Aspirin

Angiotensin converter enzyme-inhibitor

☐ Intensive therapy ■ Conventional therapy

Figure 2.5 Predefined intensive multifactorial intervention treatment goals in Steno-2 Study (*upper panel*) and incidence of events after a mean of 13.3 years (7.8 years of intensive multifactorial intervention and an additional 5.5 years of follow-up; *lower panel*). A comprehensive reduction of traditional risk factors for type 2 diabetes mellitus resulted in a striking >50% reduction of CV events (26). *Abbreviations*: CV, cardiovascular; MI, myocardial infarction.

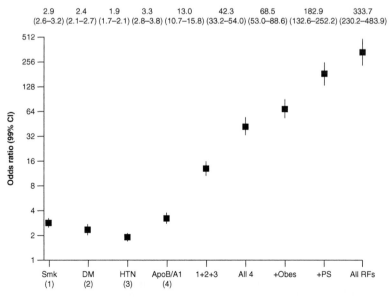

Figure 2.6 Risk of acute myocardial infarction associated with exposure to multiple risk factors in the INTERHEART Study. The risk for a subject with all risk factors is 512 times higher than that for a subject without any risk factor (27). *Abbreviations*: DM, diabetes mellitus; HTN, hypertension; Obes, abdominal obesity; PS, psychosocial factors; RF, risk factor; Smk, smoking.

RISK SCORES AND GLOBAL RISK ASSESSMENT

Although the individual traditional risk factors are significantly associated with the development of CVD, their predictive and discriminative power is, on the whole, limited when used alone. Indeed, the distribution of individual risk factors between those with and without CVD overlaps substantially.

In the Women's Health Study, although increased LDL-cholesterol levels were associated with incident CV events, 46% of these events occurred in women with LDL-cholesterol levels below 130 mg/dL (29).

In analyses of data collected from more than 122,000 patients enrolled in clinical trials with diagnoses of coronary heart disease, including myocardial infarction, unstable angina, and percutaneous coronary intervention (30), 15% of women and almost 20% of men did not have any of the four major traditional modifiable CV risk factors. In addition, more than 50% of women and 60% of men had zero or only one of these risk factors.

Thus, given the limited predictive power of individual risk factors for the development of CVD, an alternative strategy has been developed to quantify the risk and also determine the appropriateness of interventions; this strategy relies on deriving scores based on the combination of multiple risk factors found to be significantly predictive of CV events in large populations of individuals. Risk factors are assessed globally using predictive equations. The latter are derived from multivariable modeling of various weighted traditional risk factors and provide a probability estimate of developing CVD in a given time period. Risk factor interactions are, indeed, complex, involving joint effects, threshold levels, and multiplicative interactions that can magnify CV risk, and require a more complex and comprehensive approach to risk assessment.

A routine technique to estimate the utility of these risk assessment strategies is the use of receiver operating characteristic (ROC) curve analysis. The area under the ROC curve (AUC), which corresponds to c-statistics, estimates the probability that the risk function will assign a higher value to those who will develop an event compared with those who will not. Thus, it assesses how well a risk factor, or a combination of risk factors, can discriminate between affected and unaffected persons, with a value of 0.5 (or 50%) corresponding to no better than chance and a value of 1.0 being perfect discrimination. AUC values in the range of 0.7–0.9 are considered good while values greater than 0.9 are considered excellent for discrimination. The c-statistic for individual risk factors such as lipid values and blood pressure generally ranges between 0.6 and 0.7 when used alone, which is suboptimal for clinical purposes.

The AUC values and c-statistics are important in establishing how well risk factors scores improve disease prediction as compared with single risk factors, also giving important information to assess cost–benefit ratios of diagnostic interventions.

The Framingham Risk Score

The Framingham risk score (FRS) (7) is an easy-to-apply and clinically relevant scoring system that is derived using the following risk factors: age, sex, total cholesterol, HDL-cholesterol, blood pressure, and cigarette smoking.

The FRS was derived from a large population of men and women recruited in the Framingham Heart Study, who were initially free of clinical CVD. The FRS was originally based on continuous values of variables, but subsequently a simplified point scoring system based on categories of age, total cholesterol (or LDL-cholesterol), HDL-cholesterol, systolic blood pressure, diabetes, and smoking status, with separate algorithms for men and women was developed (7).

FRS provides an estimate of the 10-year risk of coronary events including angina pectoris, myocardial infarction, and coronary death (7). Although FRS has been validated in many populations, including Caucasians, Americans, and African Americans, its accuracy was shown to be somewhat limited in some more recent studies, in particular in European and Asian populations. Indeed, in a systematic review of 27 studies using the FRS, the predicted-to-observed risk ratio ranged from an underprediction of 0.43 in a high-risk population to an overprediction of 2.87 in a low-risk population (31).

There are several reasons for the lower accuracy of risk prediction recently observed with the FRS. These include the significant fall in the CV risk in Western populations in the decades that followed the Framingham Study, the difference in CVD prevalence in populations that are different from those in which the Framingham Study was conducted, and the exclusion of ethnicity as a factor that significantly influences the risk.

On the other hand, the FRS offers some advantages that have led to its broad endorsement as the primary method for CV risk assessment in the United States and in other countries. First, the FRS has been evaluated in a large number of studies and in diverse settings. Risk scores derived from FRS have also been developed to predict 30-year and lifetime risk, although these latter scores require further validation. More recently, a multivariable risk function for the assessment of CVD risk has been derived from the FRS (1).

Importantly, the FRS can be easily applied in an office-based setting with both paper and computer-based tools to facilitate its use. For these reasons the FRS is recommended by several expert panels of various scientific societies and study groups as a valid tool for the global assessment of CV risk in apparently healthy individuals.

The SCORE Project

In 2003, the ESC guidelines on CVD prevention presented a new global risk assessment algorithm called SCORE (Systematic COronary Risk Evaluation) (32). This risk function was developed based on data from more than 200,000 patients pooled from 12 European cohorts.

Focus Box 2.3

Scores based on the combination of multiple risk factors have been developed and validated in large prospective studies to ensure global risk assessment in individual patients.

The SCORE algorithm incorporates the same traditional risk factors included in FRS, but it is calibrated for European populations and predicts the 10-year risk of a first fatal CV event, caused by myocardial infarction, stroke, and aortic aneurysm. A unique aspect of the SCORE system is that separate equations have been derived for high-risk and low-risk regions of Europe, as well as for coronary artery disease and non-coronary CVD (Fig. 2.7). It should be noted that the SCORE algorithm estimates the risk for fatal atherosclerotic events only; that is, it does not consider non-fatal events. There are now several country-specific versions of the SCORE system.

The QRISK Risk Score

The QRISK risk score was derived from a large UK primary care population and included age, gender, smoking status, systolic blood pressure, the ratio of total cholesterol to HDL-cholesterol, body mass index, family history of coronary heart disease, a measure of social deprivation, and treatment with antihypertensive drugs as the risk factors (33). Subsequently, the QRISK2 risk score was developed to further improve risk prediction, by including ethnicity, diabetes mellitus, rheumatoid arthritis, renal disease, and atrial fibrillation as additional risk factors (34).

However, due to its complexity this risk score is less attractive for use in clinical practice; furthermore, it has not been validated

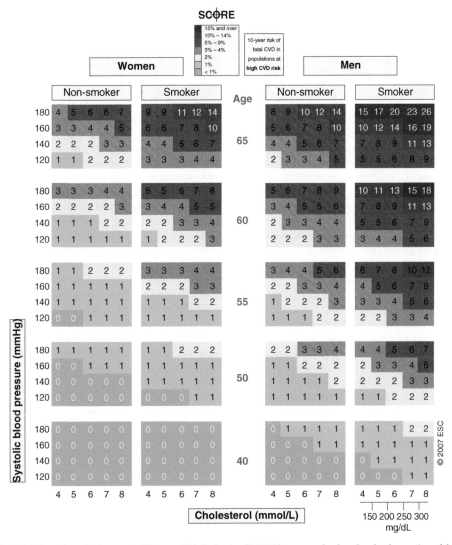

Figure 2.7 Example of risk charts from the Systematic COronary Risk Evaluation (SCORE) program developed under the auspices of the European Society of Cardiology. These charts are extremely helpful in making a quick assessment of cardiovascular risk based on the traditional risk factors (29). *Abbreviation*: CVD, cardiovascular disease.

in independent populations. Moreover, it was derived from routine datasets, rather than from prospective research studies, which were used to derive the FRS and the SCORE risk equations.

The PROCAM Risk Function

The PROCAM (PROspective CArdiovascular Munster) risk function estimates the probability of developing hard endpoints (coronary death or first myocardial infarction) within 10 years; it includes age, systolic blood pressure, LDL- and HDL-cholesterol, triglycerides, smoking, diabetes mellitus, and family history of myocardial infarction as risk factors (35).

The risk function was developed on the basis of a Cox proportional hazards model from a sample of 5,389 German men included in the PROCAM study who were free of any CVD at baseline, between 1979 and 1985. However, as it is derived from a cohort of middle-aged men, it has limited applicability to women and men above the age of 65 years. Therefore, a new PROCAM risk score has recently been developed based on a Weibull function, thus making it possible to carry out risk assessment in the general population (36).

The CUORE Risk Charts

The CUORE risk charts were developed to evaluate the global CV risk from data on 7,056 men and 12,574 women who were free of CVD and were enrolled from the north, center, and south of Italy between the mid-1980s and the mid-1990s (37). The patients were followed up for a mean period of 10 years for total and cause-specific mortality and non-fatal cerebrovascular and coronary events.

Specifically, the risk charts include diabetes mellitus, smoking habit, age, systolic blood pressure, and total cholesterol as categorical variables and apply separately to men and women aged 40–69 years. The CUORE risk charts were found to compare well with the SCORE system when applied to European populations at low risk for CV mortality (38).

PERSONAL PERSPECTIVE

The identification of traditional risk factors is the first milestone in the prevention of CVD. A second milestone is the notion that it is not enough to consider individual risk factors; it is important to measure global risk factors in order to tailor the intensity of risk factor control in individual patients. This approach has allowed us to identify: (i) patients at low risk in whom the main goal is to encourage appropriate lifestyle changes; (ii) patients at high risk in whom it is necessary, in addition to optimization of lifestyle, to achieve strict targets with regard to treatment of hypertension, dyslipidemia, and diabetes; (iii) patients at intermediate risk in whom, again, it is important to optimize lifestyle, while they remain in a gray area with regard to optimal medical treatment. Accordingly, future challenges include: (i) appropriate reclassification of patients now considered at intermediate risk and (ii) identification of patients who are at high risk of developing an acute CV event in the short term.

Intermediate risk constitutes a gray zone in CV risk assessment although up to one-third of all CV events occur in this category of risk. It would therefore be extremely useful to appropriately reclassify patients on the basis of further investigations. Advances in our understanding of the biology of atherosclerosis might allow the use of new biomarkers to sharpen the assessment of CV risk. For instance, high levels of C-reactive protein (CRP) are associated with all risk factors identified by the INTERHEART study, including those not accounted for by current risk algorithms (27). The possibility of quickly capturing these elusive risk components, such as diet, physical activity, and depression, that are difficult to measure directly might contribute to the ability of CRP to appropriately reclassify subjects at intermediate risk of CV events by traditional risk algorithms into a higher or lower risk category. Accordingly, in the recent JUPITER (Justification for the Use of Statins in Primary Prevention: an Intervention Trial Evaluating Rosuvastatin) trial, patients at intermediate risk, according to traditional risk factors, but with CRP levels >2 mg/L had a better CV outcome when randomized to statin when compared with those on placebo (39). Bio-imaging (including assessment of coronary calcium score or carotid intima-media thickness) also appears to be able to reclassify patients at intermediate CV risk. However, how CRP levels and bio-imaging can be used in clinical practice to guide treatment in individuals classified as being at intermediate risk remain to be better established.

Finally, among high-risk patients it would be highly desirable to identify subjects who harbor vulnerable plaque prone plaques that are likely to cause a CV event in the short term. However, we are probably far from this ambitious goal, as the vast majority of thin-capped plaques, which might be identified using bio-imaging, heal spontaneously without causing symptoms (40,41), and plaque erosion is difficult to detect prior to thrombus formation.

Focus Box 2.4 Tools to Assess Global Cardiovascular Risk
Framingham risk score
SCORE project
QRISK risk score
PROCAM risk function
CUORE risk charts

Focus Box 2.5
Up to one-third of cardiovascular events occur in subjects who are at intermediate global risk. This is a gray zone in cardiovascular risk assessment. So appropriate reclassification of patients in this gray zone is needed. Although C-reactive protein is a promising biomarker to this end, further studies using other biomarkers or bio-imaging techniques are warranted.

REFERENCES

1. D'Agostino RB Sr, Vasan RS, Pencina MJ, et al. General cardiovascular risk profile for use in primary care: the Framingham Heart Study. Circulation 2008; 117: 743–53.
2. Grundy SM. Primary prevention of coronary heart disease: integrating risk assessment with intervention. Circulation 1999; 100: 988–98.
3. Sacks FM, Pfeffer MA, Moye LA, et al. The effect of pravastatin on coronary events after myocardial infarction in patients with average cholesterol levels. Cholesterol and Recurrent Events Trial investigators. N Engl J Med 1996; 335: 1001–9.
4. The Long-Term Intervention with Pravastatin in Ischaemic Disease (LIPID) Study Group. Prevention of cardiovascular events and death with pravastatin in patients with coronary heart disease and a broad range of initial cholesterol levels. N Engl J Med 1998; 339: 1349–57.
5. Juul-Moller S, Edvardsson N, Jahnmatz B, et al. Double-blind trial of aspirin in primary prevention of myocardial infarction in patients with stable chronic angina pectoris. The Swedish Angina Pectoris Aspirin Trial (SAPAT) Group. Lancet 1992; 340: 1421–5.
6. Cesaroni G, Forastiere F, Agabiti N, et al. Effect of the Italian smoking ban on population rates of acute coronary events. Circulation 2008; 117: 1183–8.
7. Wilson PW, D'Agostino RB, Levy D, et al. Prediction of coronary heart disease using risk factor categories. Circulation 1998; 97: 1837–47.
8. Jackson R, Lawes CM, Bennett DA, et al. Treatment with drugs to lower blood pressure and blood cholesterol based on an individual's absolute cardiovascular risk. Lancet 2005; 365: 434–41.
9. Teo KK, Ounpuu S, Hawken S, et al. Tobacco use and risk of myocardial infarction in 52 countries in the INTERHEART study: a case-control study. Lancet 2006; 368: 647–58.
10. He J, Vupputuri S, Allen K, et al. Passive smoking and the risk of coronary heart disease–a meta-analysis of epidemiologic studies. N Engl J Med 1999; 340: 920–6.
11. Lanza GA, Sestito A, Sgueglia GA, et al. Current clinical features, diagnostic assessment and prognostic determinants of patients with variant angina. Int J Cardiol 2007; 118: 41–7.
12. Vasan RS, Larson MG, Leip EP, et al. Impact of high-normal blood pressure on the risk of cardiovascular disease. N Engl J Med 2001; 345: 1291–7.
13. Lewington S, Clarke R, Qizilbash N, et al. Age-specific relevance of usual blood pressure to vascular mortality: a meta-analysis of individual data for one million adults in 61 prospective studies. Lancet 2002; 360: 1903–13.
14. Mancia G, De Backer G, Dominiczak A, et al. Guidelines for the management of arterial hypertension: The Task Force for the Management of Arterial Hypertension of the European Society of Hypertension (ESH) and of the European Society of Cardiology (ESC). Eur Heart J 2007; 28: 1462–536.
15. Whitworth JA. World Health Organization (WHO)/International Society of Hypertension (ISH) statement on management of hypertension. J Hypertens 2003; 21: 1983–92.
16. Chobanian AV, Bakris GL, Black HR, et al. The seventh report of the Joint National Committee on prevention, detection, evaluation, and treatment of high blood pressure: the JNC 7 report. JAMA 2003; 289: 2560–72.
17. Neaton JD, Blackburn H, Jacobs D, et al. Serum cholesterol level and mortality findings for men screened in the Multiple Risk Factor Intervention Trial Research Group. Arch Intern Med 1992; 152: 1490–500.
18. Expert Panel on Detection, Evaluation, and Treatment of High Blood Cholesterol in Adults. Executive Summary of the Third Report of the National Cholesterol Education Program (NCEP) Expert Panel on Detection, Evaluation, and Treatment of High Blood Cholesterol in Adults (Adult Treatment Panel III). JAMA 2001; 285: 2486–97.
19. Grundy SM, Cleeman JI, Merz CN, et al. Implications of recent clinical trials for the National Cholesterol Education Program Adult Treatment Panel III guidelines. Circulation 2004; 110: 227–39.
20. Haffner SM, Lehto S, Ronnemaa T, et al. Mortality from coronary heart disease in subjects with type 2 diabetes and in nondiabetic subjects with and without prior myocardial infarction. N Engl J Med 1998; 339: 229–34.
21. Ryden L, Standl E, Bartnik M, et al. Guidelines on diabetes, pre-diabetes, and cardiovascular diseases: executive summary the Task Force on Diabetes and Cardiovascular Diseases of the European Society of Cardiology (ESC) and of the European Association for the Study of Diabetes (EASD). Eur Heart J 2007; 28: 88–136.
22. WHO Consultation. Definition, diagnosis and classification of diabetes mellitus and its complications. Geneva: World Health Organ, 1999.
23. Genuth S, Alberti KG, Bennett P, et al. Follow-up report on the diagnosis of diabetes mellitus. Diabetes Care 2003; 26: 3160–7.
24. Rodbard HW, Blonde L, Braithwaite SS, et al. American Association of Clinical Endocrinologists medical guidelines for clinical practice for the management of diabetes mellitus. Endocr Pract 2007; 13(Suppl 1): 1–68.
25. IDF Clinical Guidelines Task Force. Global Guideline for Type 2 Diabetes. Brussels: International Diabetes Federation, 2005.
26. Gaede P, Lund-Andersen H, Parving HH, et al. Effect of a multifactorial intervention on mortality in type 2 diabetes. N Engl J Med 2008; 358: 580–91.
27. Yusuf S, Hawken S, Ounpuu S, et al. Effect of potentially modifiable risk factors associated with myocardial infarction in 52 countries (the INTERHEART study): case-control study. Lancet 2004; 364: 937–52.
28. Wormser D, Kaptoge S, Di Angelantonio E, et al. Separate and combined associations of body-mass index and abdominal adiposity with cardiovascular disease: collaborative analysis of 58 prospective studies. Lancet 2011; 377: 1085–95.
29. Ridker PM, Rifai N, Rose L, et al. Comparison of C-reactive protein and low-density lipoprotein cholesterol levels in the prediction of first cardiovascular events. N Engl J Med 2002; 347: 1557–65.
30. Khot UN, Khot MB, Bajzer CT, et al. Prevalence of conventional risk factors in patients with coronary heart disease. JAMA 2003; 290: 898–904.
31. Brindle P, Beswick A, Fahey T, et al. Accuracy and impact of risk assessment in the primary prevention of cardiovascular disease: a systematic review. Heart 2006; 92: 1752–9.
32. De Backer G, Ambrosioni E, Borch-Johnsen K, et al. European guidelines on cardiovascular disease prevention in clinical practice. Third Joint Task Force of European and Other Societies on Cardiovascular Disease Prevention in Clinical Practice. Eur Heart J 2003; 24: 1601–10.
33. Hippisley-Cox J, Coupland C, Vinogradova Y, et al. Derivation and validation of QRISK, a new cardiovascular disease risk score for the United Kingdom: prospective open cohort study. BMJ 2007; 335: 136.

34. Hippisley-Cox J, Coupland C, Vinogradova Y, et al. Predicting cardiovascular risk in England and Wales: prospective derivation and validation of QRISK2. BMJ 2008; 336: 1475–82.

35. Assmann G, Cullen P, Schulte H. Simple scoring scheme for calculating the risk of acute coronary events based on the 10-year follow-up of the prospective cardiovascular Munster (PROCAM) study. Circulation 2002; 105: 310–15.

36. Assmann G, Schulte H, Cullen P, et al. Assessing risk of myocardial infarction and stroke: new data from the Prospective Cardiovascular Munster (PROCAM) study. Eur J Clin Invest 2007; 37: 925–32.

37. Giampaoli S, Palmieri L, Donfrancesco C, et al. Cardiovascular risk assessment in Italy: the CUORE Project risk score and risk chart. Ital J P Health 2007; 4: 102–9.

38. Donfrancesco C, Palmieri L, Cooney MT, et al. Italian cardiovascular mortality charts of the CUORE project: are they comparable with the SCORE charts? Eur J Cardiovasc Prev Rehabil 2010; 17: 403–9.

39. Ridker PM, Danielson E, Fonseca FA, et al. Rosuvastatin to prevent vascular events in men and women with elevated C-reactive protein. N Engl J Med 2008; 359: 2195–207.

40. Mann J, Davies MJ. Mechanisms of progression in native coronary artery disease: role of healed plaque disruption. Heart 1999; 82: 265–8.

41. Stone GW, Maehara A, Lansky AJ, et al. A prospective natural-history study of coronary atherosclerosis. N Engl J Med 2011; 364: 226–35.

3 The role of genomics and proteomics in identifying subjects at risk of clinical manifestations of coronary atherosclerosis and their future clinical applications

Carlos L. Alviar and Pedro R. Moreno

OUTLINE

Genomic medicine has provided tremendous advantage in the identification of subjects at increased risk of cardiovascular disease, in particular atherosclerotic heart disease. Several genes and loci have been identified with the use of advanced technologies, while significant scientific efforts are currently being directed towards the investigation of these and other markers. In the same way, proteomics and metabolomics research have provided considerable evidence about specific biomarkers that are linked to atherosclerosis. In this chapter we will first provide an overview of the different techniques in genomics and proteomics that are currently being used in biomedical research and their applications in cardiovascular medicine. Then, we will describe specific genetic markers linked to coronary atherosclerosis with a review of the evidence behind them. Finally we will review the proteomic markers associated with higher risk of coronary heart disease and we will discuss those biomarkers that have the most robust evidence as risk factors of coronary atherosclerosis, and the limitations in the interpretation of proteomics in atherosclerosis.

INTRODUCTION

Despite a significant reduction in the mortality rates from cardiovascular disease (CVD) in Western countries during the last half century (1), it continues to be the leading cause of death worldwide. With 16.7 million deaths per year, it represents almost one-third of the total global deaths (2). As a result, better risk stratification and aggressive therapy at the prevention level are important priorities for global health improvement.

Classical risk-prediction models compile traditional risk factors such as age, diabetes, gender, smoking, and others to estimate events. However, as most of these factors are widely prevalent, such algorithms lack accuracy and may not correctly estimate the real odds of having a cardiac event (3,4). The presence of heart disease in young individuals with no identifiable traditional risk factor is a clear example of risk-prediction failure with current strategies. Thus, new prediction and risk stratification models are evolving with the aim of better predicting heart disease. Genomic and proteomic biomarker evaluation offers novel alternatives for cardiovascular risk estimation (5–7). This chapter provides the reader with a systematic approach on the use of genomics and proteomics for the assessment of individuals with an increased risk of coronary heart disease (CHD). The chapter is divided into four sections. The first section is devoted to definition and clinical relevance; the second section is concerned with the available evidence on

specific biomarkers. The third section summarizes the role of genomics and proteomics in clinical practice and primary prevention. The last section section recaps key learning points and the authors' perspectives, in addition to outlining future directions of this topic in the practice of cardiology.

DEFINITIONS AND METHODOLOGY OF GENOMICS, PROTEOMICS, AND METABOLOMICS

A biomarker is defined as "a characteristic that is objectively measured and evaluated as an indicator of normal biologic processes, pathogenic processes, or pharmacologic responses to a therapeutic intervention" (8). These biomarkers might represent different molecular compounds including nucleic acids and genes (genomics), protein and peptides (proteomics), and metabolites (metabolomics). Figure 3.1 illustrates the process of gene expression, from DNA replication and transcription to translation, and depicts the areas of analysis of these three different disciplines, also known as the "omics."

The analysis of the genome includes the identification of DNA sequences and the mapping of specific genes of a living organism (9). However, only 1.5% of the 3 billion DNA base pairs that comprise the human genome represent coding sequences that can be translated into proteins. Moreover, as 99.5% of the DNA sequence is identical between different individuals, the key is to identify variations in the remaining 0.5% of the genome. Such variations include two important elements: single nucleotide polymorphisms and copy-number variants (10). These can be identified by DNA isolation, DNA cloning, polymerase chain reaction, DNA blotting, DNA autoradiography, restriction fragment length polymorphisms, fluorescence in situ hybridization (for chromosomal analysis), spectral karyotyping, somatic cell hybridzation, Southern blot, Southwestern blot, and Northern blot.

In contrast to the genome, the analysis of the proteome is performed on proteins expressed in specific cells. These proteins are involved in physiological, pathological, or adaptive processes (11). The field of proteomics can be divided into structural, expression, and interaction proteomics (12). Proteomics emerged as a technique to complement the information given by genomic analysis in biological processes. It was created to overcome the limitations of genomics associated with the fact that genetic expression is not always related to a particular protein or peptidic end-product reflecting a physiological or pathological process within the cell or tissue (13). For example, a particular DNA segment can produce different proteins by a phenomenon called alternative splicing. Thus, proteomics

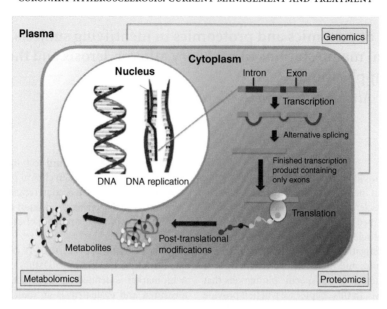

Figure 3.1 The "omic" disciplines: Gene expression in an eukaryotic cell and the process evaluated by genomics, proteomics, and metabolomics. First, the double-stranded DNA undergoes replication of the coding segment including the exons (DNA segments to be expressed) and the introns (DNA segments that will not be ultimately expressed). Then, the DNA segment is transcribed into mRNA with both the exons and the introns. Genomics involves the study of the processes up to this point. At this point the mRNA undergoes alternative splicing and a shorter mRNA segment that includes only the exons is ready to be translated into a popypeptide. Subsequently, the translated protein undergoes post-translational changes that modify the structure of the molecule. Proteomics analyzes such compounds and their structure. Finally, these proteins and other compounds, which are by-products of the enzymatic reactions or biological pathways, are released as metabolites and are analyzed by metabolomics.

complements genomics by providing a more accurate evaluation of specific markers of a biological process (12). Along the same lines, proteomics can contribute to the identification of target molecules that are involved in a particular pathologic process (13). Most importantly, proteomics can also analyze post-translational changes in proteins, thereby providing more accurate information on the biological process. An example that is relevant to atherosclerosis is post-translational modification leading to the formation of advanced glycation end-products (14). An additional advantage of proteomics is that it might allow the sequencing of entire genomes, with the subsequent identification of rare variants that would lead to improved risk prediction (15).

The different laboratory techniques used in proteomics are summarized in Table 3.1. The most commonly used technique is mass spectometry, where proteins from a particular sample are metabolized into small peptides, allowing for quantitative and qualitative analysis by high-performance liquid chromatography (HPLC) (16,17). Figures 3.2 and 3.3 illustrate the different steps involved in the identification of new biomarkers by proteomic analysis. Despite the great potential of mass spectrometry in proteomics, the application of this technique for cardiovascular risk prediction in clinical trials is still ongoing and requires more investigation.

The analysis of the metabolome (secretome) is based on the end-products of the different biological pathways. These end-products include low molecular weight compounds, not encoded

Focus Box 3.1

Intracellular processes involved in the pathophysiology of atherosclerosis are regulated by gene expression of DNA segments associated with pathophysiological pathways, which are then translated into proteins and finally converted into metabolites. Genomics, proteomics, and metabolomics can assess the different molecules involved in these stages, thus providing an opportunity for risk stratification assesment and implementation of possible interventions in individuals at risk of coronary artery disease.

by DNA, from a cell or tissue that reflect the dynamic processes underlying biological homeostasis. Metabolomics studies the final chemical signatures of pathways mediated by genomics and proteomics. Metabolites are usually the substrates and by-products of intracellular processes and enzymatic reactions. The importance of metabolomics derives from the fact that these metabolites are an accurate reflection of the phenotypic activity, while genomics and proteomics provide detailed information only about the genotype. Moreover, as the number of target molecules in genomics (about 25,000 genes) and proteomics (100,000 transcript products or 1 million proteins) is significantly high, the relatively small number of metabolites (around 6500) makes it easier to integrate the information provided by this science (18). The independence from direct genetic regulation makes it a useful complement to

Table 3.1 Different Laboratory Techniques Used for Proteomic Analysis

Name	Type of technique	Method employed	Comments
Mass spectrometry imaging (MSI or mass spec)	Imaging	Tissue is obtained and molecules are identified and located in specific areas matched by histology.	Excellent for peptides that can be ionized. Used for pharmacological molecules with the potential of measuring metabolites or proteins that have been modified in the tissue by drugs or cellular processes. When used in tissues with complex molecular structures, it might reduce the quality of the measurements.
Time of flight-secondary ion mass spectrometry (TOF-SIMS)	Imaging	Same as mass spec.	Very appropriate for identifying lipid molecules in a particular set of tissue, tissues; requires less preparation due to a reduction in the mass range.
Surface-enhanced laser desorption/ ionization-time of flight (SELDI-TOF)	Gel-free	Separates proteins from other tissue components with the use of microlaser beams.	Less intricate to perform, especially for large tissue specimens. However, a lower resolution is obtained, especially for peptides with high molecular weight.
Liquid chromatography coupled with tandem mass spectrometry	Gel-free	Protein separation using hydrophilic methods that do not involve the use of a gel.	Integration of peptide separation and identification with the use of sophisticated devices and algorithms in a mass spectrometer allows better protein separation in complex samples.
Two-dimensional difference gel electrophoresis (2D-DIGE)	Gel-based	Proteins are marked with fluorescent dyes before they are separated by 2D gel electrophoresis. Then the gel is scanned at the excitation wavelength of each dye in order to identify each molecule individually.	The main objective is to accurately identify protein abundance (accurate quantitative analysis) in tissues or individuals.
Two-dimensional electrophoresis	Gel-based	Molecules are separated based on electric charge or molecular weight using polyacrylamide gels.	Allows the analysis of the entire set of molecules in a particular sample, but mostly provides a semi-quantitative analysis.

genomics and proteomics. Few studies have analyzed the role of metabolomics in CVD (19). One of the first studies demonstrated a greater than 90% predictive power for coronary artery disease (CAD) in patients with a major lipid region analyzed by nuclear magnetic resonance spectra (20). However, another study trying to replicate these findings reported a lower predictive power of 63–80% (21). These differences highlight the variability of metabolites and the difficulty in reproducing metabolic signatures between different patient cohorts. Similarly, other studies have identified several metabolites as predictors of CAD. For example, low levels of citric acid, 4-hydroxyproline, and aspartic acid, while as well as elevated levels of lactate, urea, glucose, and valine, have prognostic value for CAD prediction (22–24). For the purpose of this chapter, we will only include a detailed description of genomics and proteomics in predicting CAD. The role of meatbolomics in CVD has been reviewed elsewhere (19).

CLINICAL RELEVANCE OF GENOMICS AND PROTEOMICS IN CARDIOVASCULAR MEDICINE

Atherosclerosis is a dynamic process, with intercalating periods of quiescence and activity, in which plaque inflammation

Focus Box 3.2

Atherosclerosis is a complex and dynamic process that involves multiple pathophysiologic pathways. The identification of specific genomic and proteomic biomarkers related to these pathways would represent the most appropriate approach for risk stratification. These markers will provide valuable information for risk assessment that is not affected by the dynamic nature of the disease. At this point, these specific markers are being evaluated for CAD risk assessment, especially in asymptomatic subjects.

and growth occurs (25). As a result, the risk prediction models used for cross-sectional evaluations might fail to accurately stratify individuals at risk. Thus, a more suitable approach would be to carry out periodic longitudinal assessment to detect changes in plaque homeostasis that represent an increase in the risk of coronary events (26). Genomic and proteomic analysis might help to fill this gap, by providing stationary markers of risk prediction that are not necessarily affected by the dynamic nature of atherosclerosis formation.

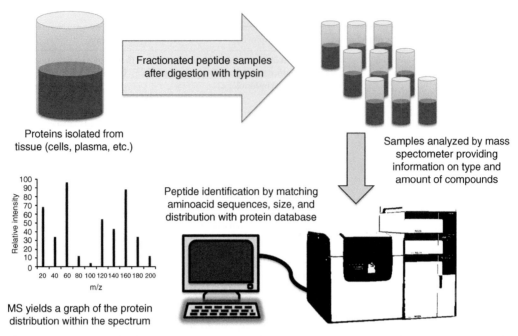

Proteins isolated from
tissue (cells, plasma, etc.)

Fractionated peptide samples
after digestion with trypsin

Samples analyzed by mass
spectrometer providing
information on type and
amount of compounds

Peptide identification by matching
aminoacid sequences, size, and
distribution with protein database

MS yields a graph of the protein
distribution within the spectrum

Figure 3.2 Processes involved in the identification of proteins and peptides as potential biomarkers using mass spectroscopy (MS).

Novel genomic and proteomic biomarkers may contribute to the understanding of the natural history of the atherosclerotic plaque and would help to identify periods of disease activity related to the prediction of coronary events. Similarly, in the study of atherosclerotic heart disease, the spectrum of genes, proteins, or molecular compounds that could be defined as biomarkers is significantly extensive. These include biomarkers for thrombosis, inflammation, lipoprotein metabolism, calcification, vascular remodeling, neovascularization, oxidative stress, defective efferocytosis, and cell death (27). Therefore, the identification of markers specifically associated with each of these processes may be needed for specific risk prediction.

CURRENT STATUS OF GENOMICS IN CVD
Family studies have widely proven that CVD has a significant genetic component, which is estimated to be up to 40% (28–30). In the absence of traditional risk factors, family history may be the only predictor for CHD, especially in cases of early presentation (29,31). However, only a minor percentage of atherosclerotic heart disease is secondary to monogenic disorders. This is the case for familial hypercholesterolemia, which results from defects in the low density lipoprotein (LDL) receptor, or Tangier disease, which results from defects in ATP-binding cassette transporters (30). Thus, the single-gene approach traditionally tested in knockout experimental models provides evidence that applies only to that gene or pathway in particular (15).

Similar to the vast majority of heritable cardiovascular disorders, atherosclerosis follows a polygenic pathway influenced by environmental interactions (32,33). A good example is the synergistic interaction between smoking and the E4 apolipoprotein E allele that has been proven to increase the risk of CVD (34). The polygenic nature of atherosclerosis requires a more global approach to assess mutations in different genes using association studies, meta-analysis, and linkage analysis. Nonetheless, specific genetic regions are fundamental when studying atherosclerosis. This is the case for the 3q26–27 and 2q34–37 loci containing genes involved in glucose and lipid metabolism, as reported by Chiodini and Lewis (35). Also, copy-number variants involved in other molecular pathways such as genetic alterations in *apolipoprotein (a)*, *apolipoprotein E*, *CXADR*, and *DAB2IP* might also determine the specific risk of coronary events in individuals carrying such alterations (Table 3.2) (32). However, this approach has several limitations, including lack of accuracy and statistical power, as evidenced by the conflicting results and the failure to yield strong conclusions from different researchers and study populations. To overcome such limitations, the candidate gene approach and the agnostic genomic approach were developed.

The candidate gene approach is usually hypothesis driven and targets the classical pathways that are known to be involved in atherosclerosis. These include genes involved in lipoprotein metabolism, vascular inflammation, neovascularization, and vascular wall homeostasis (36). The objective of this approach is to determine if variants of the genes in those pathways, typically referred to as single nucleotide polymorphisms (SNPs), are associated with cardiovascular events or subclinical disease (26). Different genetic mutations have been identified using this method. For instance, in the lipoprotein metabolism pathway the presence of one or more

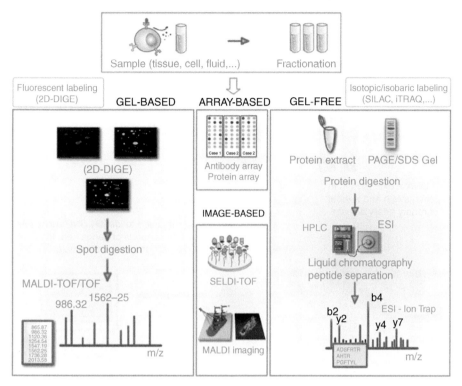

Figure 3.3 Four major proteomics approaches are outlined. Difference gel electrophoresis (DIGE) represents an improvement in comparative two-dimensional electrophoresis (2DE). Samples of proteins from two experimental conditions are labeled with two fluorescent dyes, mixed together, and run on a single 2DE gel to reduce variability and improve the sensitivity and reproducibility of the 2DE process. *Abbreviations:* ESI, electrospray ionization; HPLC, high-performance liquid chromatography; iTRAQ, isobaric tags for relative and absolute quantification; MALDI, matrix-assisted laser desorption/ionization; PAGE, polyacrylamide gel electrophoresis; SELDI-TOF, surface-enhanced laser desorption/ionization-time of flight; SDS, sodium dodecylsulfate; SILAC, stable isotope labeling by amino acids in cell culture. *Source:* Adapted from Ref. 62.

Table 3.2 Recent Advances in Ischemic Heart Disease Genomics

Gene or locus	Condition	Experimental methods	Effect size (OR) (single allele)	Effect size (OR) (multiple alleles)	Ref.
9p21.3 (*CDKN2A,* *CDKN2B*)	MI	GWAS	1.2–1.4	1.6–2.0	(32–34,37,39)
	AAA		1.31	1.74	
	Intracranial aneurysm		1.29	1.72	
	PAD		1.14	–	
LPA	CAD	GWAS, candidate gene, resquencing	1.7–1.9	2.5–4.0	(17,81)
	Enhanced aspirin response		2.2[a]	–	
APOE	CAD, dyslipidemia	GWAS, candidate gene, resquencing	1.1–1.4	1.2–1.6	(44,45)
CYP2C19	Stent thrombosis(`2–`5 alleles)	GWAS, candidate gene, resquencing	3.5	4.6	(70,71)
	Bleeding (`17 allele)		1.8	3.2	
21q21(*CXADR*)	Venticular fibrillation	GWAS	1.5–1.8	–	(43)
DAB2IP	Early onset MI	GWAS	1.18	–	(39)
	AAA		1.21	–	
	PE		1.20	–	
	PAD		1.14	–	

[a]The odds ratio represents the increased risk for CAD in rs3798220 carriers. The enhanced risk was completely abrogated by aspirin therapy.

Abbreviations: AAA, abdominal aortic aneurysm; *APOE,* apolipoprotein E; CAD, coronary artery disease; CYP, hepatic cytochrome; GWAS, genome-wide association studies; MI, myocardial infarction; OR, odds ratio; PAD, peripheral artery disease; PE, pulmonary embolism.

Source: Adapted from Ref. 32.

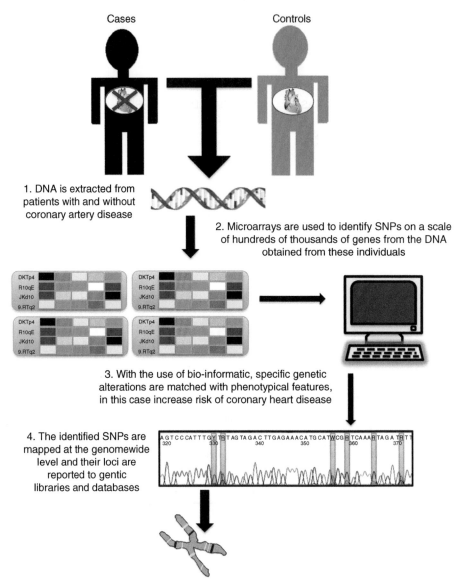

Figure 3.4 Schematic representation of the execution of genome-wide association studies. *Abbreviation*: SNP, single-nucleotide polymorphism.

of the ε4 alleles of *APOE* has been proven to be associated with increased risk of CAD (37). Mutations in LPA that lead to increasing plasma levels of lipoprotein(a) are related to a higher risk of CAD (38). Similarly, mutations in the *PCSK9* gene, which are associated with decreased plasma levels of LDL, are associated with reduced rates of coronary events (39). Conversely, the quest for other SNPs as candidate genes for other atherosclerotic pathways has not been as rewarding as the lipoprotein arena. This is related to the lack of success in the attempts to replicate candidate gene studies in these other pathways. Therefore, newer techniques for candidate gene studies are looking for SNPs located in the proximity of the candidate genes related to atherosclerosis

formation, and their correlation with linkage disequilibrium in these sequences (40). This approach is expected to increase the prognostic yield of genetic studies of atherosclerosis.

The agnostic (a term derived from the Greek word άγνωστο, meaning **unknown**) genetic approach is based on genome-wide association studies (GWAS) using as many genes as possible (Fig. 3.4). It is not based on a hypothesis and is designed to screen the genome of an entire cohort and the genes associated with CAD in these subjects. It addresses the variability of genes between individuals and patterns of linkage disequilibrium across the genome (41). The execution of GWAS requires a large number of individuals with an adequate number of controls for

Table 3.3 Single-Nucleotide Polymorphisms Associated with Coronary Disease That Have Been Identified and Replicated in Genome-Wide Association Studies

Single-nucleotide polymorphism	Locus	Pathway influenced by the genetic product of the locus	Supporting evidence (author (Ref.))
rs11206510	1p32	Cholesterol regulation	Kathiresan et al. (97)
rs9818870	3q22.3	Cellular homeostasis	Erdmann et al. (98)
rs1746048	10q11	White blood cells activation	Samani et al. (42); Kathiresan et al. (97)
rs10757278	9p21.3	Cell cycle homeostasis	Helgadottir et al. (47); Samani et al. (42); Wellcome Trust Case Control Consortium (99); Coronary Artery Disease Consortium (100); Kathiresan et al. (97)
rs12526453	6p24	Inhibits phosphoprotein phosphatase inhibitor	Kathiresan, S. *et al.* (97)
rs599839	1p13.3	Intercellular communication; p53-mediated growth suppression; metabolic regulator in adipose tissue and muscle	Willer et al. (101); Samani et al. (42); Wellcome Trust Case Control Consortium (99); Coronary Artery Disease Consortium (100); Kathiresan et al. (97)
rs9982601	21q22	Electrolyte transport, intracellular anabolism, neuromuscular regulation	Kathiresan et al. (97)
rs3184504	12q24	Membrane receptor and cytoplasmic pathways	Gudbjartsson et al.(102)
rs1122608	19p13	Endocytosis	Kathiresan et al. (97)
rs6725887	2q33	Ribosomal formation	Kathiresan et al. (97)
rs3008621	1q41	Diapedesis	Samani et al. (42); Coronary Artery Disease Consortium (100); Kathiresan et al. (97)
rs501120	10q11.2	Not known	Samani et al. (42); Coronary Artery Disease Consortium (100)

comparison, and a rigorous statistical analysis. These studies are performed by extracting DNA from white blood cells (WBCs) that will subsequently undergo genotyping, using microarrays of anywhere between 500,000 and 1 million SNPs across the genome. Using bio-informatics, the information from the locus of interest may then be used to identify specific alterations related to the increase in the risk of cardiovascular events (42). GWAS have identified around 35 SNPs in loci related to atherosclerosis, as shown in Table 3.3 (41). Such genetic loci usually increase the risk of CAD by 10–40% per allele. However, several of these alleles are also found in the general population, suggesting that the population-attributable risk can be substantial (42).

The current predictive utility of the SNPs involved in these genetic variants is still limited when compared with traditional risk factors such as diabetes or smoking (43,44). Such limitations are most likely secondary to the small relative risk and odds ratios found in genetic studies, compared with the more robust results from the studies analyzing clinical risk factors. It is also important to keep in mind that the impact of genetic variations might also vary according to the environmental factors to which an individual is exposed (45). As a result GWAS might play a role in the understanding of disease pathways and in improving prediction of events based on genetic susceptibility analysis in the setting of specific environmental factors. This might require improved methods for the assessment of environmental exposures and the inclusion of larger cohorts of patients.

SPECIFIC GENETIC MARKERS FOR CORONARY ATHEROSCLEROSIS

Several studies have focused on identifying chromosomal segments and loci with prognostic value. A particular allele, the

chromosome 9p21, showed an increased risk stratification value when added to traditional risk factors (42,46–48). Numerous studies have evaluated the role of this chromosome in CAD risk prediction (Fig. 3.5). Among them two meta-analyses reported the association of the chromosome 9p21.3 with CAD risk (49,50). Additionally, McPherson et al. showed that two SNPs (rs10757274 and rs1333049) located on chromosome 9p21 were associated with an increased risk of CAD of 15–20% in heterozygotes and 30–40% in homozygotes (46). These authors studied a small cohort of cases and controls but validated their results by analyzing this association in three larger studies, the Copenhagen City Heart Study, the Dallas Heart Study, and the Ottawa Heart Study-3. Talmud et al. found that the SNP (rs10757274) located on chromosome 9p21.3 contributed to a more accurate reclassification for risk estimation. However, it did not add significant information on top of the Framingham risk score to predict cardiovascular events (51). Similarly, in the Atherosclerosis Risk in Communities study on 10,000 patients, adding the same 9p21.3 allele to traditional risk factors modestly improved risk estimation, only in the low-intermediate and intermediate-high categories (52). Nonetheless, in a larger cohort of 22,000 female individuals, the same SNP (rs10757274) on chromosome 9p21.3 was associated with higher cardiovascular risk, but did not improve prediction when added to the classical risk factors (53). The discrepancies in the outcomes from these studies may be related to gender differences and variations in the follow-up period (10.2 years as compared with 14.6 years). Moreover, the presence of biochemical enhancers may also erratically influence gene expression at the molecular level (54).

Using a case-control approach, Samani et al. performed genotyping in patients with and without CAD from both The

Cardiovascular death

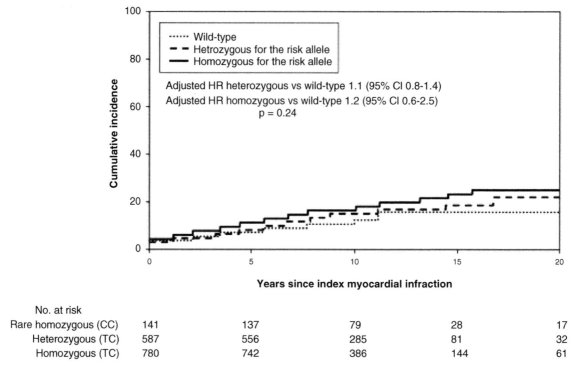

Figure 3.5 Cumulative incidence of cardiovascular events after early-onset myocardial infarction by the allele rs1333040 from the 9p21.3 locus. Kaplan-Meier cumulative incidence curve of cardiovascular death. *Abbreviations*: CI, confidence interval; HR, hazard ratio. *Source*: Addapted from Ref. 103.

Wellcome Trust Case Control Consortium and the German Myocardial Infarction Family Study. They reported a strong association of chromosome 9p21.3 (SNP, rs1333049) with CAD in both cohorts. The combined analysis of both studies identified seven additional chromosomal loci associated with CAD ($P < 1.3 \times 10^{-6}$, probability >80%) (42). Notably, a recent meta-analysis that included both prospective and retrospective studies confirmed that both SNPs (rs10757274 and rs1333049) on chromosome 9p21.3 were strongly associated with CAD risk in Caucasians (50). A larger prospective study analyzing 11,550 cases and 11,205 controls from nine European studies reported that only four loci were independent risk factors of CAD, and they include:

1. 1p13.3 (rs599839)
2. 1q41 (rs17465637)
3. 10q11.21 (rs501120)
4. 2q36.3 (rs2943634)

These loci, along with 9p21.3 (rs10757274 and rs1333049), cumulatively increased the risk of cardiovascular events by 15% (12–18%), per additional risk allele (Fig. 3.6) (55). Finally, as one of the limitations of GWAS is the modest statistical power, usually limited by small sample sizes, the CARDIo-GRAM Consortium was created. The aim of this study was to enhance the accuracy in detecting genomic variants related to CAD. This is the largest study designed to confirm the association of previously identified loci with CAD and identify novel genetic markers of CAD. This study combines numerous published and unpublished GWAS including 22,000 cases with CAD and 64,000 controls in subjects of European descent. By analyzing an average of 2.2 million SNPs per study in the form of a meta-analysis, these authors found that the SNP rs1333049 on chromosome 9p21.3 increased the risk of myocardial infarction by almost 30% per copy (49). Moreover, they confirmed the association of 10 of the 13 previously described loci related to CAD, and found 13 new loci that increased the risk of CAD by 6–17% per allele (56).

Although commercially available (57), genetic testing is still controversial in clinical practice (58,59). More importantly, it is yet to be established if genetic susceptibility studies will improve CVD prediction and outcomes and reduce complications (60). In order to maintain the ACCE criteria (Analytic validity, Clinical validity, Clinical utility, and associated Ethical, legal and social implications), the Centers of Disease Control and Prevention established a genetic testing model in 2004 (61). This includes the following criteria: (*i*) The ability to measure the genotype of interest both accurately and reliably. (*ii*) The ability of a genetic test to detect or predict the presence or

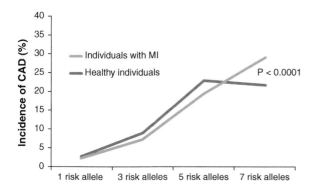

Figure 3.6 Distribution of risk alleles in individuals with and without a history of myocardial infarction (MI). As the most strongly associated loci increase (1p13.3, 1q41, 9p21, and 10q11.21), the incidence of coronary artery disease (CAD) increases and becomes significant for individuals with more number of risk alleles.

Focus Box 3.3

Atherosclerotic heart disease has a strong genetic component. The current evidence supporting the presence of specific mutations with CAD comes from the candidate gene approach and genome-wide association studies. The most robust evidence linking genetic alterations with CAD has been found to be related to genetic variations in chromosome 9p21.3. Similarly, three more chromosomal loci have been found to be associated with CAD, and they include 1p13.3, 2q36.3, and 10q11.21. Another loci, 1q41, might also provide prognostic value for CAD risk but perhaps in a less robust way. There are commercially available assays for genetic testing. Despite the early current stage, results in this area seem to be promising for CAD risk estimation, but require further prospective research before they can be recommended in clinical practice with the aim of improving current risk stratification models.

---

absence of the phenotype or clinical disease. (*iii*) The likelihood that the genetic test will lead to an improved outcome, including test and disease characteristics. (*iv*) It must take into account the impact of the genetic test results on insurance and employment, privacy and confidentiality, equity of access, and stigmatization. Other ethical aspects such as the implication of potential harms of genetic testing (including unnecessary anxiety) and the appropriate communication approach from the physician to the patients may also play a major role in the application of genetic testing in clinical practice (26).

CURRENT STATUS OF PROTEOMICS IN CVD
Proteins from atherosclerotic plaques that are the product of atherogenesis represent a potential target for cardiovascular risk prediction. Different cells or vessel wall components participate in specific stages of plaque formation and many proteins are the

reflection of these processes (27). As mentioned earlier, the lack of a completely accurate correlation between mRNA and its protein end-product is strongly influenced by alternative splicing and post-translational modifications. This supports the theory that genotyping alone is not enough to understand the complexity of a biological process or disease state (13). Therefore, the analysis of the proteome, also known as secretome, represents an appropriate complementary approach for the study of biomarkers (62).

The proteome can be studied by analyzing cell- or tissue-derived proteins from direct extraction or by studying circulating plasma proteins that reflect tissue composition (Fig. 3.7). Due to the heterogeneous cellular composition of atherosclerotic plaques, a whole tissue-derived proteomic analysis from a particular lesion might not be completely feasible. Moreover, the complexity of the pathways in atherosclerosis makes it difficult to accurately assess particular biomarkers when assessing whole tissue specimens. Therefore, research efforts have focussed on identifying isolated molecules from specific cellular or tissue extracts that can provide information on specific pathways (63). Among these methods, novel techniques such as laser capture micro-dissection (LCM) allow the extraction of specific tissue components with no background noise or contamination from other tissues or cellular components. However, as LCM might produce only minimal amounts of the protein of interest, its interpretation might be limited.

SPECIFIC PROTEOMIC MARKERS FOR CORONARY ATHEROSCLEROSIS
When targeting specific cellular components in proteomic studies, several cell lines have been studied. Examples of this include the analysis of vascular smooth muscle cells and their regulation by phosphorylation of chaperones (64), endothelial cells and their activation by pro-inflammatory cytokines (65), platelets and their dense granules fractions (66), and the adipocyte with the fatty acid-binding protein as a marker of cardiovascular risk (67). Circulating cells have also been targeted as another approach to identify biomarkers related to atherothrombosis risk (68). This includes molecules released or contained in red blood cells, platelets, and leukocytes, as outlined in Table 3.4.

Tissue-derived proteomic studies aiming to understand the composition of atherosclerotic plaques have been performed in carotid specimens. Duran et al. evaluated the proteomic profile of human carotid plaques with different levels of complexity, including normal segments, non-complicated plaques, and complicated plaques with thrombus. They cultured the vascular segments in a protein-free medium and analyzed the secreted proteins (supernatants) by two-dimensional gel electrophoresis. These authors identified several proteins from the atherosclerotic segments, including apolipoprotein A-I precursor, apolipoprotein B-100, transthyretin (prealbumin, amyloidosis type I), fibrinogen beta chain precursor, among others, and reported that the more complicated the lesion, the higher the number of secreted proteins (69). More recently, Lepeda et al. studied the proteomic characteristics of 19 stable and 29 unstable plaques in carotid arteries (70). They identified 33 different polypeptides by matrix-assisted laser

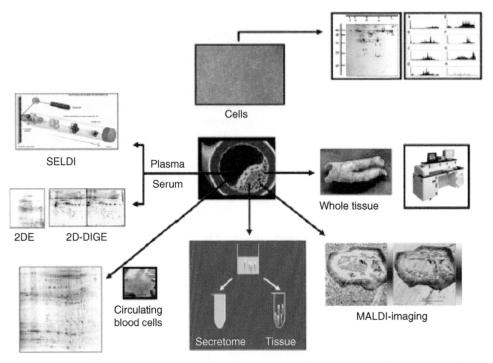

Figure 3.7 Proteomic strategies for the study of atherothrombosis. *Abbreviations*: 2DE, two-dimensional electrophoresis; DIGE, difference gel electrophoresis; MALDI, matrix-assisted laser desorption/ionization; SELDI, surface-enhanced laser desorption/ionization. *Source*: From Ref. 62.

desorption/ionization mass spectrometry using the NCBI database. They found that unstable plaques had higher amounts of ferritin light subunit, SOD2, and fibrinogen fragment D, while stable plaques showed an abundance of protective enzymes SOD3 and GST, as well as small heat shock proteins HSP27 and HSP20, annexin fA10, and Rho GDI. Interestingly, they observed that most of these proteins played a regulatory role in the inflammation and oxidative stress pathways, highlighting the importance of such an inflammatory *milieu* inside the atheroma (70). Another potential target for plasma proteomics includes microparticles derived from tissue components. They are released after cellular activation during different biological or disease processes. Mayr et al. recently demonstrated how some specific microparticles released from carotid plaque macrophages could be measured in plasma in combination with IgG (71). Such molecules have the potential to identify plaques with increased inflammation and, therefore, predict the risk of cardiovascular events (71).

The study of plasma-derived biomarkers related to CAD is more difficult when compared with tissue or cellular proteomes. One of the main reasons for this is that 90% of the plasma is composed of major proteins, primarily albumin and immunoglobulins, while 9% is composed of 12 other proteins as shown in Figure 3.8. Hence, the challenge is to identify the remaining 1% of proteins, also known as the "deep proteome" (72). To overcome this challenge, techniques that help to deplete the abundant major polypeptides have been developed. These techniques, which include SELDI-TOF platforms, protein precipitation, and protein

arrays, are described briefly in Table 3.1. They have allowed the identification of different biomarkers for CAD risk estimation. Among these, the more relevant ones are high-sensitive C-reactive protein (hs-CRP), WBC, IL-18, and TNF-α, as they were found to be inversely correlated with fibrous cap thickness, therefore increasing the risk of plaque rupture and coronary events (73). Notably, hs-CRP, also postulated as a modulator of plaque neovascularization (74), appeared to be the only independent predictor by regression analysis (75). Additionally, in terms of plasma biomarkers for therapeutic response, vitamin D binding protein has been associated with low response to aspirin, and probably with poor coronary outcomes (76). Two other important biomarkers of CAD risk are myeloperoxidase (77) and Lp-PLA2. The former acts as a potential marker of plaque vulnerability (78) whereas the latter plays a key role in expansion of the necrotic core (79). Additionally, CD40L, monocyte chemoattractant protein-1, various adhesion molecules, fibrinogen chain isoform-1, apolipoprotein A-IV, and haptoglobin 2 have been found to be elevated in hypercholesterolemic patients, but their levels decreased significantly after treatment with statins (80). Of note, it has been shown that the haptoglobin 2-2 genotype is more strongly related to a phenotype of higher plaque vulnerability (81). Some potential biomarkers of CHD identified by proteomic techniques are summarized in Table 3.5.

Despite the cumulative data on biomarkers, the clinical evidence for successful primary prevention through modification of these molecules, in particular hs-CRP, is still limited as outcomes

Table 3.4 Intracellular Pathways with End-Products Possibly Implied in the Pathogenesis of Atherosclerosis Studies

Intracellular pathway	Specific functions involved	Potential protein marker of increased atherosclerotic risk	Source
Nucleic acid processing	DNA regulation, proteasome, and molecular chaperones	Prohibitin	Neutrophils
		Hsp70, PDI	Neutrophils
		Cyclophilin A, glucose-regulated protein 78 kDa, Hsp70, Hsp47, PDI, Hsp27, proteasome 26S ATPase subunit 6	Platelets
		Chaperonin-containing TCP1, Hsp8	Erythrocytes
Cell metabolism	Enzymes involved in redox processes, hydrolases, and glycolysis as well as the transport of proteins from the Golgi apparatus, iron and ion transport, small lipophilic substances, and water	Carbonic anhydrase IV, Mn-SOD, MPO	Neutrophils
		Enolase	Neutrophils
		Coronin 7	Neutrophils
		Lactoferrin	Neutrophils
		Lipocalin (NGAL)	Neutrophils
	Proteins involved in the regulation of H_2O_2 and nitric oxide generation and intracellular lipid regulation	Lysophospholipase, monoglyceride lipase	Platelets
		SLP-2, AH receptor-interacting protein	Platelets
		Peroxiredoxin, peroxiredoxin 2, dimethyl arginase 2	Platelets
		Sorcin	Platelets
		Catalase, peroxiredoxin 1, peroxiredoxin 3	Erythrocytes
		Flotilin 1	Erythrocytes
Inflammation	Leukines and inflammatory mediators regulation, leukotriene hydrolysis, antibacterial molecules, MCH-I structure, chemokines to attract white blood cells, Toll-like receptor structure	Leukotriene A4, hydrolase, hCAP-18	Leukocytes (mostly neutrophils)
Intracellular signals and second messengers	Cell signaling	β2-microglobulin	Neutrophils
	Proteases and protease inhibitors	Connective tissue activating peptide	Neutrophils
	Protein kinases and small G proteins	Toll-interacting protein	Platelets
		14-3-3zeta, chondroitin sulfate synthase	Neutrophils
		Leukocystatin, cathepsin G, lysozyme, collagenase, chitotriosidase, leukocyte anti-elastase	Neutrophils
Cellular structure	Cytoskeletal structure and regulation, contractile proteins (actin accesory protein and actin-binding protein), tyrosine binding domain, binding proteins	14-3-3zeta, Rho-GDP-dissociation inhibitor Ly-GDI	Platelets
		RAP-1B, Ras suppressor protein 1	Platelets
		Cofilin 1, Gesolin, tropomyosin 3, TCP-1	Neutrophils
		HIP-55, ADAP (SLAP-130), Crk-L, β-arrestin, Huntingtin interacting protein 1 c-Src, Ran-GAP, ILK-1, p38 MAP kinase, RKIP, PIP5KI-α, calgranulin B, HINT1, PINCH, PAK 2	Platelets
		VASP, annexin III, annexin V, caspase-6, programmed cell death 10	
		Ankyrin 1, tropomyosin 3, EPB49, TCP-1	Erythrocytes
Other pathways	Proteasome structure	Proteasome alpha subunit 1 isoform 1, proteasome beta 1 subunit	Erythrocytes
	Direct platelet function	Coagulation factor XIII A chain	Platelets

from trials have generated a lot of controversy (82–86). Thus, the current trend is to use a multimarker approach that combines different molecules. This approach might more accurately reflect the myriad of pathways involved in the etiology of atherosclerosis, rather than an isolated process. For instance, Wang et al. evaluated 10 biomarkers in approximately 3,000 individuals who were followed up for about 7 years (84). They reported that B-type natriuretic peptide and urinary albumin excretion were predictors of both cardiovascular events and cardiovascular mortality while CRP, renin levels, and homocysteine acted as all-cause mortality predictors. Similarly, Zethelius et al. demonstrated that four biomarkers (N-terminal pro-B-type natriuretic peptide, CRP, cystatin, and troponin) significantly improved the prediction of myocardial infarction and death after 10 years of follow-up in elderly men (85). Unfortunately, although the combination of biomarkers into a common risk score enhanced risk estimation, it has not translated into a significant increment in the c-statistic results, which is a measure of the test's ability to discriminate individuals with disease from those without disease (84). In the same way, it is important to highlight that the utility of the multimarker approach might be limited when the biomarkers measured are the product of pathways that are correlated with clinical characteristics that are already being measured, such as lipoprotein alterations or inflammation (87).

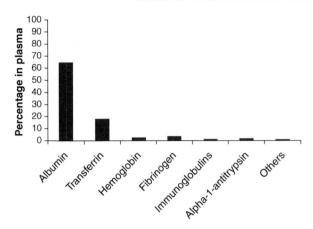

Figure 3.8 Predominant peptides found in the plasma of subjects with atherosclerosis.

Despite its promising results, proteomics faces several challenges. Among them the main technical limitation is the need for depletion of the abundant proteins in the plasma to obtain the less common molecules, also known as the "deep proteome," as mentioned earlier. Also, the human proteome comprises hundreds of thousands of circulating proteins that result from post-translational modification and alternative splicing as explained earlier. As a result, proteomics represents a more complex and difficult field when compared with the smaller human genome which contains about 30,000–40,000 genes (26,88). Hence, the search for proteomic biomarkers associated with an increased risk of coronary disease warrants the identification of new molecules that are not related to known candidate risk factors. For this purpose, an agnostic approach is perhaps the most appropriate as it might act as an unbiased way to recognize novel pathophysiologic pathways (26). Unfortunately, the agnostic approach in proteomics has not been as successful when compared with the agnostic approach for GWAS in genomics. It is hoped that as proteomic technologies evolve, along with improvements in collection, storage, preservation, and control-matching strategies, the

Table 3.5 Potential Proteomic Markers of Atherosclerotic Risk

High amounts of these proteins indicate increased atherosclerotic risk	Low amounts of these proteins indicate increased atherosclerotic risk (possible protective role)	Potential marker of atherosclerotic risk (marker vs. protective factor?)
Tropomyosin isoform	Soluble tumor necrosis factor-like weak inducer of apoptosis	Paraoxonase
Ferritin light chain	Rho GDP	CapG (gelsolin family)
Fortilin, tumor protein	Integrin-II	Cofilin 1
Cyclophilin B	Platelet-activating factor acetylhydrolase	Cathepsin H
Heat shock protein 90	Apolipoprotein D	Gelsolin
Glutathione S-transferase	Heat shock protein 27	Plasminogen activator inhibitor-1
Apoptosis-linked gene-2		Grb-2-like adaptor protein
Laminin-binding protein		Cathepsin D
Cathepsins D, L, S		Peroxiredoxin 1
Gamma-chain of fibrinogen		Proteoglycans
Actin		Lysosomal thiol reductase
Vimentin		Collagenase
Heavy chain of IgD		Interferon-gamma inducible Protein
Liver LKB-interacting protein		Dissociation inhibitor-alpha
Serum albumin		CapZ
Plasminogen activator inhibitor-2		Metalloproteinase-1
Elongation factor EF-1		
Apolipoprotein AI		
Protein disulfide isomerase		
HSP70		
HSP60		
Stomatin-like protein 2		
Tyrosine 3-monooxygenase		
Signal sequence receptor		
Annexin V		
Enolase I		
Beta-2-microglobulin		
A-adipocyte fatty acid-binding protein		
Superoxide dismutase		
Catalase		
Macrophage capping protein		
Alpha-1 antitrypsin		
Apolipoprotein B-100		
Lipoprotein Gln I		

Focus Box 3.4

The analysis of the proteome can provide useful information for the understanding of atherosclerosis development and the identification of individuals at risk of CAD. This can be accomplished by studying the secretome (proteome) from tissue or cellular components or from plasma samples. The most appropriate approach seems to be a combination of multiple biomarkers for risk stratification. The biomarkers linked to CAD with the strongest evidence include hs-CRP, Lp-PLA2, myeloperoxidase, among others. However, further evidence is needed before these biomarkers can accurately be applied in clinical practice for CAD risk prediction.

success of new biomarker identification will increase exponentially, yielding a more precise predictive and prognostic value (89,90).

Finally, before a biomarker assay can be used for risk prediction, it has to be validated using the Clinical Laboratory Improvement Amendments standards. The biomarker must meet the standards of accuracy, precision, analytical sensitivity, analytical specificity, reportable range of test results, and reference intervals. Most importantly, it must be clinically validated in patients with well-characterized clinical profiles (91). The process of performing multiple, parallel-protein measurements on the same specimen by a multidisciplinary approach is known as "multiplex assays" and requires extensive validation (92). Despite the fact that the FDA has approved the use of multiplex assays, consisting primarily of lateral flow immunoassays used for point-of-care evaluation (93), there are no multiplex assays currently available for CHD risk estimation in asymptomatic individuals.

In conclusion, the identification of proteomic biomarkers is a complex and time-consuming process and the expression of hundreds of proteins involved in atherogenesis might have a prognostic value for CAD prediction. Nonetheless, despite the valuable information provided by plasma and tissue biomarkers in alerting the clinician about patients with increased risk of CAD, further research is still needed to establish a clear role in coronary risk stratification.

CONCLUSION

The fields of genomics and proteomics in cardiovascular medicine are evolving to increase the ability to eventually predict coronary events. Both strategies may be of relevance in predicting events in populations lacking traditional risk factors. However, it is still unclear whether these data enhance the discriminatory and predictive value of currently available risk models. Hence, further prospective research is needed to completely elucidate the role of these biomarkers in coronary events (86). A modest increase in the predictive value was observed with biomarkers. Other statistical methods, such as the reclassification index or the integrated discrimination improvement, may increase the predictive value of novel biomarkers (94–96). Genomics and proteomics represent

promising techniques that provide valuable information for the understanding of atherosclerosis responsible for future cardiovascular events.

PERSONAL PERSPECTIVE

During the current era in which personalized medicine is rapidly growing, genomics and proteomics might play a major role in better selecting preventive and therapeutic approaches for specific conditions and patients. Moreover, in polygenic diseases such as atherosclerosis, the sequencing of the human genome, along with current advances in diagnostic techniques, has allowed us to accurately identify genomic and proteomic biomarkers that are indicative of an increased risk of CAD. Therefore, the role of the cardiovascular specialist is to recognize the applicability of these genetic techniques in clinical practice, by understanding the latest diagnostic methods and accurately interpreting them in each clinical scenario. As a result, physicians will be able to tailor the most appropriate treatment and implement specific preventive strategies for their patients. In the near future, we will incorporate gene therapy directed at specific genes involved in the pathogenesis, progression, and complications of atherosclerosis. At this point, however, the main utility of genomics and proteomics lies in the early detection of individuals at risk of CAD, which increases according to the estimated risk determined by the "omics" biomarkers.

REFERENCES

1. Roger VL, Go AS, Lloyd-Jones DM, et al. Heart disease and stroke statistics–2011 update: a report from the American Heart Association. Circulation 2011; 123: e18–e209.
2. Lloyd-Jones D, Adams RJ, Brown TM, et al. Heart disease and stroke statistics–2010 update: a report from the American Heart Association. Circulation 2010; 121: e46–e215.
3. Wilson PW, D'Agostino RB, Levy D, et al. Prediction of coronary heart disease using risk factor categories. Circulation 1998; 97: 1837–47.
4. Kullo IJ, Ballantyne CM. Conditional risk factors for atherosclerosis. Mayo Clin Proc 2005; 80: 219–30.
5. Morrison AC, Bare LA, Chambless LE, et al. Prediction of coronary heart disease risk using a genetic risk score: the Atherosclerosis Risk in Communities Study. Am J Epidemiol 2007; 166: 28–35.
6. Khoury MJ, Jones K, Grosse SD. Quantifying the health benefits of genetic tests: the importance of a population perspective. Genet Med 2006; 8: 191–5.
7. Cortese DA. A vision of individualized medicine in the context of global health. Clin Pharmacol Ther 2007; 82: 491–3.
8. Biomarkers Definitions Working Group. Biomarkers and surrogate endpoints: preferred definitions and conceptual framework. Clin Pharmacol Ther 2001; 69: 89–95.
9. Daniel L Hartl EWJ. Genetics: Analysis of Genes and Genomes. Boston: Jones and Bartlett Publishers, 2005.
10. Manolio TA. Genomewide association studies and assessment of the risk of disease. N Engl J Med 2010; 363: 166–76.
11. Malmstrom J, Lee H, Aebersold R. Advances in proteomic workflows for systems biology. Curr Opin Biotechnol 2007; 18: 378–84.
12. Graves PR, Haystead TA. Molecular biologist's guide to proteomics. Microbiol Mol Biol Rev 2002; 66: 39–63; table of contents.

13. Martinez-Pinna R, Martin-Ventura JL, Mas S, et al. Proteomics in atherosclerosis. Curr Atheroscler Rep 2008; 10: 209–15.

14. Schmidt AM, Yan SD, Wautier JL, Stern D. Activation of receptor for advanced glycation end products: a mechanism for chronic vascular dysfunction in diabetic vasculopathy and atherosclerosis. Circ Res 1999; 84: 489–97.

15. Tuomisto TT, Binder BR, Yla-Herttuala S. Genetics, genomics and proteomics in atherosclerosis research. Ann Med 2005; 37: 323–32.

16. Anderson NL, Anderson NG, Haines LR, et al. Mass spectrometric quantitation of peptides and proteins using Stable Isotope Standards and Capture by Anti-Peptide Antibodies (SISCAPA). J Proteome Res 2004; 3: 235–44.

17. Keshishian H, Addona T, Burgess M, Kuhn E, Carr SA. Quantitative, multiplexed assays for low abundance proteins in plasma by targeted mass spectrometry and stable isotope dilution. Mol Cell Proteomics 2007; 6: 2212–29.

18. Bain JR, Stevens RD, Wenner BR, et al. Metabolomics applied to diabetes research: moving from information to knowledge. Diabetes 2009; 58: 2429–43.

19. Goonewardena SN, Prevette LE, Desai AA. Metabolomics and atherosclerosis. Curr Atheroscler Rep 2010; 12: 267–72.

20. Brindle JT, Antti H, Holmes E, et al. Rapid and noninvasive diagnosis of the presence and severity of coronary heart disease using 1H-NMR-based metabonomics. Nat Med 2002; 8: 1439–44.

21. Kirschenlohr HL, Griffin JL, Clarke SC, et al. Proton NMR analysis of plasma is a weak predictor of coronary artery disease. Nat Med 2006; 12: 705–10.

22. Sabatine MS, Liu E, Morrow DA, et al. Metabolomic identification of novel biomarkers of myocardial ischemia. Circulation 2005; 112: 3868–75.

23. Barba I, de Leon G, Martin E, et al. Nuclear magnetic resonance-based metabolomics predicts exercise-induced ischemia in patients with suspected coronary artery disease. Magn Reson Med 2008; 60: 27–32.

24. Vallejo M, Garcia A, Tunon J, et al. Plasma fingerprinting with GC-MS in acute coronary syndrome. Anal Bioanal Chem 2009; 394: 1517–24.

25. Fuster V, Moreno PR, Fayad ZA, Corti R, Badimon JJ. Atherothrombosis and high-risk plaque: part I: evolving concepts. J Am Coll Cardiol 2005; 46: 937–54.

26. Kullo IJ, Cooper LT. Early identification of cardiovascular risk using genomics and proteomics. Nat Rev Cardiol 2010; 7: 309–17.

27. Moreno PR, Sanz J, Fuster V. Atherosclerosis. Curr Mol Med 2006; 6: 437–8.

28. Kullo IJ, Ding K. Mechanisms of disease: The genetic basis of coronary heart disease. Nat Clin Pract Cardiovasc Med 2007; 4: 558–69.

29. Williams RR, Hunt SC, Heiss G, et al. Usefulness of cardiovascular family history data for population-based preventive medicine and medical research (the Health Family Tree Study and the NHLBI Family Heart Study). Am J Cardiol 2001; 87: 129–35.

30. Lusis AJ, Fogelman AM, Fonarow GC. Genetic basis of atherosclerosis: part I: new genes and pathways. Circulation 2004; 110: 1868–73.

31. Murabito JM, Pencina MJ, Nam BH, et al. Sibling cardiovascular disease as a risk factor for cardiovascular disease in middle-aged adults. JAMA 2005; 294: 3117–23.

32. Damani SB, Topol EJ. Emerging genomic applications in coronary artery disease. JACC Cardiovasc Interv 2011; 4: 473–82.

33. Lusis AJ, Mar R, Pajukanta P. Genetics of atherosclerosis. Annu Rev Genomics Hum Genet 2004; 5: 189–218.

34. Humphries SE, Talmud PJ, Hawe E, et al. Apolipoprotein E4 and coronary heart disease in middle-aged men who smoke: a prospective study. Lancet 2001; 358: 115–9.

35. Chiodini BD, Lewis CM. Meta-analysis of 4 coronary heart disease genome-wide linkage studies confirms a susceptibility locus on chromosome 3q. Arterioscler Thromb Vasc Biol 2003; 23: 1863–8.

36. Johansen CT, Hegele RA. Predictive genetic testing for coronary artery disease. Crit Rev Clin Lab Sci 2009; 46: 343–60.

37. Utermann G, Hees M, Steinmetz A. Polymorphism of apolipoprotein E and occurrence of dysbetalipoproteinaemia in man. Nature 1977; 269: 604–7.

38. Clarke R, Peden JF, Hopewell JC, et al. Genetic variants associated with Lp(a) lipoprotein level and coronary disease. N Engl J Med 2009; 361: 2518–28.

39. Cohen JC, Boerwinkle E, Mosley TH Jr, Hobbs HH. Sequence variations in PCSK9, low LDL, and protection against coronary heart disease. N Engl J Med 2006; 354: 1264–72.

40. Ng SB, Turner EH, Robertson PD, et al. Targeted capture and massively parallel sequencing of 12 human exomes. Nature 2009; 461: 272–6.

41. Ding K, Kullo IJ. Genome-wide association studies for atherosclerotic vascular disease and its risk factors. Circ Cardiovasc Genet 2009; 2: 63–72.

42. Samani NJ, Erdmann J, Hall AS, et al. Genomewide association analysis of coronary artery disease. N Engl J Med 2007; 357: 443–53.

43. D'Agostino RB Sr, Vasan RS, Pencina MJ, et al. General cardiovascular risk profile for use in primary care: the Framingham Heart Study. Circulation 2008; 117: 743–53.

44. Gail MH. Discriminatory accuracy from single-nucleotide polymorphisms in models to predict breast cancer risk. J Natl Cancer Inst 2008; 100: 1037–41.

45. Thomas D. Gene–environment-wide association studies: emerging approaches. Nat Rev Genet 2010; 11: 259–72.

46. McPherson R, Pertsemlidis A, Kavaslar N, et al. A common allele on chromosome 9 associated with coronary heart disease. Science 2007; 316: 1488–91.

47. Helgadottir A, Thorleifsson G, Manolescu A, et al. A common variant on chromosome 9p21 affects the risk of myocardial infarction. Science 2007; 316: 1491–3.

48. Genome-wide association study of 14,000 cases of seven common diseases and 3,000 shared controls. Nature 2007; 447: 661–78.

49. Preuss M, Konig IR, Thompson JR, et al. Design of the Coronary ARtery DIsease Genome-Wide Replication And Meta-Analysis (CARDIoGRAM) Study: A Genome-wide association meta-analysis involving more than 22 000 cases and 60 000 controls. Circ Cardiovasc Genet 2010; 3: 475–83.

50. Humphries SE, Drenos F, Ken-Dror G, Talmud PJ. Coronary heart disease risk prediction in the era of genome-wide association studies: current status and what the future holds. Circulation 2010; 121: 2235–48.

51. Talmud PJ, Cooper JA, Palmen J, et al. Chromosome 9p21.3 coronary heart disease locus genotype and prospective risk of CHD in healthy middle-aged men. Clin Chem 2008; 54: 467–74.

52. Brautbar A, Ballantyne CM, Lawson K, et al. Impact of adding a single allele in the 9p21 locus to traditional risk factors on reclassification of coronary heart disease risk and implications for

lipid-modifying therapy in the Atherosclerosis Risk in Communities study. Circ Cardiovasc Genet 2009; 2: 279–85.

53. Paynter NP, Chasman DI, Buring JE, et al. Cardiovascular disease risk prediction with and without knowledge of genetic variation at chromosome 9p21.3. Ann Intern Med 2009; 150: 65–72.

54. Harismendy O, Notani D, Song X, et al. 9p21 DNA variants associated with coronary artery disease impair interferon-gamma signalling response. Nature 2011; 470: 264–8.

55. Samani NJ, Deloukas P, Erdmann J, et al. Large scale association analysis of novel genetic loci for coronary artery disease. Arterioscler Thromb Vasc Biol 2009; 29: 774–80.

56. Schunkert H, Konig IR, Kathiresan S, et al. Large-scale association analysis identifies 13 new susceptibility loci for coronary artery disease. Nat Genet 2011; 43: 333–8.

57. Hunter DJ, Khoury MJ, Drazen JM. Letting the genome out of the bottle–will we get our wish? N Engl J Med 2008; 358: 105–7.

58. Khoury MJ, McBride CM, Schully SD, et al. The Scientific Foundation for personal genomics: recommendations from a National Institutes of Health-Centers for Disease Control and Prevention multidisciplinary workshop. Genet Med 2009; 11: 559–67.

59. McGuire AL, Burke W. An unwelcome side effect of direct-to-consumer personal genome testing: raiding the medical commons. JAMA 2008; 300: 2669–71.

60. Rosenberg S, Elashoff MR, Beineke P, et al. Multicenter validation of the diagnostic accuracy of a blood-based gene expression test for assessing obstructive coronary artery disease in nondiabetic patients. Ann Intern Med 2010; 153: 425–34.

61. Haddow JE, Palomaki GE. ACCE: A model process for evaluating data on emerging genetic tests. New York: Oxford University Press, 2004.

62. Tunon J, Martin-Ventura JL, Blanco-Colio LM, et al. Proteomic strategies in the search of new biomarkers in atherothrombosis. J Am Coll Cardiol 2010; 55: 2009–16.

63. Blanco-Colio LM, Martin-Ventura JL, Vivanco F, et al. Biology of atherosclerotic plaques: what we are learning from proteomic analysis. Cardiovasc Res 2006; 72: 18–29.

64. Boccardi C, Cecchettini A, Caselli A, et al. A proteomic approach to the investigation of early events involved in the activation of vascular smooth muscle cells. Cell Tissue Res 2007; 329: 119–28.

65. Gonzalez-Cabrero J, Pozo M, Duran MC, et al. The proteome of endothelial cells. Methods Mol Biol 2007; 357: 181–98.

66. Hernandez-Ruiz L, Valverde F, Jimenez-Nunez MD, et al. Organellar proteomics of human platelet dense granules reveals that 14-3-3zeta is a granule protein related to atherosclerosis. J Proteome Res 2007; 6: 4449–57.

67. Xu A, Wang Y, Xu JY, et al. Adipocyte fatty acid-binding protein is a plasma biomarker closely associated with obesity and metabolic syndrome. Clin Chem 2006; 52: 405–13.

68. Martinez-Pinna R, Barbas C, Blanco-Colio LM, et al. Proteomic and metabolomic profiles in atherothrombotic vascular disease. Curr Atheroscler Rep 2010; 12: 202–8.

69. Duran MC, Mas S, Martin-Ventura JL, et al. Proteomic analysis of human vessels: application to atherosclerotic plaques. Proteomics 2003; 3: 973–8.

70. Lepedda AJ, Cigliano A, Cherchi GM, et al. A proteomic approach to differentiate histologically classified stable and unstable plaques from human carotid arteries. Atherosclerosis 2009; 203: 112–8.

71. Mayr M, Grainger D, Mayr U, et al. Proteomics, metabolomics, and immunomics on microparticles derived from human atherosclerotic plaques. Circ Cardiovasc Genet 2009; 2: 379–88.

72. Righetti PG, Castagna A, Antonioli P, Boschetti E. Prefractionation techniques in proteome analysis: the mining tools of the third millennium. Electrophoresis 2005; 26: 297–319.

73. Martin-Ventura JL, Blanco-Colio LM, Tunon J, et al. Proteomics in atherothrombosis: a future perspective. Expert Rev Proteomics 2007; 4: 249–60.

74. Turu MM, Slevin M, Matou S, et al. C-reactive protein exerts angiogenic effects on vascular endothelial cells and modulates associated signalling pathways and gene expression. BMC Cell Biol 2008; 9: 47.

75. Li QX, Fu QQ, Shi SW, et al. Relationship between plasma inflammatory markers and plaque fibrous cap thickness determined by intravascular optical coherence tomography. Heart 2010; 96: 196–201.

76. Lopez-Farre AJ, Mateos-Caceres PJ, Sacristan D, et al. Relationship between vitamin D binding protein and aspirin resistance in coronary ischemic patients: a proteomic study. J Proteome Res 2007; 6: 2481–7.

77. Wong ND, Gransar H, Narula J, et al. Myeloperoxidase, subclinical atherosclerosis, and cardiovascular disease events. JACC Cardiovasc Imaging 2009; 2: 1093–9.

78. Meuwese MC, Stroes ES, Hazen SL, et al. Serum myeloperoxidase levels are associated with the future risk of coronary artery disease in apparently healthy individuals: the EPIC-Norfolk Prospective Population Study. J Am Coll Cardiol 2007; 50: 159–65.

79. Serruys PW, Garcia-Garcia HM, Buszman P, et al. Effects of the direct lipoprotein-associated phospholipase A(2) inhibitor darapladib on human coronary atherosclerotic plaque. Circulation 2008; 118: 1172–82.

80. Alonso-Orgaz S, Moreno L, Macaya C, et al. Proteomic study of plasma from moderate hypercholesterolemic patients. J Proteome Res 2006; 5: 2301–8.

81. Kalet-Litman S, Moreno PR, Levy AP. The haptoglobin 2-2 genotype is associated with increased redox active hemoglobin derived iron in the atherosclerotic plaque. Atherosclerosis 2010; 209: 28–31.

82. Stefanadis C, Toutouzas K, Tsiamis E, et al. Relation between local temperature and C-reactive protein levels in patients with coronary artery disease: effects of atorvastatin treatment. Atherosclerosis 2007; 192: 396–400.

83. Khawaja FJ, Bailey KR, Turner ST, et al. Association of novel risk factors with the ankle brachial index in African American and non-Hispanic white populations. Mayo Clin Proc 2007; 82: 709–16.

84. Wang TJ, Gona P, Larson MG, et al. Multiple biomarkers for the prediction of first major cardiovascular events and death. N Engl J Med 2006; 355: 2631–9.

85. Zethelius B, Berglund L, Sundstrom J, et al. Use of multiple biomarkers to improve the prediction of death from cardiovascular causes. N Engl J Med 2008; 358: 2107–16.

86. Koenig W, Khuseyinova N. Biomarkers of atherosclerotic plaque instability and rupture. Arterioscler Thromb Vasc Biol 2007; 27: 15–26.

87. Pepe MS. An interpretation for the ROC curve and inference using GLM procedures. Biometrics 2000; 56: 352–9.

88. Venter JC, Adams MD, Myers EW, et al. The sequence of the human genome. Science 2001; 291: 1304–51.

89. Rifai N, Gillette MA, Carr SA. Protein biomarker discovery and validation: the long and uncertain path to clinical utility. Nat Biotechnol 2006; 24: 971–83.

90. Cooper LT Jr, Onuma OK, Sagar S, et al. Genomic and proteomic analysis of myocarditis and dilated cardiomyopathy. Heart Fail Clin 2010; 6: 75–85.

91. Granger CB, Van Eyk JE, Mockrin SC, Anderson NL. National Heart, Lung, And Blood Institute Clinical Proteomics Working Group report. Circulation 2004; 109: 1697–703.

92. Kingsmore SF. Multiplexed protein measurement: technologies and applications of protein and antibody arrays. Nat Rev Drug Discov 2006; 5: 310–20.

93. Rosen S. Lateral Flow Immunoassay. New York: Humana Press, 2009.

94. Ware JH. The limitations of risk factors as prognostic tools. N Engl J Med 2006; 355: 2615–7.

95. Cook NR. Use and misuse of the receiver operating characteristic curve in risk prediction. Circulation 2007; 115: 928–35.

96. Pencina MJ, D'Agostino RB Sr, D'Agostino RB Jr, Vasan RS. Evaluating the added predictive ability of a new marker: from area under the ROC curve to reclassification and beyond. Stat Med 2008; 27: 157–72; discussion 207–12.97.

97. Kathiresan S, Voight BF, Purcell S, et al. Genome-wide association of early-onset myocardial infarction with single nucleotide polymorphisms and copy number variants. Nat Genet 2009; 41: 334–41.

98. Erdmann J, Grosshennig A, Braund PS, et al. New susceptibility locus for coronary artery disease on chromosome 3q22.3. Nat Genet 2009; 41: 280–2.

99. Wellcome Trust Case Control Consortium. Genome-wide association study of 14,000 cases of seven common diseases and 3,000 shared controls. Nature 2007; 447: 661–78.

100. Coronary Artery Disease Consortium. Large scale association analysis of novel genetic loci for coronary artery disease. Arterioscler Thromb Vasc Biol 2009; 29: 774–80.

101. Willer CJ, Sanna S, Jackson AU, et al. Newly identified loci that influence lipid concentrations and risk of coronary artery disease. Nat Genet 2008; 40: 161–9.

102. Gudbjartsson DF, Bjornsdottir US, Halapi E, et al. Sequence variants affecting eosinophil numbers associate with asthma and myocardial infarction. Nat Genet 2009; 41: 342–7.

103. Ardissino D, Berzuini C, Merlini PA, et al. Influence of 9p21.3 genetic variants on clinical and angiographic outcomes in early-onset myocardial infarction. J Am Coll Cardiol 2011; 58: 426–34.

4 Identification of the patient at risk: Current role of biomarkers and evolving avenues for research

Gerard Pasterkamp, Imo Hoefer, and Dominique de Kleijn

OUTLINE

Novel biomarkers could facilitate the diagnosis of subclinical cardiovascular disease or aid risk stratification in patients with clinically manifest disease. In addition, such biomarkers could find other important applications as surrogate endpoints that could accelerate the approval process for new drugs. In addition to circulating biomarkers, ongoing studies are exploring plaque biomarkers that can be exploited in imaging modalities and "omics" studies will provide new insights into the biomarker properties of circulating cells. Microparticle proteins are still at the stage of identification of the different proteomes. In this chapter we summarize the current knowledge in the field and highlight both future avenues for research and potential clinical applications.

INTRODUCTION

There is intense ongoing research to identify novel biomarkers that might facilitate the diagnosis of subclinical cardiovascular disease (CVD) or aid risk stratification in those with clinically manifest disease. However, the potential value of such biomarkers could find important applications beyond the areas of prevention and diagnosis. For instance, the pathway for the introduction of a new drug into clinical practice requires major investment in large-scale clinical trials. Biomarkers that might help in the prediction of ultimate efficacy in large populations

---

Focus Box 4.1

Novel biomarkers could facilitate the diagnosis of subclinical CVD or aid risk stratification in those with clinically manifest disease

There are other potentially important applications beyond the areas of prevention and diagnosis

One such area is the identification of patients at high risk of future clinical events for inclusion in clinical studies, thus improving statistical power and cost effectiveness

---

Focus Box 4.2

Recent biomarker discoveries have not always been driven by hypothesis-driven research and often the function of the proposed target is unknown

These new discovery tracks will result in new insights into the pathophysiology of atherosclerotic disease

However, the proof of added predictive value over established risk factors and biomarkers and the impact on treatment strategies will dictate clinical utility

---

but whose potential can be estimated based on preliminary studies in small groups of unselected patients would accelerate the introduction of new pharmaceutical products. In addition, novel biomarkers could identify a group of patients with a very high risk of future clinical events who might be targeted for inclusion in clinical studies to improve statistical power to detect potential efficacy in a more cost-effective fashion.

Over the last two decades a significant number of new circulating biomarkers with predictive value for cardiovascular events have been validated in clinical studies. These biomarkers were representative of different pathophysiological pathways that, on theoretical grounds, might have been expected to play a role in the occurrence of adverse cardiovascular events. Differences in the level of expression of such biomarkers were considered to be surrogates for future risk. Markers of inflammation, oxidative stress, endothelial dysfunction, and platelet activation have all been tested for potential predictive value for future events (1). More recent biomarker discoveries have not always been driven by hypothesis-driven research and often the function of the proposed target is unknown (2). These discoveries have been stimulated by the availability of "omics" technologies that facilitate the detection of large numbers of differentially expressed genes and proteins among patient groups. This technology has resulted in a wave of reports with newly identified markers. However, the decision to pursue a target is still based on the available knowledge of the mechanism of action that is often deficient. These new discovery tracks will result in new insights into the pathophysiology of atherosclerotic disease. However, before incorporation into daily clinical practice, robust evidence will be needed that any such markers will have added predictive value in addition to that provided by pre-existing risk factors and that this increment in predictive value will change treatment strategies.

CLINICAL RELEVANCE

For many circulating biomarkers the predictive value for adverse events is clearly established. Table 4.1 summarizes the results of trials of classical biomarkers and indicates their proposed mechanism of action. However, the added predictive value of both relatively established and newer markers in addition to traditional risk factors seems to be relatively limited. The new biomarkers generally fail to add clinically relevant value when it comes to discrimination, calibration, or reclassification (1,3). Another general issue in biomarker research relates to the question of whether the measurement of a specific marker will influence patient management. Some have questioned the need for new markers of risk of coronary artery

Table 4.1 An Overview of Biomarkers That Have Been Evaluated in a Clinical Setting

Initiation and progression	
Inflammation and lipid accumulation	
C-reactive protein	Ridker et al. Am J Cardiol 2003; 92: 17K–22K (review)
Matrix metalloprotease-9	Sundstrom et al. Curr Opin Lipidol 2006; 17: 45–53 (review)
Interleukin-6	Lobbes et al. Atherosclerosis. 2006; 187: 18–25 (review)
Intreleukin-8	Apostolakis et al. Cardiovasc Res 2009; 84: 353–60 (review)
s-ICAM	Hulthe et al. Clin Sci 2002; 103: 123–9
Serum amyloid A	Ogasawara et al. Atherosclerosis 2004; 174: 349–56
CD40L	Lievens et al. Thromb Haemost 2009; 102: 206–14 (review)
Lipoprotein-associated phospholipase A2	Mallat et al. Circulation 2010; 122: 2183–200 (review)
Myeloperoxidase	Brennan et al. N Engl J Med 2003; 349: 1595–604
Adiponectin	Fontana et al. Diabetes 2007; 56: 1010–13
Soluble ST-2	Shimpo et al. Circulation 2004; 109: 2186–90
Osteopontin	Georgiadou et al. Eur J Clin Invest 2010; 40: 288–93
Growth differentiation factor 15	Wollert et al. Circulation 2007; 115: 962–71
Pregnancy associated plasma protein A	Lund et al. Circulation 2003; 108: 1924–6
(ox)LDLc	Kannel et al. Ann Intern Med 1979; 90: 85–91
HDLc	Gordon et al. Circulation 1989; 79: 8–15
Apo B lipoprotein 100	Lamarche et al. Circulation 1996; 94: 273–8
Apo A1	Lamarche et al. Circulation 1996; 94: 273–8
Homocysteine	Homocysteine Studies Collaboration. JAMA 2002; 288: 2015–22
Lipoprotein A	Danesh et al. Circulation 2000; 102: 1082–5 (review)
Thrombosis on rupture	
Fibrinogen	Danesh et al. JAMA 2005; 294: 1799–809
Von Willebrand factor	Whincup et al. Eur Heart J 2002; 23: 1764–70 (review)
Soluble ICAM	Lawson et al. Pharmacol Rep 2009; 6: 22–32 (review)
D-dimer	Danesh et al. Circulation 2001; 103: 2323–7
PAI-1	Ridker et al. Circulation 2004; 109(25 Suppl 1): IV6–19 (review)
Cardiovascular injury/remodeling	
N-terminal brain natriuretic peptide	Wang et al. N Engl J Med 2004; 350: 655–63
(high-sensitive) Troponin	Omland et al. N Engl J Med 2009; 361: 2538–47
Copeptin	Khan et al. Circulation 2007; 115: 2103–10
Other	
Cystatin C (kidney failure, fibrosis)	Shlipak et al. N Engl J Med 2005; 352: 2049–60
Glycated hemoglobin (diabetes)	Jorgenson et al. Circulation 2004; 110: 466–70

disease (CAD) when traditional risk factors already account for a major part of the population attributable risk (4). However, the continuous search for new biomarkers is mainly driven by the fact that optimal risk prediction, at an individual level, is required to allow, on the one hand, tailoring of treatment to a specific patient, and, on the other hand, selection of high-risk patients for drug intervention trials. In addition, new biomarkers might provide novel insights into the pathophysiological mechanisms of atherosclerotic disease. Finally, while the predominant focus has been on the predictive value of biomarkers in asymptomatic subjects, the value of biomarkers in patients with established vascular occlusive disease remains relatively unexplored (5). In patients with manifest CVD, often already treated with statins, the predictive value of the established risk factors for future events is limited (5). However, this patient population has been targeted as an appropriate one to investigate the potential efficacy of novel anti-atherosclerotic drugs.

CURRENT STATUS

It is important to recognize that biomarkers (defined as measurable biological substances) are only one potential method to identify the risk of future events in asymptomatic subjects or in patients at risk of a future event. Imaging and functional tests are also the subject of intense research in the field of risk stratification. In this chapter we will focus on biochemical markers but other diagnostic modalities and imaging techniques will be extensively discussed elsewhere in this book.

We will briefly discuss pertinent aspects of some of the circulating markers that have been widely tested in clinical settings. More extensive reviews can be found in the excellent literature available in the public domain (Table 4.1).

The ongoing search for new biomarkers that predict progression of atherosclerotic disease has met with relatively limited success. One potential explanation relates to the fact that most proposed targets are related to inflammation and are not specific markers for disease progression in the vasculature.

In biomarker research, most attention has been focused on targets that can be easily measured in circulating blood and that play a role in lipid metabolism, inflammatory processes, or coagulation (Table 4.1). One of the most studied circulating biomarkers is C-reactive protein (CRP), an acute phase protein that is raised in any inflammatory condition. CRP is predictive of

Focus Box 4.3

The value of biomarkers in patients with established vascular occlusive disease remains relatively unexplored although the predictive value of the established risk factors for future events is limited in this population

Most proposed circulating biomarkers reflect inflammatory or proteolytic activity and are based on current imperfect concepts of plaque initiation, progression, and rupture

Potential candidates, more specific for disease progression, include Lp-PLA

cardiovascular events but the evidence for a causal relationship with the disease is lacking. In fact, Mendelian randomization studies using the human genome as the basis of randomization showed that CRP is not likely to be causally related with the development of vascular disease (6). There are some potential candidates that could be more specific for atherosclerotic disease. For example, lipoprotein-associated phospholipase A2 (Lp-PLA2) is specifically expressed in the atherosclerotic vasculature. The function of Lp-PLA2 has been extensively reported in the literature. Lp-PLA2 is an interesting biomarker since it has predictive value independent of traditional risk factors (for an overview, see Ref. 7). Interestingly, while the predictive value of Lp-PLA2 is evident in patients suffering from stable CAD, it does not have predictive value for future events in patients presenting with acute coronary syndromes. This emphasizes the relevance of identifying patient subgroups where specific biomarkers could have more added value.

EVOLVING AVENUES FOR RESEARCH

There is another more provocative explanation for the limited value of newly discovered biomarkers that predict atherosclerotic disease progression: the mechanisms of biological action evoked to explain the relationship between the biomarker and disease have mostly been based on concepts that have not been proven in longitudinal human studies. Atherosclerosis is a disease that develops over decades and the natural history of the progression toward luminal occlusion is unknown. Current concepts exploring the mechanisms that contribute to the initiation and progression of atherosclerotic disease have been mainly based on cross-sectional pathological observations and studies in genetically modified animal models with a specific focus on determinants of the "vulnerable plaques." The concept of the vulnerable plaque and its role in the pathogenesis of atherosclerotic disease progression have also driven the biomarker discovery field. It is likely that the limited knowledge on the natural history of the pathogenesis of vascular occlusive disease progression in man may hamper the discovery of biomarkers that can serve as a surrogate for adverse events in the coronary, cerebral, or peripheral circulation.

In the following sections of this chapter we will discuss some evolving avenues in biomarker research: they relate to discoveries in the field of plaques, circulating cells, and microparticles. In this chapter we will not consider markers derived from genome-wide association studies (GWAS) as the number of targets identified in GWAS studies is rapidly increasing and reviewing the current status would result in a list of candidate targets that is far from complete. However, we would like to briefly mention the growing interest in pharmacogenomics as a tool for the identification of patients with deviating responses to medication. For instance, the identification of genomic markers that influence efficacy and adverse reactions has resulted in relabeling of warfarin and clopidogrel (8).

ATHEROSCLEROTIC PLAQUE BIOMARKERS

The vulnerable plaque concept, with its emphasis on pathological and biochemical differences between stable and unstable, rupture-prone plaques, has an inherent limitation in that it is based on cross-sectional and retrospective studies of ruptured plaques. Key components of the vulnerable plaque, such as inflammation and a large lipid core, are also frequently observed in asymptomatic patients and are, in fact, a common phenomenon throughout the entire atherosclerotic vascular tree. Looking objectively at most of the proposed circulating biomarkers, however, it is evident that most, such as those reflecting inflammatory or proteolytic activity, are based on current, certainly incomplete, concepts of plaque initiation, progression, and rupture.

Cross-sectional atherosclerotic tissue banks may help us to generate hypotheses regarding both the mechanisms of atherogenesis and disease progression. However, for prediction studies follow-up is required and therefore atherosclerotic tissue banks with a longitudinal study design might facilitate the discovery of plaque markers that are predictive for future cardiovascular events. Given the fact that atherosclerosis is a systemic disease and that plaque composition in different vascular beds displays many common features, one could hypothesize that local plaque characteristics, at a particular time point, might provide information with the potential to predict plaque progression in other territories of the vascular tree. Therefore, atherosclerotic plaques obtained during vascular surgery might contain predictive markers for future cardiovascular events in other vascular territories.

The Athero-Express study—an ongoing prospective cohort study with a longitudinal study design, initiated in 2002, in a population of more than 2500 patients—correlates characteristics of plaques removed during surgery with secondary cardiovascular manifestations during a three-year follow-up. First, it was shown that plaque composition appeared to be an independent predictor of restenosis after carotid endarterectomy (9). It was also shown that patients with more stable plaque phenomena had an increased risk for the development of restenosis compared with patients with unstable plaque phenomena. This was the first demonstration that atherosclerotic plaques, obtained by vascular surgery, could provide predictive information about the outcome of the procedure. However, in terms of its objective, the Athero-Express study went a significant step further. We searched for plaque proteins and

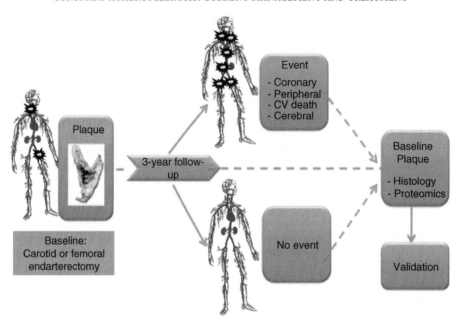

Figure 4.1 Study design of the Athero-Express study. Patients undergo carotid or femoral endarterectomy and plaques are stored for analyses. All patients undergo a 3-year follow-up. Plaque characteristics are compared for patients who suffered from a secondary event during follow-up versus patients who remained event-free. A unique aspect of the study is that it is used to locate plaque markers that reflect the instability of plaques elsewhere in the vascular system.

histological characteristics that were predictive for adverse events in all vascular territories. Plaques obtained by carotid or femoral surgery procedures were examined for markers that could also predict myocardial infarction, aneurysm formation, peripheral artery disease, or stroke (Fig. 4.1). Analysis of the proteome of atherosclerotic plaques from patients with and without secondary cardiovascular manifestations revealed osteopontin (OPN) as one of the potential predictive plaque markers (10). Validation of this marker in a large cohort indeed demonstrated that patients in the highest quartile of plaque OPN levels had a fourfold increased risk for secondary cardiovascular events, compared with patients in the lowest quartile of plaque OPN levels. This predictive power was not evident from OPN measurements in the blood. We also observed that high plaque expression levels of fatty acid binding protein 4 as well as MMP-8 were predictive for events during follow-up (11,12). The observed increased risk was independent of traditional risk factors. Studying the net reclassification index we observed that patients could be better reclassified into higher or lower risk groups using these plaque markers on top of the established risk factors (Fig. 4.2). More recently it was demonstrated that the presence of intra-plaque bleeding in a single culprit lesion was associated with a twofold increase in risk of secondary manifestations of atherosclerotic disease during follow-up. Also the presence of intra-plaque vessels was associated with an increase in event rate (13).

Unfortunately, these predictive markers have a limitation: they can be measured only after surgical dissection of atherosclerotic tissue and only at one time point. The effect of treatment or

Focux Box 4.4

Atherosclerotic tissue banks with a longitudinal study design might facilitate the discovery of plaque markers that are predictive for future cardiovascular events

Patients with "stable" plaques are more prone to restenosis than those with "unstable" plaques

Tissue but not circulating osteopontin levels have predictive value for future clinical events

intervention cannot be monitored and therefore the clinical utility of predictive plaque markers is limited. Still, the observation that one small dissected plaque cross-section reveals information regarding the risk of secondary manifestations at three-year follow-up opens up potential new avenues for research. Potential candidate predictors of plaque progression/clinical events, such as intra-plaque hemorrhage and plaque neovascularization, have emerged from the Athero-Express study. Plaque imaging may serve as a surrogate marker for the risk of future clinical events that is stronger than, for instance, intima media thickness. For example, plaque hemorrhage can be detected using MRI while high-resolution contrast-enhanced ultrasound may be a useful tool to visualize intra-plaque vessel formation.

CIRCULATING BLOOD CELL MARKERS
More recently, circulating cells such as white blood cells and platelets have gained attention as markers of disease progression (Table 4.2). At present most research is focused on the

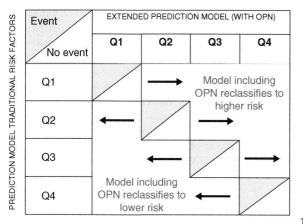

PREDICTION MODEL TRADITIONAL RISK FACTORS	EXTENDED PREDICTION MODEL (WITH OPN)			
Event \ No event	Q1	Q2	Q3	Q4
Q1		→	Model including OPN reclassifies to higher risk	
Q2	←		→	
Q3		←		→
Q4	Model including OPN reclassifies to lower risk		←	

PREDICTION MODEL TRADITIONAL RISK FACTORS	EXTENDED PREDICTION MODEL (WITH OPN)			
Event \ No event	Q1	Q2	Q3	Q4
Q1	5 / 73	0 / 16	1 / 1	1 / 1
Q2	3 / 27	8 / 31	8 / 9	6 / 7
Q3	0 / 1	3 / 18	10 / 33	14 / 20
Q4	0 / 0	0 / 0	6 / 15	39 / 41

Total patients = 397: Cases = 104, Controls = 293. Due to OPN, reclassification improvement in cases was (30 correctly shifted up −12 incorrectly shifted down)/104 = 17.3%. Reclassification improvement in controls = (61 correctly shifted down −54 incorrectly shifted up)/293 = 2.4%. This results in a total NRI due to OPN of 17.3+2.4 = 19.7%

Figure 4.2 A risk model was built including only the traditional risk factors (vertical axis). Based on this risk model patients were divided into quartiles of increasing risk from Q1 to Q4. Subsequently, the plaque marker osteopontin (OPN) was measured in carotid plaques and included in the model. Patients were again divided into quartiles based on the risk for secondary manifestations of the disease (horizontal axis). The blue boxes represent the patients who suffered from an event during follow-up (cases). The white boxes represent the patients who did not suffer from an event during follow-up (controls). The green and red numbers indicate the number of patients who were reclassified (correctly and incorrectly, respectively) in a lower or higher risk category. Using this method, one can calculate the number of cases and controls that were correctly and wrongly reclassified in another risk quartile after adding OPN in the model. In this case OPN resulted in an improvement in the net reclassification index (NRI) of 19.7%.

Table 4.2 Peripheral Blood Mononuclear Cells Predicting Cardiovascular Disease Progression

Cell type	Disease	Biomarkers	Observation	Predictive value	Reference
EPC	CHF	ac-LDL, lectin	Reduced numbers	Cardiovascular death, cardiovascular hospitalization	Balconi et al. J Cardiac Fail 2009; 15: 747
	CAD	ac-LDL, lectin	Reduced numbers	CAD severity	Kinz et al. Am Heart J 2006; 152: 19025
	Healthy men >21 years	ac-LDL, lectin	Reduced numbers	Increased FRS	Hill et al. N Engl J Med 2003; 348: 593
	CAD	CD34+KDR+	Reduced numbers	MACE	Schmidt-Lucke et al. Circulation 2005; 111: 2981
	CAD	CD34+KDR+	Reduced numbers	Cardiovascular death, cardiovascular hospitalization	Werner et al. N Engl J Med 2005; 353: 999
Lymphocytes	CAD	CD3+CD4+CD28-	Increased numbers	CAD severity	Alter et al. Int J Cardiol 2009; 135: 27
	ESRD	CD3+CD4+CD28-	Increased numbers	Atherosclerosis	Betjes et al. Nephrol Dial Transplant 2010; 25: 3640
	Diabetes	CD3+CD4+CD28-	Increased numbers	MACE	Giubilato et al. (16)
	CHF	Osteopontin+CD4+	Increased numbers	CHF severity	Soejima et al. Circ J 2007; 71: 1879
Monocytes	CHF	CD14+CD6+	Increased numbers	CHF severity, creatinine	Barisione et al. Dis Markers 2010; 28: 115
	ESRD	CD14+CD16+	Increased numbers pre-dialysis	MACE	Heine et al. Kidney Int 2008; 73: 622
	ESRD	CD14+CD16+	Increased numbers	Cardiovascular death	Ulrich et al. (20)
	AMI	CD 14+CD16+CX3CR1 +	Increased numbers	Late lumen loss	Liu et al. Circ J 2010; 74: 2585
	CAD	CD14+LLR2+, CD14+LLR4+	Increased numbers	CAD severity	Mizoguchi et al. Coron Artery Dis 2007; 18: 31

Abbreviations: EPC, endothelial progenitor cell; CHF, chronic heart failure; ac-LDL, acetylated low-density lipoprotein; CAD, coronary artery disease; ESRD, end-stage renal disease; AMI, acute myocardial infarction; FRS, Framingham risk score; MACE, major adverse coronary event.

protein products that are generated by the cell with little effort directed at exploiting the wealth of information potentially available from the biomarker factory: the circulating cell. Inflammatory cells are directly involved in the pathogenesis and progression of atherosclerosis and CVD and therefore have a high potential for risk prediction. During their transit through the vasculature, cells are exposed to the systemic consequences of risk factors and to local inflammatory and proteolytic processes. Many cells come into close contact with the atherosclerotic lesion and may end up in the plaque or the perivascular tissue. A considerable proportion will re-enter the circulation, imprinted with information from this interaction. The advent of improved cell sorting and cytometry techniques have made cell-based information more accessible and paved the way for potential applications in the field of CVD. Platelet-activation tests have already been shown to identify patients who are less responsive to platelet-aggregation inhibitors and those with a higher risk of cardiac events during follow-up (14). Using flow cytometry, many cell-based markers can be assessed simultaneously, allowing the identification of subgroups of cells. Simple or complicated panels of cell-based markers that may be used to identify the individual patient at risk can be studied, although many challenges need to be overcome. Such panels require extra attention and thorough analyses to preclude interdependence of the included markers. The majority of studies to date have focused on relatively simple panels, for example, by using flow cytometry for surface marker expression analysis. While there are countless variations of possible marker combinations, subpopulations of cells have attracted special interest in CVD patients.

Endothelial progenitor cells (EPCs) have been ascribed a central role in vascular homeostasis. As such, EPCs have been correlated with various diseases involving the vasculature. Several methods have been established to quantify EPCs, for example, flow cytometry analysis or enumeration assays. Studies have observed inverse relationships between EPC numbers and cardiovascular risk factors or the Framingham risk score (FRS). Compared other risk factors, EPC numbers have been shown to be second only to age as a predictor of advanced CAD. Other studies have demonstrated that a decreased number of circulating EPCs is correlated with subsequent cardiovascular events (15). In addition to the as yet unknown additive predictive value over classical risk factors, EPC characterization and quantification remain a matter of debate, limiting cross-validation and hence their use as a potential biomarker.

Among the immune cells directly involved in atherosclerosis, T-cells and CD4+CD28− T-cells in particular have moved into focus. In contrast to conventional CD4+CD28+ T-helper cells, CD4+CD28− cells are terminally differentiated, pro-inflammatory, and cytotoxic. CD4+CD28− cells preferentially accumulate in unstable atherosclerotic plaques rather than stable ones and consequently have been correlated with acute coronary syndromes. Moreover, CD4+CD28− numbers are independently associated with the extent of CVD in stable angina and end-stage renal disease patients and high CD4CD28− cell

counts are independent predictors of secondary cardiovascular events (16). The relative insensitivity of CD4+CD28− cell numbers to acute cardiovascular events, remaining stable for up to 3 months after myocardial infarction, is an important advantage for future biomarker applications (17).

Because of their pivotal role in atherosclerosis, monocytes are potential candidates in the search for cell-based biomarkers. Previous studies have linked monocyte numbers, surface marker expression, and functionality with the extent of CVD and the likelihood of future events (18,19). More recently, CD14+CD16+ (or CD16+ monocytes) have attracted much interest, specifically in patients suffering from kidney failure. CD16+ monocytes are, like CD4+CD28− T-cells, considered to have a strong pro-inflammatory phenotype and be directly involved in CVD progression. In chronic heart failure patients, CD16+ monocytes are significantly increased compared to with controls, positively correlating with the severity of clinical symptoms according to the NYHA classification. Further subclassification by adding known markers is likely to occur. Preliminary studies indicate the predictive value of CD16+ monocyte subpopulations in combination with high expression of angiotensin-converting enzyme (20).

As outlined above, it seems unlikely that a single biomarker will add significantly to the established risk factors. One potential deficit of predictive markers to date might be the fact that their discovery has been based on relatively simple assumptions, for example, that characteristics of leukocytes in their "circulation" mode predict their reaction when they come into contact with atherosclerotic plaques. An alternative approach could be to mimic the atherosclerotic environment ex vivo to force the cells to switch to their "plaque" mode. First steps have been taken in this direction by measuring the response of peripheral blood cells toward Toll-like receptor-activating agents (e.g., Pam3Cys, LPS). TLR-2 and TLR-4 have been shown to be directly involved in atherogenesis and hence represent a logical starting point. Moreover, the expression of TLR-2 and TLR-4 in peripheral blood monocytes are independent predictors of atherosclerotic disease and cardiovascular events (21). Advanced "omics" technologies offer the potential to establish novel multimarker scores, integrating genetic information, mRNA and miRNA expression data, and protein and metabolite levels. Studying cell-based biomarkers is difficult since there are no large biobanks that have stored cell fractions in large numbers of patients. The first initiatives have been undertaken in private–public consortia in the Netherlands where cell-based markers are being explored

---

Focus Box 4.5

The notion that the characteristics of leukocytes in their "circulation" mode predict their reaction when they come into contact with atherosclerotic plaques is simplistic

Techniques that mimic the atherosclerotic environment ex-vivo and force the cells to switch to their "plaque" mode may provide novel insights

in large numbers of patients undergoing coronary catheterization. It is expected, however, that more biobanks with white and red blood cell fractions will be initiated in order to explore the potential of this biological source which can be considered as the factory of most circulating biomarkers.

MICROPARTICLES

Microparticles are circular membrane vesicles that can be found in different biological fluids such as plasma, urine, saliva, and breast milk. Microparticles include exosomes that range in size between 50 and 100 nm, have lipid rafts, and contain protein, RNA, and miRNA. Exosome-like vesicles (30–90 nm) do not contain lipid rafts. Exosomes and exosome-like vesicles differ from the much bigger (<100–1000 nm) microvesicles, membrane particles, ectosomes, and apoptotic bodies in their mechanism of release.

Exosomes and exosome-like vesicles are derived by the fusion of multivesicular bodies with the plasma membrane while the larger membrane particles originate from the surface membrane after activation or apoptosis (22).

Although first considered to be involved in cellular garbage disposal, it is now widely accepted that exosomes play an important role in processes such as coagulation, tissue injury, and inflammation (Fig. 4.3) (23).

Several functions of microparticles have been associated with CVD. Coagulation has been related to monocyte microparticles that are enriched in tissue factor after activation of lipopolysaccharide (24). These monocyte microparticles bind activated platelets to initiate the coagulation cascade. Before the tissue factor can initiate coagulation, the vesicle needs to bind to membranes expressing P-selectin to activate the encrypted tissue factor (23). It has been shown that microparticle-linked tissue factor is increased after ST elevation myocardial infarction (25), pointing to hypercoagulability after injury; however, evidence is still needed to establish the role of microparticle-linked tissue factor in the initiation of cardiovascular events.

In stem cell biology, it has been suggested that bone-marrow stem cell differentiation depends on signals delivered from injured cells by microparticles. In CVD regenerative medicine, the so-called paracrine hypothesis has gained much attention and is supported by recent experimental data (26). It has been shown that mesenchymal stem cell-conditioned medium (MSC-CM) enhances cardiomyocyte and/or progenitor

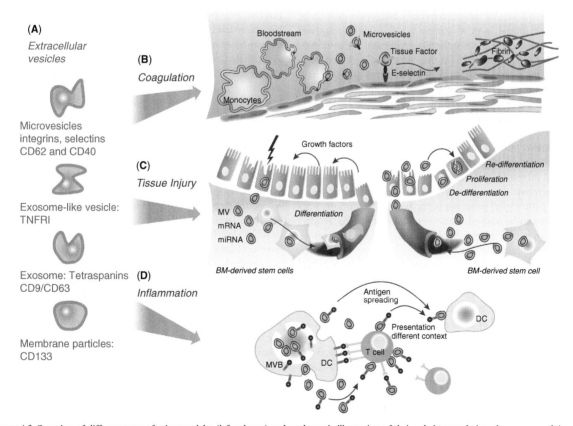

Figure 4.3 Overview of different types of microparticles (left column) and a schematic illustration of their role in coagulation, the response of tissue to injury and inflammation.

survival after hypoxia-induced injury (26). In both murine and
porcine models of myocardial ischemia reperfusion it was
shown that MSC-CM reduces infarct size (27) and this therapeutic action was independent of the cell source for the MSCs.
Purification of this MSC-CM resulted in the identification of
exosomes as the cardioprotective factor in MSC-CM (28). The
experimental evidence that exosomes can act as a "natural
polypill" in order to rescue ischemic tissue is strong. This
observation suggests that the exosomes encompass content that
may reveal new biomarker properties. This is of interest since
different cell types may release exosomes resulting in differential exosome profiles in the patient's blood.

Inflammatory processes contribute to the progression of atherosclerotic disease and subsequent events. Microparticles may be
involved in several ways as conveyors of immune responses
between immune cells affecting the pro- and/or anti-inflammatory
property of the targeted cells. In this context, it is interesting to
note that microparticles from platelets and macrophages have
been found in the lipid core of atherosclerotic plaques and that
increased levels of plasma microparticles have been observed in
cardiovascular pathology (29,30).

CIRCULATING MICROPARTICLES AS BIOMARKERS

Microparticles are involved in important processes relevant to
CVD and increased levels have been associated with the risk of
CVD. Microparticles might therefore contain information about
ongoing pathological processes in the body. Furthermore, microparticles can be isolated from frozen human plasma, rendering cardiovascular plasma biobanks as valuable sources to
identify and validate new biomarkers.

To date, blood-derived micro(mi)RNAs present in microparticles have attracted a lot of attention, especially in the field of
cancer prognosis and diagnosis, but cardiovascular miRNAs are
emerging. The role of microparticle proteins for diagnosis and
prognosis in the field of CVD is relatively unexplored.

miRNA has been extensively studied because its isolation
from blood is relatively easy, using RNA extraction methods on
(frozen) plasma or serum, and because of the use of array technology and established quantitative PCR for discovery and
validation. miRNAs are ~22-nucleotide long non-coding RNA
molecules that regulate a variety of cellular processes including
cell differentiation, cell cycle progression, and apoptosis, and
are present in plasma and serum within microparticles.

For example, miR423-5p has been identified as a marker that
correlated with the presence of heart failure (31). Myocardial
damage including myocardial infarction is associated with a
high level of cardiomyocyte-specific microRNAs-208b and -499
in the circulation (32). Although miRNA levels are comparable
with troponin increase, the number of patients is still low and
further validation is needed.

For atherosclerosis, circulating levels of miR-126, miR-17,
miR-92a, and the inflammation-associated miR-155 were significantly reduced in patients with CAD compared with healthy
controls (33), pointing to circulating miRNAs as possible atherosclerotic disease markers. Again numbers are low and markers need to be validated. The prognostic value of miRNAs in the
prediction of cardiovascular events also remains unexploited.

In addition to miRNAs, microparticles also contain significant amounts of proteins.

Studies are focusing on the proteomes of different particles. Platelet-derived microparticles are the most abundant
type of microparticle in the human blood and were the first
to be analyzed. Little et al. (34) described the proteome of
ectosomes and exosomes and observed correlations with age
and gender. They concluded that this proteome might be a
useful and reliable source of biologically relevant disease
biomarkers.

FUTURE PERSPECTIVES

New biomarkers are being explored both in plasma and in non-
plasma-based material. Ongoing studies are exploring plaque biomarkers that can be exploited in imaging modalities and "omics"
studies will provide new insights into the biomarker properties of
circulating cells. Microparticle proteins are still at the stage of
identification of the different proteomes. Their potential as biomarkers for disease is recognized but still unexplored. We antici-
pate that in the next few years microparticles will rapidly emerge
as an important source of markers with diagnostic and prognostic
value in the field of CVD.

Another issue is how to proceed with the applications of
newly developed biomarkers in a clinical setting? Should we
search for one "holy grail" or start integrating the knowledge
acquired from the different "omics" fields in an attempt to
develop algorithms including multiple biomarkers? The discoveries in the field of genomics, proteomics, and metabolomics suffer from limitations such as multiple testing, which
may result in false positive observations, and they require
extensive validation studies. Still, it may possible that multimarker panels will improve predictive power specifically
when they reflect different biological pathways. Moreover,
the use of bioinformatics will facilitate unbiased analyses and
reveal whether patient subgroups exist in which biomarker
signatures are highly predictive for events. With the newly
available discovery platforms and increasing calculation
power, we expect that the coming decade will result in
algorithms for risk prediction that require upgrading on a
regular basis, indicating that this field is not prepared for
stabilization.

REFERENCES

1. Wang TJ. Assessing the role of circulating, genetic, and imaging biomarkers in cardiovascular risk prediction. Circulation 2011; 123: 551–65.

2. Loscalzo J. Association studies in an era of too much information. Circulation 2007; 116: 1866–70.

3. Wang TJ, Gona P, Larson MG, et al. Multiple biomarkers for the prediction of first major cardiovascular events and death. N Engl J Med 2006; 355: 2631–9.

4. Nilsson PM, Nilsson JA, Berglund G. Population-attributable risk of coronary heart disease risk factors during long-term follow-up: the Malmo Preventive Project. J Intern Med 2006; 260: 134–41.

5. Arsenault BJ, Barter P, DeMicco DA, et al. Prediction of cardiovascular events in statin-treated stable coronary patients by lipid and nonlipid biomarkers. J Am Coll Cardiol 2011; 57: 63–9.

6. Zacho J, Tybjaerg-Hansen A, Jensen JS, et al. Genetically elevated C-reactive protein and ischemic vascular disease. N Engl J Med 2008; 359: 1897–908.

7. Mallat Z, Lambeau G, Tedgui A. Lipoprotein-associated and secreted phospolipases A2 in cardiovascular disease: roles as biological effectors and biomarkers. Circulation 2010; 122: 2183–200.

8. Wang L, McLeod HL, Weinshilboum RM. Genomics and drug response. N Engl J Med 2011; 364: 1144–53.

9. Hellings WE, Moll FL, De Vries JP, et al. Atherosclerotic plaque composition and occurrence of restenosis after carotid endarterectomy. JAMA 2008; 299: 547–54.

10. de Kleijn DPV, Moll FL, Hellings WE, et al. Local atherosclerotic plaques are a source of prognostic biomarkers for adverse cardiovascular events. Arterioscler Thromb Vasc Biol 2010; 30: 612–9.

11. Peeters W, de Kleijn DP, Vink A, et al. Adipocyte fatty acid binding protein in atherosclerotic plaques is associated with local vulnerability and is predictive for the occurrence of adverse cardiovascular events. Eur Heart J 2011; 32: 1758–68.

12. Peeters W, Moll FL, Vink A, et al. Collagenase matrix metalloproteinase-8 expressed in atherosclerotic carotid plaques is associated with systemic cardiovascular outcome. Eur Heart J 2011; 32: 2314–25.

13. Hellings WE, Peeters W, Moll FL, et al. Composition of carotid atherosclerotic plaque is associated with cardiovascular outcome: a prognostic study. Circulation 2010; 121: 1941–50.

14. Breet NJ, van Werkum JW, Bouman HJ, et al. Comparison of platelet function tests in predicting clinical outcome in patients undergoing coronary stent implantation. JAMA 2010; 303: 754–62.

15. Povsic TJ, Goldschmidt-Clermont PJ. Endothelial progenitor cells: markers of vascular reparative capacity. Ther Adv Cardiovasc Dis 2008; 2: 199–213.

16. Giubilato S, Liuzzo G, Brugaletta S, et al. Expansion of CD4+CD28 null T-lymphocytes in diabetic patients: exploring new pathogenetic mechanisms of increased cardiovascular risk in diabetes mellitus. Eur Heart J 2011; 32: 1214–26.

17. Dumitriu IE, Araguas ET, Baboonian C, Kaski JC. CD4+CD28 null T cells in coronary artery disease: when helpers become killers. Cardiovasc Res 2009; 81: 11–9.

18. Nasir K, Guallar E, Navas-Acien A, Criqui MH, Lima JAC. Relationship of monocyte count and peripheral arterial disease: results from the National Health and Nutrition Examination Survey 1999-2002. Arterioscler Thromb Vasc Biol 2005; 25: 1966–71.

19. Athanassopoulos P, Vaessen LMB, Balk AHMM, et al. Altered chemokine receptor profile on circulating leukocytes in human heart failure. Cell Biochem Biophys 2006; 44: 83–101.

20. Ulrich C, Heine GH, Seibert E, Fliser D, Girndt M. Circulating monocyte subpopulations with high expression of angiotensin-converting enzyme predict mortality in patients with end-stage renal disease. Nephrol Dial Transplant 2010; 25: 2265–72.

21. Kuwahata S, Fujita S, Orihara K, et al. High expression level of toll-like receptor 2 on monocytes is an important risk factor for arteriosclerotic disease. Atherosclerosis 2010; 209: 248–54.

22. Théry C, Ostrowski M, Segura E. Membrane vesicles as conveyors of immune responses. Nat Rev Immunol 2009: 581–93.

23. Tushuizen ME, Diamant M, Sturk A, Nieuwland R. Cell-derived microparticles in the pathogenesis of cardiovascular disease: friend or foe? Arterioscler Thromb Vasc Biol 2011; 31: 4–9.

24. Del Conde I, Shrimpton CN, Thiagarajan P, López JA. Tissue-factor-bearing microvesicles arise from lipid rafts and fuse with activated platelets to initiate coagulation. Blood 2005; 106: 1604–11.

25. Huisse MG, Ajzenberg N, Feldman L, Guillin MC, Steg PG. Microparticle-linked tissue factor activity and increased thrombin activity play a potential role in fibrinolysis failure in ST-segment elevation myocardial infarction. Thromb Haemost 2009; 101: 734–40.

26. Gnecchi M, He H, Noiseux N, et al. Evidence supporting paracrine hypothesis for Akt-modified mesenchymal stem cell-mediated cardiac protection and functional improvement. FASEB J 2006; 20: 661–9.

27. Timmers L, Lim SK, Arslan F, et al. Reduction of myocardial infarct size by human mesenchymal stem cell conditioned medium. Stem Cell Res 2007; 1: 129–37.

28. Lai RC, Arslan F, Tan SS, et al. Derivation and characterization of human fetal MSCs: an alternative cell source for large-scale production of cardioprotective microparticles. J Mol Cell Cardiol 2010; 48: 1215–24.

29. Leroyer AS, Tedgui A, Boulanger CM. Role of microparticles in atherothrombosis. J Intern Med 2008; 263: 528–37.

30. Simak J, Gelderman MP. Cell membrane microparticles in blood and blood products: potentially pathogenic agents and diagnostic markers. Transfus Med Rev 2006; 20: 1–26.

31. Tijsen AJ, Creemers EE, Moerland PD, et al. MiR423-5p as a circulating biomarker for heart failure. Circ Res 2010; 106: 1035–9.

32. Corsten MF, Dennert R, Jochems S, et al. Circulating MicroRNA-208b and MicroRNA-499 reflect myocardial damage in cardiovascular disease. Circ Cardiovasc Genet 2010; 3: 499–506.

33. Fichtlscherer S, De Rosa S, Fox H, et al. Circulating microRNAs in patients with coronary artery disease. Circ Res 2010; 107: 677–84.

34. Little KM, Smalley DM, Harthun NL, Ley K. The plasma microparticle proteome. Semin Thromb Hemost 2010; 36: 845–56.

5 Stable and unstable atherosclerotic disease: Definitions, clinical manifestations, and pathophysiology

John A. Ambrose and Joel A. Lardizabal

OUTLINE

In the last 25 years, our understanding of the causes of unstable atherosclerotic myocardial syndromes has evolved, leading to major improvements in prevention and treatment. The paramount roles of plaque rupture/erosion with subsequent platelet and fibrin deposition represent the immediate cause of occlusive and non-occlusive coronary thrombi in unstable syndromes. Understanding these processes has resulted in various therapeutic options that target the vessel wall, the various components of arterial thrombus, and/or the arterial lumen. This chapter will consider the various definitions and clinical manifestations of stable and unstable coronary atherosclerotic syndromes and correlate them to their pathophysiology.

GENERAL CONCEPTS OF CORONARY PATHOPHYSIOLOGY

Slow and Rapid Atherosclerotic Progression

Atherosclerosis can progress both slowly and rapidly in any given individual. Slow and rapid progression may occur in several cycles over several decades, and this progression is accelerated in patients with known risk factors for coronary artery disease (CAD). Early atherosclerosis is a slow process resulting in an increase in intimal thickness owing to the uptake of oxidized low-density lipoprotein cholesterol by intra-intimal macrophages followed by the migration and proliferation of smooth muscle cells. As the intima thickens, vasa vasorum already present in the adventitia grow into the intima to provide nourishment. These thin-walled vessels are prone to hemorrhage, which represents one of the mechanisms for rapid atherosclerotic progression. As the red cell membrane is lipid-rich, hemorrhage can be a mechanism for rapid lipid accumulation as well. The second mechanism for rapid atherosclerotic progression is intraluminal thrombus formation as a result of plaque rupture or plaque erosion (1,2).

Neither of these mechanisms necessarily produces symptoms (Fig. 5.1). These processes ultimately lead to either asymptomatic progression of CAD or stable/unstable coronary syndromes. There are several factors that determine the result and the interplay of these processes is complex. The rate of atherosclerotic progression; the presence, amount, rate of deposition, and composition of the intraluminal thrombus; embolization of the thrombus to the distal microvascular bed; vasoconstriction at or distal to the lesion; the final degree of luminal narrowing; and the ability to acutely recruit collaterals are all important factors that determine the outcome (3). An acute coronary syndrome (ACS) would likely result from rapid luminal occlusion with an intraluminal thrombus. Non-occlusive or subtotally occlusive thrombi

usually cause many cases of non-ST elevation ACS, while totally occlusive thrombi cause most cases of ST elevation myocardial infarction (MI). Non-ST elevation MI has several possible causes related to this process, including intermittent total coronary occlusion, distal embolization of the thrombus, and permanent total occlusion of either a small artery or an artery in the "silent" area of the heart as measured by the ECG, such as the posterolateral wall. Later sections will discuss the causes for acute MI other than those mentioned above.

Supply/Demand Imbalance

Symptomatic CAD is the result of an imbalance in myocardial blood supply and oxygen demand. Stable symptoms in coronary atherosclerotic disease occur when demand outstrips supply, as would occur with exercise or other forms of stress. Stable clinical symptoms in the absence of coronary atherosclerosis from such diverse causes as aortic stenosis, left ventricle hypertrophy, uncontrolled hypertension, and cardiac "syndrome X" result from a similar imbalance.

Unstable symptoms, as observed in unstable angina (UA), non-ST, or ST elevation MI, represent the other extreme of this supply/demand imbalance. In these instances, supply is greatly reduced or absent at rest. The reduction in blood supply or the supply/demand imbalance is intermittent in UA, but usually prolonged for several hours or permanent in ST elevation MI.

ANGINA PECTORIS

Angina pectoris is a clinical syndrome that is commonly defined as chest discomfort and related symptoms resulting from myocardial ischemia, which occurs when there is a mismatch between myocardial oxygen supply and demand. Global or regional myocardial ischemia is most often associated with significant narrowing of one or more epicardial coronary arteries during the atherosclerotic process (4).

Typical angina is a diffuse discomfort felt across the chest that may radiate to the neck, jaw, and/or down the left arm, which share the same dermatomal distribution as the heart. Ischemic pain is typically described as tightness, pressure, burning, aching, strangling, or fullness (Fig. 5.2). Qualities such as sharp, stabbing, pricking, or needle-like pain are generally not angina-related, especially when the pain is pleuritic, positional, or reproducible with palpation (5). However, patients with diabetes mellitus, the very elderly, or females may present with atypical symptoms partly related to autonomic and sensory nervous dysfunction.

The Canadian Cardiovascular Society grading system (Table 5.1) is widely used to quantify the severity of angina (6).

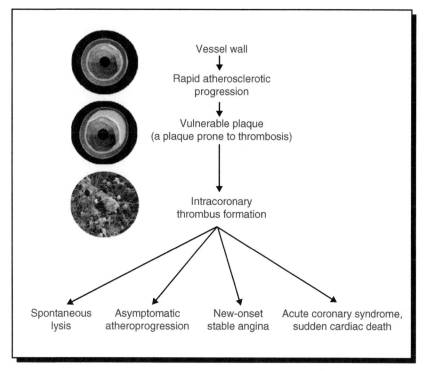

Figure 5.1 The current concept of rapid atherosclerotic progression and potential manifestations.

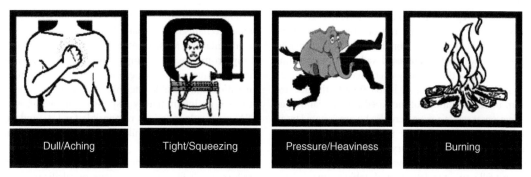

Figure 5.2 A visual tool of typical descriptors used to help patients in characterizing the quality of classic angina pectoris.

Table 5.1 The Canadian Cardiovascular Society Grading System for Angina Pectoris

Grade I	*Ordinary physical activity does not cause angina.* Activities such as walking and climbing stairs do not cause angina. Angina can be caused by strenuous, rapid, or prolonged exertion at work or recreation
Grade II	*Slight limitation of ordinary activity.* Walking or climbing stairs rapidly, walking uphill, walking or climbing stairs after meals, or in cold or windy conditions, under emotional stress, or a few hours after waking up. Walking more than two blocks on the level and climbing more than one flight of ordinary stairs at a normal pace and in normal conditions
Grade III	*Marked limitation of ordinary physical activity.* Walking one or two blocks on the level and climbing one flight of stairs in normal conditions and at a normal pace
Grade IV	*Inability to carry on any physical activity without discomfort.* Anginal syndrome may be present at rest

Source: Adapted from Ref. 6.

Angina pectoris is often associated with other symptoms such as shortness of breath, fatigue, lightheadedness, diaphoresis, and clamminess, which may result from ischemia-related diastolic dysfunction and/or a reduction in cardiac output. Unexplained dyspnea is particularly worrisome because of a markedly higher risk of mortality in these patients (7).

While traditionally referred to as "chest pain," angina pectoris from myocardial ischemia is most commonly described by patients as discomfort rather than pain. Chest pain is generally classified into three categories: typical, atypical, or non-anginal. Typical or definite angina is defined as (a) substernal chest discomfort with a characteristic quality and duration that is (b) provoked by exertion or emotional stress and (c) relieved by rest or nitroglycerin. Atypical or probable angina has only two of the three characteristics of typical angina. Non-anginal or non-cardiac chest pain meets none or only one of the criteria for typical angina (8). Classifying chest pain into these categories is important because it has a huge influence on the likelihood of CAD in symptomatic patients. For example, in young men aged 30–39 years presenting with chest pain, the likelihood of CAD is 76% if symptoms are typical, 34% if atypical, and only 4% if non-anginal in quality. Although the overall risk is much lower in young women of the same age group, the likelihood of CAD follows the same pattern: 26%, 12%, and 2% for typical, atypical, and non-anginal symptoms, respectively (Table 5.2).

STABLE ANGINA

Chronic stable angina (CSA) refers to a clinical presentation in which signs and symptoms of myocardial ischemia occur in a predictable manner, reproduced at a certain level of exertion or emotional stress, and relieved with rest or nitroglycerin. Most cases of CSA are thought to result from the slow and progressive accumulation of plaque within the vessel wall, eventually leading to luminal narrowing of the coronary artery that is severe enough to cause a significant imbalance of blood flow to the affected myocardium under conditions of increased myocardial oxygen demand. New-onset stable angina may also be precipitated by an acute progression of CAD, related to the same processes of plaque hemorrhage or intracoronary thrombus formation. In these situations, the degree of narrowing is such that symptoms are present but fall under the definition of stable angina.

In addition to the fixed luminal stenosis, vasomotor impairment and endothelial dysfunction also accompany the atherosclerotic changes in the affected vessel. During high-demand periods (e.g., exertion), elevated catecholamine levels normally cause generalized coronary vasodilatation to increase myocardial blood supply. The diseased artery, however, is unable to dilate and may actually undergo paradoxical vasoconstriction because of vasomotor and endothelial dysfunction. Blood flow is thus diverted preferentially to the areas of normal vasculature, and perfusion to the region supplied by the stenotic artery may become even more compromised, a phenomenon referred to as "coronary steal."

Depending on the degree of perfusion deficit and the amount of myocardium at risk, the resulting ischemia initially causes diastolic dysfunction of the ventricle, followed by systolic dysfunction, wall motion abnormalities, and electrocardiographic (ECG) changes, before anginal symptoms are even experienced. With rest or coronary vasodilator therapy, myocardial ischemia slowly improves over a period of several minutes, followed by resolution of symptoms, ECG abnormalities, systolic dysfunction, and diastolic dysfunction, generally in that particular order. However, most ischemic episodes are asymptomatic. Up to 80% of episodes of significant ST depression during ambulatory ECG monitoring are not associated with any symptoms (9).

UNSTABLE ANGINA

The quality of chest discomfort in UA is typically similar to CSA, but is markedly increased in intensity and frequency, as well as more prolonged in duration. Recent onset of severe angina or the presence of symptoms at rest is also classified as UA. While mechanical occlusion of coronary flow with an imbalance in myocardial supply/demand is the overall mechanism involved in both UA and CSA, the underlying pathophysiologic mechanisms are usually different, hence the dissimilarities in presentation. Most cases of UA or ACS are caused by the abrupt, complete, or incomplete occlusion of a coronary vessel due to plaque rupture or erosion, with subsequent thrombus formation and possible intermittent vasospasm. Underlying all of this is an inflammatory response of the vessel wall. Unlike CSA, most culprit lesions responsible for UA (and other ACS manifestations) are only mildly or moderately obstructive prior to the acute event.

In general, the atherosclerotic plaque responsible for CSA is predominantly fibrous, collagenous, or calcific in composition, with negligible lipid content. This is observed in the majority of CSA cases where rapid atheroprogression is not responsible for

Table 5.2 The Pretest Likelihood of Significant CAD in Symptomatic Patients According to Age and Gender

Age (years)	Non-anginal chest pain		Atypical angina		Typical angina	
	Men (%)	Women (%)	Men (%)	Women (%)	Men (%)	Women (%)
30–39	4	2	34	12	76	26
40–49	13	3	51	22	87	55
50–59	20	7	65	31	93	73
60–69	27	14	72	51	94	86

Source: Adapted from Ref. 8.

the symptomatology. On the other hand, the plaque that predisposes to UA usually contains a large lipid-rich soft core with high levels of inflammatory activity, making it highly thrombogenic. In addition, the fibrous cap overlying the lipid pool is markedly thinned and stressed, making the atheroma particularly vulnerable to disruption (10). There is, however, a great overlap in plaque morphology and the degree of inflammation between CSA, UA, and even asymptomatic plaques (11), such that definitive identification of the vulnerable plaque remains a challenge.

EVOLUTION IN THE NOMENCLATURE OF UNSTABLE CORONARY SYNDROMES

Our understanding of unstable coronary syndromes has changed dramatically since the 1980s, and the last 30 years have witnessed the evolution of different terminologies and definitions that have been used to classify and categorize these conditions.

Before the 1970s, there was very little appreciation for the pathogenesis of UA, which was then referred to by several names, including "preinfarction angina," "status anginosis," and "acute coronary insufficiency." The term "unstable angina" was adopted in the early 1970s to encompass the conditions characterized by severe transient myocardial ischemia. At the time, MI was classified as either transmural or non-transmural, based on pathologic criteria (12). By the end of the decade, it was generally recognized that occlusive coronary thrombus was the cause of most cases of transmural MI (13). This concept was definitively established by DeWood et al. in 1980, who found occlusive thrombus in over 80% of patients undergoing coronary angiography in the first few hours of evolving Q-wave MI (14).

In the 1980s, MI was generally re-categorized clinically based on ECG findings into either Q-wave or non-Q-wave infarctions. The prevailing opinion at that time was that a Q-wave MI represented a transmural infarct, and a non-Q-wave MI was indicative of a non-transmural infarction. Beginning in 1985, our group published a series of papers investigating the angiographic features potentially implicated in the pathophysiology of UA and non-Q-wave MI (15–17). We found that in individuals with an identifiable angina or infarct-related vessel about 70% with either syndrome had a severe lesion in a major coronary artery that was eccentric and/or irregular. It was postulated that this represented plaque rupture and/or intraluminal thrombus formation. At the same time, Falk (18) and Davies and Thomas (19) separately published a series of autopsy studies in patients who died from MI or sudden cardiac death (SCD). It was noted that UA leading to MI, fatal MI, and SCD were all linked by the presence of intraluminal coronary thrombus formation. These observations suggested a new paradigm that most ACSs were interrelated, with UA, non-Q-wave MI, Q-wave MI, and a majority of SCD cases representing acute non-occlusive or occlusive thrombotic syndromes.

In the late 1980s and early 1990s, the Q-wave/non-Q-wave categorization of MI was supplanted by a new ECG-based classification system (ST or non-ST elevation MI), which was thought to have more clinical relevance in terms of patient management. ST elevation MI represented total occlusion of a coronary artery that is associated with a worse prognosis, thereby requiring emergent revascularization. Also, during this period, the Braunwald classification (20) was initially proposed and subsequently validated, stratifying UA into risk categories based on its severity, timing, and the clinical circumstances in which it occurs (Table 5.3) (21). In the 1990s, a better understanding emerged regarding the relationship between coronary thrombus, embolization, and mild elevations in cardiac biomarkers, sometimes referred to as "myocardial infarctlets" (22). During this period, it became commonplace to classify ACS into either ST or non-ST elevation ACS, the latter referring to both UA and non-ST elevation MI.

Significant changes in terminology and a greater understanding of the pathophysiology of MI occurred at the turn of the twenty-first century. Initially, a consensus statement from the United States, Europe, and the World Health Organization (23,24) highlighted the importance of cardiac biomarkers in the diagnosis of MI, with troponin designated as the preferred biomarker. As a result, any patient with a clinical syndrome consistent with UA and an elevated troponin level was reclassified as

Table 5.3 The Braunwald Classification of Unstable Angina (UA)

Severity	Clinical circumstances		
	(A) Develops in the presence of an extracardiac condition that intensifies myocardial ischemia (secondary UA)	(B) Develops in the absence of an extracardiac condition (primary UA)	(C) Develops within 2 weeks after acute myocardial infarction (postinfarction UA)
I. New onset of severe angina or accelerated angina (no rest pain)	IA	IB	IC
II. Angina at rest within past month but not within preceding 48 hr (angina at rest, subacute)	IIA	IIB	IIC
III. Angina at rest within 48 hr (angina at rest, acute)	IIIA	IIIB	IIIC

Source: Adapted from Ref. 20.

Table 5.4 Clinical Classification of the Different Types of Myocardial Infarction Based on the Universal Definition

Type 1	Spontaneous myocardial infarction related to ischemia due to a primary coronary event such as plaque erosion and/or rupture, fissuring, or dissection
Type 2	Myocardial infarction secondary to ischemia due to either increased oxygen demand or decreased supply, for example, coronary artery spasm, coronary embolism, anemia, arrhythmias, hypertension, or hypotension
Type 3	Sudden unexpected cardiac death, including cardiac arrest, often with symptoms suggestive of myocardial ischemia, accompanied by presumably new ST elevation, new left bundle branch block, or evidence of fresh thrombus in a coronary artery by angiography and/or at autopsy, but death occurring before blood samples could be obtained, or at a time before the appearance of cardiac biomarkers in the blood
Type 4a	Myocardial infarction associated with percutaneous coronary intervention
Type 4b	Myocardial infarction associated with stent thrombosis as documented by angiography or at autopsy
Type 5	Myocardial infarction associated with coronary artery bypass grafting

Source: Adapted from Ref. 25.

having definite MI. However, as troponin assays became more sensitive, elevated levels of this biomarker were commonly found in individuals with various conditions but without other clinical evidence suggesting MI. This created a dilemma as to whether or not these cases should be classified as true infarctions.

In 2007, a universal definition of MI (25) was proposed to provide a standardized and more precise definition of the condition for use in current clinical practice and health care delivery systems, as well as epidemiology and clinical trials. Infarction was divided into five types based on pathophysiology rather than on pathologic or ECG changes (Table 5.4). The definition of MI required (a) a rise and fall of troponin, levels and (b) clinical evidence of ischemia, including chest pain or its equivalent, ECG change, non-invasive evidence such as new wall motion abnormalities, or angiographic evidence of thrombus. Of particular interest was the distinction between type 1 and 2 MI. Type 1 MI included those with an epicardial lesion indicating primary plaque disruption/erosion with thrombus—the typical non-ST or ST elevation MI as the underlying cause (terminology still considered appropriate to describe MI). On the other hand, type 2 MI had a different pathophysiological basis for the imbalance between supply and demand, such as might be observed with severe hypertension, hypotension, tachyarrhythmias, etc. This distinction might explain why not all patients with an infarction have an obvious infarct-related artery or an infarct-related lesion. Our group has found that culprit lesions are generally not seen in type 2 MI (26).

It remained unclear as to what proportion of patients with a rise and fall of troponin levels fulfill the universal definition of MI. In a prospective study, Javed et al. reported that in less than 30% of individuals with an elevated troponin level, an MI could be diagnosed using the universal definition (Fig. 5.3) (27). In most cases with an elevated troponin level, there was no clinical evidence for MI and the etiology of the "troponin leak" was multifactorial, which included hypertension, congestive heart failure, etc. As troponin assays become even more sensitive in the future, the specificity of troponin will decrease even further.

It should also be recognized that a diagnosis of type 1 MI can occur without typical atherosclerotic disease. While the limitations of angiography in defining the amount of atherosclerosis

may be responsible in some cases, the etiology of most other cases is multifactorial.

UNUSUAL CAUSES OF ACUTE CORONARY SYNDROMES
There are several etiologies of ACS, some of which are non-atherosclerotic in nature. A discussion of all potential etiologies is beyond the scope of this chapter (Table 5.5). However, in this section, we discuss the most important causes that are considered to be of significant clinical relevance.

Dynamic Large-Vessel Obstruction
Prinzmetal or variant angina is a condition where intense focal spasm of an epicardial coronary artery segment occurs, causing significant blood flow occlusion that can trigger UA and its associated symptoms (28). A circadian pattern is usually observed, with most episodes occurring in the early morning. Unlike CSA, it usually occurs without a preceding increase in myocardial oxygen demand, and patients may be younger and have fewer cardiac risk factors. The precise pathogenesis of Prinzmetal angina is poorly understood, but it is postulated that the focal coronary spasm is due to a dysfunctional endothelium that leaves the medial smooth muscle vulnerable to the effects of vasoconstricting catecholamines, thromboxane A2, serotonin, histamine, and endothelin.

There is a large subset of patients with vasospastic angina where the focal coronary spasm occurs at or just distal to a coronary segment where there is evidence of significant obstructive atherosclerotic disease, and it is suggested that these patients may have worse prognostic outcomes (29). In general, a majority of episodes of vasospastic angina resolve spontaneously without clinical sequelae. However, prolonged vasospasm can also occur, particularly in patients with underlying coronary obstruction, which may lead to MI, ventricular tachyarrhythmias, high-grade heart blocks, or sudden cardiac death.

Stimulant-Induced Coronary Vasospasm
The commonly abused stimulants—cocaine and methamphetamine—have also been shown to induce epicardial coronary vasospasm, which may result in myocardial ischemia and show signs and symptoms that are indistinguishable from

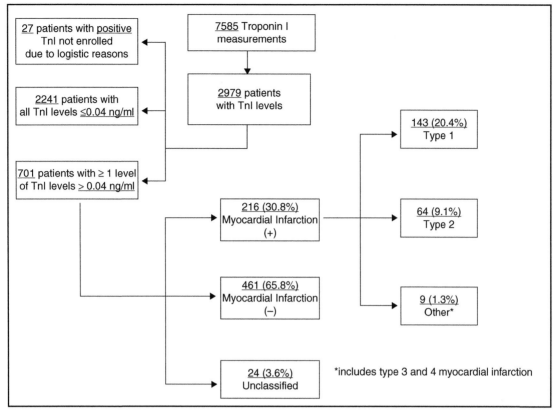

Figure 5.3 Incidence of the different types of myocardial infarction based on the universal definition in patients presenting with elevated troponin (Tn) levels. *Source*: Adapted from Ref. 27.

Table 5.5 Uncommon Causes of Unstable Angina and Acute Coronary Syndromes

---

Coronary embolization
Coronary ostial occlusion from aortic arteritis, aortic dissection, or aortic valve tumor/thrombus/vegetation
Anomalous coronary artery insertion
Coronary artery dissection
Coronary vasospasm, spontaneous or drug-related (e.g., cocaine, methamphetamines)
Coronary aneurysm
Kawasaki disease and other causes of coronary arteritis
Blunt trauma
Takotsubo syndrome
Cardiac syndrome X
Hypertrophic cardiomyopathy
Amyloidosis
Hypercoagulable states

---

atherosclerotic UA or acute MI. These substances block the presynaptic reuptake of the vasoconstricting neurotransmitters norepinephrine and dopamine, leading to sympathetic activation and either macrovascular and/or microvascular spasm. A direct contractile effect of these drugs on the vascular smooth muscle has also been demonstrated. Furthermore, cocaine and methamphetamine increase myocardial oxygen demand by raising the heart rate, blood pressure, and myocardial contractility in a dose-dependent fashion. Typical angiographic findings in those presenting with an ACS are that of coronary spasm in an epicardial vessel with no demonstrable (or only minimal) CAD. Cocaine and methamphetamine, however, may also accelerate coronary atherosclerosis. Most patients presenting with UA due to substance-induced coronary vasospasm do not develop MI and have a good overall prognosis, at least for the acute event (30).

Cardiac Syndrome X

Cardiac syndrome X (CSX) is defined by the triad of exercise-induced angina, objective evidence of ischemia on exercise stress testing, and normal (or minimally diseased) epicardial coronary arteries on angiography. This syndrome predominantly affects women and can also present with features of atypical chest pain. The mechanisms underlying the disorder are multifactorial. Purported causes include endothelial dysfunction with reduced nitric oxide production, impairment in non-endothelium-dependent microvascular dilation, exaggerated vasoconstrictive response to sympathetic stimulation, or exercise-induced coronary vasospasm (31). Short-term prognosis for patients with CSX appears to be excellent. Long-term data, however, shows that even in the documented absence of obstructive coronary disease on angiography, up to 16% of these patients may have subsequent major adverse cardiac events within 5 years (32).

Spontaneous Coronary Dissection

Arterial dissection is defined as separation of the layers of the vessel wall, creating a false lumen between the intima and the media, or between the media and the adventitia. Bleeding into the false lumen of a dissected coronary artery causes impingement of the true lumen and reduction in myocardial blood flow, which can lead to an unstable coronary syndrome or sudden cardiac death. While the vast majority of coronary artery dissections are traumatic in etiology (e.g., cardiac catheterization, cardiac surgery, chest injury), they can also occur spontaneously. Spontaneous coronary dissection is rare and occurs predominantly in young women, particularly in the peripartum period. During labor and the peripartum period, there is an increase in the levels of eosinophils, which contain collagenase, peroxidase, major basic protein, and acid phosphatase. When released, these lytic enzymes may break down the medial–adventitial layers, thus contributing to coronary dissection. The hormonal and hemodynamic changes associated with pregnancy are accompanied by alterations in the elastic and collagenous components of the coronaries that further predispose to spontaneous dissection (33,34). Other conditions associated with the development of spontaneous coronary dissections include atherosclerosis, hypertension, congenital abnormalities of the arterial wall (e.g., Marfan syndrome, Ehlers–Danlos syndrome, lysyl oxidase deficiency), and connective tissue diseases (e.g., polyarteritis nodosa, systemic lupus, eosinophilic arteritis, antiphospholipid syndrome), as well as certain medications (e.g., oral contraceptives, cyclosporine, 5-flurouracil, fenfluramine, stimulants) and vigorous exercise (e.g., weightlifting) (35,36).

Stress Cardiomyopathy

There has been an increasing awareness of a unique cause of elevated troponin in patients presenting with ACS-like symptoms but with apparently normal epicardial coronary arteries on angiography. Stress cardiomyopathy, also known as apical ballooning or takotsubo syndrome, was originally described as acute regional left ventricle (LV) systolic dysfunction that mimics acute MI in patients who meet the following criteria: (a) transient LV apical ballooning, (b) no significant angiographic CAD, and (c) no other known cause of cardiomyopathy (37). Other variants, such as mid-cavitary or basal LV wall motion abnormalities, have also been described (38). The syndrome occurs almost exclusively in postmenopausal women, and is frequently associated with an acute inciting event such as severe emotional, psychological, or physical stress. Most patients present with chest discomfort, ECG abnormalities, and

elevated cardiac biomarkers. The syndrome accounts for 1–5% of patients presenting with acute MI (39), although the actual incidence may be higher because of under-recognition (40). The precise pathophysiologic mechanisms are unclear, but catecholamine-mediated processes appear to be implicated. Patients with takotsubo syndrome have been shown to have impaired endothelial function, heightened vasoconstriction, and excessive catecholamine release in response to acute mental stress, implying that abnormal vasoreactivity and sympathetic responses may be key to its pathogenesis (41). A large proportion of patients develop acute heart failure, but the overall prognosis is generally excellent with relatively rapid and complete resolution of cardiac dysfunction in over 90% of cases (42).

CONCLUSIONS

Our understanding of the process of atherosclerosis, the pathogenesis of coronary disease, the mechanisms underlying the different coronary syndromes, and the clinical spectrum of potential presentations has expanded exponentially over the past 30 years. This has been appropriately accompanied by the constant re-evaluation of the methods and systems using which stable and unstable coronary disease conditions have been defined. The numerous reinventions of the nomenclature and classification schemes are, in general, reflective of the advancements in therapies and management strategies. This process is dynamic and ongoing, and further refinements are likely in the future as a result of scientific progress.

REFERENCES

1. Kolodgie FD, Gold HK, Burke AP, et al. Intraplaque hemorrhage and progression of coronary atheroma. N Engl J Med 2003; 349: 2316–25.
2. Virmani R, Burke AP, Farb A, Kolodgie FD. Pathology of the vulnerable plaque. J Am Coll Cardiol 2006; 47(8 Suppl): C13–18.
3. Ambrose JA. In search of the "vulnerable plaque": can it be localized and will focal regional therapy ever be an option for cardiac prevention? J Am Coll Cardiol 2008; 51: 1539–42.
4. Lardizabal JA, Deedwania PC. The anti-ischemic and anti-anginal properties of statins. Curr Atheroscler Rep 2011; 13: 43–50.
5. Lee TH, Cook EF, Weisberg M, et al. Acute chest pain in the emergency room. Identification and examination of low-risk patients. Arch Intern Med 1985; 145: 65.
6. Campeau L. Grading of angina pectoris. Circulation 1976; 54: 5223.
7. Abidov A, Rozanski A, Hachamovitch R, et al. Prognostic significance of dyspnea in patients referred for cardiac stress testing. N Engl J Med 2005; 353: 1889–98.
8. Gibbons RJ, Abrams J, Chatterjee K, et al. ACC/AHA 2002 guideline update for the management of patients with chronic stable angina–summary article: a report of the American College of Cardiology/American Heart Association Task Force on Practice Guidelines (Committee on the Management of Patients With Chronic Stable Angina). Circulation 2003; 107: 149–58.
9. Cohn PF, Fox KM, Daly C. Silent myocardial ischemia. Circulation 2003; 108: 1263–77.
10. Falk E, Shah PK, Fuster V. Coronary plaque disruption. Circulation 1995; 92: 657–71.

11. van der Wal AC, Becker AE, Koch KT, et al. Clinically stable angina pectoris is not necessarily associated with histologically stable atherosclerotic plaques. Heart 1996; 76: 312–6.

12. Epstein SE, Redwood DR, Goldstein RE, et al. Angina pectoris: pathophysiology, evaluation, and treatment (NIH Conference). Ann Intern Med 1971; 75: 263–96.

13. Chandler AB, Chapman I, Erhardt LR, et al. Coronary thrombosis in myocardial infarction. Report of a workshop on the role of coronary thrombosis in the pathogenesis of acute myocardial infarction. Am J Cardiol 1974; 34: 823–33.

14. DeWood MA, Spores J, Notske R, et al. Prevalence of total coronary occlusion during the early hours of transmural myocardial infarction. N Engl J Med 1980; 303: 897–902.

15. Ambrose JA, Winters SL, Stern A, et al. Angiographic morphology and the pathogenesis of unstable angina pectoris. J Am Coll Cardiol 1985; 5: 609–16.

16. Ambrose JA, Winters SL, Arora RR, et al. Coronary angiographic morphology in myocardial infarction: a link between the pathogenesis of unstable angina and myocardial infarction. J Am Coll Cardiol 1985; 6: 1233–8.

17. Gorlin R, Fuster V, Ambrose JA. Anatomic-physiologic links between acute coronary syndromes. Circulation 1986; 74: 6–9.

18. Falk E. Unstable angina with fatal outcome: dynamic coronary thrombosis leading to infarction and/or sudden death. Autopsy evidence of recurrent mural thrombosis with peripheral embolization culminating in total vascular occlusion. Circulation 1985; 71: 699–708.

19. Davies MJ, Thomas A. Thrombosis and acute coronary-artery lesions in sudden cardiac ischemic death. N Engl J Med 1984; 310: 1137–40.

20. Braunwald E. Unstable angina: a classification. Circulation 1989; 80: 410–4.

21. van Miltenburg-van Zijl AJ, Simoons ML, Veerhoek RJ, et al. Incidence and follow-up of Braunwald subgroups in unstable angina pectoris. J Am Coll Cardiol 1995; 25: 1286–92.

22. Abdelmeguid AE, Topol EJ. The myth of the myocardial 'infarctlet' during percutaneous coronary revascularization procedures. Circulation 1996; 94: 3369–75.

23. Alpert JS, Thygesen K, Antman E, et al. Myocardial infarction redefined—a consensus document of The Joint European Society of Cardiology/American College of Cardiology Committee for the redefinition of myocardial infarction. J Am Coll Cardiol 2000; 36: 959–69.

24. Luepker RV, Apple FS, Christenson RH, et al. Case definitions for acute coronary heart disease in epidemiology and clinical research studies: a statement from the AHA Council on Epidemiology and Prevention; AHA Statistics Committee; World Heart Federation Council on Epidemiology and Prevention; the European Society of Cardiology Working Group on Epidemiology and Prevention; Centers for Disease Control and Prevention; and the National Heart, Lung, and Blood Institute. Circulation 2003; 108: 2543–9.

25. Thygesen K, Alpert JS, White HD, et al. Joint ESC/ACCF/AHA/WHF Task Force for the Redefinition of Myocardial Infarction. Universal definition of myocardial infarction. J Am Coll Cardiol 2007; 50: 2173–95.

26. Ambrose JA, Loures-Vale A, Javed U, Buhari C, Aftab W. Angiographic correlates in Type 1 and Type 2 MI by the universal definition. JACC Imaging 2012; 5: 463–4.

27. Javed U, Aftab W, Ambrose JA, et al. Frequency of elevated troponin I and diagnosis of acute myocardial infarction. Am J Cardiol 2009; 104: 9–13.

28. Prinzmetal M, Goldman A, Shubin H, et al. Angina pectoris II. Am Heart J 1959; 57: 530–43.

29. Rovai D, Bianchi M, Baratto M, et al. Organic coronary stenosis in Prinzmetal's variant angina. J Cardiol 1997; 30: 299–305.

30. McCord J, Jneid H, Hollander JE, et al. Management of cocaine-associated chest pain and myocardial infarction: a scientific statement from the American Heart Association Acute Cardiac Care Committee of the Council on Clinical Cardiology. Circulation 2008; 117: 1897–907.

31. Kaski, JC. Pathophysiology and management of patients with chest pain and normal coronary arteriograms (cardiac syndrome X). Circulation 2004; 109: 568.

32. Gulati M, Cooper-DeHoff RM, McClure C, et al. Adverse cardiovascular outcomes in women with nonobstructive coronary artery disease: a report from the Women's Ischemia Syndrome Evaluation Study and the St James Women Take Heart Project. Arch Intern Med 2009; 169: 843–50.

33. Kamran M, Guptan A, Bogal M. Spontaneous coronary artery dissection: case series and review. J Invasive Cardiol 2008; 20: 553–9.

34. Kansara P, Graham S. Spontaneous coronary artery dissection: case series with extended follow up. J Invasive Cardiol 2011; 23: 76–80.

35. El-Sherief K, Rashidian A, Srikanth S. Spontaneous coronary artery dissection after intense weightlifting. Catheter Cardiovasc Interv 2011; 78: 223–7.

36. Ito H, Taylor L, Bowman M, et al. Presentation and therapy of spontaneous coronary artery dissection and comparisons of postpartum versus nonpostpartum cases. Am J Cardiol 2011; 107: 1590–6.

37. Tsuchihashi K, Ueshima K, Uchida T, et al. Transient left ventricular apical ballooning without coronary artery stenosis: a novel heart syndrome mimicking acute myocardial infarction. Angina Pectoris-Myocardial Infarction Investigations in Japan. J Am Coll Cardiol 2001; 38: 11–8.

38. Hurst RT, Prasad A, Askew JW, et al. Takotsubo cardiomyopathy: a unique cardiomyopathy with variable ventricular morphology. JACC Cardiovasc Imaging 2010; 3: 641–9.

39. Kurowski V, Kaiser A, von Hof K, et al. Apical and midventricular transient left ventricular dysfunction syndrome (tako-tsubo cardiomyopathy): frequency, mechanisms, and prognosis. Chest 2007; 132: 809–16.

40. Strunk B, Shaw RE, Bull S, et al. High incidence of focal left ventricular wall motion abnormalities and normal coronary arteries in patients with myocardial infarctions presenting to a community hospital. J Invasive Cardiol 2006; 18: 376–81.

41. Martin EA, Prasad A, Rihal CS, et al. Endothelial function and vascular response to mental stress are impaired in patients with apical ballooning syndrome. J Am Coll Cardiol 2010; 56: 1840–6.

42. Madhavan M, Rihal CS, Lerman A, Prasad A. Acute heart failure in apical ballooning syndrome (TakoTsubo/stress cardiomyopathy): clinical correlates and Mayo Clinic risk score. J Am Coll Cardiol 2011; 57: 1400–1.

6

Clinical evaluation of the patient with chest pain
Attilio Maseri

OUTLINE

The chapter describes the most common features of anginal pain and discusses its mechanisms, its very variable location and radiation as well as its total absence in some cases. It presents a description of the typical patterns of recurrence of painful episodes which characterize distinct anginal syndromes and provide clues about the respective underlying causes and the differential diagnosis. It discusses the diagnosis of acute myocardial ischemia and of its underlying causes, together with the determinants of prognosis in anginal syndromes. Finally it presents the problem of the recurrence of angina in patients with previous coronary revascularization or angiography and the evaluation and risk stratification of acute chest pain in the emergency department.

INTRODUCTION

Chest pain is the symptom that most often brings patients with episodes of acute myocardial ischemia to medical attention in outpatient and emergency departments. The symptoms may recur with transient recurrent episodes having a stable pattern suggestive of *chronic stable angina*, a recent onset and rapidly worsening pattern suggestive of *unstable angina*, or with acute prolonged pain suggestive of an *acute myocardial infarction*.

The relative frequency of these traditionally recognized presentations has gradually changed over the years because of the growing awareness that recent onset chest pain is a potential harbinger of major cardiac events and that the risk associated with such a presentation can be reduced by prompt detection and correction of underlying "culprit" coronary artery stenoses. Thus, most patients are now seen in the emergency departments of hospitals at the time of their first complaint of chest pain (and diagnosed as acute infarction when markers of myocardial necrosis are positive). Yet up to 15% of all males and 30% of all females subjected to angiography are found to have no flow-limiting stenoses. Accordingly, patients first seen with an uncomplicated history of chronic stable angina, lasting over 2 months, are encountered less frequently, and the possibility that symptoms may be due to variant angina or microvascular coronary dysfunction is often not even considered. However, recurrent angina, in patients who have already undergone coronary angiography and revascularization procedures, has become more and more frequent. Therefore, it appears useful to review the natural presentation of the various typical patterns of angina as the very first manifestation of ischemic heart disease (IHD), as they were observed in the pre-interventional era, because this can provide a rational basis for the assessment and management of the growing number of patients presenting with recurring anginal episodes after previous angiography or intervention, with and without new or residual flow-limiting coronary stenosis, or with "normal" angiograms.

Patients presenting with acute chest pain to the emergency department without an established pattern of recurrence will be dealt with at the end of this chapter, following the discussion of the mechanism of pain and diagnostic and prognostic principles in stable and unstable angina and in their respective subgroups.

The location, radiation, intensity, and duration of anginal pain vary considerably among patients, but in any given patient, the location and radiation of pain tend to remain the same in successive episodes, especially when ischemia involves the same myocardial region (4); thus their pattern of recurrence becomes recognized and reported by the patient. A careful enquiry about the pattern of recurrence of symptoms can provide valuable diagnostic clues to the underlying causes of myocardial ischemia.

Indeed, angina is a broad syndrome (Fig. 6.1A–D) (1), just like anemia, as transient myocardial ischemia can be caused by different mechanisms in the presence of variable severity and extension of coronary atherosclerosis, which is not a necessary nor a sufficient diagnostic feature by itself of ischemic cardiac pain: many patients with angina caused by transient ischemia have angiographically "normal" coronary arteries while some with extensive atherosclerosis do not have ischemic episodes or angina. In turn, flow-limiting coronary stenoses, acute thrombosis, epicardial coronary artery constriction, and microvascular constriction each can be caused by a variety of mechanisms. Too often the diagnosis of stable or unstable angina is used, by itself, without additional diagnostic descriptors, and the diagnosis of angina and "normal" coronary arteries is made lumping together variant and microvascular angina which have an obviously different prognosis and treatment.

Therefore, the initial clinical diagnosis of stable or unstable angina is incomplete without consideration of: (*i*) previous history of IHD; (*ii*) pattern of attacks; (*iii*) their usual triggers and effort tolerance; (*iv*) duration of pain; and (*v*) response to acute nitrates.

The demonstration, during a painful episode, of transient ischemic electrocardiogram (ECG) changes is indicative of a cardiac origin of the pain and, in most cases, of ischemic causes. Conversely, the absence of ECG changes suggests non cardiac causes, although it does not completely rule out an ischemic origin. The final diagnosis should be made on the basis of the demonstration of myocardial ischemia and a comprehensive assessment of all available diagnostic criteria rather than the result of any single test.

This chapter will cover seven topics:

1. A description of the most common features of anginal pain;
2. A discussion of the mechanisms of ischemic cardiac pain and its very variable location and radiation as well as its total absence in some cases;

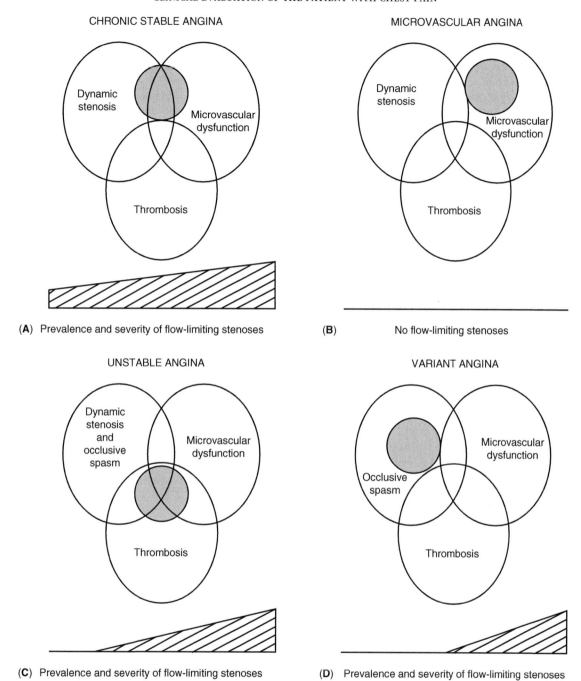

Figure 6.1 Pathogenetic components of stable and unstable anginal syndromes. Chronic stable angina (A) is caused by flow-limiting coronary artery steno-ses of variable severity and number, but residual coronary flow reserve can be modulated by dynamic changes in peristenotic smooth muscle tone (dynamic stenoses) or by microvascular dysfunction. Microvascular angina (B) is caused by coronary microvascular dysfunction. Unstable angina (C) is caused bv a variable combination of thrombosis, dynamic stenoses, occlusive spasm and microvascular dysfunction occurring not only in the presence of flow-limiting coronary artery stenoses, but also in their absence. Variant angina (D) is caused by occlusive epicardial coronary artery spasm, which may occur not only at the site of flow-limiting stenoses of variable severity, but also in angiographically normal segments. The actual causes of thrombosis and vasoconstrictor response and of microvascular dysfunction may be multiple, possibly different from those contributing to stable syndromes. *Source*: From Ref. 1, Chapter 16 pp. 454–455.

3. A description of the typical patterns of recurrence of painful episodes which characterize distinct anginal syndromes and provide clues about the respective underlying causes and the differential diagnosis;
4. The diagnosis of acute myocardial ischemia and of its underlying causes;
5. The determinants of prognosis in anginal syndromes;
6. The recurrence of angina in patients with previous coronary revascularization or angiography;
7. The evaluation and risk stratification of the patient with acute chest pain in the emergency department.

CLINICAL FEATURES OF ANGINAL PAIN

As described in masterly fashion by Heberden, in its most typical presentation, anginal pain is retrosternal with a crushing, squeezing, or burning character. It may radiate to the throat, neck or ulnar side of the left arm, extend down to the little finger and, occasionally, to the interscapular region or epigastrium. Less frequently, it radiates to both arms, or to the right arm or to the jaw and teeth. The variations are numerous and over 300 variants, including radiation to the left leg, the wrist or the jaw have been reported. In some patients the pain may be reproducibly confined exclusively to only one of these areas. Angina pectoris may also be associated with a strangling sensation in the upper chest and neck. The intensity of the discomfort can vary greatly, from a mild feeling of retrosternal fullness or tingling in only one dermatome to pain that is excruciating and unbearable. The duration of anginal episodes

is never seconds or hours, but a few minutes and usually recurs with similar features. The total lack of pain (and also of any other symptom) represents one extreme of the spectrum of the possible clinical presentations of myocardial ischemia. Although in general the more severe and long lasting the pain, the more severe the ischemia, the relationship between the severity of myocardial ischemia and pain is extremely variable: indeed even myocardial infarction (MI), may be painless in over 20% of cases (2). Conversely, severe pain may also occur even in the absence of detectable transient regional ventricular dysfunction and ECG changes when ischemia is caused by sparse, small coronary artery constriction.

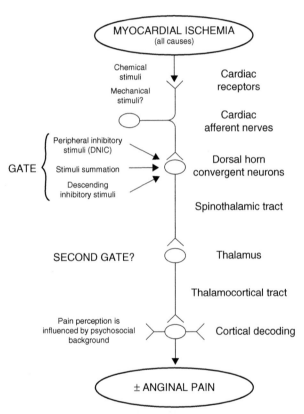

Figure 6.2 Afferent neural pathways involved in the transmission of cardiac ischemic pain. Cardiac sensory receptors may be stimulated by chemical or mechanical stimuli. Afferent impulses project to dorsal horn convergent neurons where their progression toward supraspinal centers is modulated by peripheral or descending stimuli (the "gate" theory). Further modulation of cardiac afferent stimuli might occur in the thalamus. Pain perception takes place when cardiac afferent stimuli are decoded in the cortex and is strongly influenced by the psychosocial background. Afferent fibers from different cardiac areas and from other visceral and somatic areas converge on the same ascending neurons. The existence of specific neurons involved in only the transmission of pain (the "specificity" hypothesis) is, so far, unproven. The intense excitation of polymodal fibers, also involved in autonomic nervous control, was proposed as an alternative hypothesis (the "intensity" hypothesis). *Source:* From Ref. 1, Chapter 14, p. 411.

Focus Box 6.1

Neither the location or radiation of ischemic cardiac pain nor its absence is related to the actual cause of ischemia which is often unrelated to the extension and severity of coronary atherosclerosis. Conversely, the pattern of angina attacks with the circumstances during which they tend to recur, their duration, and response to nitrates together with the electrocardiogram changes during the attack can provide indications on their ischemic nature and clues about the underlying cause of ischemia. The association with signs of acute left ventricular failure or obvious arrhythmias indicates severe, extensive ischemia

---

Focus Box 6.2

Because of the large convergence of several afferent neurons coming from different visceral organs and from somatic dermatomes on a very limited number of ascending neurons, cardiac pain can be perceived as coming from several dermatomes and radiating to various other dermatomes. In addition, also non cardiac stimuli can cause pain with similar features to those of cardiac ischemic pain. Blockade of ascending afferent impulses may totally prevent the perception of pain

PHYSIOLOGICAL BASIS OF ANGINAL PAIN PERCEPTION

The anatomical and physiological basis of visceral pain perception can be summarized as follows (Fig. 6.2) (3).

1. Noxious stimuli excite bipolar neurons, situated in thoracic sympathetic ganglia which have a peripherally directed axon, innervating the heart, and a centrally directed axon, connecting with the spinal dorsal horn neurons.
2. Transmission of these potentially painful messages from the dorsal horn to the thalamus is modulated (and may be also blocked) by afferent and descending impulses from supraspinal centers; transmission of impulses from the thalamus to the cortical centers may also be modulated by afferent and descending impulses.
3. Perception of these afferent impulses that reach the cortex is related to their decoding as a conscious unpleasant experience.

Noxious Stimuli

Available information suggests that adenosine is a chemical mediator of pain, but pain can also be caused by mechanical stimulation of epicardial coronary arteries.

Evidence of Chemical Stimulation in Man

Intracoronary infusion of adenosine consistently causes pain identical to that experienced during transient myocardial ischemia in daily life.

Selective blockade of A1 adenosine receptors by bamiphylline reduced anginal pain without affecting its vasodilator effects, thus suggesting that the algogenic effects of adenosine are mediated predominantly by A1 receptors (4).

Stimulation of the afferent nerve fibers by adenosine occurs during ischemia, whenever oxygen supply becomes inadequate to meet the demands, as the intramyocardial concentration of adenosine increases markedly.

Transmission and Modulation of Cardiac Afferent Stimuli

Cardiac afferent impulses travel through unmyelinated or small myelinated fibers in the cardiac sympathetic nerves to the upper five thoracic sympathetic ganglia where these neurons originate, and from there the impulses travel to the dorsal horn neurons through the white rami communicantes, the gray rami (although to a minor extent), and the upper thoracic dorsal roots. Afferent impulses traveling through vagal fibers could explain the referred pain in the jaw, head, and neck which was found to become more common when sympathectomy was used to cure intractable angina.

The convergence of afferent nervous impulses from both visceral and somatic sensory nerves to the same few dorsal horn neurons provides a plausible explanation for the very variable somatic component of visceral pain.

Convergence of Cardiac Afferent Stimuli on Dorsal Horn Spinal Neurons

In about 70% of anginal patients, the selective infusion of adenosine into the right coronary artery elicited pain identical to that experienced when it was infused into the left coronary artery. In all patients, the adenosine-induced pain was similar to that experienced during anginal attacks occurring in daily life. This indicates that, man afferent stimuli from different myocardial regions often converge onto the same dorsal neurons. In the remaining 30%, the distribution of pain during adenosine infusion into the right coronary artery was different to that experienced during infusion into the left coronary artery. The location and radiation of pain was reported to be the same in about 70% of patients who had two episodes of myocardial infarction, one anterior and one inferior, but it was clearly different in the remaining 30% (5). Differences in the location and radiation of anginal pain during successive attacks in the same patient may, therefore, be clues to the occurrence of ischemia in different areas of the heart.

The transmission of nociceptive messages is modulated, to a very considerable extent, as early as the first relays in the dorsal horn spinal neurons. The "gate control" theory proposed by Melzack and Wall was an attempt to summarize this notion in schematic form. According to this theory, the condition, either open or closed, of the "gate" at the level of the dorsal horn neurons depends on both afferent and descending nervous impulses and determines whether a specific nociceptive message reaches supraspinal centers.

Summation of subliminal nociceptive messages, from the same or different dermatomes, has been shown to result in the stimulation of neurons converging at the dorsal horn. Thus, episodes of cardiac ischemic pain may be more intense in patients with chronic pain originating from other visceral or somatic structures.

Modulation of Cardiac Afferent Stimuli in Anginal Patients

In patients with angina, the modulation of cardiac afferent impulses at the site of neurons converging on the dorsal horn is indicated by the observations that (i) esophageal stimulation lowers the anginal threshold during exercise, thus suggesting the occurrence of summation of subliminal stimuli, and (ii) transcutaneous electrical nerve stimulation, dorsal column stimulation, or carotid sinus massage or stimulation can raise the anginal threshold. Diabetic neuropathy may contribute to reduced pain perception in some patients.

The nociceptive messages reaching the spinal dorsal horn and modulated at that site by the gate system, project to the thalamus along the spinothalamic tract and from the thalamus to the cortex. The ascending pathways of nociceptive messages beyond the thalamus are not precisely known, but during anginal pain, thalamic and cortical activation are detectable by regional cerebral blood flow measurements.

The conscious perception of pain is related to the cortical decoding of afferent stimuli as unpleasant. The intensity of pain is influenced not only by the intensity of the afferent impulses reaching the cortex but also by the individual's personality, emotional status, and previous experience of pain. Nociceptive messages can apparently be modulated in supraspinal centers by inhibition or facilitation of their transmission, opioids, and cortical subjective attitudes such as stoicism and denial. Both the complaint and the protective reaction elicited by pain are likely to be profoundly affected by an individual's personal, social, and cultural backgrounds.

Onset of Myocardial Ischemia, Appearance of Anginal Pain, and Silent Ischemia

In patients with variant angina, in whom the onset of ischemia is easily identified by the dramatic elevation of the ST-segment on the ECG, a minimal duration (more than 3 min) and severity of ischemia (more than 7 mmHg increase in left ventricular

end-diastolic pressure) are observed before the development of anginal pain; but severe and prolonged episodes can be totally asymptomatic. Also, in acute infarction pain may appear minutes and even hours after the onset of ST segment elevation and is absent in about 20% of cases. Only some of these patients with painless ischemia suffer from diabetes.

Conversely, in patients with chronic stable angina undergoing exercise stress testing, pain often precedes (or occurs simultaneously) with the onset of ischemic ST-segment depression, particularly when ischemia is caused by small coronary vessel dysfunction. During stress testing, pain may also be completely absent despite marked ST segment depression, perfusion defects, and transient contractile dysfunction. During Holter monitoring about 70% of episodes are silent, particularly those that are shorter and less severe. Conversely, pain may be very severe in patients with microvascular angina, even in the absence of transient regional contractile dysfunction (Fig. 6.3).

CHARACTERISTIC PATTERNS OF ANGINAL PAIN RECURRENCE IN DISTINCT ANGINAL SYNDROMES: A CLUE TO THE UNDERLYING MECHANISMS OF ISCHEMIA

A stable pattern of recurrence of ischemic episodes, provoked by effort or emotion with or without pain, over at least the past two months, suggests chronic stable causes of transient ischemic episodes: *chronic stable angina*. Conversely, recent onset and/or rapid worsening of effort tolerance, severity, and duration of ischemic episodes suggest unstable causes: *unstable angina*. Within both stable and unstable subsets of patients a more detailed analysis of the pattern of the ischemic episodes identifies major clinical subgroups with specific ischemic causes (Table 6.1).

Within each of these subgroups, a number of variants have been described, reflecting a variable. A combination of the four basic pathogenetic mechanisms is illustrated in Figure 6.1 and differences in their individual etiological causes: (i) various mechanisms of plaque formation, growth, and evolution; (ii) various mechanisms of epicardial coronary artery spasm and microvascular constriction; (iii) intensity of various mechanisms and time course of thrombogenic stimuli and thrombotic response.

A rationale for specific treatment and prevention of each anginal syndrome would require a precise understanding of its potentially multiple causal mechanisms and identification of their specific diagnostic descriptors.

Chronic Stable, Predominantly Effort-related Angina

In these patients, angina episodes are predominantly effort related, relieved promptly (within about 5 min) by rest or sublingual nitrates, with an unchanged pattern of recurrence

---

Focus Box 6.3

In summary, the relationship between ischemia and anginal pain may be seen as a bell-shaped distribution in which patients with totally painless ischemia are at one extreme and patients with microvascular angina are at the other. For each individual patient the relationship varies in time because of the dynamic modulation of the perception of pain, possibly related to the gating system of afferent impulses and their central decoding

Thus, myocardial ischemia, regardless of its cause, can be (*i*) painful, with one of the many variations on the Heberden theme; (*ii*) painless, but symptomatic because of dyspnea (due to transient left ventricular failure), palpitation or syncope (due to transient arrhythmias) or (*iii*) totally silent, with no clinical manifestation, usually identified by transient ischemic changes on the ECG

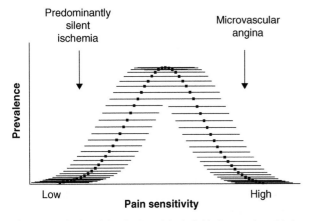

Figure 6.3 Bell-shaped distribution of the individual perception of ischemic pain. At one extreme are patients with only silent myocardial ischemia and at the other are those with microvascular angina and no detectable ischemic dysfunction. The oscillations indicate the variability of an individual's perception of pain in time. Diabetic patients are more often to the left of the curve, those with microvascular angina to the right. *Source*: From Ref. 1, Chapter 16, p. 452.

Table 6.1 Major Clinical Patterns of Angina

a. Chronic stable, predominantly effort-related angina
a.1. Microvascular angina
b. Unstable angina, predominantly at rest
b.1. Variant angina

during the preceding two months. It may be the first presentation of IHD and may remain stable for several years in spite of multivessel coronary disease. Two extreme subgroups of patients can be recognized from the pattern of recurrence of angina episodes:

- Patients in whom angina predictably develops whenever levels of effort of broadly similar intensity are exceeded, and in whom pain is promptly relieved by rest; greater levels of effort cannot be tolerated. The constancy of the angina threshold indicates a fixed reduction of coronary blood flow reserve, caused by fixed flow limiting coronary stenoses as the only cause of angina. Such predictable, effort-related, angina is rare and is completely cured by removal of

coronary flow-limiting stenoses. However, some of these patients, for unknown reasons may occasionally become unstable or develop an acute MI, and at present cannot be distinguished from those who will remain stable.

- Patients who, besides reporting an upper effort threshold of angina that they cannot exceed even during their "good days," also complain of angina episodes occurring, unpredictably, for efforts usually well tolerated and even at rest. They have a mixed form of chronic stable angina (6), and the variability of the angina threshold indicates that ischemic episodes are a result of a combination of increased demand and a coincidental transient reduction of

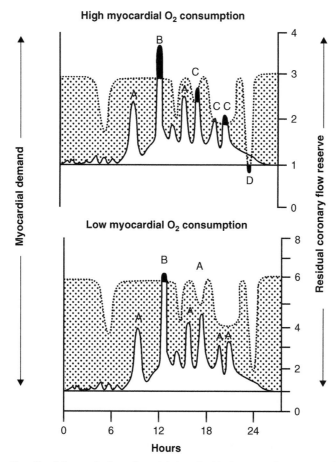

Figure 6.4 Chronic stable angina: effect of basal flow on the dynamic modulation of residual coronary flow reserve and ischemic threshold. In the scheme depicted in the upper panel, basal flow during 24 h is double of that depicted in the lower panel because of a higher basal MVO$_2$. The maximal residual coronary flow allowed by the most critical stenosis is the same in both the upper and lower panels but, in the upper panel, flow can increase only three times above baseline, as against six times in the lower panel. For a similar increase in myocardial demand (white area, points A) and a similar reduction of coronary flow reserve (striped area), ischemia is less likely to occur (points C and D) when basal flow is low. The increase in MVO$_2$ may be insufficient to cause ischemia (A) because it does not exceed maximal residual coronary flow reserve. Myocardial demand may exceed maximal residual coronary flow reserve (B) but ischemia is more severe when basal MVO$_2$ is high. Basal flow can be reduced by decreasing MVO$_2$ and by correcting anemia and hypoxemia when present. The dynamic modulation of residual coronary flow reserve can be eliminated by preventing dynamic stenoses and inappropriate microvascular constriction. Maximal residual coronary flow can be increased by collateral development or by revascularization procedures. *Source*: From Ref. 1, Chapter 16, p. 467.

coronary blood flow reserve, caused by vasoconstriction at the site of a stenosis (dynamic stenosis) or in small distal vessels. In patients with mixed chronic stable angina removal of the culprit coronary stenosis may not prevent occasional angina episodes caused by vasoconstriction (Fig. 6.4). The triggers of dynamic coronary stenosis may be different from those of variant angina and different from those responsible for microvascular constriction.

Microvascular Angina

In some patients angina is characterized by episodes, usually precipitated by effort or emotion, of much longer duration than those caused by a flow-limiting stenosis (sometimes 15–30 min), that are not promptly relieved by rest and respond poorly to sublingual nitrates. Indeed in these patients, sublingual nitrates were shown to worsen effort tolerance during exercise stress testing (7). The dipyridamole test is typically positive in these patients because it reproduces their typical pain, usually with diagnostic ECG changes, sometimes with myocardial perfusion defects, but without detectable new ventricular wall motion abnormalities (8). These alterations possibly result from a mechanism of focal microvascular blood flow steal and patchy adenosine release (9). These patients also often have an enhanced perception of pain (10,11) and respond unpredictably to high doses of calcium antagonists and beta blockers. Thus, treatment is largely empirical and should focus on patient reassurance and on very prompt use of acute nitrates at the very onset of the pain, which may abort the episode. Some of these patients also describe occasional episodes at rest that are usually long lasting and poorly responsive to nitrates with only mild to moderate ST segment depression on the ECG. Finally, microvascular dysfunction has been described in several other non coronary conditions such as primary myocardial disease, as well as in acute atherosclerotic ischemic syndromes (12,13) and Takotsubo syndrome (14).

Available evidence suggests that inappropriate constriction of pre-arteriolar coronary vessels, mediated by alpha adrenergic stimulation, neuropeptide Y (NPY) release, circulating or locally produced autacoids, or endothelial dysfunction can cause occasional, transient reductions of distal flow, initially compensated by adenosine release and consequent distal arteriolar dilatation. Compensatory arteriolar dilation may be insufficient in preventing ischemia in the myocardium perfused by the most constricted pre-arteriolar vessels (which are not exposed to adenosine). Such constriction is likely to occur proximally to arterioles (which are promptly dilated by adenosine released by ischemic myocytes. As pre-arteriolar vessels may not be all constricted to the same extent), ischemia may be focal, patchily distributed, predominantly in the subendocardium (which is more vulnerable to ischemia) and may not result in detectable regional contractile dysfunction, when it is compensated by the contraction of adjacent, normally perfused, and contracting myocytes. However, increased adenosine concentration in focal areas may be sufficient to stimulate pain receptors.

Unstable Angina, Predominantly at Rest

The sudden onset or the sudden exacerbation of angina, with severe and protracted attacks typically occurring spontaneously at rest, caused by a transient critical reduction of coronary blood supply, are indications of unstable causes of acute coronary obstruction, with the potential to result in persistent occlusion and, therefore, demand prompt medical attention and aggressive management, particularly in the presence of ischemic ECG changes. For patients admitted to the hospital or seen in an emergency department, positive circulating markers of myocardial necrosis, typically troponin elevation, is diagnostic of acute, recent myocardial necrosis, indicative of prolonged severe ischemic episodes, and hence a threat of impending acute total occlusion and infarction.

Coronary instability is traditionally attributed to the development of thrombogenic plaques, often in association with rupture, possibly related to focal or multifocal inflammatory mechanisms, which tend to evolve toward rapid stenosis progression or a complete, persistent thrombotic–vasospastic occlusion, and MI in the short term (Fig. 6.5) (15). However, in some cases it may also be caused by persistent coronary spasm or intense widespread microvascular constriction, in the absence of coronary stenoses, or in association with stenoses and thrombosis as discussed above (Fig. 6.5) and in the absence of elevated markers of inflammation (16).

Variant Angina

This syndrome was identified by Prinzmetal from the observation that some patients who reported a pattern of episodes of angina at rest, particularly in the early morning hours, of a few minutes' duration, sometimes occurring in clusters of 2–3 episodes within 1 or 2 hours, associated with ST segment elevation on the ECG and usually with preserved effort tolerance. He postulated a transient increase of "tonus" at the site of a subcritical stenosis, which occluded the artery causing transmural myocardial ischemia, because the notion of coronary spasm was not accepted at the time (17). Subsequently, variant angina was reported also in patients with angiographically normal coronary arteries and defined as the "variant of the variant!" (18) and in patients with severe coronary stenoses (19,20). Yet nowadays, often the possibility of spasm is only considered in patients with angina and "normal" angiograms (as the detection of a stenosis would provide, by itself a plausible explanation for angina!).

In patients with the typical chronic presentation, the development of occlusive spasm appears related to a local postreceptoral hyperreactivity of the coronary smooth muscle to a wide variety of constrictor stimuli, acting on distinct receptors, may result in local or diffuse occlusion of a coronary artery, and may also involve multiple sites (multifocal spasm). It appears more widely reported among Japanese patients, most often with normal coronary angiograms (21), possibly because such patients are more

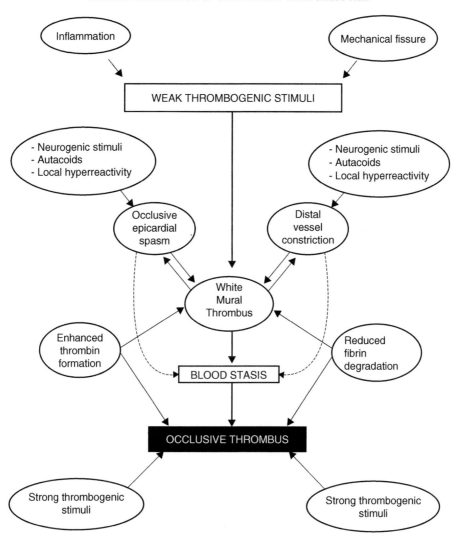

Figure 6.5 Vicious circles leading to the formation of a thrombus at the site of coronary occlusion. An occlusive red thrombus can form rapidly within minutes at the site of a highly thrombogenic injury (as in the copper coil dog model). An occlusive white thrombus can form only very gradually at the site of a weak, persisting thrombogenic stimulus (as in the electric wire dog model). In the presence of a mural thrombus, occlusive thrombosis may be the result of vicious circles, in which proximal or distal coronary constriction creates blood stasis, with consequent formation of an occlusive red thrombus. The triggers of the vicious circle and the "gain" of its components can have a variable importance and prevalence in different groups of patients. For example, an enhanced thrombotic tendency can be caused, on the one hand, by all the alterations that lead to an enhanced thrombin formation and, on the other, by all the alterations that reduce fibrinolysis. *Source*: From Ref. 1, Chapter 9, p. 280.

often subjected to provocative tests than those with obstructive coronary disease. The causes of the local hyperactivity is still unknown, but many patients exhibit waxing and waning of anginal episodes, which become more frequent during stressful periods and less frequent during serene phases of life; remissions of months may be followed by relapses. Some patients develop episodes of ventricular tachycardia and fibrillation during or at the end of ischemic episodes, (or complete atrioventricular block when associated with inferior ST segment elevation) caused by sudden transient spastic coronary occlusion, usually

during waxing phases and such malignant arrhythmias during anginal attacks are a typical diagnostic feature of variant angina (22) Most patients respond to high doses of calcium antagonists and to long-acting nitrates before going to bed but some patients are refractory (23). In my personal experience gathered in Pisa, London, and Rome this typical presentation represented about 1% of those admitted for IHD but the occurrence of isolated, occasional spasm may be more common. A combination of epicardial and small coronary artery spasm was also reported (24,25). The trigger of these various manifestations of spasm may be multiple; thus distinctive features should be carefully noted in order to focus research on carefully characterized, phenotypically homogeneous groups of patients.

Diagnosis of Myocardial Ischemia and Its Underlying Causes

The diagnostic process should proceed in two steps: (*i*) the demonstration of ischemia; (*ii*) the search for its causes.

The clinical diagnosis of anginal pain is straightforward when careful questioning of patients who appear to be reliable historians reveals a pattern of recurrence of pain typical of one of the anginal syndromes described above and summarized in Table 6.2. In these patients the first diagnostic step is the documentation of ischemia, its location, extension, severity, and prognostic implications. When the evidence for myocardial ischemia is not available, the diagnosis may be uncertain, particularly in patients who are poor historians or report a very recent onset of symptoms, thus removing the possibility of identifying a pattern of recurrence.

Potential differential diagnoses and diagnostic tests should be considered separately for each pattern of clinical presentation and suspected anginal syndromes.

Diagnostic Tests
The clinical diagnosis of anginal syndromes must be confirmed by the demonstration of:

1. *An ischemic origin of pain indicated by:* diagnostic transient ischemic ST segment changes on the 12 lead ECG or Holter recordings; transient defects in regional myocardial perfusion assessed by radionuclide or by nuclear magnetic resonance technology; transient left ventricular wall motion abnor-

malities (which are absent in microvascular angina because of the focal nature of ischemia). Episodes of transient ST segment elevation are indicative of transmural myocardial ischemia due to transient coronary occlusion, when short and repeated, and when associated with a negative stress test, most likely caused by spasm.

2. *The actual causes of ischemia can be demonstrated by coronary angiography showing:* a flow-limiting stenosis (fixed or dynamic), in patients with fixed or variable effort tolerance; an irregular stenosis with or without superimposed thrombosis, suggestive of unstable plaque, in patients with unstable angina; an occlusive or subocclusive coronary spasm at the site of a subcritical, or of a critical stenosis or in a normal coronary segment, (occurring spontaneously or following a provocative test and relieved by intracoronary nitrates), in patients with variant angina; the absence of flow limiting coronary stenosis, in patients with microvascular angina, "soft" suggestion of microvascular flow impairment is provided by the observation of a slow contrast medium progression in some coronary artery branches in patients with acute coronary syndromes and in some of those with microvascular "stable" angina.

It should be stressed once more that there is no unequivocal correlation between coronary atherosclerosis and angina, as many patients with coronary atherosclerosis do not present

---

Table 6.2 Pattern of Recurrence of Anginal Episodes Typical of Each Distinct Anginal Syndrome

Fixed threshold chronic stable exertional angina: episodes develop predictably only whenever a given level of effort is exceeded and are promptly relieved by rest

Mixed chronic stable angina: episodes occur with a stable pattern but occasionally also for efforts usually well tolerated and even at rest as a result of a variable residual coronary flow reserve (modulated by a dynamic stenosis or by inappropriate coronary prearteriolar coronary constriction)

Microvascular angina: episodes usually induced by effort or emotion, or by a positive dipyridamole test without associated contractile dysfunction, characterized by severe pain of long duration, not promptly relieved by rest or by acute nitrates

Unstable angina: episodes are of recent onset or worsening, occurring at rest, usually with impaired effort tolerance and of prolonged duration suggestive of an impending infarction

Variant angina: episodes occur spontaneously at rest, of 3–10 min. duration, typically in the early morning hours or at night, usually with preserved effort tolerance sometimes associated with palpitations and syncope (which, when occurring in association with an anginal attack are very suggestive of occlusive spasm)

Focus Box 6.4

The diagnostic gold standard of myocardial ischemia is:

Metabolic evidence of ischemia is provided by the detection in the coronary sinus of an increased concentration of lactic acid during pacing-induced ischemia in patients with a flow limiting stenosis in the left coronary system which drains into the coronary sinus (but could not be applicable with right coronary stenosis!). A definite demonstration of ischemia is also provided by the simultaneous development, together with ischemic ECG changes of perfusion defects and contraction abnormalities in the same myocardial segments. Finally the magnitude of ischemic alterations in any test is an important diagnostic component

In patients with microvascular angina a definite diagnosis can only be obtained by the detection of ischemic metabolites washed into the coronary sinus at the very end of pacing induced ischemia, because during ischemia the release of lactic acid from a few small areas with reduced perfusion is diluted by the large amount of blood coming from normally perfused myocardium. By contrast, at the end of pacing, the return of flow to ischemic foci can drain the high concentration of ischemic products accumulated during ischemia (25). A very positive dipyridamole or myocardial stress test, without wall motion abnormalities are also convincing clinical diagnostic evidence

with transient ischemia and angina, whereas others without or with angiographically detectable plaques may have variant or microvascular angina.

Diagnosis of Chronic Stable Angina

The effort test can document objectively not only the development of ischemia but also the level of residual coronary flow reserve and effort tolerance. Other provocative tests fail to indicate the level of residual coronary flow reserve and effort tolerance which have major therapeutic and prognostic implications. Conversely, the location, extension, and severity of ischemia can be best documented by perfusion imaging or by the assessment of regional myocardial dysfunction, (which provides also critical prognostic information on preexisting baseline contractile impairment.

For patients with mixed angina and a positive stress test at a low workload, the repetition of the test following acute nitrates could reveal the contribution of dynamic stenoses, by producing a dramatic improvement of effort tolerance. The sensitivity and specificity of ischemic ECG changes during stress test are usually assessed versus the presence or absence of flow-limiting stenoses (in the absence of a gold standard of ischemia and they are largely influenced by the pre-test probability of disease). This form of assessment only applies for effort-induced angina which, by definition, is caused by a flow-limiting coronary stenosis, but it does not apply for variant angina (although occasionally coronary spasm can be induced also by stress tests) nor for microvascular angina. A negative maximal stress test indicates the absence of a critical coronary flow-limiting stenosis, but does not rule out variant angina, microvascular angina, mixed angina with a major vasoconstrictor component, or the presence of subcritical stenoses.

Among possible differential diagnoses of effort-induced angina are severe aortic stenosis, severe pulmonary hypertension, and hypertrophic cardiomyopathy as all of them may cause a stable pattern of effort angina. Finally severe anemia may reduce sufficiently the coronary flow reserve, particularly in the presence of moderate stenoses, and reduce the anginal threshold, because of increased heart work and myocardial demand associated with a reduced blood oxygen carrying capacity.

Coronary arteriography provides the demonstration of: (i) the location and severity of the chronic, flow-limiting stenosis, (fixed or dynamic according to the presence or absence of dilatation following intracoronary nitrates), responsible for the reduction of coronary flow reserve, and the indication for appropriate revascularization procedures; (ii) the match between the site of the stenosis and the ischemic area. Slow progression of contrast during arteriography in the absence of flow-limiting stenosis has been reported in stable and unstable patients as an indication of microvascular constriction (26).

Diagnosis of Microvascular Angina

The diagnosis of microvascular angina, suggested by the pattern of symptoms described above can be obtained by the demonstration of a positive ECG exercise test, of a positive myocardial scintigraphy or by a positive dipyridamole test, without detectable transient left ventricular dysfunction. The coronary arteries appear, by definition, free from flow-limiting coronary stenoses (because the detection of coronary stenoses would provide by itself, a plausible, generally accepted, explanation for anginal episodes). However, given the high prevalence of coronary stenoses in the general elderly population, in the presence of typical symptoms, the possible coexistence of stenoses and microvascular angina should not be excluded (and could be subsequently revealed by the persistence of symptoms following successful removal of the stenosis). Noncardiac causes to be considered are those indicated earlier in the chapter for chronic stable angina with the addition for patients who also report prolonged episodes at rest, of musculoskeletal causes, esophageal stimuli (reflux, spasm, esophagitis), and psychological disturbances.

Thus clinical symptoms play a key diagnostic role. A clearly positive dipyridamole test with the development of ST segment depression and pain without transient left ventricular contraction abnormalities, appears the most practical objective evidence. The final proof is the detection of ischemic metabolites, washed out from the ischemic zone (in which they accumulated because of the reduced flow) into the coronary sinus at the very end of pacing-induced chest pain and ST segment depression (27). They may not be detectable during pacing because of the focal nature of ischemia and of their dilution with blood coming from non-ischemic areas that are in the majority.

Diagnosis of Unstable Angina

The notion of instability is a clinical one related to the medical history and the pattern of symptoms described by the patients. With this clinical suspicion the prompt recording of a 12 lead ECG during pain or discomfort is the first diagnostic step for patients with recent onset or recent worsening of episodes of chest pain, lasting 10–20 min, recurring at rest, together with measurements of biomarkers of myocardial injury indicative of very prolonged episodes of severe ischemia. Coronary arteriography may reveal complex thrombotic lesions, but it may also be normal when caused by thrombus or spasm no longer present at the time of angiography by intense microvascular constriction. Patients with acute chest pain and hemodynamic instability, syncope or near-syncope should be immediately referred to an emergency department where diagnosis and differential diagnoses can be established.

Diagnosis of Variant Angina

In patients presenting with a typical history, the first diagnostic test is the recording of a 12 lead ECG during an episode of pain or a continuous monitoring of three or more ECG leads in those patients reporting frequent episodes of pain. Transient diagnostic elevation of the ST segment confirms the diagnosis. The ECG recorded soon after prolonged episodes may show inverted T waves, gradually returning to normal over periods of hours.

Spontaneous coronary artery spasm may be observed during coronary arteriography (before injection of nitrates) or induced by provocative tests: ergonovine (the most specific), hyperventilation or acetylcholine (the most sensitive) and relieved by intracoronary nitrates. Differential diagnosis of recurring episodes of pain at rest are esophageal reflux and/spasm (usually of longer duration and relieved by antiacid drugs), but transient ST elevation and a prompt response to acute nitrates suggests variant angina. At the very onset of symptoms, variant angina cannot be distinguished from unstable angina, unless associated with syncope (which suggests arrhythmias induced by sudden occlusive spasm (22)) or with short recurring episodes of recurring ST segment elevation. This suspicion has relevant practical consequences, as variant angina would require urgent treatment with intravenous nitrates and with high doses of calcium antagonist drugs, rather than with percutaneous coronary intervention.

Coronary angiography typically shows a subcritical stenosis in the branch perfusing the ischemic region which is the site of the spastic occlusion. However, the stenosis may also be critical and alternatively no stenosis may be detectable. Spasm may occur spontaneously (before the injection of nitrates) or following a provocative test.

Determinants of Prognosis

Prognosis and its determinants vary in the various anginal syndromes.

- *In patients with chronic stable angina,* the major determinants of prognosis are: (*i*) a history of previous coronary disease; (*ii*) the number of stenosed coronary arteries; (*iii*) the extent of baseline left ventricular dysfunction; (*iv*) the area of myocardium at risk; (*v*) the effort tolerance (The CASS registry showed that patients with three vessel coronary disease who could perform stage 5 of the BRUCE protocol, treated medically had no mortality at 4 years irrespectively of the positivity of the test (28)).

It should be considered that the number of stenosed coronary arteries is closely correlated with the extension of coronary atherosclerosis, thus removal of stenoses cannot correct completely the atherosclerotic risk. In prognostic studies and in registries, patients with previous infarction and left ventricular dysfunction should not be lumped together with those without previous history of infarction.

- *In patients with unstable angina,* the major determinants of prognosis are the same as for those with chronic stable angina with the addition of the severity, duration, and waxing nature of acute chest pain and its objective counterpart of severe prolonged ischemic episodes indicated by ECG changes and by hemodynamic evidence of acute left ventricular failure, or hypotension and/or by the elevation of indices of myocardial necrosis.

- *In patients with variant angina,* prognosis is on average better in those without coronary stenoses but infarction, and sudden death is not uncommon also in patients with angiographically normal coronaries and the major determinant is a history of syncope, which indicates the propensity for occlusive spasm-related arrhythmias, and may require the implantation of a protective device.

- *In patients with microvascular angina,* prognosis is normal in spite of the severity of symptoms (12,13). Uncertainties exist because in many studies these patients are inappropriately lumped together with those presenting with variant angina and angiographically normal coronaries, who, as stated above, may develop fatal arrhythmias and infarction, or with those that have prolonged episodes of microvascular constriction, clinically indistinguishable from unstable angina (13).

Recurrences of Angina in Patients with Previous Coronary Revascularization or Angiography with No Flow Limiting Coronary Stenoses

In patients with previous successful revascularization, the immediate suspicion suggested by the recurrence of angina is coronary stent restenosis. However, in order to limit costs and risks, the first diagnostic step should not be a new arteriography! Indeed, a rational approach requires the demonstration of ischemia by exercise stress testing and/or other tests and whether the location of ischemia corresponds to the wall perfused by the previously dilated artery or to a different segment, thus suggesting a new critical stenosis. A careful clinical history may provide basic clues for the selection of the test that could demonstrate the underlying mechanisms of ischemia, as indicated above.

In patients presenting with recurrence of angina in spite of a previous demonstration of a "normal" coronary angiogram, the first diagnostic step should not be a new arteriography in search for a newly formed stenosis, for the reasons outlined above, but the documentation of myocardial ischemia and of its causes, beginning with a careful history, and with the diagnostic strategies indicated above.

In a 3–4-year median period of follow-up of patients submitted to coronary percutaneous intervention for an acute coronary syndrome in optimal medical treatment (29), the incidence of new combined coronary events was 20%, a low figure considering that about 50% were revascularizations or progressive angina, and that only a small percentage were fatal or non fatal infarction. Of these, nearly 50% could be attributed to the progression of a mild, non culprit lesion and nearly 50% to restenoses of the culprit lesion originally treated; in 2.7% it was not possible to determine a cause. In about one half of the patients the recurrent event was progressive angina associated with moderate progression of a non culprit stenosis. Out of 595 thin-cap fibroatheromas, identified by radiofrequency intravascular ultrasonography, only 25 (4.5%) were sites of recurring events at a median follow-up at 3.4 years. The predictive value of other plaque features was similarly low. Even among plaques that had a luminal area <4 mm^2, a total plaque burden >70% and a thin-cap fibroatheroma, 78.8% were not associated with an adverse event. Thus, more specific diagnostic targets and detection techniques should be developed to increase the predictive power of coronary arteriography. Until then the efforts should be concentrated on curing the varied mechanisms of angina and on correction of risk factors rather than on the identification of plaques thought to be "at risk," particularly considering the fact that about 70% of infarct-related arteries have only minimal or mild stenoses, thus suggesting a limited beneficial value of quantifying and treating flow-limiting stenoses. At the other extreme, patients without coronary stenoses should not be dismissed as having "non anginal pain" because they may have variant or microvascular angina.

MANAGEMENT AND RISK STRATIFICATION OF ACUTE CHEST PAIN IN THE EMERGENCY DEPARTMENT

Among patients presenting with acute chest pain in emergency departments, about 20% are found to have unstable angina or MI. A small percentage of these patients have other cardiovascular or non-cardiovascular conditions (such as acute aortic dissection, pulmonary embolism, pericarditis, pneumothorax, musculoskeletal pain, or reflux esophagitis). However, most patients are discharged without a diagnosis or with a diagnosis of a non cardiac condition. Some of these might have had an ischemic chest pain as transient ischemia may leave no trace, when of short duration. Conversely, a prolonged episode of pain with negative troponin test in a six-hour sample, rules out a cardiac ischemic origin.

The probability of an ischemic origin of chest pain is greatly increased by a previous history of coronary disease, particularly if the pain is similar to that experienced during previous documented ischemic events. It should be noted that, together with chest pain, also indigestion or heart burn, nausea and vomiting, shortness of breath, and dizziness might be related to a myocardial ischemic cause. The prompt recording of a 12 lead ECG during pain or symptoms is mandatory and continuous ECG monitoring is indicated in patients with recurrent chest pain, but asymptomatic at the time of observation with a normal or unchanged baseline ECG tracing. Serum markers of myocardial necrosis should be promptly obtained and repeated after 6 hours, according to the guidelines (30).

Simultaneously with the effort to document the diagnosis of unstable angina or of acute MI, the attending physician should address the following issues:

- Does the patient have an immediately life-threatening condition, such as aortic dissection, acute pulmonary embolism, or acute left ventricular failure? A careful history (the sudden onset of chest pain suggests aortic dissection) and physical examination are essential components of the initial assessment as they are the major determinants of immediate risk and guide prompt management.

- Is the patient stable with a low risk of life-threatening conditions, so that it is safe to follow the triage options indicated by the guidelines for discharge? For all cases, the guidelines for management of patients in the emergency setting should be followed because they provide general indications, based on statistical evidence of the "average" risk and therapeutic responses. Guidelines, however, must be adapted to the individual patient, considering clinical history, age, comorbidities, and general health state according to common sense and experience.

CONCLUSIONS

This chapter is not intended to indicate "one size fit all" strategies, supported by documented average risk and therapeutic response of widely heterogeneous groups of patients, but should stimulate the treatment of patients rather than that of the disease. It is intended for readers interested in personalized patient management, beyond current baseline protocols and guidelines. It provides a rational basis for understanding the multiple features of anginal pain as a potential warning symptom of acute myocardial ischemia and of its distinct multiple pathogenetic mechanisms.

It emphasizes the importance of a careful medical history for identifying distinctive patterns of recurrence of pain, which provide clues of their underlying mechanisms of myocardial ischemia.

Indeed, it should be stressed once more that angina is a broad clinical syndrome, just like anemia, which may be caused by different mechanisms of myocardial ischemia requiring specific diagnostic tests and management and having a different prognosis (1). Thus broad, widely used classification should be applied only to a specific type of patients (for example, Canadian classification is meaningful only for patients with fixed threshold effort angina).

Yet the diagnosis of "stable" or "unstable" angina or simply of "angina" is often used as a single descriptor to define broad common diagnostic and therapeutic strategies, largely based on coronary arteriographic evidence of severity and extent of atherosclerosis and on the average result of tests, registries, and trials. Thus, chest pain non associated with coronary stenoses is often considered of non cardiac origin or patients with "angina" and normal coronary arteries are lumped together without a distinction between "variant angina," which carries a risk of infarction and sudden death, and "microvascular angina" which does not carry appreciable risk of major cardiac events. Even the etiology of variant angina and epicardial coronary artery constriction are likely to be multiple (31).

The widespread "one size fits all" approach is the result of: (i) the physician inclination to have clear cut diagnostic categories, based on easily obtainable descriptors; (ii) the faster and faster pace imposed on the medical profession, with waiting lists getting longer and longer and time to ask questions and to listen to patients getting shorter and shorter. Thus the clinical evaluation of patients is replaced, rather than complemented, by tests.

A return to paying due attention to distinctive features of presentation reported by patients, rather than adopting broad common descriptors, is also useful in order to focus research on the specific pathophysiology of the varied mechanisms of ischemia suggested by distinctive features observed in "special" patients groups, which should then become the basis of personalized patient care. The importance of "anecdotal" cases was recently re-evaluated (32).

REFERENCES

1. Maseri A. Ischemic Heart Disease - A rational basis for clinical practice and clinical research. Churchill Livingston, Inc, 1995. New York, Edinburgh, London, Melbourne, Tokyo.
2. Maseri A, Chierchia S, Davies G, et al. Mechanisms of ischemic cardiac pain and silent myocardial ischemia. Am J Med 1985; 79: 7.
3. Burges PR, Perl ER. Cutaneous mechanoreceptors and nociceptors. In: Iggo A, ed. Handbook of Sensory Physiology, Somatosensory System. Vol 2 Berlin: Springer-Verlag, 1973: 29.
4. Crea F, Gaspardone A, Kaski KC, Davies G, Maseri A. Relationship between stimulation site of cardiac afferent nerves by adenosine and location of cardiac pain: results of a study in patients with stable angina. J Am Coll Cardiol 1992; 20: 1498.
5. Pasceri V, Cianflone D, Finocchiaro ML, Crea F, Maseri A. Relation between myocardial infarction site and pain location in Q-wave acute myocardial infarction. Am J Cardiol 1995; 75: 224–7.
6. Maseri A, Chierchia S, Kaski JC. Mixed angina pectoris. Am J Cardiol 1985; 56: 30E.
7. Lanza GA, Manzoli A, Bia E, Crea F, Maseri A. Cute effects of nitrates on exercise testing in patients with syndrome X. Clinical and pathophysiological implications. Circulation 1994; 90: 2695–700.
8. Picano E, Lattanzi F, Masini M, Distante A, L'Abbate A. Usefulness of a high-dose dipyridamole-echocardiolgraphy test for diagnosis of syndrome X. Am J Cardiol 1987; 60: 508.
9. Maseri A, Crea F, Kaski JC, Crake T. Mechanisms of angina pectoris in syndrome X. J Am Coll Cardiol 1991; 17: 499.
10. Turiel M, Galassi AR, Glazier JJ, et al. Pain threshold and tlereance in women with syndrome X and women with stable angina pectoris. Am J Cardiol 1987; 60: 503.
11. Cannon RO, Quyyumi AA, Schenke WH, et al. Abnormal cardiac sensitivitu in patients with chest pain and normal coronary arteries. J Am Coll Cardiol 1990; 16: 1359.
12. Camici PG, Crea F. Coronary microvascular dysfunction. N Engl J Med 2007; 356: 830–40.
13. Lanza GA, Crea F. Primary coronary microvascular dysfunction: clinical presentation, pathophysiology, and management. Circulation 2010; 121: 2317–25.
14. Galiuto L, De Caterina AR, Porfidia A, et al. Reversible coronary microvascular dysfunction: a common pathogenetic mechanism in apical ballooning or tako-tsubo syndrome. Eur Heart J 2010; 31: 1319–27.
15. Maseri A, Fuster V. Is there a vulnerable plaque? Circulation 2003; 107: 2068–71.
16. Cristell N, Cianflone D, Durante A, et al.; Attilio Maseri FAMI Study Investigators. High-sensitivity C-reactive protein is within normal levels at the very onset of first ST-segment elevation acute myocardial infarction in 41% of cases: a multiethnic case-control study. J Am Coll Cardiol 2011; 58: 2654–61.
17. Prinzmetal M, Kennamer R, Merliss R, Wade T, Bor N. Angina pectoris. I. The variant form of angina pectoris. Am J Med 1959; 27: 375.
18. Cheng TO, Bashour T, Kelser GA, Weiss L, Bacos J. Variant angina of Prinzmetal with normal coronary arteriograms: a variant of the variant. Circulation 1973; 47: 476–85.
19. Maseri A, Severi S, De Nes DM, et al. "Variant" angina: one aspect of a continuous spectrum of vasospastic myocardial ischemia. Am J Cardiol 1978; 42: 1019.
20. Specchia G, De servi S, Falcone C, et al. Coronary arterial spasm as a cause of exercise-induces St-segment elevation in patients with variant angina. Circulation 1979; 59: 948.
21. Maseri A, Beltrame JF, Shimokawa H. Role of coronary vasoconstriction in ischemic heart disease and search for novel therapeutic targets. Circ J 2009; 73: 394–403.
22. Maseri A, Severi S, Marzullo P. Role of coronary arterial spasm in sudden coronary ischemic death. Ann NY Acad Sci 1982; 382: 204.
23. Lefroy DC, Crake T, Haider AW, Maseri A. Medical treatment of refractory coronary artery spasm. Cor Art Dis 1992; 3: 745.
24. Bugiardini R, Pozzati A, Ottani F, Morgangi GL, Puddu P. Vasotonic angina: a spectrum of ischemic syndromes involving functional abnormalities of the epicardial and microvascular coronary circulation. J Am Coll Cardiol 1993; 22: 417.
25. Mohri M, Kooyanagi M, Egashira K, et al. Angina pecroris caused by coronary microvascular spasm. Lancet 1998; 351: 1165–9.
26. Beltrame JF, Limaye SB, Wuttke RD, Horowitz JD. Coronary hemodynamic and metabolic studies of the coronary slow flow phenomenon. Am Heart J 2003; 146: 84–90.
27. Buffon A, Rigattieri S, Santini SA, et al. Myocardial ischemia-reperfusion damage after pacing-induced tachycardia in patients with cardiac Syndrome X. Am J Physiol Heart Circ Physiol 2000; 279: 2627–33.
28. Weiner Da, Ryan TJ, McCabe CH, et al. Prognostic importance of a clinical profile and exercise test in medically treated patients with coronary artery disease. J Am Coll Cardiol. 1984; 3: 772.
29. Stone GW, Maehara A, Lansky AJ, PROSPECT Investigators. A prospective natural-history study of coronary atherosclerosis. N Engl J Med 2011; 364: 226–35.
30. Anderson JL, Adams CD, Antman EM, et al. ACC/AHA 2007 guidelines for the management of patients with unstable angina/non-ST-elevation myocardial infarction: a report of the American College of Cardiology/American heart Association Task force on Practice Guidelines (Writing Committee to Revise the 2002 Guidelines for the Management of Patients With Unstable Angina/Non-ST-Elevation Myocardial Infarction) developed in collaboration with the American College of Emergency Physicians, the Society for Cardiovascular Angiography and Interventions, and the Society of Thoracic Surgeons endorsed by the American Association of Cardiovascular and Pulmonary Rehabilitation and the Society for Academic Emergency Medicine. J Am Coll Cardiol. 2007; 50: e1.
31. Maseri A, Davies G, Hackett D, Kaski JC. Coronary artery spasm and vasoconstriction. The case for a distinction. Circulation 1990; 81: 1983–91.
32. Stuebe AM, Level IV. Evidence–adverse anecdote and clinical practice. N Engl J Med 2011; 365: 8–9.

7

Exercise stress testing, stress echocardiography, and scintigraphy: Which tool for which patient?

Arend F.L. Schinkel and Manolis Bountioukos

OUTLINE

Exercise stress testing, stress echocardiography (SE), and myocardial perfusion scintigraphy are frequently used for the evaluation for patients with known or suspected ischemic heart disease (1). First, these techniques provide important information that is invaluable for the diagnosis of coronary artery disease (CAD). Second, they are useful in evaluating the effect of therapy in patients with CAD. Finally, stress testing provides important prognostic information that can be used to identify low-risk and high-risk patient subsets and guide clinical management (2). This chapter describes pathophysiological aspects of CAD that can be probed with stress testing. The methodology and the practical aspects of exercise stress testing, SE, and myocardial perfusion scintigraphy are described. The diagnostic accuracy of the various stress testing modalities for evaluation of CAD is discussed. The prognostic value and risk stratification are addressed. Subsequently, the advantages and limitations of the various stress testing modalities are discussed and a scheme for appropriate clinical application of these modalities is proposed.

ELECTROCARDIOGRAPHIC STRESS TESTING

Despite the development of new and more sophisticated methods, electrocardiographic (ECG) stress testing remains the baseline tool for the detection of myocardial ischemia and for assessing prognosis in patients with known or suspected CAD.

Methodology

The two most common techniques of ECG stress testing are either graded exercise on a treadmill or bicycle (supine or upright) ergometer. The electrical treadmill is the preferred modality in North America and several protocols have been developed for standardization of this procedure (Bruce, Naughton, Cornell, etc.). Bicycle ergometry is mainly used in European countries. For individuals not capable of using their lower extremities, arm ergometry is another option.

Physiology

The common element of all modalities and protocols for ECG stress testing is the gradual increase in patient's workload. The test end-points are either predefined (target heart rate or workload), or symptom-limited. Detection of ischemia with ECG stress testing is based upon the impact of exercise on heart rate, blood pressure, and contractility and the subsequent mismatch between myocardial oxygen supply and demand when one or more epicardial coronary arteries are significantly narrowed.

ECG abnormalities and angina on exercise are the end manifestations of the cascade of intracellular events that lead to myocardial ischemia (Fig. 7.1) (3). The magnitude, extent, and time of appearance of these manifestations are indicative of the severity of CAD. However, the relatively late appearance of ECG abnormalities and angina is in itself one of the major limitations of ECG stress testing, because a significant number of patients fail to exercise to the point where these events will be manifest.

Wilson et al. demonstrated that ECG stress testing outcomes depend on coronary flow reserve, which in turn does not correlate well with the angiographically documented severity of coronary artery lesions (4). Therefore, ECG stress testing has the advantage of assessing the physiological significance of an atherosclerotic plaque, which is clinically more important than the angiographic classification of a lesion. Additionally, there is evidence that the sensitivity of exercise testing increases in multi-vessel disease but substantially decreases in single-vessel, especially when vessels other than the left anterior descending artery (LAD) are involved. However, a major pitfall is that exercise ECG testing cannot localize the extent or the site of ischemia, which is vital information, especially in patients with prior percutaneous coronary intervention (PCI) or coronary artery bypass grafting (CABG).

Diagnostic Value

Although several computer algorithms have been proposed to improve accuracy, their validity to date, has not been clearly proven. The diagnostic value of ECG stress testing depends mainly on the so called 'pretest probability' of CAD for a given patient. This can be obtained by simply taking a good clinical history, and derives from the assessment of: (*i*) demographics such as age and gender, (*ii*) conventional risk factors (diabetes, smoking, hypercholesterolemia, hypertension, family history of CAD), (*iii*) resting ECG abnormalities, and (*iv*) the nature of symptoms.

ECG stress testing has the best diagnostic value in populations with an intermediate pretest probability of CAD. Patients with very low or very high pretest probability of CAD are usually excluded because a positive or negative result respectively does not alter significantly the pretest probability of CAD and has little impact on clinical decision making (5). In general, asymptomatic individuals have a low pre-test probability of significant CAD and routine ECG stress testing is not recommended. On the other hand, patients with typical angina (especially men older than 40 years and women older than 60 years) have a high pretest probability of CAD and should be referred directly for assessment of coronary anatomy. Before a patient is

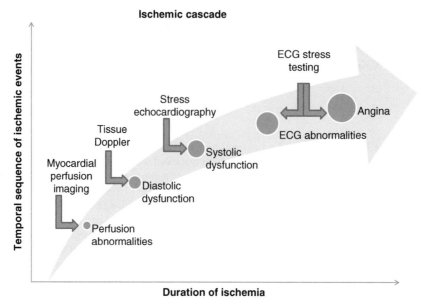

Figure 7.1 The ischemic cascade representing a sequence of pathophysiological events caused by coronary artery disease. Myocardial perfusion imaging probes an earlier event in the ischemic cascade compared with echocardiography. Exercise testing probes late events in the ischemic cascade.

referred for ECG stress testing, the low specificity in specific subgroups such as females, patients with marked resting ST-T abnormalities, and patients taking digitalis should be taken into account. In addition, ECG stress testing, where the indication is the detection of ischemia, is of no value in patients with left bundle branch block (LBBB) or ventricular-paced rhythm.

There is wide variability of reported diagnostic accuracy in literature. In an extensive meta-analysis, which compared exercise-induced ST-depression with coronary angiography, 147 consecutively published reports involving 24074 patients were included (6). This meta-analysis found a mean sensitivity of 68% (range 23–100%; SD 16%) and a mean specificity of 77% (range 17–100%; SD 17%). Obviously, patient characteristics, methodology, and definition of an abnormal ECG response were important factors that affected diagnostic accuracy in these reports.

Prognostic Value
The basic features that assess adverse prognosis of CAD are baseline poor left ventricular (LV) function and an extensive amount of jeopardized myocardium. Patients with such characteristics may benefit from coronary angiography and subsequent coronary intervention. Several clinical and ECG variables during exercise have been shown to indicate adverse prognosis; angina, especially at a low workload, poor exercise capacity, chronotropic incompetence, and abnormal blood pressure response during exercise and recovery are the most established clinical predictors. On the other hand, ST segment depression ≥1 mm, ST segment elevation in leads not corresponding to myocardial scar, multiple-lead involvement, ventricular tachycardia, and early onset or late recovery of ST changes are the most commonly used ECG predictors.

In patients with known CAD, ESC guidelines on the management of stable angina pectoris published in 2006 recommend ECG stress testing for risk stratification as an initial evaluation (Class I, level of evidence B), or after a significant change in symptom level has occurred (Class I, level of evidence C) for patients with stable angina who can exercise and who have no resting ECG abnormalities (2). It is also recommended in post-revascularization patients with a significant deterioration in symptomatic status (Class II, level of evidence B). These recommendations are summarized in Table 7.1.

The latest ESC/EACTS guidelines on myocardial revascularization (7) state that symptom-limited ECG stress testing can be safely performed 7–14 days after primary PCI for ST elevation myocardial infarction (STEMI) and as soon as 24 h after elective PCI for functional evaluation and exercise training prescription. However, based on the same guidelines, stress imaging should be preferably used instead of ECG stress testing for follow-up and management in symptomatic and asymptomatic patients after myocardial revascularization (Class IA).

After an episode of atypical chest pain, ECG stress testing can be useful before hospital discharge in patients with a non-diagnostic ECG, no signs of heart failure, and normal biomarkers. A normal early exercise testing has a high negative prognostic value (8).

Following ST-segment elevation acute myocardial infarction (MI), the role of ECG stress testing for risk assessment has decreased in recent years, due to the increasing use of primary PCI. Thus, risk assessment before discharge has become less vital. If, in spite of angiography and PCI in the infarct-related

Table 7.1 Recommendations for Selection of Stress Test Modality

	ECG stress testing	Exercise stress echocardiography	Exercise stress SPECT	Pharmacological stress echocardiography	Pharmacological stress SPECT
Patients with known or suspected CAD undergoing initial evaluation, or patients with significant change in clinical status, who are able to exercise and who have intermediate-to-high pretest probability of CAD	Class I[a]	Class IIa	Class IIa	Class IIa[b]	Class IIa[b]
Post-revascularization patients with a significant deterioration in symptomatic status	Class IIa[a]	Class IIa	Class IIa	Class IIa	Class IIa
Patients with pre-excitation syndrome, electronically paced ventricular rhythm, ≥1 mm resting ST depression, >120 ms QRS duration, which prevent accurate interpretation of ECG changes during stress	-	Class I	Class I	Class I	Class I
Patients with a non-conclusive exercise ECG who do not have a high probability of significant coronary disease and in whom the diagnosis is still in doubt	-	Class I	Class I	Class I[b]	Class I[b]
To assess functional severity of intermediate lesions on coronary angiography		Class IIa	Class IIa	Class IIa[b]	Class IIa[b]
Patients with prior revascularization (PCI or CABG) in whom localization of ischemia is important	-	Class IIa	Class IIa	Class IIa[b]	Class IIa[b]
To localize ischemia when planning revascularization options in patients who have already had coronary angiography	-	Class IIa	Class IIa	Class IIa[b]	Class IIa[b]
Patients who cannot exercise	-	-	-	Class I	Class I

Abbreviations: CABG, coronary artery bypass grafting; CAD, coronary artery disease; ECG, electrocardiogram; PCI, percutaneous coronary intervention; SPECT, single-photon emission computed tomography. Recommendations are based on Ref. 2.
[a]Patients with pre-excitation syndrome, electronically paced ventricular rhythm, ≥1 mm resting ST depression, or >120 ms QRS duration are excluded.
[b]Where local facilities do not include exercise imaging.

Focus Box 7.1

- Electrocardiography (ECG) stress testing remains the baseline tool for evaluation of coronary artery disease
- The inability to perform exercise testing is associated with an adverse prognosis
- Pretest probability of coronary artery disease is essential when interpreting an ECG stress test
- ECG stress testing provides no/limited information on the localization and extent of myocardial ischemia
- The test's sensitivity increases in multi-vessel disease, whereas it substantially decreases in single-vessel, especially non-left anterior descending artery, coronary artery disease

artery, there are concerns about inducible ischemia in the infarct or non-infarct-related area, pre-discharge or outpatient ECG stress testing within 4–6 weeks is appropriate.

As has been already mentioned, routine use of ECG stress testing in an asymptomatic population is not validated, because there are no strong data to suggest cost-effectiveness or a mortality benefit. A possible exception is asymptomatic patients at moderate or high risk of CAD who may be considered for stress testing in specific situations, such as those who work in high-risk

occupations (9). Similarly, abnormal ECG stress testing has been found to predict increased cardiovascular risk in asymptomatic individuals, especially when multiple risk factors for CAD are present (10). This kind of patients could possibly benefit from aggressive modification of risk factors. Finally, ACC/AHA guidelines for exercise testing state that it is appropriate in asymptomatic patients with diabetes who plan to start vigorous exercise (Class IIa, level of evidence: C) (11).

STRESS ECHOCARDIOGRAPHY

Echocardiography in conjunction with stress is a feasible and patient-friendly modality that has gained wide acceptance among cardiologists during the last three decades. SE is primarily used to evaluate non-invasively the presence, extent, and distribution of myocardial ischemia, as well as viability of myocardium that is dysfunctional at rest (1,2). In specific situations, Doppler echocardiography during stress helps to determine the true severity of valvular lesions and the magnitude of pulmonary artery pressure.

Methodology

As is the case with all non-invasive imaging modalities, SE is based on a gradual increase in cardiac workload. Physical exercise, compared with pharmacological stimulation, is the preferable stressor because it: (*i*) exerts a more physiological effect on blood pressure and heart rate, (*ii*) enables evaluation of patient's exercise capacity and tolerance, which are important prognostic elements of stress testing, and (*iii*) potential side effects of drug infusions are avoided. Exercise on treadmill has the advantage of an efficient increase in heart rate. However, echo images need to be acquired shortly after stress termination, thus reducing test sensitivity (increased rate of false-negative results). On the other hand, supine or upright bicycle ergometry has the advantage of enabling continuous evaluation of cardiac function during stress although the chronotropic response is not always as effective as during treadmill exercise.

Pharmacological stress is an alternative for patients who cannot exercise due to physical handicaps or temporary mobility problems. Moreover, it is the first-choice modality when the assessment of myocardial viability is the main goal. The most commonly used pharmacological agents are dobutamine and the vasodilator drugs adenosine and dipyridamole. Dobutamine is a synthetic adrenergic agonist that exerts a positive inotropic and chronotropic effect on myocardium, thus increasing myocardial oxygen demands. Adenosine produces marked coronary arteriolar vasodilation with less marked dilatation of the peripheral arterioles. Dipyridamole prevents the cellular uptake of endogenous adenosine, thereby potentiating its vasodilator effect. Standard protocols for dobutamine and dipyridamole infusion are illustrated in Figures 7.2 and 7.3. Both dobutamine and vasodilators are generally well-tolerated. Pacing either by intravenous pacemaker or by transesophageal pacing of the atrium can be used as an alternative to physical and pharmacological stressors.

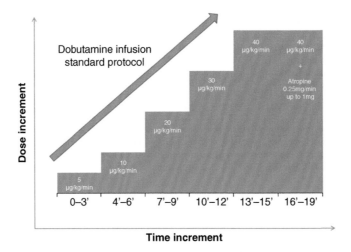

Figure 7.2 Diagram showing a commonly used protocol for pharmacological stress testing using dobutamine that can be used in conjunction with stress echocardiography or myocardial perfusion imaging.

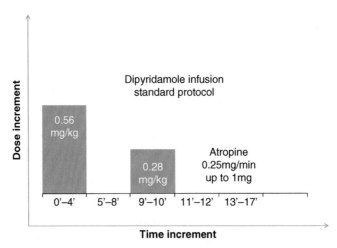

Figure 7.3 Diagram showing a commonly used protocol for pharmacological stress testing using dipyridamole that can be used in conjunction with stress echocardiography or myocardial perfusion imaging.

Tissue harmonic imaging, which is available as a standard equipment on most echocardiographic systems, offers significant improvement in test sensitivity and interobserver variability (12). Intravenous contrast agents can be used to improve endocardial border delineation and image quality if two or more segments are not well visualized (13).

The possible responses of myocardium at stress are shown in Figure 7.4. Location, magnitude and time of appearance of regional dysfunction are the main features that help to assess the anatomy, extent, and severity of coronary artery lesion(s). Interpretation is performed offline by visual inspection of myocardial thickening and endocardial excursion, with the help of dedicated software that enables direct comparison of synchronized cine-loops in quadruple format. The myocardium is divided into sixteen or seventeen segments (14) and every segment is graded from 1 to 4 for normal/hyperkinetic, hypokinetic, akinetic, and dyskinetic, respectively. Assessment of global LV shape, size, and function at rest and during stress gives additional information.

The wall motion score index derives from the division of the total score of myocardial segments by the number of segments scored. It is a semi-quantitative index that depends heavily on the skill and experience of the observer. Several approaches have been proposed in an attempt to quantify segmental myocardial performance and to narrow inter- and intraobserver variability: Automated endocardial border detection, tissue Doppler imaging that enables evaluation of myocardial displacement, and myocardial strain and strain rate that reflect segmental myocardial deformation. These techniques have been shown to be more sensitive than visual analysis alone.

Nevertheless, due to several limitations, none of them has gained widespread acceptance in everyday clinical practice.

Future Approaches to Stress Echocardiography

Real time 3D echocardiography has emerged as a promising modality to improve the already high accuracy of SE. The evolution of matrix-array transducers allows instantaneous on-line volume-rendered reconstruction and visualization of multiple 2D views, thus decreasing acquisition time during stress and permitting direct comparison of segments that would not be seen on routine 2D views (15). Furthermore, progress in computer technology and contrast agent characteristics may eventually enable the simultaneous evaluation of both myocardial perfusion and contractility during stress without the need for ionizing radiation.

Diagnostic Value

As is the case for other competing imaging modalities, the diagnostic accuracy of SE depends on several factors: (*i*) the definition of 'significant' CAD, (the higher the degree of stenosis that defines a lesion as 'significant', the better the sensitivity); (*ii*) the extent of disease (lower sensitivity for one-vessel disease, compared with multi-vessel disease); and (*iii*) the adequacy of the stress level achieved (a suboptimal workload level decreases sensitivity).

SE, when compared with other non-invasive imaging modalities, has the highest specificity with comparable sensitivities for the detection of CAD. In several meta-analyses, sensitivity ranges from 80–85% and specificity from 77–84% (16,17). There is high variability in SE performance, depending on

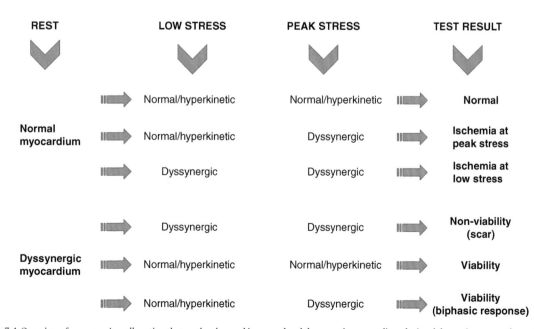

Figure 7.4 Overview of responses in wall motion that can be observed in normal and dyssynergic myocardium during dobutamine stress echocardiography.

stressors and protocols used, and on the local center's expertise. A meta-analytic comparison of different echocardiographic stressors that included studies published between 1981 and 2001 showed that transatrial pacing in conjunction with transthoracic or transesophageal echocardiography had the highest sensitivity and specificity. Among the other stressors, exercise provided the highest sensitivity, and dobutamine showed the best specificity (18). A meta-analysis of SE studies comparing dobutamine and dipyridamole revealed equal accuracies (19). However, LV concentric remodeling has been reported to remarkably reduce sensitivity of dobutamine SE (20). Finally, according to another meta-analysis in patients with LBBB, ECG stress testing and myocardial perfusion imaging were the most sensitive modalities to detect CAD (83.4% and 88.5%, respectively) in comparison with SE (74.6%), but SE had the best specificity (88.7%, vs. 60.1% and 41.2% for ECG stress testing and myocardial perfusion imaging, respectively) (21).

Prognostic Value

SE is a reliable modality for the risk stratification of patients with known or suspected CAD. A large number of studies have reported on the prognostic value of SE in various clinical settings. There is consensus that assessment of regional and global LV function during stress provides prognostic information that is incremental to that obtained with a combination of clinical variables, resting wall motion abnormalities and ECG abnormalities during stress.

Risk stratification with SE has been shown to help decision making in two important clinical settings: patients after an acute MI and patients undergoing major non-cardiac surgery. The prognosis of post-acute MI patients is adversely influenced by variables such as advanced age, poor LV function, and residual angina. The absence of viability in the infarct area and/or the presence of remote ischemia at stress are strongly predictive of future adverse outcome, independently of clinical or angiographic variables (22,23). SE is warranted for preoperative evaluation of patients with clinical predictors indicating high perioperative risk before major non-cardiac surgery. In this setting, dobutamine SE is preferred, because this kind of patients are usually unable to exercise. A positive test result with high-risk features (extensive ischemia or ischemia at low heart rates)

before vascular surgery classifies patients at high risk for perioperative and late cardiac events (24). Deferral of surgery, intensifying postponement, intensifying medical treatment and/or coronary revascularization is recommended preoperatively for these patients.

MYOCARDIAL PERFUSION IMAGING

Myocardial perfusion imaging using single-photon emission computed tomography (SPECT) is a commonly used myocardial stress test. SPECT can be used for the diagnosis, prognosis, and evaluation of myocardial function in patients with known or suspected CAD (25). Moreover, in patients with LV dysfunction due to chronic CAD, myocardial perfusion imaging can be used for the evaluation of myocardial viability. Exercise SPECT provides information on exercise test variables including workload, blood pressure response and symptoms, and information on myocardial perfusion and function. In patients who are not able to perform an exercise test, due to vascular, neurologic, or orthopedic disease, pharmacological stress testing can be performed in conjunction with SPECT.

ECG-gated myocardial SPECT acquisition has been a step forward in nuclear cardiology, and is now routinely used in most laboratories. Gated SPECT allows simultaneous assessment of myocardial perfusion and function, allowing automated quantitative assessment of wall motion and thickening, LV volumes and ejection fraction.

Methodology

Various exercise and pharmacological stress protocols can be used for myocardial perfusion imaging using SPECT. Preferably exercise stress is used, and pharmacological stress is a useful alternative in patients with limited exercise capacity. Typically image acquisition is performed after exercise and pharmacological stress and at rest. For many years, thallium-201 was the most commonly used radionuclide tracer for myocardial stress SPECT. The introduction of the technetium-99 m-labeled radionuclide tracers, sestamibi and tetrofosmin, have provided improved image quality, increased reliability of image analysis and a larger injectable dose due to a shorter half-life compared with thallium-201. Nowadays, most myocardial SPECT studies are performed using technetium-99-m-labeled radionuclide tracers. These radionuclides are distributed in the myocardium relative to myocardial blood flow. After intravenous administration of technetium-99-m-labeled radionuclide tracers, a relatively fast clearance from the blood and extracardiac structures occurs with minimal redistribution from the myocardial tissue. Regional variations in myocardial blood flow cause regional variations in radionuclide uptake and consequently perfusion defects at myocardial SPECT imaging. Various SPECT acquisition protocols have been developed. In the majority of these protocols, the radionuclide tracer is administered intravenously, shortly before or during peak stress and SPECT image acquisition is performed after 30–60 min. Generally for the resting study, a second dose of radionuclide tracer is administered at least 24 h after the stress study. Subsequently,

---

Focus Box 7.2

- Exercise or pharmacological stress echocardiography provides information on the presence, localization, and extent of myocardial ischemia
- In patients with ischemic left ventricular dysfunction low-dose dobutamine stress echocardiography can be performed to evaluate contractile reserve
- Interpretation of stress echocardiography is to some extent reader dependent; quantification of wall motion and thickening may further improve reproducibility in the near future

resting images are acquired. Before SPECT images can be interpreted, filtering and reconstruction is performed and attenuation correction can be applied.

SPECT image interpretation is usually performed semiquantitatively by visual analysis assisted by analysis of the circumferential profiles. Stress and rest tomographic images are reviewed side-by-side using a 17-segment model of the left ventricle. This model is used to correlate perfusion abnormalities, wall motion, and wall thickening to coronary territories, although a large natural variation in coronary anatomy exists. Interpretation of SPECT images includes the type of perfusion defect (fixed, reversible, or partially reversible), and the location, extent and severity of the perfusion defect. Regional and global left and right ventricular function is evaluated and lung uptake of the radionuclide tracer is assessed. Gated SPECT information is also used to recognize attenuation artifacts, which still are a major source of false-positive SPECT studies thereby improving the diagnostic accuracy.

Diagnostic Value

Myocardial perfusion SPECT has an established role in the diagnosis of patients with suspected CAD. A fixed perfusion defect usually corresponds to a previous (silent) MI, whereas a reversible perfusion defect usually corresponds to a flow-limiting stenosis in an epicardial coronary artery. Coronary angiography is the reference technique for evaluation of the epicardial coronary arteries. Multiple studies have assessed the diagnostic value of myocardial perfusion SPECT for assessment of CAD in comparison with coronary angiography. In a large study including 2560 patients, Kapur et al. (26) studied the diagnostic value of myocardial perfusion SPECT using 3 tracers and mostly using adenosine stress, and reported a sensitivity of 91% and a specificity of 87% in patients who underwent coronary angiography. An overview of literature including 62 studies demonstrated a sensitivity of 70–75% and specificity of 70–75% of exercise SPECT for the detection of CAD (27). Pharmacological stress SPECT demonstrated a sensitivity of 90% and specificity of 75–80% for dipyridamole and adenosine stress. Dobutamine stress SPECT demonstrated a sensitivity of 80–90% and a specificity ranging from 64% to 100%. When interpreting these studies, it is important to realize that coronary angiography is primarily used to asses anatomy and SPECT is primarily used to assess myocardial perfusion. Discrepancies between coronary anatomy and myocardial perfusion may occur for various reasons including endothelial function, microvessel function, and the presence of collateral circulation.

Prognostic Value

Myocardial perfusion SPECT provides powerful prognostic information and can be used for risk stratification of patients with known or suspected CAD. The presence and extent of fixed and reversible perfusion defects are important variables that have incremental prognostic value over clinical information and stress test data. Gated SPECT provides additional information including LV ejection fraction, post-stress LV ejection fraction, and post-stress ventricular dilatation which are independent predictors of outcome. Multiple studies have demonstrated that patients with a normal myocardial perfusion SPECT have a favorable prognosis. Event rates in patients with a normal SPECT study are comparable with event rates in the general population. Also, patients with known non-obstructive CAD, previous percutaneous or surgical revascularization, and normal myocardial perfusion SPECT have a good clinical outcome. A recent review of available literature including 13 studies and the total number of patients studied more than 19,000 demonstrated that the evidence for prognostic stratification of patients with known or suspected CAD is strong (28). The average follow-up of most studies ranged from 1 to 6 years. The studies consistently have demonstrated that clinical outcome after a normal SPECT is favorable and a significant relative risk is associated with an abnormal study.

Limitations

Myocardial stress imaging with SPECT has several limitations. Clearly radiation exposure related to SPECT limits the application in some patients. Attenuation artifacts may occur as a result of breast tissue or the left hemidiaphragm. Myocardial stress SPECT acquisition is not real-time, and may be disturbed by patient motion. The relatively long scanning times may limit utility for a few patients. The spatial resolution of SPECT images is limited, but in clinical practice this seems less relevant. Finally, gated SPECT acquisition can be disturbed by heart rhythm disturbances (particularly atrial fibrillation) and the presence of extensive and severe perfusion defects.

SUMMARY OF ADVANTAGES AND DISADVANTAGES OF STRESS MODALITIES

Comparison of Exercise Testing Modalities

ECG stress testing is a widely available, low-cost, and feasible modality that can be applied even in the environment of a medical office. The main limitations of ECG stress testing are the relatively low accuracy, and the inability to localize the site and extent of myocardial ischemia. Combination of exercise with imaging significantly improves accuracy, and offers additional information regarding not only the topography and

---

Focus Box 7.3

- Exercise or pharmacological stress myocardial perfusion single-photon emission computed tomography (SPECT) provides important information on the presence and extent of myocardial ischemia and previous infarction
- Electrocardiography-gated SPECT provides information on wall motion and thickening, left ventricular volumes, and ejection fraction
- Reproducibility of SPECT studies is high because visual evaluation is usually assisted by automated quantitative analysis

quantity of ischemic myocardium, but LV morphology and valvular function as well. However, compared with ECG stress testing, exercise imaging studies are more expensive and time-consuming, and, most importantly, there is a need for specialized personnel and technically advanced equipment. The strengths and weaknesses of the various stress testing modalities is presented in Table 7.2.

Comparison Between Exercise and Pharmacological Modalities

Only exercise stress testing permits the assessment of functional capacity and exercise tolerance, which are basic elements of prognostic evaluation. Pharmacological stressors are mainly used in patients who, for various reasons, cannot exercise. In addition, pharmacological stressors facilitate evaluation of myocardial viability, which is not always feasible with exercise imaging. Accuracy is higher with pharmacological stressors than with exercise stress, in case of patient characteristics that limit ST segment analysis, such as pacemaker rhythm, LBBB, LV hypertrophy or digoxin treatment. Pharmacological stressors are generally well-tolerated, but a number of side effects and contraindications may limit their use (see below).

Comparison of Pharmacological Stressors

Pharmacological stress is a useful alternative to exercise testing in patients who are unable to perform an exercise test for various reasons. The available data suggest that dobutamine SE may be more effective than vasodilator SE. Combined data from seven direct comparative studies have demonstrated that the sensitivity of dobutamine SE for diagnosis of CAD is higher as compared with vasodilator SE, whereas specificity of both stressors in conjunction with SE is similar (29). Myocardial perfusion SPECT is usually performed with exercise or vasodilator stress. Alternatively in patients who are unable to perform exercise testing and have contraindications for vasodilator stress, dobutamine stress can be performed.

In general, dobutamine side effects are easily reversed by beta-blocker infusion. Hypotension, dizziness, and non-sustained supraventricular or ventricular arrhythmias are the most common side effects of dobutamine, whereas life-threatening

arrhythmias are extremely rare, and occur predominantly in patients with poor LV function. Flushing, headache, and dyspnea are rarely reported with vasodilators and are rapidly reversed by intravenous administration of aminophylline. Vasodilators are contraindicated in patients with significant conduction defects or pulmonary obstructive disease.

Comparison Between Stress Echocardiography and Myocardial Perfusion Imaging

SE seems to have some advantages over myocardial SPECT. it is less time-consuming and ionizing-radiation free. Another basic advantage of SE is that it provides more extensive information on cardiac function and anatomy. On the other hand, myocardial perfusion imaging is a well-standardized, highly reproducible, and relatively reader-independent technique.

A systematic review of literature demonstrated that 17 direct comparative studies including a total of 1405 patients are available that have compared SE and myocardial perfusion imaging for the diagnosis of CAD in the same patients (Fig. 7.5) (1). Pooled analysis of these studies demonstrated a slightly higher sensitivity of myocardial perfusion imaging as compared with SE (84% vs. 80%, $p < 0.05$). SE had a higher specificity for the detection of CAD (86% vs. 77%, $p = 0.001$). These differences in diagnostic accuracy of these 2 imaging modalities can be partially explained by the ischemic cascade, because perfusion abnormalities occur earlier than systolic dysfunction (1).

Exercise Stress Testing, Stress Echocardiography, and Scintigraphy: Which Tool for Which Patient?

There are currently various effective modalities that can help CAD diagnosis and assessment of prognosis in patients with known or suspected CAD. Sometimes, more than one modality is suitable for a given patient. Furthermore, there is no standard method that perfectly fits in with all patients. A schematic algorithm for the selection of the appropriate test is presented in Figure 7.6. However, it must be emphasized that selection of the

Table 7.2 Diagnostic Accuracy and Cost of Exercise Stress Testing, Stress Echocardiography, and Scintigraphy for Evaluation of Coronary Artery Disease

	ECG stress testing	Stress echocardiography	SPECT
Diagnostic accuracy	+/−	++	++
Sensitivity	+/−	+	+++
Specificity	+/−	++	+
Cost	++	+	+/−

Abbreviations: ECG, electrocardiogram; SPECT, single-photon emission computed tomography.

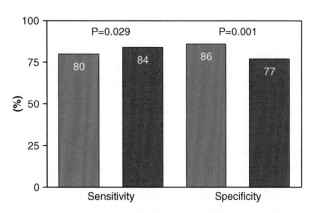

Figure 7.5 Diagnostic accuracy of stress echocardiography and myocardial perfusion imaging for the detection of coronary artery disease (blue = echocardiography, red = nuclear imaging). *Source*: Figure based on Ref. 1.

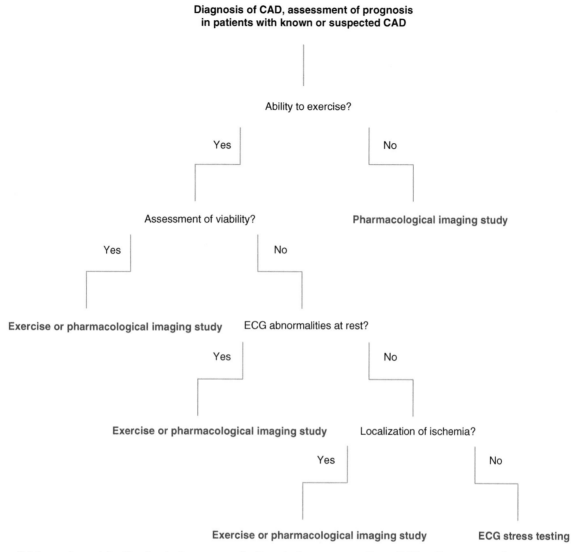

Diagnosis of CAD, assessment of prognosis in patients with known or suspected CAD

Ability to exercise?

Yes — No

Assessment of viability? — **Pharmacological imaging study**

Yes — No

Exercise or pharmacological imaging study — ECG abnormalities at rest?

Yes — No

Exercise or pharmacological imaging study — Localization of ischemia?

Yes — No

Exercise or pharmacological imaging study — **ECG stress testing**

Figure 7.6 Proposed general algorithm for selecting a stress test for diagnosis of coronary artery disease (CAD) and/or assessment of prognosis in patients with known or suspected CAD.

Focus Box 7.4

- Exercise electrocardiography testing, stress echocardiography, and myocardial perfusion single-photon emission computed tomography have proved to be particularly valuable tests for the evaluation of coronary artery disease
- Myocardial perfusion single-photon emission computed tomography is a sensitive test with somewhat lower specificity for the detection of coronary artery disease; the converse is true for stress echocardiography
- Patient characteristics, local expertise, and availability are factors that influence the choice for a stress test

right modality is heavily influenced by local availability and the specific expertise available in a center. Referring physicians must have in-depth knowledge of the advantages, limitations and pitfalls of each technique, in order to obtain the optimum benefit for their patients.

REFERENCES
1. Schinkel AF, Bax JJ, Geleijnse ML, et al. Noninvasive evaluation of ischaemic heart disease: myocardial perfusion imaging or stress echocardiography? Eur Heart J 2003; 24: 789–800.
2. Fox K, Garcia MA, Ardissino D, et al. Task Force on the Management of Stable Angina Pectoris of the European Society of Cardiology; ESC Committee for Practice Guidelines (CPG). Guidelines

on the management of stable angina pectoris: executive summary: the Task Force on the Management of Stable Angina Pectoris of the European Society of Cardiology. Eur Heart J 2006; 27: 1341–81.

3. Nesto RW, Kowalchuk GJ. The ischemic cascade: temporal sequence of hemodynamic, electrocardiographic and symptomatic expressions of ischemia. Am J Cardiol 1987; 59: 23C–30C.

4. Wilson RF, Marcus ML, Christensen BV, Talman C, White CW. Accuracy of exercise electrocardiography in detecting physiologically significant coronary arterial lesions. Circulation 1991; 83: 412–21.

5. Weiner DA, Ryan TJ, McCabe CH, et al. Exercise stress testing. Correlations among history of angina, ST-segment response and prevalence of coronary-artery disease in the Coronary Artery Surgery Study (CASS). N Engl J Med 1979; 301: 230–5.

6. Gianrossi R, Detrano R, Mulvihill D, et al. Exercise-induced ST depression in the diagnosis of coronary artery disease. A meta-analysis. Circulation 1989; 80: 87–98.

7. Piepoli MF, Corra U, Benzer W, et al. Secondary prevention through cardiac rehabilitation: from knowledge to implementation. A position paper from the Cardiac Rehabilitation Section of the European Association of Cardiovascular Prevention and Rehabilitation. Eur J Cardiovasc Prev Rehabil 2010; 17: 1–17.

8. Nyman I, Wallentin L, Areskog M, Areskog NH, Swahn E. Risk stratification by early exercise testing after an episode of unstable coronary artery disease. The RISC Study Group. Int J Cardiol 1993; 39: 131–42.

9. Laukkanen JA, Kurl S, Lakka TA, et al. Exercise-induced silent myocardial ischemia and coronary morbidity and mortality in middle-aged men. J Am Coll Cardiol 2001; 38: 72–9.

10. Gibbons LW, Mitchell TL, Wei M, Blair SN, Cooper KH. Maximal exercise test as a predictor of risk for mortality from coronary heart disease in asymptomatic men. Am J Cardiol 2000; 86: 53–8.

11. Gibbons RJ, Balady GJ, Bricker JT, American College of Cardiology/American Heart Association Task Force on Practice Guidelines. Committee to Update the 1997 Exercise Testing Guidelines. ACC/AHA 2002 guideline update for exercise testing: summary article. A report of the American College of Cardiology/American Heart Association Task Force on Practice Guidelines (Committee to Update the 1997 Exercise Testing Guidelines). J Am Coll Cardiol 2002; 40: 1531–40.

12. Sozzi FB, Poldermans D, Bax JJ, et al. Second harmonic imaging improves sensitivity of dobutamine stress echocardiography for the diagnosis of coronary artery disease. Am Heart J 2001; 142: 153–9.

13. Pellikka PA, Nagueh SF, Elhendy AA, Kuehl CA, Sawada SG. American Society of Echocardiography recommendations for performance, interpretation, and application of stress echocardiography. J Am Soc Echocardiogr 2007; 20: 1021–41.

14. Lang RM, Bierig M, Devereux RB, et al. Recommendations for chamber quantification: a report from the American Society of Echocardiography's Guidelines and Standards Committee and the Chamber Quantification Writing Group, developed in conjunction with the European Association of Echocardiography, a branch of the European Society of Cardiology. J Am Soc Echocardiogr 2005; 18: 1440–63.

15. Ahmad M, Xie T, McCulloch M, Abreo G, Runge M. Real-time three-dimensional dobutamine stress echocardiography in assessment stress echocardiography in assessment of ischemia: comparison with two-dimensional dobutamine stress echocardiography. J Am Coll Cardiol 2001; 37: 1303–9.

16. Fleischmann KE, Hunink MG, Kuntz KM, Douglas PS. Exercise echocardiography or exercise SPECT imaging? A meta-analysis of diagnostic test performance. JAMA 1998; 280: 913–20.

17. Kim C, Kwok YS, Heagerty P, Redberg R. Pharmacologic stress testing for coronary disease diagnosis: A meta-analysis. Am Heart J 2001; 142: 934–44.

18. Noguchi Y, Nagata-Kobayashi S, Stahl JE, Wong JB. A meta-analytic comparison of echocardiographic stressors. Int J Cardiovasc Imaging 2005; 21: 189–207.

19. Picano E, Molinaro S, Pasanisi E. The diagnostic accuracy of pharmacological stress echocardiography for the assessment of coronary artery disease: a meta-analysis. Cardiovasc Ultrasound 2008; 6: 30.

20. Smart SC, Knickelbine T, Malik F, Sagar KB. Dobutamine-atropine stress echocardiography for the detection of coronary artery disease in patients with left ventricular hypertrophy. Importance of chamber size and systolic wall stress. Circulation 2000; 101: 258–63.

21. Biagini E, Shaw LJ, Poldermans D, et al. Accuracy of non-invasive techniques for diagnosis of coronary artery disease and prediction of cardiac events in patients with left bundle branch block: a meta-analysis. Eur J Nucl Med Mol Imaging 2006; 33: 1442–51.

22. Carlos ME, Smart SC, Wynsen JC, Sagar KB. Dobutamine stress echocardiography for risk stratification after myocardial infarction. Circulation 1997; 95: 1402–10.

23. Sicari R, Landi P, Picano E, et al. Exercise-electrocardiography and/or pharmacological stress echocardiography for non-invasive risk stratification early after uncomplicated myocardial infarction. A prospective international large scale multicentre study. Eur Heart J 2002; 23: 1030–7.

24. Poldermans D, Fioretti PM, Forster T, et al. Dobutamine stress echocardiography for assessment of perioperative cardiac risk in patients undergoing major vascular surgery. Circulation 1993; 87: 1506–12.

25. Beller GA, Zaret BL. Contributions of nuclear cardiology to diagnosis and prognosis of patients with coronary artery disease. Circulation 2000; 101: 1465–78.

26. Kapur A, Latus KA, Davies G, et al. A comparison of three radionuclide myocardial perfusion tracers in clinical practice: the ROBUST study. Eur J Nucl Med Mol Imaging 2002; 29: 1608–16.

27. Underwood SR, Anagnostopoulos C, Cerqueira M, et al. Myocardial perfusion scintigraphy: the evidence. Eur J Nucl Med Mol Imaging 2004; 31: 261–91.

28. Gibbons RJ. Noninvasive diagnosis and prognosis assessment in chronic coronary artery disease: stress testing with and without imaging perspective. Circ Cardiovasc Imaging 2008; 1: 257–69.

29. Geleijnse ML, Marwick TH, Boersma E, et al. Optimal pharmacological stress testing for the diagnosis of coronary artery disease: a probabilistic approach. Eur Heart J 1995; 16(Suppl M): 3–10.

8 Multislice computed tomography: Role in diagnosis and risk stratification

Gert-Jan R. ten Kate, Koen Nieman, and Pim J. de Feyter

OUTLINE

Cardiac computed tomography (CT) is an X-ray-based, cross-sectional imaging technique that allows noninvasive imaging of the heart, coronary arteries, and even atherosclerotic plaque within the coronary vessel wall. Calcium scoring has high sensitivity but only moderate specificity for detecting obstructive coronary artery disease. In asymptomatic patients at intermediate risk, calcium scoring provides additional prognostic information as compared with the risk factor analysis alone. Although a zero coronary calcium score is associated with a good prognosis in asymptomatic patients, it cannot reliably rule out ischemia, as a cause for symptoms, in patients with suspected acute coronary syndromes or in patients with stable chest pain who have high risk features.

CT coronary angiography (CT-CA) can image the vessel lumen to evaluate, in a semi-quantitative fashion, the severity of obstructive coronary disease. In addition, CT allows visualization of the atherosclerotic vessel wall. Plaque volumes can be measured and plaque contents can be differentiated to a certain extent. In patients with suspected acute coronary syndrome, CT can be used to safely rule out obstructive coronary artery disease. A normal CT-CA is associated with an excellent prognosis in terms of the risk of future major adverse coronary events. In patients with dilated cardiomyopathy, an ischemic etiology can be accurately detected by using CT. Where the calcium score is zero, an ischemic etiology is highly unlikely. In asymptomatic patients at intermediate/high risk, CT-CA may help both in the assessment of prognosis in individual patients and to guide management. The ability to visualize the three-dimensional coronary anatomy makes cardiac CT an ideal technique to evaluate coronary artery anomalies.

INTRODUCTION

The increasing burden of coronary artery disease (CAD) in the Western world has provided a stimulus for the development of more efficient and patient-friendly imaging techniques. Noninvasive imaging modalities such as ultrasound, nuclear imaging, positron emission tomography and magnetic resonance imaging have undergone constant technical improvements increasing their clinical usefulness.

Computed tomography (CT), developed in the early 1970s, became a coronary imaging tool with the introduction of electron beam CT (EBCT). Due to its high temporal resolution, it allowed motion-free imaging of the coronary arteries. Although contrast-enhanced EBCT became technically feasible in clinical practice, it was mostly used for the detection and quantification of coronary artery calcification (CAC).

Noninvasive coronary angiography took off when spiral CT scanners, with multiple detector rows allowing for fast, high-quality data acquisition, and complete coverage of the heart within the time of a single breath hold, were developed. Over the past decade, technological advances such as an increase in the number of detectors coupled with better temporal resolution, have established cardiac CT as a clinically reliable technique with a resulting rapidly expansion in its use in clinical practice. However, this improvement in image quality was achieved at the expense of a gradual increase in radiation doses. More recent technical innovations have been aimed at reducing the radiation exposure without compromising image quality. Meanwhile, other applications of cardiac CT, including plaque characterization, infarct imaging, and myocardial perfusion imaging are under investigation.

In this chapter we evaluate current indications for both coronary calcium scoring and contrast-enhanced plaque imaging. To enhance understanding, relevant technical aspects of CT will be discussed where necessary.

FUNDAMENTALS OF COMPUTED TOMOGRAPHY

CT is one of the many medical applications based on tissue-dependent X-ray attenuation. During CT scanning a roentgen source mounted on the scanners gantry, rotates around the patient. The emitted roentgen beam is attenuated by absorption and scattering of photons, depending on the type and density of the traversed tissues and the energy of the photons. The remaining photons reach the detectors located at the opposite side of the gantry from which attenuation coefficients can be calculated. By combining attenuation coefficients obtained by individual detector elements, the so-called attenuation profiles are created. During rotation of the scanners gantry, a large number of attenuation profiles are obtained. By combining these profiles, the regional attenuation within the encircled plane can be calculated using sophisticated reconstruction algorithms.

To reconstruct a single image, profiles acquired during a minimum of 180-degree rotation are required. Therefore, the rotation time directly affects the temporal resolution of the scanner. In the case of dual-source CT or with the use of special reconstruction algorithms, the temporal resolution can be improved. The regional attenuation is expressed in Hounsfield units (HU), relative to the attenuation of water, which is defined as 0 HU. Regional attenuation data are displayed using a sliding gray scale, resulting in the cross-sectional CT images that are used in clinical practice. The entire data set consists of a large stack of these cross-sectional images. Secondary, post processing can create new cross-sections through the different axial slices or volume-rendered models to display the images in a three-dimensional fashion.

CT IMAGING OF THE HEART

Imaging of a moving organ such as the heart requires synchronization of the acquisition of data or the reconstruction of images to the rhythm of the heart. Most scanners are unable to scan the entire heart during a single heart cycle and therefore require acquisition of data over several heart cycles. Because of the limited temporal resolution of cardiac CT, motion-free imaging can only be accomplished during specific intervals within the cardiac cycle when the heart is relatively stationary.

There are two widely used techniques for electrocardiogram (ECG)-synchronized imaging. For prospectively ECG-triggered sequential/axial scanning (step-and-shoot), a single set of data is acquired at a time point during the selected cardiac phase while the table remains stationary. Then the table is moved to the next position to await the next acquisition. With the advent of spiral CT this method was replaced by continuous acquisition of overlapping CT data during continuous movement of the table. Based on the recorded ECG trace, the images were then retrospectively reconstructed during the desired cardiac phase. ECG-gated spiral CT is a very robust technique that allows fast coverage, flexible phase selection, and is less vulnerable to ECG irregularities. The drawback is, however, that continuous radiation exposure throughout the cardiac cycle results in considerable exposure to radiation.

Development of faster rotating CT systems with a wider coverage combined with algorithms that recognize and deal with ECG irregularities, allowed re-introduction of prospectively, ECG-triggered, axial acquisition protocols. Without compromising the image quality, this scan mode has contributed significantly to reduce the overall radiation doses associated with cardiac CT over the recent years. Modern scanners allow both the axial and spiral mode of data acquisition.

CORONARY CALCIUM IMAGING

The relation between atherosclerosis and CAC was first discovered at autopsy. With the introduction of fluoroscopy and ultrafast EBCT, it became possible to non-invasively detect and quantify CAC with results that compared favorably with postmortem microscopy and in vivo intravascular imaging (1,2). Because of its high density CAC is easy to discriminate from surrounding tissue on CT images without the need for intravascular contrast media. Although atherosclerosis is characterized by both progression and regression, the plaque seems to advance following a common pathway (3). Deposition of calcium phosphate is a manifestation of advanced atherosclerotic disease and although the relation between calcification and future coronary events is still unclear on a per plaque basis, it is evident that patients with high calcium scores in general have more extensive CAD and are at increased risk of future coronary events (4). It is assumed that CAC is a marker of disease activity in the past rather than a direct cause of future coronary events (5). Greater

amounts of CAC per lesion do, however, correlate with stenosis grade in both post mortem and EBCT studies (6).

At the time that coronary calcium quantification was developed, EBCT was the choice for cardiac imaging. In 1990, Agatston et al. introduced a method to semi-quantify the amount of calcium within the coronary arteries. It remains the most widely used method for reporting the extent of coronary calcium (7). While only 20 contiguous 3-mm slices were acquired in the original paper to cover the most proximal parts of the coronary arteries, modern scanners allow complete coverage of the heart. Structures with an attenuation value above 130 HU are considered calcified. Lesion areas are multiplied by a number that depends on the highest attenuation value measured in that lesion: 130–199 HU = 1, 200–299 HU = 2, 300–399 HU = 3, ≥400 HU = 4. The total Agatston score is the total of lesion scores (maximum density score multiplied by the lesion area in mm (2)) per slice for all slices and can be specified for each coronary vessel. Alternative algorithms quantify coronary artery calcium in terms of calcified volume or mass. The volume score is defined as the total of ≥130 HU voxels independent of further density specification. The mass score is defined as mass ((area × slice increment × mean density)/250). This score, unlike the volume score, incorporates data on tissue density based on HU specification (Fig. 8.1).

Accuracy, Reproducibility, and Monitoring Progression of CAD

The reproducibility of the calcium score is important, especially for monitoring progression of disease. Achenbach et al. found a median Agatston score variability of 7.8%, mainly influenced by image noise and the total amount of CAC; the higher the amount of calcium present, the better the reproducibility of the scan. In patients with small amounts of CAC, small overall differences in repeated measurements correspond to large relative differences (8).

The Agatston score is prone to be influenced by partial voluming, which occurs when image elements (voxels) contain more than one type of tissue and the attenuation value becomes an average of the attenuation values of those respective tissues. Because of the relatively large image elements (because of the thick slice thickness of EBCT) and dependence on the highest attenuation per lesion, partial voluming contributes to the modest reproducibility of the Agatston score. Alternative quantification methods that measure volumes or the mass of coronary calcium are less prone to partial voluming and therefore have better reproducibility (9). Nevertheless, between EBCT, single-slice spiral CT, and multi-slice CT, good correlation exists for quantification of CAC (10,11).

Prevalence and Progression of Coronary Calcium

The amount of CAC is strongly associated with age and gender. In the general population, coronary calcium is rare during the first decennia of life in both men and women. The mean total calcium scores of men between the ages of 40 and 69 years are comparable with those of women who are 10 years

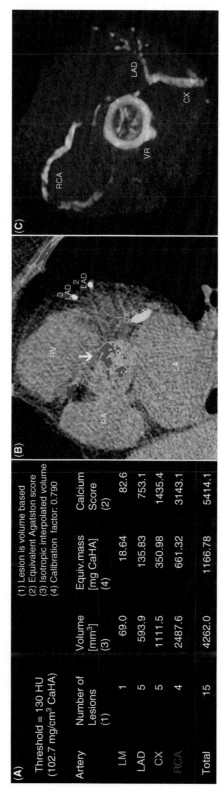

Figure 8.1 Calcium, because of its high attenuation co-efficient, is readily discriminated from surrounding tissue in this non-enhanced scan. (A) Coronary calcium is quantified by using volume, mass, and Agatston algorithms using dedicated software. Lesions are further specified according to their location and number. (B) One of the axial slices used for calcium scoring. Software assigns a pink coloration to regions with attenuation factors >130 HU. After selecting a lesion, one can specify the coronary artery for further analysis. Note the high attenuation area caused by the leaflets of the prosthetic aortic valve implanted in this patient (*arrow*). (C) Volume rendered image of the same patient showing high density structures such as diffuse coronary calcifications and valve structures. *Abbreviations:* CX, circumflex coronary artery; LA, left atrium; LAD, left anterior descending coronary artery; RCA, right coronary artery; RV, right ventricle; VR, valvular ring.

older, consistent with the later onset of CAD in women. Before the age of 60 years, men have approximately twice the amount of CAC as compared with women. At older ages, gender differences gradually diminish (Fig. 8.2) (12).

The degree of CAC is also influenced by ethnicity. Caucasians not only have the highest prevalence of CAC, but also have the highest disease severity. In blacks and Hispanics, the disease prevalence was lower (22% and 15%, respectively) as compared with whites after adjustment for coronary risk factors. Age, male gender, and hypertension were significant predictors of the presence of CAC in all ethnic groups (13). High-risk populations such as patients who suffer from diabetes mellitus or familial hypercholesterolemia have higher levels of CAC and a larger total plaque burden (14,15).

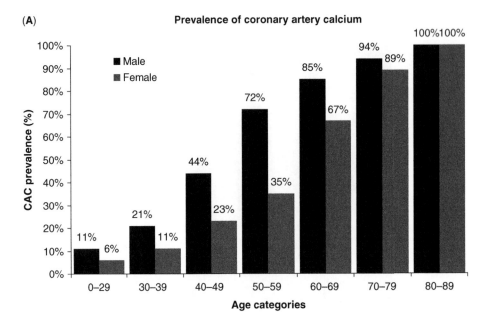

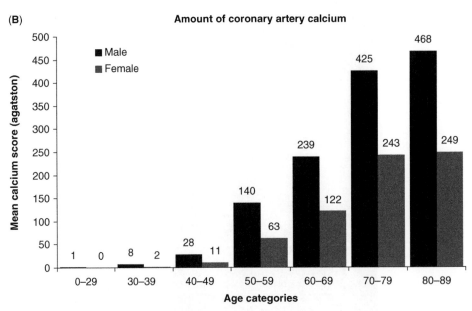

Figure 8.2 Prevalence and degree of coronary artery calcification (CAC) in 1,396 male and 502 female subjects by using electron beam computed tomography. Patients were all asymptomatic for coronary artery disease at the time of inclusion. Source: Adapted from Janowitz et al. (12). (A) Note the increasing prevalence of CAC in both men and women with age. The prevalence of CAC is almost double in men as compared with women until the age of about 60 years when differences diminish. (B) Total CAC is higher in men than in women for all age groups. Note the 10-year time lag for CAC between women and men in their seventh decade of life.

Diagnostic Use of Coronary Calcium Imaging

Most patients with obstructive CAD have detectable calcium on non-enhanced CT images. In patients with stable chest pain and a low-to-intermediate probability of disease a negative calcium scan virtually excludes severe obstructive CAD (16). A positive calcium score, however, does not imply the presence of obstructive disease, although the odds increase with a higher calcium score. Furthermore, studies in symptomatic low-risk patients show that the absence of CAC is associated with an excellent prognosis (17). Studies in high-risk populations (undergoing invasive angiography) have shown that a considerable proportion of patients have obstructive disease in the absence of calcium. In such patients with a high pretest probability a non-enhanced CT scan may not suffice to exclude CAD.

In the context of an acute coronary syndrome (ACS), culprit lesions fairly often contain little or no calcium. Most patients will have calcified plaque in other vessels, which explains the high accuracy of the calcium scan to exclude acute coronary disease. However, given the availability of CT angiography nowadays, and the potentially severe consequences of a missed myocardial infarction, few physicians will settle for a negative calcium scan to exclude an ACS in clinical practice.

Risk (Re-) Stratification in Asymptomatic Patients

Considering the global magnitude of coronary heart disease and the fact that in nearly half the patients, unheralded cardiac death or a non-fatal myocardial infarction is the first clinical manifestation of coronary disease, calcium imaging is considered a potentially valuable tool for cardiovascular risk stratification. Currently used risk prediction models such as the Framingham Risk Score (FRS) or the European SCORE are based on several well-known risk factors including age, gender, low-density lipoprotein, high-density lipoprotein, blood pressure, diabetes mellitus, and smoking (18). Based on, for instance the FRS, individuals can be classified as low (<10%), intermediate (10–20%), or high risk (>20%) of suffering an adverse coronary event in the next 10 years.

The long-term prognostic power of classical risk prediction is well established. However, individual risk factor exposure may change over time resulting in patient-specific exposure profiles that are difficult to measure and could lead to misclassification of risk. Therefore, using results from population-based studies to guide individual patient management decisions could lead to inaccurate assessment of prognosis and potentially result in over or under treatment.

The calcium score can be used for risk re-stratification of asymptomatic individuals. The incremental value of calcium scoring over traditional risk assessment was demonstrated in several prognostic studies (Fig. 8.3). Erbel et al. demonstrated that calcium scoring achieved significantly better results for C-statistics as compared with traditional risk factor analysis for both men and women: 0.68 for the FRS, 0.74 for the log (CAC+1), and 0.75 for the combination of FRS and log (CAC+1). After 5 years, individuals at intermediate risk (by clinical risk score) and a low calcium score (<100) had an event rate similar to low-risk individuals, while those with a high calcium score (>400) had an event rate comparable with high-risk individuals (19). Currently, calcium scoring in low- or high-risk individuals is generally discouraged. Whether widespread calcium screening will affect clinical outcome and whether this warrants the tremendous societal costs, remains a topic of debate that needs to be evaluated in large-scale trials before it can be recommended.

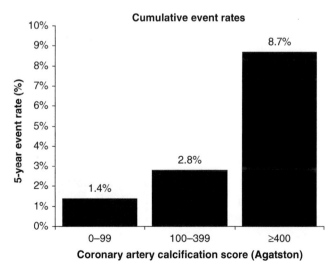

Figure 8.3 The Heinz Nixdorf Recall Study investigated the prognostic power of coronary artery calcification (CAC) scoring as compared with the traditional risk factor analysis. The incidence of hard events (nonfatal myocardial infarction and coronary death) was evaluated in 4,129 subjects without overt coronary artery disease at baseline. Note the difference in event rates between CAC strata for patients at intermediate risk (10–20%) according to the Framingham Risk Score. *Source:* Adapted from Ref. 19.

CONTRAST-ENHANCED CT CORONARY IMAGING

By injecting the contrast medium, coronary lumen can be distinguished from the surrounding tissues on CT images, allowing the detection of obstructive CAD. Because of the low native attenuation of pericardial fat CT angiography also allows visualization of the atherosclerotic vessel wall of the epicardial coronary arteries, depicting both calcified and non-calcified tissues. Contrast-enhanced CT coronary angiography (CT-CA) is more elaborate as compared with the non-enhanced calcium imaging. Iodinated contrast medium (60–100 ml) is injected intravenously for opacification of the coronary lumen and other blood-filled cardiac structures of interest. Sufficiently high image quality requires dedicated acquisition and reconstruction protocols, which is associated with a higher radiation dose. Image quality benefits from a regular rhythm and a slow heart rate, which can be achieved medically with the use of beta-blocker, sinus node blockers, or other medication. Dual-source CT reduces the necessity for routine beta-blockade. Contemporary scan protocols allow for routine CT angiography at doses below 5 mSv (Fig. 8.4) (20–22).

Evaluation of Obstructive Coronary Artery Disease

Four- and 16-slice CT scanners lacked sufficient robustness for non-invasive coronary angiography to be accepted in clinical practice (23). However, with the introduction of 64-slice CT technology, the evaluation of all clinically relevant branches of the coronary tree became feasible. In a multicenter, multi-vendor study, Meijboom et al. reported a sensitivity of 99% and a negative predictive value of 97% of CT angiography in comparison with invasive coronary angiography in a group of patients at intermediate to high risk of significant CAD. Specificity was moderate at 64% with a positive predictive value of 86%. Sensitivity and specificity were similar for patients presenting with unstable or stable symptoms (24).

Most technical validation studies included non-evaluable vessel segments into the analysis, grading them as clinically significant in accordance with the intention-to-diagnose principle. As a result, reported sensitivities are relatively high at the expense of specificity, especially if the number of non-evaluable segments is substantial. With continuing improvements in image quality, the number of non-assessable coronary segments has decreased significantly. In recent studies CT-CA was reported to have a specificity of 87–98% and a sensitivity of 94–95% (25). Although reported accuracy is high, residual disagreement persists on the significance of individual lesions partly related to the limited spatial and temporal resolution of CT-CA as compared with invasive coronary angiography (ICA). A recent meta-analysis by Von Ballmoos et al. demonstrated that contemporary dose-saving acquisition techniques had no adverse effect on the diagnostic accuracy of cardiac CT in comparison with invasive angiography (26).

The images obtained by noninvasive and invasive coronary angiography are fundamentally different. Invasive angiograms are moving shadows of a contrast-filled coronary artery from a single projection angle, while CT creates cross-sectional images of lower spatial resolution depicting the coronary and surrounding tissues at a single time instant or a single heart cycle at the best. For this reason invasively detected disease is quantified

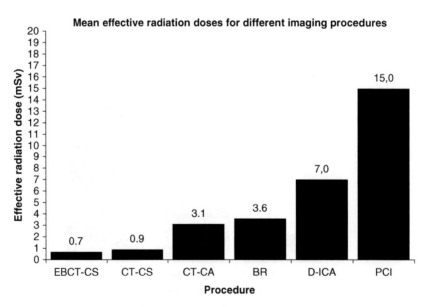

Figure 8.4 Reported mean effective radiation doses for different imaging procedures, including computed tomography (CT) applications by contemporary prospectively triggered axial scan modes. The mean estimated annual level of background radiation in the USA was added for reference purposes. *Abbreviations*: BR, estimated annual background radiation in USA; CT-CA, CT coronary angiography; CT-CS, CT calcium scoring; D-ICA, diagnostic invasive coronary angiography; EBCT-CS, electron beam CT; PCI, percutaneous coronary intervention. Source: Adapted from Ref. 20–22.

as diameter stenosis, while CT reports area stenosis. Given the limited spatial resolution of CT, obstructive disease is generally assessed in a visual manner using categories of obstructive severity: 0% diameter stenosis (normal), <25% stenosis (minimal), 25–49% stenosis (mild), 50–69% stenosis (moderate), 70–99% stenosis (severe), and 100% stenosis (occluded). Moderate lesions are defined as 'possible flow limiting' whereas severe lesions are defined as 'probable flow limiting' (27). Lesions that narrow the coronary artery lumen diameter by 50% or more are considered angiographically significant.

Software that allows for (semi-)automatic stenosis quantification has become available. The accuracy of these algorithms in comparison with invasive angiography is affected by the fundamental differences between both techniques, limited spatial resolution, and image artifacts on CT. Improved accuracy of automatic quantification algorithms over the human eye has not been convincingly demonstrated. Besides, CT probably does not require perfect agreement with invasive angiography to be meaningful in clinical practice. Discrepant stenosis quantification by CT and conventional angiography receives remarkable attention, whereas its importance for clinical outcome is rather uncertain. However, the ability to non-invasively assess coronary plaque in addition to lumen obstructions shows promise for improved risk assessment (28). Currently, decision making is more and more affected by the ischemic consequences of obstructive CAD. It is conceivable that the lumen area measurements (as by CT) better correlate with coronary flow than the projectional lumen diameter.

Plaque Imaging

As previously mentioned, contrast-enhanced CT allows appreciation of the atherosclerotic vessel wall. In the proximal coronary arteries, CT detects most atherosclerotic plaques, particularly when some degree of calcification is present. Plaques that were considered to be predominantly calcified, fibrous, or lipid-rich by intravascular ultrasound (IVUS) imaging, have different CT attenuation values with thresholds varying among studies. In fact, the measured attenuation of individual plaques is affected by many (imaging) factors, limiting the differentiation to calcified and non-calcified plaque tissue in clinical practice (Fig. 8.5).

Detection of High-Risk Plaque

The potential use of CT to identify vulnerable plaque has been the subject of intense research in recent years (Fig. 8.6). Several studies have evaluated the appearance of unstable coronary lesions on cardiac CT using intravascular imaging techniques as a comparator. Well-known features of culprit lesions in patients who suffered an ACS can be reliably identified by CT angiography, including large plaque volume, low plaque attenuation values, outward vessel remodelling, and spotty calcification (Table 8.1) (29). Detection of lipid pools and plaque rupture by CT has incidentally been described. Other plaque features associated with plaque vulnerability on invasive imaging techniques are more difficult to visualize by CT, including the thickness of the fibrous cap that covers the liponecrotic

pool. Imaging of macrophages using small iodine particles has recently been demonstrated in atherosclerotic aortas of rabbits. An alternative and perhaps more sensitive approach to image plaque inflammation combines CT with nuclear imaging techniques. The uptake of 18-F fluorodeoxyglucose by macrophages, and subsequent decrease of activity after statin treatment has been demonstrated in carotid arteries (30).

Hulten et al. determined the prognostic value of CT-CA in a meta-analysis comprising almost 10,000 symptomatic patients, showing that the annualized event rates for combined major adverse coronary events (death, myocardial infarction, unstable angina, or revascularization) was higher (1.41%) for patients with non-obstructive plaque compared with those with completely normal CT scans (0.17%). For obstructive CAD, the annual event rate was highest (8.84%) (Fig. 8.7) (31).

Plaque Quantification

Voros et al. recently published a meta-analysis of 33 studies comparing CT-CA to IVUS. For vessel lumen area, plaque area, percent area stenosis, and plaque volume, the weighted mean difference was determined. CT-CA showed excellent diagnostic accuracy for the detection of coronary plaques with an area under the curve for receiver operating characteristics analysis of 0.94, a sensitivity of 0.90, and a specificity of 0.92. For quantitative analysis, CT slightly overestimated lumen area by 7%, presumably caused by partial voluming that can lead to overestimation of the size of high-density volumes such as the opacified coronary artery lumen. Both plaque area and volume were similar on CT and IVUS (32). Quantification of the coronary plaque is challenging due to poor definition of the outer vessel boundaries. Substantial inter-observer variability of more than 30% in terms of plaque volume has been reported with a 64-slice CT.

There is currently little data on the natural progression of plaque on coronary CT angiography in terms of size or characteristics or the effect of therapeutic interventions.

Clinical Utility of CT Angiography

CT-CA has several potential advantages when compared with other non-invasive imaging tests without the potential drawbacks of ICA. CT-CA can be performed quickly, is less expensive than ICA, and is not associated with the discomfort and risks of this invasive procedure. The high negative predictive value of CT allows CAD to be reliably excluded as a cause of symptoms. The diagnostic performance of the various stress tests is variable, particularly when compared with ICA. While functional tests and anatomical tests provide complementary information in patients with chest pain symptoms, CT angiography is increasingly replacing stress testing in the context of stable angina pectoris. Several consensus statements now support the use of coronary CT angiography in symptomatic patients at low-to-intermediate probability, particularly when stress tests cannot be performed or produce equivocal results (33). Randomized controlled trials of the effectiveness and safety of cardiac CT compared with functional testing are currently ongoing.

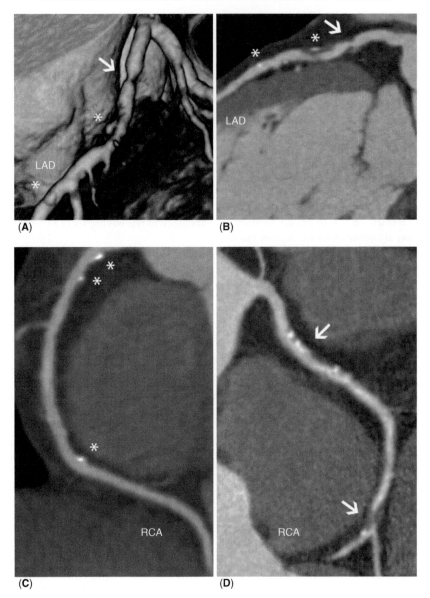

Figure 8.5 Examples of different plaque characteristics on contrast enhanced computed tomography coronary angiography. Panels A and B referring to the same patient. (**A**) Volume rendered image showing a non calcified plaque (arrow), a mixed plaque (proximal asterix) and a calcified plaque (distal asterix). (**B**) Multi-planar reconstruction of the left anterior descending coronary artery (LAD) showing the bright appearance of coronary artery calcification in calcified and mixed plaque. (**C**) Spotty calcifications of the right coronary artery (RCA) without significant luminal narrowing. (**D**) Mixed plaque in the proximal RCA (*arrow*), distally the lumen is obstructed. Note the spotty calcification after the obstruction.

Given the ability to depict the complete three-dimensional coronary anatomy, coronary CT angiography is particularly effective in depicting anomalous coronary anatomy (34). Although coronary artery anomalies are rare, they can be responsible for cardiovascular morbidity and even mortality. Coronaries coursing between the aorta and pulmonary artery can become compressed with serious implications; such anomalies can be readily diagnosed by CT (Fig. 8.8). Use of low-radiation scan protocols is particularly pertinent in young patients with suspected coronary anomalies.

Triage of Acute Chest Pain

Patients suspected of an ACS with normal initial biochemical markers and a normal or uninterpretable ECG, pose a major diagnostic and logistic challenge. Although the majority have symptoms that will ultimately prove to be non-cardiac in origin,

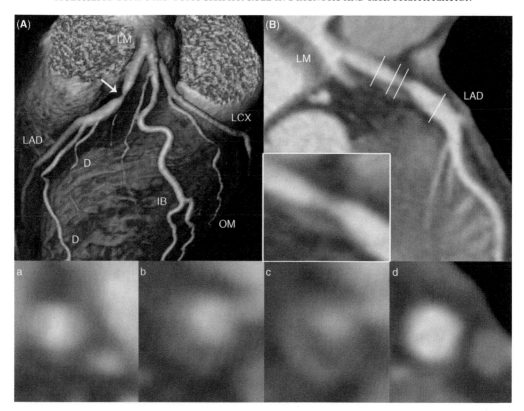

Figure 8.6 Contrast enhanced computed tomography coronary angiography showing a non-calcified, hemodynamically significant lesion in a patient with atypical chest pain and electrocardiogram changes. The patient was immediately transferred for percutaneous revascularization, which resolved the symptoms (**A**) Volume rendered image showing the left coronary system with an isolated lesion in the proximal LAD (segment 6). In the remainder of the coronary arteries no atherosclerosis was detected, total coronary artery calcification (*Agatston*) was zero. (**B**) Multi-planar reconstruction of the diseased coronary artery segment showing positive arterial remodeling at the lesion site. Note the increase in luminal diameter distal to the lesion. (a,b,c,d) Axial projections at different locations along the coronary artery. Note the small lumen that remains in panel c and the large plaque volume containing a liponecrotic pool characterized by its low density (*dark surface*). *Abbreviations*: D, diagonal branch; IB, intermediate branch; LAD, left anterior descending coronary artery; LCX, left circumflex coronary artery; LM, left main coronary artery; OM, obtuse marginal coronary artery.

Table 8.1 Plaque Morphology

	Sensitivity (%)	Specificity (%)	PPV (%)	NPV (%)
Positive remodeling	84	78	79	83
Spotty calcifications	25	100	100	56
Contrast-enhanced rim	25	100	100	57
Combination of all	50	93	86	62

Pflederer et al. analyzed the typical morphological characteristics of atherosclerotic plaques in acute coronary syndrome patients as compared with lesions found in patients with stable angina pectoris (stable lesions) using computed tomography coronary angiography. Spotty calcifications embedded within non-calcified plaque components or a contrast-enhanced rim around the respective lesions were only found in the culprit lesions of acute coronary syndrome patients but never in stable lesions.
Abbreviations: NPV, negative predictive value; PPV, positive predictive value.
Source: Adapted from Ref. 29.

effective triage of patients with suspected ACS has the potential to reduce mortality.

One of the first studies investigating the efficacy of CT-CA for diagnosing ACS was conducted by Sato et al. using 4- and 16-slice CT. Information on stenosis grade (≥75%), low-attenuation plaque, and myocardial perfusion defects was used for the CT diagnosis of ACS resulting in a sensitivity and specificity of 96% and 89%, respectively (35). By lowering the threshold on luminal narrowing to 50% or more and without using additional CT information, Hoffman et al. found a sensitivity and negative

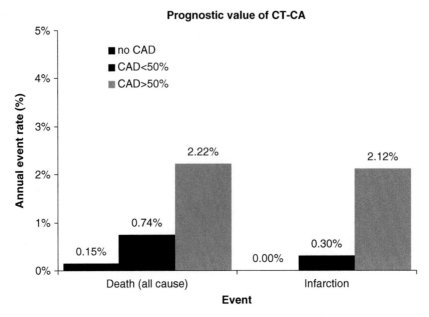

Figure 8.7 Adverse cardiovascular events are rare among patients without CAD by CT-CA. All cause death and myocardial infarction are less rare along strata with increasing severity of CAD. Although normal CT-coronary angiograms are correlated with excellent prognosis for symptomatic patients evaluated for suspected CAD, a positive scan is not strongly predictive of future major coronary events. *Abbreviations*: CAD, coronary artery disease; CT-CA, computed tomography-coronary angiography; *Source*: Adapted from Ref. 31.

predictive value for ACS of 77% and 98%, respectively. None of the patients without CAD on CT-CA were diagnosed with an ACS (50% of the study population). By contrast, specificity and positive predictive value of detected CAD was moderate to low because many patients had plaque on CT-CA without a clinical diagnosis of ACS (positive predictive value 17 %, specificity 54%) (36).

The accuracy of CT for the diagnosis of ACS or the prediction of major adverse coronary events during the following 30 days proved to be comparable or even better as compared with stress nuclear imaging (37). In a follow-up study by Schlett et al., patients presenting with acute chest pain and a normal CT scan had no major adverse events over the next two years. The event rate was, as expected, higher for patients with obstructive CAD (30%), but was also higher for those with non-obstructive coronary plaque (5%) (38).

Coronary CT imaging has the potential to be an important tool for the diagnostic workup of patients with suspected ACS. From the available data, it can be concluded that patients without detectable plaque on CT-CA can be discharged safely whereas patients with obstructive coronary disease should be triaged to observation and additional diagnostic investigation. Non-obstructive plaque appears to be associated with a small number of ACS and later adverse events. The logistic and economic consequences of using CT for triage of patients with acute chest pain are currently under investigation.

Dilated Cardiomyopathy

CAD is considered the main cause of dilated cardiomyopathy (DCM) in about two-thirds of patients. DCM as a result of myocardial ischemia usually involves multiple coronary arteries and such lesions generally have extensive calcification. Therefore, the absence of coronary calcium virtually excludes ischemic heart disease as the primary etiology (39,40). Ghostine et al. compared CT-CA with ICA for the initial evaluation of patients with DCM. CT-CA was able to detect significant underlying ischemic heart disease with great accuracy. Overall, sensitivity, specificity, PPV, and NPV were 90, 97, 93, and 95%, respectively (41). Cornily et al. found excellent sensitivity and a high negative predictive value of CT-CA when restricted to patients with a calcium score of less than 1000. In this group of patients CT-CA identified all but one patient without CAD, and could potentially avoid invasive angiography in 21 out of 27 patients (42).

In conclusion, a zero calcium score can be used to safely rule out ischemic disease in DCM of unknown origin. CT angiography may be of use in patients with a low-intermediate calcium score, its utility will be limited in patients with a very high calcium score.

Risk (re-) Stratification in Asymptomatic Patients

The use of contrast-enhanced CT for the detection of occult CAD in asymptomatic patients is controversial and discouraged

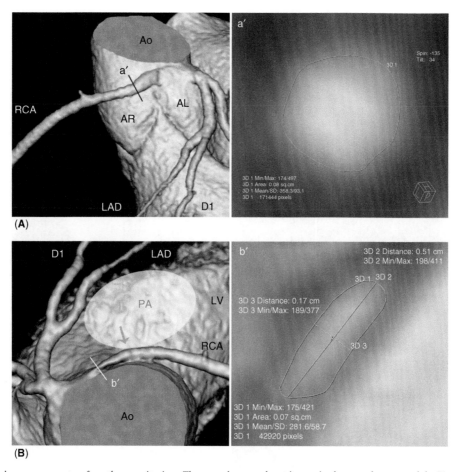

Figure 8.8 Anomalous coronary artery from the opposite sinus. The anomalous vessel part is coursing between the aorta and the PA typical of malignant anomalies. (**A**) Volume rendered image showing the highest density structures only, being the contrast enhanced blood pool within the coronary arteries, aorta, and left ventricle. Note the aberrant coronary ostium of the RCA at the AL and the normal coronary dimensions in this projection illustrated by panel a′. (**B**) Superior view of RCA revealing a sharp decrease of luminal diameter at its ostium. Distal to the arrow the coronary artery lumen is round. The PA was drawn schematically to accentuate the inter-arterial course of this coronary artery anomaly that makes it more vulnerable for lateral compression. The ovoid shape of the RCA can be quantified by the asymmetry ratio (smallest/largest diagonal) as illustrated in panel b′. *Abbreviations*: Ao, aorta; AR/AL, anterior right and anterior left aortic cusps; D1, first diagonal; LAD, left anterior descending coronary artery; PA, pulmonary artery; RCA, right coronary artery.

in international consensus statements (43). The radiation exposure associated with CT-CA is a major reason for this. However, current dose-saving algorithms have resulted in a marked reduction of radiation exposure. In the near future this may expand the use of CT-CA for coronary risk assessment in asymptomatic patients that are at intermediate or high risk of future coronary events (Fig. 8.9).

Hadamitzky et al. retrospectively analyzed outcomes of 451 asymptomatic patients who underwent CT-CA with regard to the prevalence of obstructive CAD and the incidence of subsequent cardiac events after a mean duration of follow-up of 27.5 months. All patients were referred by a cardiologist who ordered the test generally because of elevated cardiovascular risk profiles. According to the FRS, 150 patients (33%) had low cardiovascular risk, 252 (56%) had intermediate risk, and

49 (11%) had high risk. Although there was no significant difference in the FRS between patients with and without cardiac events, the event rate in patients with obstructive CAD (3.1%) was significantly higher than the event rate in patients without obstructive CAD (0.2%). In this cohort of patients, 83% had CAD, 23% had obstructive CAD, and 10 % had lesions suitable for percutaneous coronary intervention. CT-CA could reclassify two-thirds of patients regarding their risk for future symptomatic CAD. From the intermediate risk group 75% of patients and from the high-risk group 59% of the patients could be reclassified to the low-risk group. Patients without obstructive CAD on CT-CA had a very low risk of future coronary events during the study follow-up (44).

Neefjes et al. determined the calcium score and coronary plaque burden in 101 asymptomatic statin-treated patients

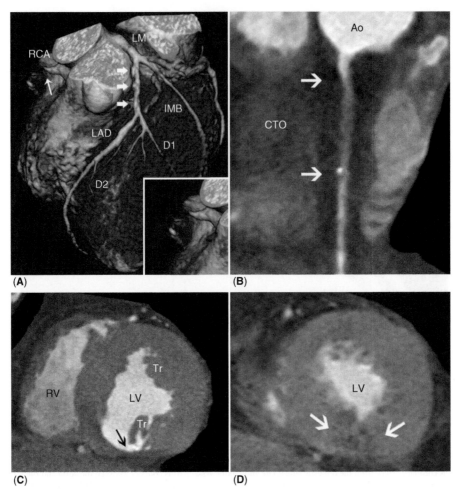

Figure 8.9 Images of an asymptomatic male patient in his fifties referred for computed tomography-coronary angiography because of his high-risk profile (diabetes mellitus). The absence of symptoms is likely due to neuropathy associated with the diabetic status of the patient. (A) Volume rendered image showing both the left and right coronary systems in this patient with three-vessel disease. Just distal to the ostium of the RCA the lumen is completely occluded (arrow + magnification). The LAD contains multiple calcified and mixed plaques (arrows). (B) Multi planar reconstruction of the RCA visualizing the occlusion that is 3.5 cm in length. Distal from the occlusion the lumen is retrogradely filled as can be seen by the local (hypo) enhancement. (C) Short axis view; as a result of the occlusion the dependant myocardium turned into scar tissue resulting in local thinning of the ventricular wall (arrow). (D) Short axis view at a more apical level showing regional hypo enhancement (between arrows) suggestive of local perfusion defects at the borderzone of the infarction. *Abbreviations*: Ao, aorta; CTO, chronic total occlusion; D1/D2, first and second diagonal; IMB, intermediate branch; LAD, left anterior descending coronary artery; LM, left main coronary artery; LV, left ventricle; RCA, right coronary artery; RV, right ventricle; Tr, trabecularization.

with heterozygous familial hypercholesterolemia and compared the results with a control group of patients with low probability of CAD having non-anginal chest pain. The median total calcium score was significantly higher in patients with familial hypercholesterolemia as compared with the control group. In addition, their coronary plaque burden was significantly higher despite intense statin treatment. However, in 15% of cases no atherosclerosis was detected.

In high-to-intermediate risk populations without symptoms, both CT-calcium scoring and CT-CA could be of major importance for determining prognosis and guiding patient treatment (14). Zero calcium could be used to exclude substantial coronary artery plaque and will be associated with a good prognosis. High calcium scores implicate vast progression of disease and are associated with calcium-related blooming artifacts. These patients may benefit from maximum medical treatment without further contrast-enhanced scanning. Patients with intermediate amounts of coronary calcium could, however, benefit from CT-CA to further evaluate coronary artery plaque progression and their individual risk profile.

To further evaluate the prognostic potential of CT-CA in comparison with, and in addition to, traditional risk prediction models, prospective research is needed, ideally without disclosure of the CT results.

CONCLUSIONS

Coronary calcium can be readily detected on cardiac CT scans. The CT calcium score is associated with the burden of atherosclerosis and predicts adverse events. In low-intermediate probability patients with stable chest complaints, calcium excludes obstructive CAD in the vast majority of patients. In asymptomatic individuals, calcium scoring can be helpful for reclassification of those at intermediate risk, in whom there is uncertainty regarding instituting preventive measures.

Coronary CT angiography correlates well with invasive angiography with an excellent sensitivity for the detection of obstructive CAD. Overestimation of disease may occur in the presence of extensive calcification. Remaining inconsistencies between invasive and non-invasive angiography can be explained by differences in methodology and image quality, but are generally of limited clinical relevance.

CT also allows for the detection of coronary plaque, measurement of the extent of coronary lesions, differentiation of calcified and non-calcified components, and potential identification of plaque features associated with plaque instability.

Cardiac CT is gradually finding a role in clinical practice, mainly for the exclusion of obstructive CAD in patients with stable symptoms. The ability to safely triage patients with acute chest pain is also a promising indication. In patients with dilated cardiomyopathy, calcium scanning and CT angiography can be of clinical use to exclude ischemic heart disease as the underlying etiology. Further research is needed to evaluate the incremental prognostic value of CT angiography in asymptomatic individuals.

PERSONAL PERSPECTIVE

Atherosclerosis imaging by CT will benefit from further technical refinements. Improved spatial, temporal, and contrast resolution will improve identification and differentiation of plaques. Automatic plaque segmentation and quantification software with improved accuracy and reproducibility will be developed to assess the overall contrast-enhanced, coronary plaque burden. Molecular imaging by nuclear or other imaging techniques may open new avenues for non-invasive plaque characterization. Other potential technical developments that may benefit atherosclerosis imaging by CT are dual-energy or spectral CT, although cardiac motion obviously poses a problem. Already cardiac CT for evaluation of obstructive CAD in symptomatic patients is gaining ground. Demand for personalized medicine and prevention, combined with decreasing radiation doses will undoubtedly increase the clinical use of cardiac CT also in asymptomatic individuals.

REFERENCES

1. Simons DB, Schwartz RS, Edwards WD, et al. Noninvasive definition of anatomic coronary artery disease by ultrafast computed tomographic scanning: a quantitative pathologic comparison study. J Am Coll Cardiol 1992; 20:1118–26.
2. Soeda T, Uemura S, Morikawa Y, et al. Diagnostic accuracy of dual-source computed tomography in the characterization of coronary atherosclerotic plaques: Comparison with intravascular optical coherence tomography. Int J Cardiol 2011; 148: 313–8.
3. Stary HC, Chandler AB, Dinsmore RE, et al. A definition of advanced types of atherosclerotic lesions and a histological classification of atherosclerosis. A report from the Committee on Vascular Lesions of the Council on Arteriosclerosis, American Heart Association. Circulation 1995; 92: 1355–74.
4. Arad Y, Goodman KJ, Roth M, Newstein D, Guerci AD. Coronary calcification, coronary disease risk factors, C-reactive protein, and atherosclerotic cardiovascular disease events: the St. Francis Heart Study. J Am Coll Cardiol 2005; 46: 158–65.
5. Blankenhorn DH, Stern D. Calcification of the coronary arteries. Am J Roentgenol Radium Ther Nucl Med 1959; 81: 772–7.
6. Kragel AH, Reddy SG, Wittes JT, Roberts WC. Morphometric analysis of the composition of coronary arterial plaques in isolated unstable angina pectoris with pain at rest. Am J Cardiol 1990; 66: 562–7.
7. Agatston AS, Janowitz WR, Hildner FJ, et al. Quantification of coronary artery calcium using ultrafast computed tomography. J Am Coll Cardiol 1990; 15: 827–32.
8. Achenbach S, Ropers D, Mohlenkamp S, et al. Variability of repeated coronary artery calcium measurements by electron beam tomography. Am J Cardiol 2001; 87: 210–13; A8.
9. Callister TQ, Cooil B, Raya SP, et al. Coronary artery disease: improved reproducibility of calcium scoring with an electron-beam CT volumetric method. Radiology 1998; 208: 807–14.
10. Becker CR, Kleffel T, Crispin A, et al. Coronary artery calcium measurement: agreement of multirow detector and electron beam CT. AJR Am J Roentgenol 2001; 176: 1295–8.
11. Ghadri JR, Goetti R, Fiechter M, et al. Inter-scan variability of coronary artery calcium scoring assessed on 64-multidetector computed tomography vs. dual-source computed tomography: a head-to-head comparison. Eur Heart J 2011; 32: 1865–74.
12. Janowitz WR, Agatston AS, Kaplan G, Viamonte M Jr. Differences in prevalence and extent of coronary artery calcium detected by ultrafast computed tomography in asymptomatic men and women. Am J Cardiol 1993; 72: 247–54.
13. Bild DE, Detrano R, Peterson D, et al. Ethnic differences in coronary calcification: the Multi-Ethnic Study of Atherosclerosis (MESA). Circulation 2005; 111: 1313–20.
14. Neefjes LA, Ten Kate GJ, Rossi A, et al. CT coronary plaque burden in asymptomatic patients with familial hypercholesterolaemia. Heart 2011.
15. Rivera JJ, Nasir K, Choi EK, et al. Detection of occult coronary artery disease in asymptomatic individuals with diabetes mellitus using non-invasive cardiac angiography. Atherosclerosis 2009; 203: 442–8.
16. Dedic A, Rossi A, Ten Kate GJ, et al. First-line evaluation of coronary artery disease with coronary calcium scanning or exercise electrocardiography. Int J Cardiol. 2011.
17. Sarwar A, Shaw LJ, Shapiro MD, et al. Diagnostic and prognostic value of absence of coronary artery calcification. JACC Cardiovasc Imaging 2009; 2: 675–88.
18. Wilson PW, D'Agostino RB, Levy D, et al. Prediction of coronary heart disease using risk factor categories. Circulation 1998; 97: 1837–47.
19. Erbel R, Mohlenkamp S, Moebus S, et al. Coronary risk stratification, discrimination, and reclassification improvement based on quantification of subclinical coronary atherosclerosis: the Heinz Nixdorf Recall study. J Am Coll Cardiol 2010; 56: 1397–406.

20. Chen J, Einstein AJ, Fazel R, et al. Cumulative exposure to ionizing radiation from diagnostic and therapeutic cardiac imaging procedures: a population-based analysis. J Am Coll Cardiol 2010; 56: 702–11.

21. McCollough CH. Patient dose in cardiac computed tomography. Herz 2003; 28: 1–6.

22. Mettler FA Jr, Huda W, Yoshizumi TT, Mahesh M. Effective doses in radiology and diagnostic nuclear medicine: a catalog. Radiology 2008; 248: 254–63.

23. Nieman K, Oudkerk M, Rensing BJ, et al. Coronary angiography with multi-slice computed tomography. Lancet 2001; 357: 599–603.

24. Meijboom WB, Meijs MF, Schuijf JD, et al. Diagnostic accuracy of 64-slice computed tomography coronary angiography: a prospective, multicenter, multivendor study. J Am Coll Cardiol 2008; 52: 2135–44.

25. Nasis A, Leung MC, Antonis PR, et al. Diagnostic accuracy of non-invasive coronary angiography with 320-detector row computed tomography. Am J Cardiol 2010; 106: 1429–35.

26. von Ballmoos MW, Haring B, Juillerat P, Alkadhi H. Meta-analysis: diagnostic performance of low-radiation-dose coronary computed tomography angiography. Ann Intern Med 2011; 154: 413–20.

27. Austen WG, Edwards JE, Frye RL, et al. A reporting system on patients evaluated for coronary artery disease. Report of the Ad Hoc Committee for Grading of Coronary Artery Disease, Council on Cardiovascular Surgery, American Heart Association. Circulation 1975; 51(4 Suppl): 5–40.

28. Arbab-Zadeh A, Hoe J. Quantification of coronary arterial stenoses by multidetector CT angiography in comparison with conventional angiography methods, caveats, and implications. JACC Cardiovasc Imaging 2011; 4: 191–202.

29. Pflederer T, Marwan M, Schepis T, et al. Characterization of culprit lesions in acute coronary syndromes using coronary dual-source CT angiography. Atherosclerosis 2010; 211: 437–44.

30. Hyafil F, Cornily JC, Rudd JH, et al. Quantification of inflammation within rabbit atherosclerotic plaques using the macrophage-specific CT contrast agent N1177: a comparison with 18F-FDG PET/CT and histology. J Nucl Med 2009; 50: 959–65.

31. Hulten EA, Carbonaro S, Petrillo SP, Mitchell JD, Villines TC. Prognostic value of cardiac computed tomography angiography: a systematic review and meta-analysis. J Am Coll Cardiol 2011; 57: 1237–47.

32. Voros S, Rinehart S, Qian Z, et al. Coronary atherosclerosis imaging by coronary CT angiography current status, correlation with intravascular interrogation and meta-analysis. JACC Cardiovasc Imaging 2011; 4: 537–48.

33. Mark DB, Berman DS, Budoff MJ, et al. ACCF/ACR/AHA/NASCI/SAIP/SCAI/SCCT 2010 expert consensus document on coronary computed tomographic angiography: a report of the American College of Cardiology Foundation Task Force on Expert Consensus Documents. Catheter Cardiovasc Interv 2010; 76: E1–42.

34. Ten Kate GJ, Weustink AC, de Feyter PJ. Coronary artery anomalies detected by MSCT-coronary angiography in the adult. Neth Heart J 2008; 16: 369–75.

35. Sato Y, Matsumoto N, Ichikawa M, et al. Efficacy of multislice computed tomography for the detection of acute coronary syndrome in the emergency department. Circ J 2005; 69: 1047–51.

36. Hoffmann U, Bamberg F, Chae CU, et al. Coronary computed tomography angiography for early triage of patients with acute chest pain: the ROMICAT (Rule Out Myocardial Infarction using Computer Assisted Tomography) trial. J Am Coll Cardiol 2009; 53: 1642–50.

37. Gallagher MJ, Ross MA, Raff GL, et al. The diagnostic accuracy of 64-slice computed tomography coronary angiography compared with stress nuclear imaging in emergency department low-risk chest pain patients. Ann Emerg Med 2007; 49: 125–36.

38. Schlett CL, Banerji D, Siegel E, et al. Prognostic value of CT angiography for major adverse cardiac events in patients with acute chest pain from the emergency department 2-year outcomes of the ROMICAT trial. JACC Cardiovasc Imaging 2011; 4: 481–91.

39. Budoff MJ, Shavelle DM, Lamont DH, et al. Usefulness of electron beam computed tomography scanning for distinguishing ischemic from nonischemic cardiomyopathy. J Am Coll Cardiol 1998; 32: 1173–8.

40. Abunassar JG, Yam Y, Chen L, D'Mello N, Chow BJ. Usefulness of the Agatston score = 0 to exclude ischemic cardiomyopathy in patients with heart failure. Am J Cardiol 2011; 107: 428–32.

41. Ghostine S, Caussin C, Habis M, et al. Non-invasive diagnosis of ischaemic heart failure using 64-slice computed tomography. Eur Heart J 2008; 29: 2133–40.

42. Cornily JC, Gilard M, Le Gal G, et al. Accuracy of 16-detector multislice spiral computed tomography in the initial evaluation of dilated cardiomyopathy. Eur J Radiol 2007; 61: 84–90.

43. Taylor AJ, Cerqueira M, Hodgson JM, et al. ACCF/SCCT/ACR/AHA/ASE/ASNC/NASCI/SCAI/SCMR 2010 appropriate use criteria for cardiac computed tomography. A report of the American College of Cardiology Foundation Appropriate Use Criteria Task Force, the Society of Cardiovascular Computed Tomography, the American College of Radiology, the American Heart Association, the American Society of Echocardiography, the American Society of Nuclear Cardiology, the North American Society for Cardiovascular Imaging, the Society for Cardiovascular Angiography and Interventions, and the Society for Cardiovascular Magnetic Resonance. J Am Coll Cardiol 2010; 56: 1864–94.

44. Hadamitzky M, Meyer T, Hein F, et al. Prognostic value of coronary computed tomographic angiography in asymptomatic patients. Am J Cardiol 2010; 105: 1746–51.

9 Magnetic resonance imaging: Role in diagnosis and risk stratification

Pier Giorgio Masci and Jan Bogaert

OUTLINE

Cardiac magnetic resonance imaging (MRI) has emerged as an increasingly useful diagnostic technique that does not involve the use of ionizing radiation, for the evaluation of patients with diverse presentations of coronary artery disease. It enables a multifaceted approach to the complexity of heart disease by exploiting an array of imaging techniques. In the acute setting of acute myocardial infarction MRI enables precise characterization of ischemic injury by differentiating reversible from irreversible damage and accurately characterizes microvascular injury. In the chronic setting, detection of ischemia and viability assessment by cardiac MRI can play a pivotal role in risk stratification. In this chapter we provide an overview of the technique, its strengths and limitations, and its role in the various presentations of coronary disease.

INTRODUCTION

Over the past few decades, cardiac magnetic resonance imaging (MRI) has emerged as an accurate diagnostic technique for the evaluation of patients with proven or suspected coronary artery disease (CAD). Of note, cardiac MRI enables a multifaceted approach to the complexity of heart disease by exploiting an array of diverse imaging techniques. In the acute setting of CAD, that is, acute myocardial infarction (MI), a comprehensive cardiac MRI study allows precise characterization of the extent and nature of ischemic myocardial injury. It provides detail on the degree of ventricular dysfunction, can differentiate reversible from irreversible injury, and quantify the extent of microvascular injury. In the chronic setting of CAD, cardiac MRI can provide, in a single examination, information on ventricular function, inducible ischemia, and myocardial viability that otherwise requires the use of several different imaging modalities. In the future, cardiac MRI may become the preferred modality for risk stratification.

APPLICATIONS

Role of Cardiac MRI in Acute CAD—the Study of Jeopardized Myocardium

The study of acute ischemic myocardial damage has to take into account the complexity of events occurring in an evolving MI. As a reperfused infarct evolves, the myocardium first becomes edematous, thereafter hyperemia, hemorrhage and inflammation appear, and are followed by the processes of repair. Thus, an acute infarct goes through a series of inflammatory and healing stages with replacement of the dead myocardium by collagenized scar tissue. Cardiac MRI is an ideal imaging tool for an accurate in-vivo depiction of the abovementioned pathophysiological phenomena by using its array of techniques (Figs. 9.1 and 9.2).

Characterization of Myocardium (Area) at Risk

In the past years, a growing body of evidence has been accumulated on the value of T2-weighted imaging in detecting myocardium (or area) at risk, that is, the ischemic myocardium at the time of coronary occlusion (Fig. 9.3). This sequence is particularly sensitive to free water content enabling accurate visualization of the myocardial edema caused by acute ischemic damage. Experimentally, Aletras et al. (1) demonstrated that the hyperintense edematous region depicted on T2-weighted imaging two days after a reperfused infarction corresponded to the area at risk demarcated at the time of the ischemic episode. Additionally, in this canine model of reperfused infarction (90 minute of coronary occlusion), the extent of myocardium at risk was significantly larger than that of ultimately infarcted myocardium. This indicated that the edematous region visualized by T2-weighted imaging comprised both reversibly and irreversibly damaged myocardium (i.e., jeopardized myocardium). This technique has been recently validated in comparison with single-photon emission computed tomography (SPECT) in patients with reperfused ST-segment elevation MI. In particular, the myocardium at risk determined during coronary occlusion, using [99-m] Tc-tetrofosmin SPECT on the day of infarction, was closely similar to that yielded by T2-weighted imaging 7 days after the acute event. Besides the fact that T2-weighted imaging is completely non-invasive and ionizing radiation-free, this technique holds the advantage that the area at risk can be determined retrospectively. Considering that myocardial edema is a consistent feature of acute ischemia, T2-weighted imaging has been used to identify patients with unstable angina or evolving MI in the emergency department. Finally, T2-weighted imaging allows depiction of post-reperfusion myocardial hemorrhage which appears as a hypointense region (caused by the paramagnetic effects of breakdown products of hemogloblin) within the core of the jeopardized myocardium. Recent studies have shown that myocardial hemorrhage post-infarction is associated with an adverse outcome (2).

Characterization of Myocardial Infarction

Contrast-enhanced cardiac MRI with late gadolinium enhancement (LGE) technique is an accurate modality to visualize and quantify irreversible ischemic damage in the context of myocardium at risk (3). This procedure consists of performing T1-weighted inversion-recovery sequence between 10 and 20 minutes after the bolus injection of gadolinium-based

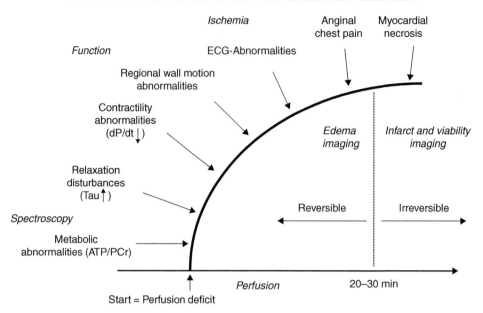

Figure 9.1 Ischemic cascade and the role of magnetic resonance imaging (MRI) techniques. MRI is of value to assess the ischemic cascade at different levels (shown in italics). *Abbreviations*: ECG, electrocardiogram.

contrast agent (CA). Although the mechanisms of LGE are yet to be fully elucidated, there is convincing evidence that on LGE imaging, the time-varying enhancement is broadly different in infarcted and normal myocardium. Basically, in the infarcted myocardium the wash-in and wash-out phases of CA are consistently delayed as compared with the normal myocardium so that on late post-contrast imaging CA concentration is higher in the infarcted myocardium. With an appropriate setting, the normal myocardium appears hypointense (dark) whereas the infarcted myocardium appears hyperintense (bright) as depicted in a typical example (Fig. 9.3). Several patho-physiological factors have been implicated in the 'late' accumulation of CA in the infarcted tissue, namely residual blood flow (anterograde and/or collateral flow) to the infarcted region, the extent of patency of the coronary microsculature and the distribution volume. The latter is of particular importance since gadolinium is an extracellular CA (i.e., distributed principally in the interstitial space). Thus, in normal myocardium with densely packed myocytes, the tissue volume is predominantly intracellular (75–80%), resulting in a low concentration of gadolinium per voxel of myocardial tissue. Acute myocardial necrosis causes an increase in distribution volume due to interstitial edema and membrane rupture resulting in increased gadolinium concentration, shortened T1 relaxation, and thus hyperenhancement (Fig. 9.4). However, the extent of LGE is significantly influenced by the time elapsed between the MI and the post-contrast imaging. Kim et al. have demonstrated an overestimation of infarct size at 3 days post infarction, disappearing when studies were repeated at 8 weeks (3). Although this can be partially explained by volume loss due to infarct shrinkage up to four-fold decrease between 4 days and 6 weeks post-infarction, recent studies

showed a significant decrease in the extent of enhancement between day 1 and day 7 post infarction, suggesting an overestimation of the extent of irreversible damage on very early imaging (day 1) (4). In a pioneering study, Reimer and Jennings showed that during the first four days after coronary occlusion, the true infarct volume almost doubles due to edema and accumulation of inflammatory cells (5). Therefore, it seems conceivable that LGE imaging overestimates the extent of infarction in the early days after an acute event because of an increase in extracellular volume that is not related to myocardial necrosis. Thanks to the high spatial resolution of the LGE technique and the marked difference in signal intensity between normal and necrotic myocardium, the extent of MI can be quantified with excellent accuracy and reproducibility. In addition, the degree of involvement of the wall (subendocardial or transmural) can be accurately depicted along with the potential involvement of small but functionally important cardiac structures, such as papillary muscles and the right ventricular wall. In particular, the current established techniques for right ventricular (RV) infarct detection underestimate the true incidence of RV ischemic injury. In a recent study, we observed RV edema and LGE in the acute phase in as many as 75% and 54%, respectively, of patients with inferior left ventricular (LV) infarction (Fig. 9.3) (6). Interestingly, RV wall edema and LGE were observed in 33% and 11%, respectively, of patients with an acute anterior LV infarction. This is due to the fact that a considerable portion of the anterolateral RV free wall is perfused by small branches of the left anterior descending (LAD) coronary artery. In another study, we demonstrated that patients with anterior MI experience more pronounced post-infarction LV remodeling and dysfunction than those with non-anterior MI due to a greater

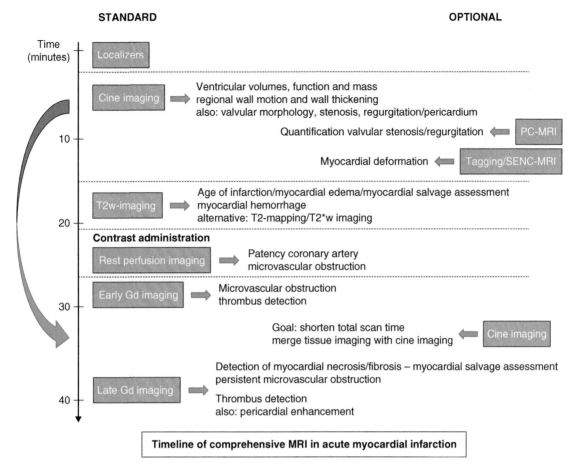

Figure 9.2 Timeline of comprehensive magnetic resonance imaging (MRI) examination in a patient with acute myocardial infarction. The standard sequences are shown on the left, the optional sequences on the right. To shorten total imaging time cine imaging can be performed following contrast administration. *Abbreviations:* Gd, gadolinium; PC-MRI, phase-contrast MRI; SENC-MRI, sensitivity-encoding MRI; T2*w imaging, T2-weighted imaging.

magnitude of myocardial necrosis without any independent contribution related to the location of infarction (7). In addition, the ability of post-contrast LGE imaging to depict myocardial necrosis as small as 1 g renders this technique ideal for depicting post-percutaneous coronary intervention (PCI) MI (8). Two types of LGE patterns due to PCI-related myocardial necrosis have been described, that is, "adjacent" myonecrosis in the neighborhood of the stent related to side-branch occlusion, and "distal" myonecrosis due to distal embolization of plaque material. Moreover, contrast-enhanced imaging is an extremely accurate technique to diagnose LV thrombus formation, which is a potentially serious complication of infarction. Mollet et al. (9) reported that LGE imaging identified LV thrombosis in a substantially higher proportion of patients than transthoracic echocardiography. Other studies have confirmed the high sensitivity and specificity of contrast-enhanced MRI in depicting LV thrombus in comparison with transthoracic or transesophageal echocardiography.

In reperfused acute MI, contrast-enhanced MRI also allows accurate assessment of the presence and extent of microvascular obstruction (MVO). Indeed, it is important to keep in mind that although primary PCI is effective in achieving rapid and sustained patency of the infarct-related artery, a considerable proportion of ST-segment elevation MI patients (up to 50%) show impaired myocardial reperfusion due to MVO (10). On contrast-enhanced imaging, MVO typically appears as a subendocardially located hypointense area within the hyperenhanced myocardium (i.e., infarcted myocardium). To fully appreciate the extent of MVO, contrast-enhanced imaging should be performed as soon as possible after CA administration in order to minimize the diffusion of gadolinium molecules into the MVO zone, which results in an underestimation of this phenomenon (Fig. 9.2) (11). The occurrence of MVO is independently associated with the lack of functional recovery, adverse ventricular remodeling and worse patient outcome (12,13). MRI will facilitate the assessment, in randomized

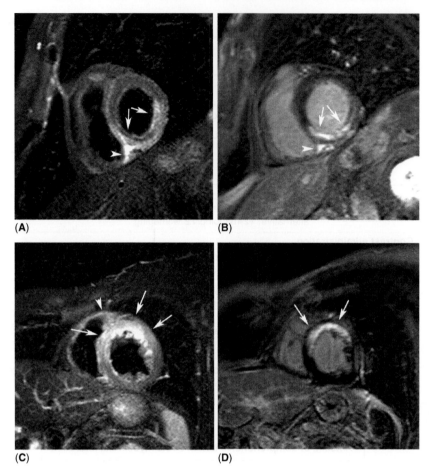

Figure 9.3 Combined T2-weighted magnetic resonance imaging (MRI) (A,C) and late gadolinium enhancement (LGE) MRI (B,D) in acute myocardial infarction. Patient with an acute reperfused inferior left ventricular infarction (A,B), and a second patient with an acute reperfused anteroseptal infarction (C,D). Edema imaging, using T2-weighted imaging, shows increased signal intensity in the area at risk (*arrows*, A,C). Moreover, the extension of edema into the right ventricular free wall can be visualized (*arrowheads*, A,C). LGE MRI enables to accurately depict the presence, circumferential and transmural extent of necrosis (*arrows*, B,D), and the extension toward the right ventricular inferior wall (*arrowhead*, B).

controlled trials, of techniques and drugs that may prove beneficial in this setting.

To sum up, in patients with acute MI, a comprehensive cardiac MRI study performed in the first week after the acute event can provide an accurate estimate of myocardium at risk, microvascular damage and the extent of infarction (Fig. 9.2). Additionally, myocardial salvage can be derived by subtracting the infarct size from the amount of myocardium at risk. Myocardial salvage is independently associated with early ST-segment resolution (14), and is an independent predictor of adverse LV remodeling and major cardiac events (i.e., cardiac deaths, non-fatal MI) at intermediate follow-up (14,15). Although the volume of myocardium at risk exceeds that of irreversibly damaged myocardium, they are closely related (14). Typically, edema involves the entire width of the myocardial wall, whereas the transmural spread of necrosis is variable. Interestingly in an MRI study by Francone et al. (16), it was shown that increasing ischemic time does not affect the extent of myocardium at risk

but results in an increasing infarct size and subsequently decreased myocardial salvage. In particular, salvaged myocardium was markedly reduced after 90 min of coronary occlusion. Early mechanical reperfusion and maintenance of antegrade or collateral flow independently preserves myocardial salvage primarily through a reduction of the extent of transmural infarction. Myocardial salvage corrects the extent of MI by area at risk rendering this index particularly attractive as a surrogate end-point for testing novel or adjunctive reperfusion strategies (17).

Cardiac MRI in Patients with Acute Chest Pain
Accumulating data support an increasing role for cardiac MRI in the evaluation of patients with acute chest pain. American Heart Association guidelines recommend a non-invasive approach in those patients with low likelihood for MI or with severe co-morbidities. Similarly, European Society of Cardiology guidelines recommend non-invasive

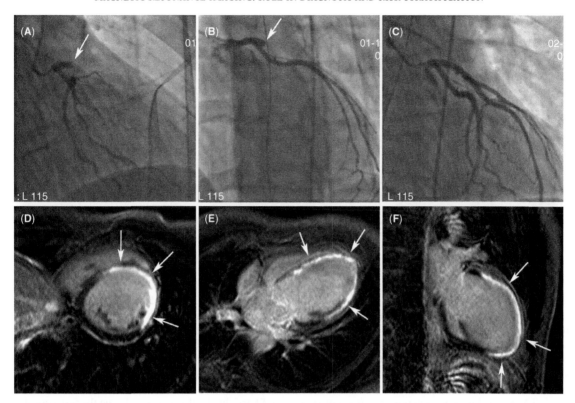

Figure 9.4 Traumatic occlusion of the LAD coronary artery, following a scooter accident, in a 35-year-old man. Coronary angiography before (**A,B**) and after PCI (**C**) shows total occlusion of the proximal LAD (*arrows*, **A,B**), with restoration of patency post PCI and stent placement (c). LGE MRI in cardiac short-axis (D), horizontal long-axis (E) and vertical long-axis (F) planes shows extensive, nearly complete transmural infarction (*arrows*, D–F) involving more than 50% of the left ventricle.

imaging testing in patients with acute chest pain but serial negative troponins and a normal or non-diagnostic electrocardiogram (ECG). Although the diagnosis of ST-segment elevation MI is straightforward, the majority of patients with acute chest pain admitted to the emergency department do not have an acute coronary syndrome. This scenario is further complicated by the universal definition of MI based on merican College of Cardiology/European Society of Cardiology consensus document, which suggested troponin measurements and the ECG as the cornerstone tests for diagnosing acute MI. As a matter of fact, troponins are a sensitive but poorly specific marker of ischemic myocardial damage since an increase in troponin is caused by any condition provoking myocyte necrosis. Additionally, troponin increase is limited to a relatively narrow time window reducing their sensitivity in subacute infarction. Similarly, ECG changes overlap between ischemic and non-ischemic heart disease, and a small infarction may not result in typical ECG abnormalities. In these circumstances, comprehensive cardiac MRI examination is of great value in diagnosing and, eventually, differentiating acute MI from other similar clinical entities such as perimyocarditis, Takotsubo cardiomyopathy, or acute aortic disease. In the latter condition, however, it should be kept in mind that cardiac computed tomography is the preferential

Focus Box 9.1

a. Cardiac magnetic resonance imaging (MRI) has evolved as one of the preferred imaging modalities to study the entire spectrum of patients with coronary artery disease, ranging from those presenting with acute coronary syndromes and evolving myocardial infarction (MI) to those with chronic coronary artery disease

b. In patients with acute MI, cardiac MRI offers full characterization of the jeopardized myocardium along with the assessment of the consequences on ventricular function and detection of life-threatening mechanical complications. In particular, T2-weighted and post-contrast late gadolinium enhancement imaging allow accurate assessment of the amount of myocardium at risk and the extent of myocardial necrosis, respectively. The combination of the two techniques allows a precise quantification of the salvaged myocardium, an ideal surrogate end-point to test the effectiveness of reperfusion strategies

c. MRI in the early phase of acute MI may overestimate the extent of myocardial damage

d. In patients presenting with acute chest pain, cardiac MRI is useful in the diagnosis of less common causes of myocardial damage such as myopericarditis or Takotsubo cardiomyopathy

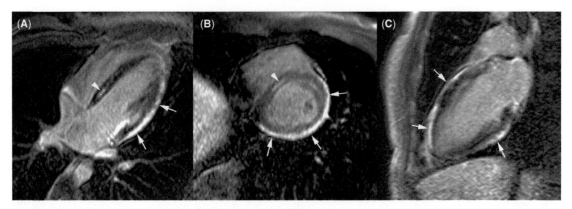

Figure 9.5 Myocarditis in a 21-year-old man. Late gadolinium enhancement magnetic resonance imaging in horizontal long-axis (A), short-axis (B), and vertical long-axis (C) image plane. Strong enhancement is seen in the subepicardial part of the entire lateral left ventricular wall, extending to the anterior as well to the inferior wall (*arrows*, A–C). Moreover, focal midmyocardial enhancement is present in the basal part of the ventricular septum (*arrowhead*, A,B).

imaging technique. In patients presenting with acute chest pain, troponin elevation but a normal coronary angiogram, cardiac MRI may yield findings typical for acute myocarditis in as many as 30–50% of the cases (Fig. 9.5). In Takotsubo cardiomyopathy, which is characterized by typical chest pain, ECG changes, and normal coronary angiography, cardiac MRI may uncover akinesia or dyskinesia of the LV apex and edema on T2-weighted imaging, whereas the pattern of myocardial LGE, when present, is typically different from that of myocarditis or acute MI. However, it has to be kept in mind that only few clinical trials have addressed the value of cardiac MRI in patients with acute chest pain admitted to the emergency department. Of note, Kwong et al. (18) reported that contrast-enhanced MRI (T2-weighted imaging was not performed) had a sensitivity of 84% and specificity of 85% for the diagnosis of an acute coronary syndrome in patients with chest pain, normal, or raised troponin but without ST-segment elevation. Other authors (19), by adding T2-weighted imaging to the study protocol improved the overall accuracy of cardiac MRI in detecting acute MI yielding a sensitivity of 85% and specificity of 96%. Based on the data by Kwong et al. (18), cardiac MRI is feasible in an emergency department setting since only 11% of patients were excluded from analysis (5% because of claustrophobia). However, in routine clinical practice there are several constraints limiting the application of cardiac MRI in patients presenting to medical attention because of acute chest pain, such as limited capability to accommodate studies in an emergency setting.

Role of Cardiovascular Magnetic Resonance in Chronic CAD
Detection of Inducible Myocardial Ischemia
Cardiac MRI has gained acceptance as an accurate, reproducible, and radiation-free technique to assess inducible myocardial ischemia by means of two main modalities, namely stress-perfusion and stress-function cardiac MRI.

Stress-Perfusion Cardiac MRI
The principle of the most common approach of stress-perfusion cardiac MRI consists of monitoring the wash-in kinetics of gadolinium-based CA into the myocardium during pharmacologically induced hyperemic state (adenosine or dipyridamole). This technique relies on the differences in signal intensity between ischemic and non-ischemic myocardium as depicted by T1-weighted pulse sequence during the first-pass of CA. In particular, the ischemic myocardium is visualized as a dark region (hypointense) as compared with normally perfused (hyperintense) myocardium (Fig. 9.6). Several requirements are mandatory to ensure good accuracy in detecting inducible myocardial ischemia by stress-perfusion cardiac MRI. Considering that the first-pass of CA lasts about 5–15 seconds, the T1-weighted pulse sequence has to be fast (i.e., high temporal resolution) but must permit optimal coverage of the left ventricle. In addition, signal- and contrast-to-noise ratios have to be sufficiently high to reliably differentiate normally and hypo-perfused myocardium. Finally, good spatial resolution is required to differentiate subendocardial from transmural perfusion defects. At present this technique has been well validated (20,21), showing similar or even better accuracy as compared with routinely used techniques such as SPECT imaging. In the largest perfusion-stress cardiac MRI study conducted in 18 centers in Europe and USA, the perfusion imaging yielded an area-under-curve of 0.86 (sensitivity and specificity of 86 and 67%, respectively) (21). In a meta-analysis including 24 studies (1516 patients), perfusion imaging demonstrated a sensitivity of 91% (CI 88–94%) and a specificity of 81% (CI 77–85%) (22). In comparison with $^{13}NH_3$- labeled positron emission tomography as the reference standard, sensitivity and specificity for ischemia detection by stress-perfusion MRI were 91% and 94%, respectively, and for detection of ≥50% diameter stenoses, sensitivity and specificity were 87% and 85%, respectively. Adenosine and dipyridamole are the most commonly used vasodilator agents in stress-perfusion

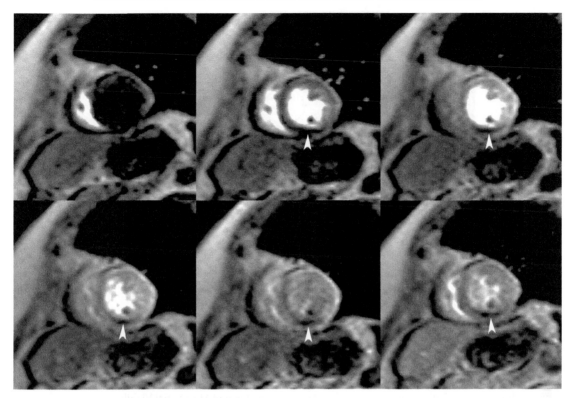

Figure 9.6 Adenosine stress-perfusion defect in inferior left ventricular wall in a 70-year-old woman with in-stent restenosis following percutaneous coronary intervention of right coronary artery and left circumflex coronary arteries. Six time frames are shown starting at the arrival of contrast in the right ventricular cavity (*left upper panel*), till the moment of the second pass (*right lower panel*). The perfusion defect (*arrowhead*) becomes visible as soon as the normal myocardium enhances, while the myocardium supplied by the stenotic coronary artery is visible as hypo-intense myocardium that fills-in (and enhances) slowly. In this case, there was a long persistence of the perfusion defect.

cardiac MRI. Adenosine induces maximal hyperemia during the third minute of infusion (0.14 mg/min/kg) and has a particularly short half-life (10 seconds) resulting in an excellent safety profile (1 infarction in 9000 examinations, no death). Dipyridamole causes indirect coronary vasodilatation by inhibiting the re-uptake and catabolism of adenosine, and the infusion regime of 0.56 mg/kg for 4 min yields the peak of vasodilatation at 2–4 minutes. Dipyridamole is catabolized by the liver and its half-life is in the range of 6 hours requiring the administration of its antidote (i.e., aminophylline) at the end of stress-perfusion. However, due to its prolonged half-life, dipyridamole stress cardiac MRI provides the possibility to combine the analysis of LV wall motion with myocardial perfusion improving the specificity of the stress test. A modified protocol using higher dose of dipyridamole (0.84 mg/kg administered in 6 minutes) similarly to that used in dipyridamole stress-echocardiography has been proposed.

Whereas in daily clinical practice, stress-induced perfusion defects are usually assessed visually based on the presence of a subendocardial or transmural hypo-intense rim during the first-pass of CA, semi-quantitative or quantitative approaches have become available, slowly finding their way into clinical practice. A relatively simple semi-quantitative method, used by several groups, is the assessment of the myocardial perfusion reserve (MPR) or MPR index in patients with CAD, which is defined as the ratio of regional myocardial blood flow under hyperemic conditions to that under resting conditions, and has been validated against other techniques such as coronary fractional flow reserve measurements. Al-Saadi et al. (20) found a significant difference in MPR between ischemic and normal myocardial segments (1.08 ± 0.23 and 2.33 ± 0.41, $p < 0.001$). Using a cut-off value of 1.5, the diagnostic sensitivity, specificity, and diagnostic accuracy for the detection of coronary artery stenosis ($\geq 75\%$) were 90%, 83%, and 87%, respectively. Using fractional flow reserve in addition to the degree of stenosis on coronary angiography as reference standard, an MPR index cut-off value of 1.5 was able to distinguish hemodynamically relevant from non-relevant coronary lesions with a sensitivity of 88% and specificity of 90%.

Stress-Function Cardiac MRI

Although it is possible to perform exercise stress-function MRI using a specific MRI-compatible cycle ergometer, functional stress testing is usually performed during dobutamine

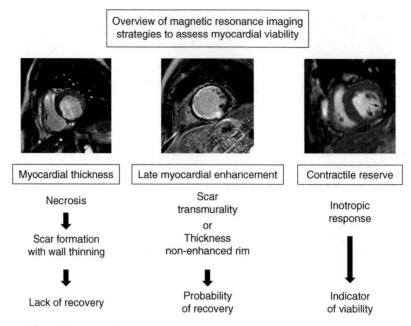

Figure 9.7 Overview of magnetic resonance imaging strategies to assess myocardial viability.

(± atropine) administration. Dobutatime-stress cardiac MRI consists of the assessment of regional wall motion during the infusion of increasing dose of dobutamine, paralleling the protocol used in stress echocardiography. The great advantage of dobutamine-stress cardiac MRI as compared with echocardiography resides in the absence of restriction due to image quality yielding an excellent reproducibility (23). In particular, several studies have demonstrated the superiority of high-dose stress dobutamine MRI to high-dose dobutamine stress echocardiography in detecting patients with significant CAD (≥50% diameter stenosis) (24). Patients with poor echo windows derive particular benefit from MRI stress testing. The better MRI image quality was deemed responsible for the higher accuracy (86% vs. 72.7%). During the stress testing, myocardium supplied by a normal coronary artery will show a progressive increase in myocardial contractility. By contrast, myocardium supplied by a flow-limiting coronary stenosis will become ischemic when the increase in coronary blood supply is insufficient to match the increased demand in oxygen, resulting in wall motion abnormalities. Over the last few years, some pivotal studies highlighted also the prognostic value of dobutamine-stress MRI by reporting an excellent outcome in patients with negative stress imaging (25). Of note, the predictive value of major adverse cardiac event was similar for stress-perfusion and dobutamine cardiac MRI (25). Besides detection of flow-limiting coronary stenoses in patients suspected of obstructive CAD, another application for stress function imaging is the differentiation between viable and non-viable dysfunctional myocardium in patients with chronic CAD.

Assessment of Myocardial Viability
Transient sub-lethal ischemia rapidly impairs contractile function, and this dysfunction can persist for hours after the restoration of normal match between oxygen demand and supply. This phenomenon is known as myocardial stunning, and repeated episodes of ischemia may result in cumulative stunning contributing to chronic post-ischemic LV dysfunction. Myocardial hibernation is a concept derived by the clinical observation that patients with post-ischemic LV dysfunction before revascularization improved ventricular function after coronary by-pass. A severe reduction of coronary flow reserve is observed both in stunning and hibernation, and the functional recovery of hibernated myocardium is associated with restoration of an adequate flow reserve. It is important to emphasize that most of our knowledge on the clinical utility of pre-operative assessment of myocardial viability in patients with chronic LV post-ischemic dysfunction is based on retrospective studies. These indicate that viability testing includes information regarding in-hospital or 1-year prognosis when added to clinical and angiographic data. However, recently a sub-study of the STICH trial suggests that the assessment of myocardial viability by SPECT in patients with chronic LV dysfunction did not identify patients with a different survival benefit from by-pass as compared with guideline-based medical therapy (26). The different approaches to assess myocardial viability and a timeline for a comprehensive examination are shown in Figures 9.6 and 9.7.

Dobutamine-stress cardiac MRI at low-dose of dobutamine (5–10 μg kg min⁻¹) increases contractility in dysfunctional but viable segments whereas at higher doses (up to 40 µg kg min^{-1} plus atropine) contractility may decrease reflecting inducible myocardial ischemia. The so called "biphasic response" is highly predictive of post-operative functional recovery. LV segments with transmural scar usually do not show functional recovery in contrast to those without significant scarring. Dobutamine stress MRI has a good specificity (83%, range 70–95%) but moderate sensitivity (74%, range 50–89%), values that are in line with those of dobutamine echocardiography (27).

Contrast-enhanced cardiac MRI enables accurate detection of replacement myocardial fibrosis due to a previous MI. This is due to the fact that in fibrotic scars, similar to what is observed in acutely necrotic myocardium, the intracellular space is markedly reduced in favor of extracellular space yielding an accumulation of gadolinium-based contrast media in the scarred myocardium. As a result, on post-contrast LGE imaging the scarred myocardium appears hyperintensive whereas the signal of normal myocardium is "nulled" and appears black. In patients with stable CAD myocardial LGE frequently occurs in dysfunctional segments and is associated with nonviability on SPECT imaging or dobutamine echocardiography, whereas absence of LGE correlates with measures of viability irrespective of resting function. In particular the likelihood of improvement in regional contractility after revascularization is inversely related to the transmural extent of hyperenhancement (28). In dysfunctional segments without hyperenhancement 78% had improved contractility post-revascularization as compared with only 2% of segments with scar tissue extending >75% of the LV wall. These findings resulted in a paradigm shift, that is, the absence of LGE in a thinned (<5 mm) and dysfunctional myocardium, previously assumed to be non-viable myocardium, and can potentially be associated with restoration of normal function after revascularation. Post-contrast LGE technique has an excellent sensitivity (97%, range 91–100%) but a relatively low specificity (68%, range 51–85%) (29). The relatively low specificity can be ascribed to several factors: (*i*) short-term follow-up between revascularization and assessment of LV function (time course of hibernating myocardium functional recovery can require up to 14 months), (*ii*) false positive results including those due to procedural injury, (*iii*) incomplete revascularization, and (*iv*) tethering to adjacent scarred segments.

Diagnosis of Unrecognized Myocardial Infarction

Patients with unrecognized infarction have a prognosis comparable or even worse than patients with diagnosed MI. Previous studies indicate that more than one fourth of apparently healthy patients (age >30 years) have an unrecognized infarction based on abnormal Q-wave on ECG. However, by definition the ECG is unable to detect old non-Q wave infarction and, in addition, pathological Q-wave can be observed in non-ischemic cardiomyopathy. LV wall motion abnormalities may not occur unless the infarcted region exceeds at least 20% of myocardial wall thickness.

Similarly SPECT is unable to identify infarcts involving less than 10 g of tissue. Thus, the prevalence of unrecognized MI is underestimated and several studies have shown, using contrast-enhanced MRI as a morphologic in-vivo validation technique, that the ECG significantly underestimates the true prevalence of myocardial scarring due to prior MI. Importantly, the presence of prior MI as detected by LGE imaging was independently associated with major adverse cardiac events beyond the clinical and angiographic determinants, LV volumes, and function (30). Typically, the ECG has a particularly low sensitivity but a good specificity in detecting healed MI, and those patients with positive ECG criteria for healed MI have larger MIs, lower LV ejection fraction, and a poorer wall motion score compared with those without ECG evidence of MI. Interestingly, the comparison of contrast-enhanced LGE imaging and ECG in patients with a prior MI has prompted to reconsider our previous knowledge regarding the ECG abnormalities in patients with healed MI. First, Q-wave infarction is not associated with the transmural spread of infarction but rather with MI size. Second, ECG-derived estimates of infarct size correlate modestly with LGE extent resulting in an overestimating small infarcts and underestimating large infarcts. Importantly, the lateral LV territories are electrically silent and therefore may show little ECG alterations. Recently, a consensus statement of a multi-specialist team has assessed the correspondence between ECG and contrast-enhanced MRI findings in patients with Q-wave infarction (31). The consensus defined the infarct locations based on LGE imaging by using the name of the more involved wall or segment of the left ventricle, and then correlated these findings with the pattern of abnormal Q-wave and Q-wave equivalent. Although four out of six ECG patterns had good sensitivity (>80%) and specificity (>90%) in correctly assigning the location of infarct location, however, the lateral and mid-anterior ECG patterns yielded a sensitivity of only 66% (Fig. 9.8).

PERSONAL PERSPECTIVE AND EVOLVING INDICATIONS

In the last decade, cardiac MRI has gained acceptance in the cardiology community as an accurate and reproducible diagnostic imaging modality in patients with CAD. As a matter

Focus Box 9.2

a. Stress perfusion and stress function cardiac magnetic resonance imaging (MRI) are highly valuable but currently still underused techniques to study patients with chronic coronary artery disease with excellent diagnostic accuracy
b. Post contrast LGE and low dose dobutamine cardiac MRI enable an accurate evaluation of myocardial viability
c. Post contrast late gadolinium enhancement cardiac MRI is an ideal technique to detect silent myocardial infarction outperforming the other diagnostic modalities

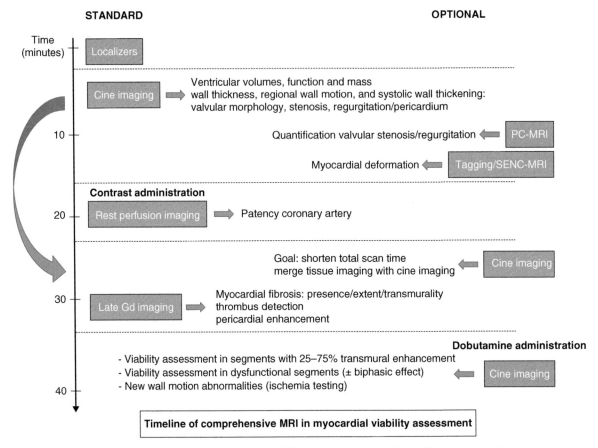

Figure 9.8 Timeline of comprehensive magnetic resonance imaging (MRI) examination in myocardial viability assessment. The standard sequences are shown on the left, the optional sequences on the right. To shorten total imaging time cine imaging can be performed following contrast administration. *Abbreviations*: Gd, gadolinium; PC-MRI, phase-contrast MRI; SENC-MRI, sensitivity-encoding MRI.

of fact, the better awareness of clinical cardiologists about the potential of cardiac MRI, the increased availability of magnetic resonance scanners and skilled operators along with the evidence-based indications for performing this kind of imaging studies are rapidly filling the gap between cardiac MRI and the other imaging modalities. In particular, in patients with acute MI, a comprehensive cardiac MRI study enables an accurate and reproducible assessment of both reversible and irreversible ischemic myocardial damage. Notably, the further development of post-processing software for more reliable, reproducible, and easier automatic detection and characterization of the ischemic myocardial damage will likely improve the usage of cardiac MRI in patients with acute MI. In the setting of chronic CAD, myocardial ischemia detection by stress-perfusion imaging will benefit from techniques and post-processing analysis aiming at quantifying the myocardial blood flow. In the near future, clinical studies are needed to test the value of post-contrast LGE imaging in predicting global LV function recovery and prognosis after coronary revascularization in patients with ischemic LV dysfunction.

REFERENCES
1. Aletras AH, Tilak GS, Natanzon A, et al. Retrospective determination of the area at risk for reperfused acute myocardial infarction with T2-weighted cardiac magnetic resonance imaging. Histopathological and displacement encoding with stimulated echoes (DENSE) functional validations. Circulation 2006; 113: 1865–70.
2. Ganame J, Messalli G, Dymarkowski S, et al. Impact of myocardial hemorrhage on left ventricular function and remodelling in patients with reperfused acute myocardial infarction. Eur Heart J 2009; 30: 662–70.
3. Kim RJ, Fieno DS, Parrish TB, et al. Relationship of MRI delayed contrast enhancement to irreversible injury, infarct age, and contractile function. Circulation 1999; 100: 1992–2002.
4. Engblom H, Hedström E, Heiberg E, et al. Rapid initial reduction of hyperenhanced myocardium after reperfused first myocardial infarction suggests recovery of the peri-infarction zone. One-year follow-up by MRI. Circ Cardiovasc Imaging 2009; 2: 47–55.

5. Reimer KA, Jennings RB. The changing anatomic reference base of evolving myocardial infarction. Underestimation of myocardial collateral blood flow and overestimation of experimental anatomic infarct size due to tissue edema, hemorrhage and acute inflammation. Circulation 1979; 60: 866–76.

6. Masci PG, Francone M, Desmet W, et al. Right ventricular ischemic injury in patients with acute ST-segment elevation myocardial infarction. Characterization with cardiovascular magnetic resonance. Circulation 2010; 122: 1405–12.

7. Masci PG, Ganame J, Francone M, et al. Relationship between location and size of myocardial infarction and their reciprocal influences on post-infarction left ventricular remodelling. Eur Heart J 2011.

8. Porto I, Selvanayagam JB, Van Gaal WJ, et al. Plaque volume and occurrence and location of periprocedural myocardial necrosis after percutaneous coronary intervention. Insights from delayed-enhancement magnetic resonance imaging, thrombolysis in myocardial infarction myocardial perfusion grade analysis, and intravascular ultrasound. Circulation 2006; 114: 662–9.

9. Mollet NR, Dymarkowski S, Volders W, et al. Visualization of ventricular thrombi with contrast-enhanced magnetic resonance imaging in patients with ischemic heart disease. Circulation 2002; 106: 2873–76.

10. Niccoli G, Burzotta F, Galiuto L Crea F. Myocardial no-reflow in humans. J Am Coll Cardiol 2009; 54: 281–92.

11. Bogaert J, Kalantzi M, Rademakers FE, Dymarkowski S, Janssens S. Determinants and impact of microvascular obstruction in successfully reperfused ST-segment elevation myocardial infarction. Assessment by magnetic resonance imaging. Eur Radiol 2007; 17: 2572–80.

12. Hombach V, Grebe O, Merkle N, et al. Sequelae of acute myocardial infarction regarding cardiac structure and function and their prognostic significance as assessed by magnetic resonance imaging. Eur Heart J 2005; 26: 549–57.

13. Wu KC, Zerhouni EA, Judd RM, et al. Prognostic significance of microvascular obstruction by magnetic resonance imaging in patients with acute myocardial infarction. Circulation 1998; 97: 765–72.

14. Masci PG, Ganame J, Strata E, et al. Myocardial salvage by CMR correlates with LV remodeling and early ST-segment resolution in acute myocardial infarction. J Am Coll Cardiol Imaging 2010; 3: 45–51.

15. Eitel I, Desch S, Fuernau G, et al. Prognostic significance and determinants of myocardial salvage assessed by cardiovascular magnetic resonance in acute reperfused myocardial infarction. J Am Coll Cardiol 2010; 55: 2470–9.

16. Francone M, Bucciarelli-Ducci C, Carbone I, et al. Impact of primary coronary angioplasty delay on myocardial salvage, infarct size, and microvascular damage in patients with ST-segment elevation myocardial infarction. Insight from cardiovascular magnetic resonance. J Am Coll Cardiol 2009; 54: 2145–53.

17. Desmet W, Bogaert J, Dubois C, et al. High-dose intracoronary adenosine for myocardial salvage in patients with acute ST-segment elevation myocardial infarction. Eur Heart J 2011; 32: 867–77.

18. Kwong RY, Schussheim AE, Rekhraj S, et al. Detecting acute coronary syndrome in the emergency department with cardiac magnetic resonance imaging. Circulation 2003; 107: 531–7.

19. Curry RC, Shash K, NagurneyJT, et al. Cardiac magnetic resonance with T2-weighted imaging improves detection of patients with acute coronary syndrome in the emergency department. Circulation 2008; 118: 837–44.

20. Al-Saadi N, Nagel E, Gross M, et al. Noninvasive detection of myocardial ischemia from perfusion reserve based on cardiovascular magnetic resonance. Circulation 2000; 101: 824–34.

21. Schwitter J, Wacker CM, Van Rossum AC, et al. MR-Impact: comparison of perfusion-cardiac magnetic resonance with single-photon emission computed tomography for the detection of coronary artery disease in a multicentre, multivendor, randomized trial. Eur Heart J 2008; 29: 480–9.

22. Nandalur KR, Dwamena BA, Choudhri AF, Nandalur MR, Carlos RC. Diagnostic performance of stress cardiac magnetic resonance imaging in the detection of coronary artery disease. A meta-analysis. J Am Coll Cardiol 2007; 50: 1343–53.

23. Paetsch I, Jahnke C, Ferrari VA, et al. Determination of interobserver variability for identifying inducible left ventricular wall motion abnormalities during dobutamine stress magnetic resonance imaging. Eur Heart J 2006; 27: 1459–64.

24. Nagel E, Lehmkuhl HB, Bocksch W, et al. Noninvasive diagnosis of ischemia-induced wall motion abnormalities with the use of high-dose dobutamine stress MRI: comparison with dobutamine stress echocardiography. Circulation 1999; 99: 763–70.

25. Jahnke C, Nagel E, Gebker R, et al. Prognostic value of cardiac magnetic resonance stress tests: Adenosine stress perfusion and dobutamine stress wall motion imaging. Circulation 2007; 115: 1769–76.

26. Bonow RO, Maurer G, Lee KL, et al. STICH Trial Investigators. Myocardial viability and survival in ischemic left ventricular dysfunction. N Engl J Med 2011; 364: 1617–25.

27. Kaandorp TAM, Lamb HJ, Van Der Wall EE, De Roos A, Bax JJ. Cardiovascular MR to assess myocardial viability in chronic ischaemic LV dysfunction. Heart 2005; 91: 1359–65.

28. Kim RJ, Wu E, Rafael A, et al. The use of contrast-enhanced magnetic resonance imaging to identify reversible myocardial dysfunction. N Engl J Med 2000; 343: 1445–53.

29. Camici PG, Prasad SK, Rimoldi OE. Stunning, hibernation, and assessment of myocardial viability. Circulation 2008; 117: 103–14.

30. Kwong RY, Chan AK, Brown KA, et al. Impact of unrecognized myocardial scar detected by cardiac magnetic resonance imaging on event-free survival in patients presenting with signs or symptoms or coronary artery disease. Circulation 2006; 113: 2733–43.

31. Bayés de Luna A, Wagner G, Birnbaum Y, et al. A new terminology for left ventricular walls and location of myocardial infarcts that present Q wave based on the standard of cardiac magnetic resonance imaging. A statement for healthcare professionals from a committee appointed by the International Society for Holter and Noninvasive electrocardiography. Circulation 2006; 114: 1755–60.

10 PET-CT: Role in diagnosis and potential to predict the response to revascularization

Angela S. Koh and Marcelo F. Di Carli

OUTLINE

Despite advances in therapy and prevention strategies, coronary artery disease (CAD) remains highly prevalent worldwide. This has stimulated continued expansion and refinement of our non-invasive armamentarium for guiding diagnosis and management of CAD. The integration of positron emission tomography (PET) with multidetector CT scanners provides a unique opportunity to delineate cardiac and vascular anatomic abnormalities, and their physiological consequences in a single setting. It allows detection and quantification of the burden and the extent of calcified and non-calcified plaques, quantification of vascular reactivity and endothelial health, identification of flow-limiting coronary stenoses, and assessment of myocardial viability. In this chapter, we will review technical considerations regarding the clinical use of PET/CT in cardiovascular disease, and the potential application of this integrated imaging strategy for diagnosis and management of CAD.

TECHNICAL CONSIDERATIONS

Several technical advantages account for the improved image quality and diagnostic ability of PET compared with single photon emission CT (SPECT). First, the application of routine measured (depth independent) attenuation correction helps to decrease false positive scans from soft tissue attenuation. Of note, artifacts due to errors in attenuation correction are common and have been reported in 30–60% of cases with PET/CT (1,2). These artifacts are usually related to the misalignments between emission and CT transmission datasets caused by the patient, cardiac, and/or respiratory motion (2,3), and may lead to false regional defects in some cases (4). The development of dedicated software for routine correction of misalignments between transmission and emission images has helped to reduce the frequency of artifacts and improve diagnostic accuracy. Second, PET has higher spatial and contrast resolution (heart-to-background ratio) that allows improved detection of small perfusion defects, thereby decreasing false negatives and increasing sensitivity. New detector technology for PET has led to continued improvement in the overall count detection sensitivity and spatial resolution (5). Increased detector sensitivity combined with optimization of scanner electronics and improved image reconstruction algorithms have substantially improved overall image quality and allow decreased patient doses compared with prior generation PET systems. Third, PET has high temporal resolution, which allows dynamic imaging of radiotracer kinetics and absolute quantification of myocardial perfusion (in mL/min/g of tissue). Fourth, the optimization of list mode imaging has been particularly important for cardiac imaging because it enables multiple image reconstructions (see imaging protocols below) from a single image acquisition, thereby facilitating a more comprehensive examination. Finally, the emergence of integrated PET/CT technology as the dominant configuration of clinical scanners holds great promise for cardiac imaging as it permits combined examinations delineating both the anatomic extent of epicardial coronary atherosclerosis and the physiological consequence of these lesions assessed by myocardial perfusion PET imaging. The integration of PET and magnetic resonance imaging (MRI) scanners may further expand the possibilities for the combined characterization of myocardial tissue architecture and physiology (6).

Radiopharmaceuticals for Clinical PET Imaging

Table 10.1 describes PET imaging agents that have been used to evaluate myocardial perfusion imaging in humans. Rubidium-82 is a potassium analog with kinetic properties similar to those of Thallium-201 (7). It is approved by the U.S. Food & Drug Administration (FDA) for cardiac imaging. Because it is a generator product, Rubidium-82 is the most widely used radionuclide for assessment of myocardial perfusion with PET. Its parent radionuclide is Strontium-82, which has a physical half-life of 26 days. Consequently, the Strontium-82/Rubidium-82 generator is replaced every 4 weeks. The short physical half-life of Rubidium-82 (76 sec) and the rapid reconstitution of the generator allow for fast sequential perfusion imaging and laboratory throughput, thereby maximizing clinical efficiency.

[13]N-ammonia requires an on-site cyclotron and radiopharmacy synthesis capability. It is also FDA-approved for cardiac imaging. It has a physical half-life of ~10 min. The first pass myocardial extraction of ^{13}N-ammonia is high, although, like other extractable tracers (e.g., Rubidium-82), it decreases at higher blood flow rates. Regional myocardial retention of ^{13}N-ammonia may be heterogeneous—the lateral wall of the left ventricle (LV) tends to have lower activity than that of other segments. ^{13}N-ammonia images may also be occasionally degraded by intense liver and/or lung (especially in heart failure patients) activity, which can interfere with the evaluation of the inferior and lateral walls, respectively.

[62]Cu-PTSM is produced from elution of Zinc-62 generators. It is not FDA-approved for clinical use. It has a physical half-life

Table 10.1 Radiopharmaceuticals for Cardiac PET Imaging

PET Radiopharmaceutical	Production	Clinical application	Regulatory status	Physical half-life
[15]O-water	Cyclotron	Myocardial perfusion	Investigational	~2 min
[13]N-ammonia	Cyclotron	Myocardial perfusion	FDA approved	~10 min
Rubidium-82	Strontium-82/Rubidium-82 generator	Myocardial perfusion	FDA approved	~76 sec
[62]Cu-PTSM	Zinc-62/Copper-62 generator	Myocardial perfusion	Investigational	~10 min
[18]F-Flurpiridaz	Cyclotron	Myocardial perfusion	Investigational	~110 min
^{18}F-FDG	Cyclotron	Myocardial metabolism	FDA approved	~110 min

Abbreviations: FDA, Food and Drug Administration; PET, positron emission tomography.

of ~10 min. [62]Cu-PTSM has a single-pass extraction similar to ^{13}N-ammonia, with a markedly prolonged myocardial retention and rapid blood-pool clearance (8–10). In experimental animals, the myocardial activity appears to correlate with microsphere determined blood flow, although as with other extractable tracers there is a plateau in its net extraction at relatively higher flows (11,12). One disadvantage of [62]Cu-PTSM is the relatively short physical half-life of the parent radioisotope ([62]Zn, t1/2 = 9.1 hr), necessitates daily delivery of [62]Zn/[62]Cu generators, limiting practical application. Nonetheless, this agent is still under clinical investigation.

[15]O-water is a cyclotron-product with a physical half-life of ~2 min. It is not FDA-approved for clinical use. It is a freely diffusible agent with very high myocardial extraction across a wide range of myocardial blood flows (7). The degree of extraction is independent of the flow and is not affected by the metabolic state of the myocardium (7). Because it is a freely diffusible tracer, however, imaging is challenging due to its high concentration in the blood pool requiring additional post-processing to visualize the myocardium. Its use is limited to research applications.

[18]F-flurpiridaz is a pyridaben derivative that binds to the mitochondrial complex 1 inhibitor (13). Animal and human studies demonstrate homogeneous myocardial uptake with very good activity ratios between myocardium and blood, liver, and lungs. It shows a very high first-pass extraction across a wide range of myocardial blood flows (13–15). Phases I and II clinical studies have been completed. The FDA has recently approved plans for Phase III studies, which are currently under way. One potential advantage of this agent is that its flourine-18 radiolabel will allow unit dose distributions, similar to fluorodeoxyglucose (FDG) for cardiac metabolism, which will facilitate broader access to cardiac PET imaging. Further, the long physical half-life of fluorine-18 label (~110 min) permits its use in combination with exercise stress testing.

^{18}F-FDG is a glucose analog that is transported into myocytes by specific glucose transporters (GLUT-1 and GLUT-4). Inside the myocyte, FDG undergoes phosphorylation and becomes essentially trapped (16). As discussed above, the relatively longer physical half-life of F-18 allows sufficient time for production of ^{18}F-FDG and distribution by commercial radiopharmacies. It is also FDA approved for evaluation of myocardial viability.

Imaging Protocols

Figure 10.1 illustrates state-of-the-art imaging protocols for evaluation of myocardial perfusion and viability. The use of list mode imaging allows multiple image reconstructions from a single image dataset (i.e., summed, electrocardiogram (ECG) gated, and multi-frame or dynamic) for a comprehensive physiological examination of the heart. With this approach, image acquisition starts with the bolus injection of the radiopharmaceutical and continues for 6–7 min after Rubidium-82 and ~10–20 min after ^{13}N-ammonia injections. Stress testing is most commonly performed with pharmacological agents (e.g., vasodilators or dobutamine), but exercise is also possible (17), especially with ^{13}N-ammonia which has a longer half-life than Rubidium-82.

After completion of rest and stress PET imaging, patients who are not known *a priori* to have CAD will generally undergo low dose scan to ascertain the presence of coronary artery calcium score. This scan is less helpful in patients with known CAD and is generally omitted. In selected patients undergoing sequential coronary CT angiography (CT-CA), they generally receive sublingual nitroglycerin to maximize coronary vasodilation and β-adrenergic blocking agents to slow the heart rate to approximately 60 bpm or lower in order to maximize image quality. Prospective ECG-triggering or ECG-triggered tube current modulation results in lower radiation exposures, but requires slow, regular heart rates. For details of CT-CA imaging protocols, please refer to Chapter 8.

In patients who also need viability imaging, regional glucose uptake is then assessed with ^{18}F-FDG (a marker of exogenous glucose uptake), providing an index of myocardial metabolism and, thus, cell viability.

Radiation Dosimetry

Table 10.2 summarizes the radiation dosimetry of PET radiotracers and protocols used for clinical imaging. In general, the use of relatively short-lived radiopharmaceuticals with PET results in substantially lower radiation doses to patients compared with SPECT imaging (18). For Rubidium-82, recent data suggest that the total body effective dose from a rest-stress myocardial perfusion study is ~4–5 mSv (19,20). For ^{13}N-ammonia and ^{15}O-water, total body effective dose from a rest-stress myocardial perfusion study is <3 mSv (18). When myocardial viability is necessary, imaging is required with 18F-FDG results in ~7 mSv of added radiation dose.

MYOCARDIAL PERFUSION PROTOCOL

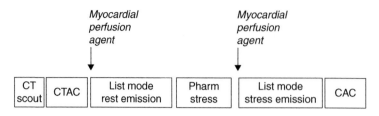

MYOCARDIAL ISCHEMIA AND VIABILITY PROTOCOL

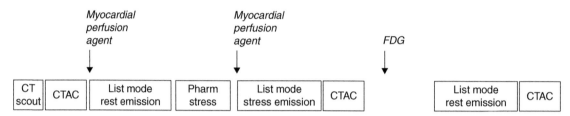

Figure 10.1 Protocols for clinical cardiac PET/CT imaging. *Abbreviations*: CAC, coronary artery calcium score; CT, computed tomography; CTAC, CT attenuation correction; FDG, fluorodeoxyglucose; PET, positron emission tomography.

Table 10.2 Radiation Dosimetry for Cardiac Positron Emission Tomography/Computed Tomography Imaging Protocols

Protocol	Average injected dose	Average whole body effective dose (mSv)	Average whole body effective dose from CTAC	Average total effective dose
[13]N-ammonia	20 mCi x 2	2.4	0.5	2.7
Rubidium-82	45 mCi x 2	3.7	0.5	4.2
[15]O-water	30 mCi x 2	2.5	0.5	3.0
^{18}F-FDG	10 mCi	7.0	0.5	7.5

Effective doses are calculated based on International Commission on Radiological Protection (ICRP) Publication 60 tissue weighting factors and average radionuclide activities specified in current American Society of Nuclear Cardiology (ASNC) guidelines. Rubidium-82 dosimetry estimated according to Ref. 20.
Except for ^{18}F-fluorodeoxyglucose, injected doses are lower when using 3-D imaging, resulting in lower whole body effective dose.

PET IMAGING FOR EVALUATION OF PATIENTS WITH KNOWN OR SUSPECTED CORONARY ARTERY DISEASE WITH PRESERVED LEFT VENTRICULAR FUNCTION
Diagnosing Obstructive CAD
Stress myocardial perfusion PET is an accurate approach to uncover flow-limiting CAD (Fig. 10.2), which is particularly well suited for patients undergoing pharmacological stress and those who are obese. Table 10.3 summarizes the published studies documenting the diagnostic accuracy of myocardial perfusion PET imaging for detecting obstructive CAD. The average weighted sensitivity for detecting at least one coronary artery with >50% stenosis is 90% (range, 83–100%), whereas the average specificity is 89% (range, 73–100%). The corresponding average positive predictive value (PPV) and negative predictive value (NPV) are 94% (range, 80–100%) and 73% (range, 36–100%), respectively, and the overall diagnostic accuracy is 90% (range, 84–98%).

Three studies have performed a direct comparison of the diagnostic accuracy of Rubidium-82 myocardial perfusion PET and Thallium-201 or ^{99m}Tc SPECT imaging in the same or

Focus Box 10.1 Positron Emission Tomography Techniques

Compared with conventional single photon-emission computed tomography (SPECT), positron emission tomography (PET) has higher spatial and contrast resolution, thereby increasing sensitivity

Attenuation correction during PET improves overall specificity

Quantitation of absolute myocardial blood flow can be achieved by dynamic PET techniques

Integrated PET-CT scanners allow evaluation of both anatomic and myocardial perfusion imaging

Wide range of PET tracers available for assessment of myocardial perfusion and metabolism

The use of relatively short-lived PET radiopharmaceuticals results in lower radiation doses compared with SPECT imaging

matched patient populations. Two older studies including a total of 283 patients reported higher sensitivity (93% vs. 76%)

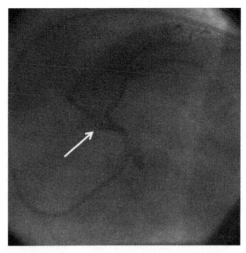

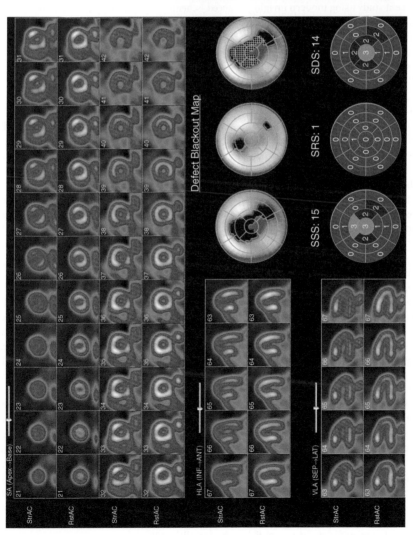

Figure 10.2 Stress and rest ^{82}Rb positron emission tomography myocardial perfusion imaging (*left*) showing multiple severe reversible perfusion defects involving the apical, anterior, and anteroseptal walls consistent with inducible ischemia in the left anterior descending coronary territory (LAD), and the inferolateral wall consistent with ischemia in the left circumflex/obtuse marginal coronary territory (LCX/OM). The blackout areas within the bull's eyes plots represent the extent of perfusion deficit and the hatched area reflects the magnitude of defect reversibility. The patient underwent prompt cardiac catheterization (*right*), which confirmed the finding of a tight stenosis in the proximal LAD (*arrow*). There was also moderate stenosis in the LCX/OM territory.

Table 10.3 Diagnostic Accuracy of Stress Myocardial Perfusion PET

Author	Patients	Women	Prior CAD	PET Radiotracer	Sens	Spec	PPV	NPV	Accuracy
Sampson (77)	102	0.42	0	^{82}Rb	0.93	0.83	0.80	0.94	0.87
Bateman (23)	112	0.46	0.25	^{82}Rb	0.87	0.93	0.95	0.81	0.89
Marwick (78)	74	0.19	0.49	^{82}Rb	0.90	1.0	1.0	0.36	0.91
Grover-McKay (79)	31	0.01	0.13	^{82}Rb	1.0	0.73	0.80	1.0	0.87
Stewart (22)	81	0.36	0.42	^{82}Rb	0.83	0.86	0.94	0.64	0.84
Go (21)	202	NR	0.47	^{82}Rb	0.93	78	0.93	0.80	0.90
Demer (80)	193	0.26	0.34	^{82}Rb/^{13}NH$_3$	83	0.95	0.98	0.60	0.85
Tamaki (81)	51	NR	0.75	^{13}NH$_3$	0.98	1.0	1.0	0.75	0.98
Gould (82)	31	NR	NR	^{82}Rb/^{13}NH$_3$	0.95	1.0	1.0	0.90	0.97
Weighted Summary	877	0.29	0.35		0.90	0.89	0.94	0.73	0.90

Abbreviations: ^{82}Rb, Rubidium-82; ^{13}NH$_3$, ^{13}N-ammonia; CAD, coronary artery disease; NPV, negative predictive value; PET, positron emission tomography; PPV, positive predictive value; Sens, sensitivity; Spec, specificity;.*Source*: From Ref. 27.

(21), or higher specificity (83% vs. 53%) (22) for PET compared with SPECT. A more recent study using modern imaging technology compared Rubidium-82 PET and ^{99m}Tc Sestamibi SPECT in two matched patient cohorts undergoing clinically indicated pharmacological-stress perfusion imaging using contemporary technology for both SPECT and PET (23). Overall diagnostic accuracy using either a 50% (87% vs. 71%) or a 70% (89% vs. 79%, respectively) angiographic threshold was higher for PET than for SPECT. Differences in diagnostic accuracy reflected primarily the increased specificity (with a marginal advantage in sensitivity) of PET vs. SPECT, and applied to both men and women, and to obese and non-obese individuals.

Role of Quantification in the Evaluation of Multivessel CAD
As discussed above, the myocardial perfusion PET approach is very accurate for the diagnosis of CAD at a patient level. However, like SPECT (24), it often uncovers only coronary territories supplied by the most severe stenosis (25). Consequently, it is relatively insensitive to accurately delineate the extent of obstructive angiographic disease especially in the setting of multivessel CAD (24,25). Two quantitative approaches help mitigate this limitation. One of them relates to PET's unique ability to assess LV function at rest and during peak stress (as opposed to post-stress with SPECT) (25). The data suggest that in normal subjects, LV ejection fraction (LVEF) increases from baseline to peak vasodilator stress (25). In patients with obstructive CAD, however, the delta change in LVEF is inversely related to the extent of obstructive angiographic CAD (Figs. 10.3 and 10.4). Patients with multivessel CAD show a drop in LVEF during peak stress even in the absence of apparent perfusion defects. By contrast, those without significant CAD or with low-risk disease show a normal increase in LVEF. Consequently, the diagnostic sensitivity of gated PET and its NPV for correctly excluding the presence of multivessel disease increase significantly (25).

The second approach is based on the ability of PET to enable absolute measurements of myocardial blood flow (in mL/min/g) and coronary flow reserve (the ratio of peak to basal myocardial blood flow). Software tools for routine quantification of myocardial

blood flow are now available. In patients with the so-called balanced ischemia or diffuse CAD, measurements of coronary flow reserve uncover areas of myocardium at risk that would generally be missed by performing only relative assessments of myocardial perfusion (Fig. 10.5) (26). Beyond diagnostic applications, these measures of coronary flow reserve have important prognostic implications as discussed later in this chapter.

Integrated PET/CT Imaging for Diagnosis and Management
As discussed in Chapter 8, CT-CA provides excellent diagnostic sensitivity for stenoses in the proximal and mid segments (>1.5 mm in diameter) of the main epicardial coronary arteries. Although the refinements implemented in the latest generation of CT technology have substantially reduced the number of non-evaluable coronary segments, the spatial resolution is still relatively limited compared with invasive angiography and the accuracy of this approach is reduced substantially in more distal coronary segments and side branches and in those associated with higher calcium burden (27). This limitation may be difficult to address because a significant improvement in spatial resolution for CT will necessarily be associated with a substantial increase in radiation dose. However, this limitation of CT-CA can be offset by the PET myocardial perfusion information that is generally not affected by the location of coronary stenoses. First clinical results appear encouraging and they support the notion that dual-modality imaging may offer superior diagnostic information with regard to identification of the culprit vessel (28–30). For example, Kajander et al. reported a significant improvement in specificity (87–100%) and PPV (81–100%) without a change in sensitivity or NPV for detection of obstructive CAD as defined by combined quantitative coronary angiography and fractional flow reserve in a cohort of patients with known or suspected CAD undergoing hybrid PET/CT-CA imaging (29). Conversely, CT-CA improves the specificity (91–100%) and PPV (86–100%) of quantitative PET imaging by allowing the differentiation of epicardial stenosis from microvascular abnormalities (29).

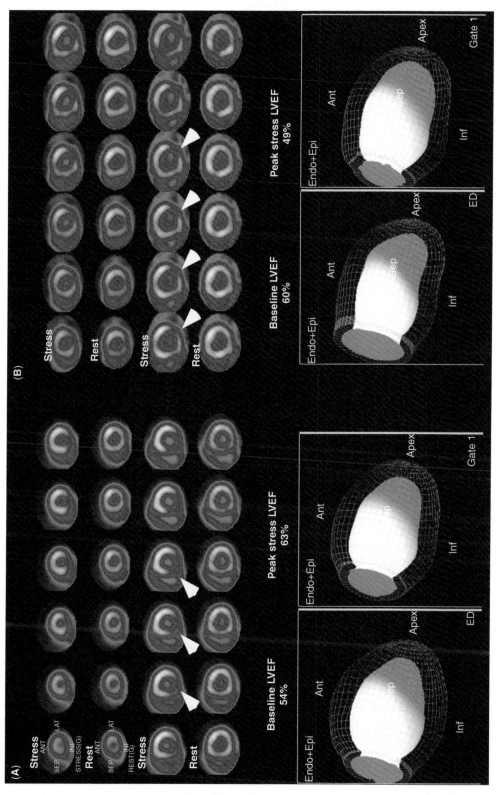

Figure 10.3 Gated rest–stress Rubidium-82 myocardial perfusion positron emission tomography (PET) images illustrating the added value of left ventricular function over the perfusion information. Panel (A) (*left*) demonstrates a normal rise in left ventricular ejection fraction (LVEF) from rest to peak stress (*arrows*) in a patient with angiographic single vessel coronary artery disease ('CAD'), showing a single perfusion defect in the inferior wall on the PET images (*arrows*). Panel (B) (*right*) demonstrates an abnormal drop in LVEF from rest to peak stress in a patient with angiographic multivessel CAD, also showing a single perfusion defect in the inferolateral wall on the PET images (*arrows*). *Source:* From Ref. 27.

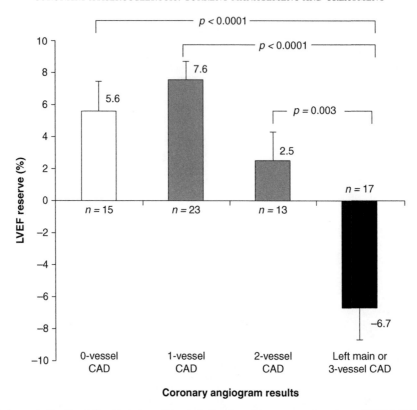

Figure 10.4 Bar graph demonstrating the relationship between the extent of angiographic coronary artery disease (CAD) (>70% stenosis) and the delta change in left ventricular ejection fraction (LVEF). *Source*: From Ref. 25.

On the other hand, the potential to acquire and quantify rest and stress myocardial perfusion, and coronary artery calcium score (CAC) using non-contrast CT within a single hybrid study may offer a unique opportunity to expand the prognostic value of stress nuclear imaging. The rationale for this integrated approach is predicated on the fact that the perfusion imaging approach is designed to uncover only obstructive atherosclerosis and, thus, insensitive for detecting subclinical disease (Fig. 10.6). The CAC score, reflecting the anatomic extent of atherosclerosis (31), may offer an opportunity to improve the conventional models for risk assessment using nuclear imaging alone especially among patients with normal perfusion. For example, recent data suggest that quantification of CAC scores at the time of stress nuclear imaging using a hybrid PET/CT approach can enhance risk predictions in patients with suspected CAD (32). Indeed, the annualized event rate in patients with normal stress PET perfusion imaging and no CAC appears substantially lower than among those with normal stress PET and a CAC ≥1,000 (32). The addition of CAC scoring within a hybrid PET/CT imaging strategy in patients with suspected CAD may serve as a more rational basis for personalizing the intensity and goals of medical therapy in a more cost-effective manner.

Risk Prediction with Myocardial Perfusion PET

The emerging prognostic data with PET perfusion imaging suggest that, as with with SPECT, the presence of normal myocardial perfusion identifies patients at relative low risk for cardiovascular events, and that the risk increases linearly with increasing extent and severity of stress perfusion defects (Figs. 10.2 and 10.7) (33–36). Furthermore, there is growing, consistent evidence that measurements of coronary flow reserve assessed by PET can also provide important prognostic information. The concept that the presence of coronary microvascular dysfunction assessed by quantitative PET portends a higher clinical risk has been demonstrated in patients with cardiomyopathy (37,38). This has also been related to increased clinical risk in patients with coronary risk factors (39). More recently, impaired flow reserve by PET in patients with known or suspected CAD has been shown to be associated with increased risk of adverse events (Table 10.4). In the largest study to date (40), the risk of cardiac death was consistently higher among patients with reduced global coronary flow reserve, irrespective of the extent of inducible ischemia and LVEF (Fig. 10.8). In risk-adjusted analysis, the lowest tertile of coronary flow reserve (<1.5) was associated with a 5.6-fold increase in the risk of cardiac death compared with

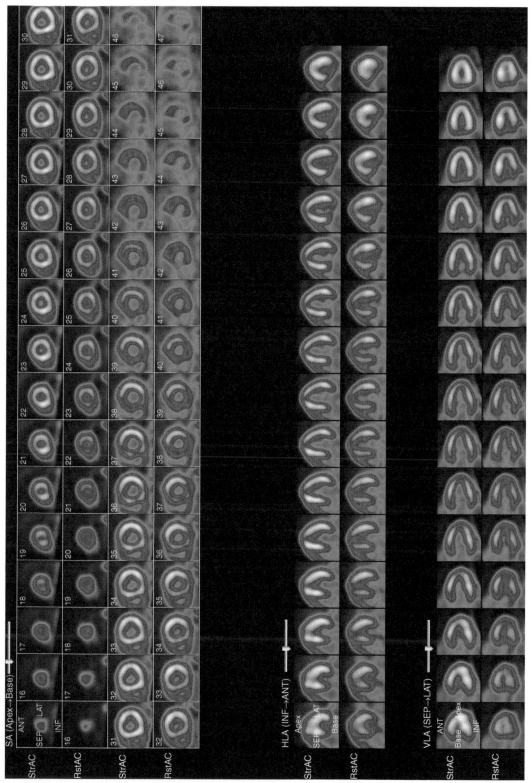

Figure 10.5 Example of a patient with transient ischemic dilatation during stress in the absence of regional perfusion defects (*left panel*). The quantitative data (*right panel*) demonstrates impaired coronary vasodilator reserve (stress flow divided by rest flow) in all three coronary artery territories. Subsequent coronary angiography demonstrated significant 3-vessel coronary artery disease. *Abbreviations*: LAD, left anterior descending coronary artery; LCX, left circumflex artery; LV, left ventricle; RCA, right coronary artery; RV, right ventricle; TOT, total.

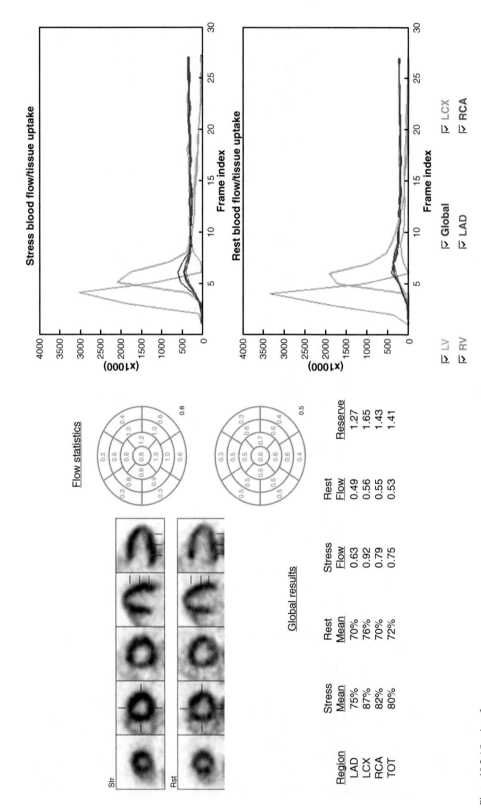

Figure 10.5 (Continued)

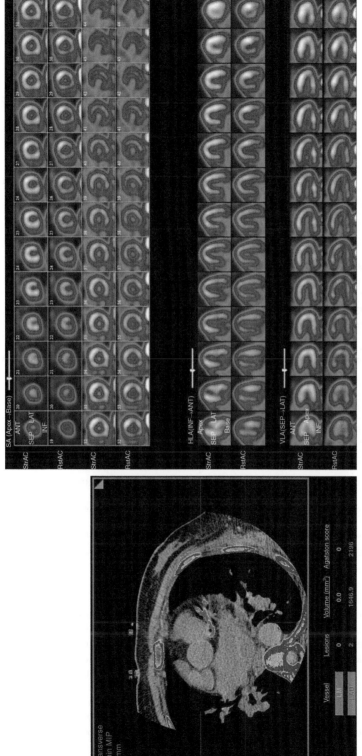

Figure 10.6 Example of a patient with relatively normal regional myocardial perfusion positron emission tomography study (*right panel*), showing rather extensive coronary artery calcium score especially involving the left anterior descending coronary artery (highlighted in pink in the *left panel*). The Agatston score was 2190. This illustrates the presence of extensive subclinical coronary atherosclerosis without flow-limiting coronary artery stenoses.

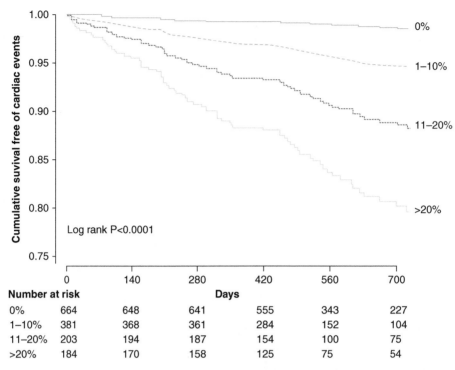

Number at risk					
0%	664	648	641	555	343	227
1–10%	381	368	361	284	152	104
11–20%	203	194	187	154	100	75
>20%	184	170	158	125	75	54

Figure 10.7 Adjusted survival curves demonstrating the risk of cardiac death and myocardial infarction with increasing extent and severity of perfusion deficit by stress positron emission tomography in patients with known or suspected coronary artery disease. *Source*: From Ref. 35.

Table 10.4 Quantitative Coronary Flow Reserve for Risk Prediction

	Herzog (83)	Slart (84)	Fukushima (85)	Ziadi (86)	Murthy (40)
Patients	256	344	224	677	2,783
Follow Up (years)	10	7	1	1	1.4
Endpoint	MACE (n = 78)	CD (n = 60)	MACE (n = 33)	CD/MI (n = 27)	CD (n = 137)
Hazard Ratio	1.6	4.1	2.9	3.3	5.6
Multivariable Adjustment	Age, sex, smoking, SSS	Age, sex	SSS, age	SSS, prior MI, LVEF	Clinical risk, LVEF, SSS, LVEF reserve
PET tracer	^{13}N-ammonia	^{13}N-ammonia	Rubidium-82	Rubidium-82	Rubidium-82

Abbreviations: CD, cardiac death; LVEF, left ventricular ejection fraction; MACE, major adverse cardiac events;MI, myocardial infarction; SSS, summed stress score .

the highest tertile (40). This information was incremental to demographic, clinical, and other important imaging variables (i.e., the extent of perfusion abnormalities and LVEF). Incorporation of coronary flow reserve measurements into cardiac death risk assessment models resulted in the reclassification of risk category of 35% of intermediate risk patients.

Identification of Revascularization Candidates with PET/CT Imaging

One of the most compelling arguments supporting a clinical role of hybrid imaging is its potential ability for optimizing management decisions. The importance of stress perfusion imaging in the hybrid imaging strategy is the ability of noninvasive estimates of inducible ischemia to identify which patients may benefit from revascularization (Fig. 10.9). Indeed, nonrandomized observational data using risk-adjustment techniques and propensity scores has demonstrated the ability of stress perfusion imaging to identify which patients may accrue a survival benefit from revascularization (41). The benefit of an ischemia-guided approach to management is further supported by invasive estimates of flow-limiting stenosis (e.g., fractional flow reserve, FFR) (42–44). In the setting of an FFR >0.75, revascularization can be safely deferred without increased

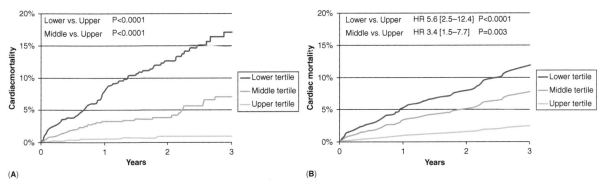

Figure 10.8 Cumulative incidence of cardiac mortality for tertiles of coronary flow reserve (CFR) presented in Kaplan-Meier format (**A**) and after adjustment for age, sex, body mass index, hypertension, dyslipidemia, diabetes mellitus, family history of coronary artery disease (CAD), tobacco use, prior CAD, chest pain, dyspnea, early revascularization, rest left ventricular ejection fraction (LVEF), summed stress score, and LVEF reserve (**B**), showing a significant association between CFR and cardiac mortality. HR indicates hazard ratio. *Source:* From Ref. 40.

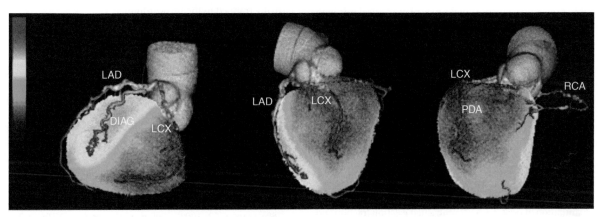

Figure 10.9 Fused 3-D reconstructions of a coronary computed tomography angiogram (CTA) and stress Rubidium-82 myocardial perfusion study obtained in the same setting, assessed through integrated positron emission tomography/CTA. The CTA demonstrated 3-vessel coronary artery disease. The fused CTA-stress myocardial perfusion images demonstrate a large area of severe stress-induced perfusion abnormality (*deep blue color*) only in the territory of the dominant left circumflex (LCX) coronary artery. *Abbreviations:* RCA, right coronary artery, DIAG, diagonal. *Source:* From Ref. 94.

patient risk, despite the presence of what visually appears to be a significant stenosis (42–44). In the recent FAME trial (42), routine use of an ischemia-guided approach (FFR) significantly reduced the rate of the composite endpoint of death, nonfatal myocardial infarction, and repeat revascularization by 28% at one year compared with an angiographically-guided strategy. The advantages of a noninvasive myocardial perfusion approach are clear—avoidance of unnecessary catheterizations that expose patients to risk and, and the potential for associated cost-savings (45,46). While CT-CA is an excellent method to exclude CAD, its ability to accurately assess the degree of luminal narrowing as a surrogate for physiological significance is only modest (29,30), and results in higher rates of downstream cardiac catheterization and revascularization than a myocardial perfusion approach (46). This is consistent with prior data

from multiple laboratories using either sequential (CT-CA followed by SPECT) (47–50) or hybrid imaging (SPECT/CT or PET/CT) (28,29,51–53) demonstrating that the PPVof CT-CA for identifying coronary stenoses producing objective evidence of stress-induced ischemia is suboptimal.

Together, these data suggest that by identifying which patients have sufficient ischemia to merit revascularization, stress perfusion imaging may play a significant role in the selection of patients for catheterization within a strategy based on identification of patient benefit. From the discussion above, this physiological data would have greater clinical impact than visually-defined coronary anatomy for revascularization decision-making. In patients with multivesel CAD, the value of hybrid imaging approach may allow better localization of the culprit stenosis and may offer a more targeted approach to revascularization.

PET IMAGING FOR EVALUATION OF PATIENTS WITH CORONARY ARTERY DISEASE AND SEVERE LV DYSFUNCTION

Rationale

Normal myocardium uses a variety of energy-producing substrates to fulfill its energy requirements (54). In the fasting state, free fatty acids (FFA) are mobilized in relatively large quantities from triglycerides stored in adipose tissue. Thus, the increased availability of FFA in plasma makes them the preferred energy-producing fuel in the myocardium (54). In the fed state, however, the increase in plasma glucose and the subsequent rise in insulin levels significantly reduce FFA release from adipose tissue and, consequently, its availability in plasma. This leads to an increased utilization of exogenous glucose by the myocardium (55).

FFA metabolism via beta-oxidation in the mitochondria is highly dependent on oxygen availability and, thus, it declines sharply during myocardial ischemia (56,57). Under this condition, studies in animal experiments (56) and in humans (58) have shown that the uptake and subsequent metabolism of glucose by the ischemic myocardium is markedly increased. This shift to preferential glucose uptake may play a critical role in the survival of functionally compromised myocytes (i.e., stunned and hibernating), as glycolytically derived high-energy phosphates are thought to be critical for maintaining basic cellular functions. Consequently, noninvasive approaches that can assess the magnitude of exogenous glucose utilization play an

---

Focus Box 10.2 Evaluation of Patients for Coronary Artery Disease

Positron emission tomography (PET) has higher diagnostic accuracy for detection of flow-limiting coronary artery disease (CAD) compared with single photon emission computed tomography (CT)

Quantitation of peak stress left ventricular ejection fraction and myocardial blood flow aid in detection of multivessel CAD

In addition to perfusion information, coronary flow reserve assessment by PET has prognostic value

Hybrid PET-CT systems with calcium scoring help to detect subclinical CAD while combined imaging with coronary CT angiography may aid in localization of culprit coronary artery stenosis

---

important role in the evaluation of tissue viability in patients with myocardial dysfunction due to CAD. For these metabolic adaptations to occur, sufficient nutrient perfusion is required to supply energy-rich substrates (e.g., glucose) and oxygen, and for removal of the byproducts of glycolysis (e.g., lactate and hydrogen ion). A prolonged and severe reduction of myocardial blood flow rapidly precipitates depletion of high-energy phosphate, cell membrane disruption, and cellular death. Therefore, assessment of regional blood flow also provides important information regarding the presence of tissue viability within dysfunctional myocardial regions.

With PET, regional glucose uptake is assessed with FDG, a marker of exogenous glucose uptake providing an index of myocardial metabolism and, thus, cell viability (59). After intravenous administration, FDG traces the initial transport of glucose across the myocyte membrane and its subsequent hexokinase-mediated phosphorylation to FDG-6-phosphate (60). Since the latter is a poor substrate for further metabolism and is rather impermeable to the cell membrane, it becomes virtually trapped in the myocardium.

PET Patterns of Myocardial Viability

The use of ^{18}F-FDG to assess regional myocardial glucose utilization (an index of tissue viability) is the most commonly used PET protocol (61). With this approach, specific abnormalities in metabolism within dysfunctional myocardium reflecting viable (perfusion-FDG mismatch) and scarred (perfusion-FDG match) myocardium have been described (Fig. 10.10). Contractile dysfunction is predicted to be reversible after revascularization in regions with a *perfusion-FDG mismatch*, and irreversible in those with reduced FDG uptake or a *perfusion-FDG match* pattern. Using these criteria, the average PPV for predicting improved segmental function after revascularization is 76% (range, 52–100%), whereas the average NPV is 82% (range, 67–100%) (61).

Predicting Improvement in Global LV Function after Revascularization

Several studies using different PET approaches have shown that the gain in global LV systolic function after revascularization is related to the magnitude of viable myocardium assessed

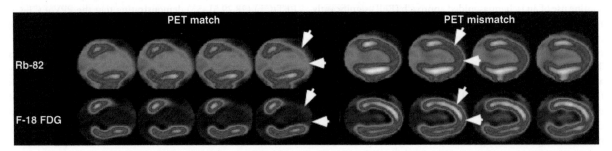

Figure 10.10 Positron emission tomography (PET) patterns of myocardial viability. The (*left panel*) demonstrates concordant reductions in myocardial perfusion (Rubidium-82) and glucose metabolism (fluorodeoxyglucose (FDG)), reflecting myocardial infarction. The (*right panel*) demonstrates preserved glucose metabolism (FDG) in a territory with decreased myocardial perfusion (Rubidium-82), reflecting complete tissue viability. *Source:* From Ref. 27.

Table 10.5 Relationship between the Extent of Myocardial Viability and the Change in LVEF after Revascularization with Positron Emission Tomography

Author	N	Criteria for viability	Pre LVEF (%)	Post LVEF (%)
Tillisch (59)	17	Mismatch ≥25% LV	30 ± 11	45 ± 14
Carrel (87)	23	Mismatch ≥17% LV	34 ± 14	52 ± 11
Vanoverschelde (88)	12	Ant wall mismatch	55 ± 7	65 ± 8
Maes (89)	20	Ant wall mismatch	51 ± 11	60 ± 10
Grandin (90)	25	Mismatch ≥20% LV	51 ± 12	63 ± 18
Schwarz (91)	24	Ant wall mismatch	44 ± 12	54 ± 9
Wolpers (92)	30	Ant wall mismatch	39 ± 10	49 ± 17
vom Dahl (93)	82	Mismatch ≥1 CAT	46 ± 9	54 ± 11

Abbreviation: CAT, coronary artery territory; LV, left ventricle; LVEF, left ventricular ejection fraction..

preoperatively (Table 10.5) (62). These data demonstrate that clinically meaningful changes in global LV function can be expected after revascularization only in patients with relatively large areas of hibernating and/or stunned myocardium (~20% of the LV mass). Similar results have been reported using estimates of myocardial scar with PET (63). The inverse relationship between the extent of scar assessed by FDG PET and the changes in LVEF after revascularization are consistent with those obtained with SPECT (64), dobutamine echocardiography (65), and contrast-enhanced MRI (66).

Predicting Improvement in Symptoms after Revascularization

In keeping with the observed changes in LV function post-revascularization, the magnitude of improvement in heart failure symptoms also correlates with the preoperative extent of viable myocardium (Fig. 10.11) (67). Further, the observed improvement in symptom status in patients with viability by PET also seems to correlate with the reduced frequency of hospital readmission for decompensated heart failure following revascularization (68). The notion that noninvasive imaging of viability can predict the degree of symptomatic improvement in heart failure patients have been confirmed in studies involving PET (69) and SPECT imaging of Tl-201 or Tc-99m sestamibi (70), and identification of contractile reserve by dobutamine echocardiography (71). Taken together, these data suggest that the extent of dysfunctional ischemic viable myocardium in heart failure patients can be used as a potential marker of the symptomatic benefit that will accrue as a result of revascularization.

Predicting Improvement in Survival after Revascularization

An issue of even greater clinical relevance is whether viability imaging may help identify patients with low ejection fraction for whom revascularization may offer a survival advantage. Early PET reports showed that patients with viable myocardium treated medically had a consistently higher event rate than those without viability (61). These data also suggested that the poor event-free survival of patients with viable myocardium undergoing medical therapy was improved significantly and consistently by early referral to revascularization (61). These initial findings

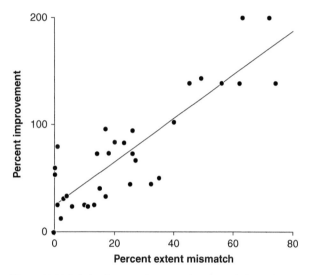

Figure 10.11 Relation between the anatomic extent of the perfusion-fluorodeoxyglucose positron emission tomography mismatch (% of the left ventricle) and the change in functional capacity after CABG in patients with severe left ventricular dysfunction (r = 0.87, p < 0.001). *Source*: From Ref. 67.

with FDG PET have been confirmed by subsequent studies using noninvasive imaging with either nuclear testing or echocardiography (72,73). A recent prospective randomized study of 428 patients with LVEF ≤35% investigated whether an FDG PET assisted management of patients with ischemic LV dysfunction altered outcomes compared with standard care (74). The study demonstrated that when management decisions adhered to the PET recommendations regarding revascularization versus medical therapy alone, outcomes were better with a PET-guided strategy (hazard ratio for the composite outcome was 0.62, 95% CI 0.42–0.93; p = 0.019) as compared with standard care (Fig. 10.12). Together, these findings imply that despite an increasing clinical risk of revascularization with worsening LV dysfunction, non-invasive imaging evidence of preserved viability may provide information on clinical benefit to balance against that risk, informing clinical decision-making.

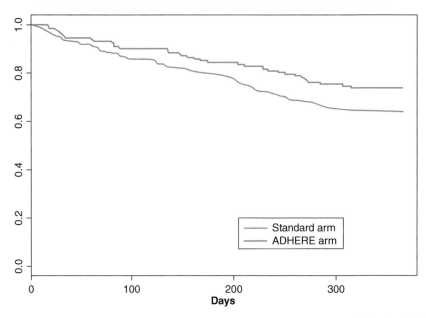

Figure 10.12 Probability of survival free of cardiac events in patients randomized to a positron emission tomography (PET)-guided approach who adhered to PET recommendations (Adhere group) versus standard care arm. Adjusted hazard ratio = 0.62, 95% CI 0.42–0.93, p = 0.019. *Source*: From Ref. 74.

The results of the prospective viability substudy of the STICH trial have casted some doubts regarding the utility of viability imaging for guiding decisions regarding revascularization in patients with ischemic LV dysfunction (75). In this substudy, 601 patients of the original STICH cohort underwent viability imaging with either Thallium-201 SPECT and/or dobutamine echocardiography. Although the presence of viable myocardium was associated with a greater likelihood of survival, the viability information did not identify patients with a survival advantage from revascularization compared with medical therapy. The strengths of the STICH viability substudy included the fact that it was the largest prospective study to date, and that medical therapy followed accepted guidelines and it was closely monitored. The study also has several weaknesses. First, it is not randomized and selection of patients for viability imaging was at the discretion of site investigators, introducing an important selection bias. Second, the definition of viability was too broad. Indeed, 81% of patients in this study were categorized as having viable myocardium, which is significantly higher than that observed in the Christmas trial (59%) using similar methodology (76) and may have obfuscated the identification of patients with potentially reversible LV dysfunction. Third, the STICH viability substudy did not include stress imaging to identify the extent of ischemic burden nor did it use information about the extent of LV remodeling to identify patients with potentially reversible LV dysfunction. Finally, the study did not include more FDG PET or cardiac MRI to assess viability.

Focus Box 10.3 Evaluation of Patients with Left Ventricular Dysfunction

Differences in regional glucose uptake as assessed by fluoro-deoxyglucose-positron emission tomography provide an assessment of myocardial metabolism and viability

Identification of hibernating and/or stunned myocardium that responds to revascularization may improve left ventricular function, symptoms, and survival

CONCLUSIONS

Cardiac PET imaging is an accurate and reproducible technique for the non-invasive evaluation of myocardial ischemia and viability. The clinical data presented highlight the ability of cardiac PET and PET-CT to detect, characterize, and quantify the extent and severity of coronary atherosclerosis. By providing concurrent quantitative information about myocardial blood flow and metabolism with coronary and cardiac anatomy, PET/CT offers the opportunity for a comprehensive non-invasive evaluation of the consequences of epicardial atherosclerosis in the myocardium, thereby helping management decisions regarding the need for potential revascularization. As we continue to define the role of PET and PET-CT in the risk stratification of patients with coronary heart disease, the future will focus on understanding more complex interactions between viability and ischemia, and the molecular changes that lead to myocyte function and regeneration.

ACKNOWLEDGEMENTS

This work was supported in part by grants from the National Institutes of Health (RC1 HL101060-01, T32 HL094301-01A1).

REFERENCES

1. Goetze S, Wahl RL. Prevalence of misregistration between SPECT and CT for attenuation-corrected myocardial perfusion SPECT. J Nucl Cardiol 2007; 14: 200–6.

2. Gould KL, Pan T, Loghin C, et al. Frequent diagnostic errors in cardiac PET/CT due to misregistration of CT attenuation and emission PET images: a definitive analysis of causes, consequences, and corrections. J Nucl Med 2007; 48: 1112–21.

3. McQuaid SJ, Hutton BF. Sources of attenuation-correction artefacts in cardiac PET/CT and SPECT/CT. Eur J Nucl Med Mol Imaging 2008; 35: 1117–23.

4. Slomka PJ, Le Meunier L, Hayes SW, et al. Comparison of myocardial perfusion 82Rb PET performed with CT- and transmission CT-based attenuation correction. J Nucl Med 2008; 49: 1992–8.

5. Humm JL, Rosenfeld A, Del Guerra A. From PET detectors to PET scanners. Eur J Nucl Med Mol Imaging 2003; 30: 1574–97.

6. Higuchi T, Nekolla SG, Jankaukas A, et al. Characterization of normal and infarcted rat myocardium using a combination of small-animal PET and clinical MRI. J Nucl Med 2007; 48: 288–94.

7. Schelbert HR. Evaluation of myocardial blood flow in cardiac disease. In: Skorton DJ, Schelbert HR, Wolf GL, Brundage BH. eds Cardiac Imaging. A Companion to Braunwald's Heart Disease. Vol 2 Philadelphia: W.B: Saunders, 1991: 1093–112.

8. Shelton ME, Green MA, Mathias CJ, Welch MJ, Bergmann SR. Kinetics of copper-PTSM in isolated hearts: a novel tracer for measuring blood flow with positron emission tomography. J Nucl Med 1989; 30: 1843–7.

9. Shelton ME, Green MA, Mathias CJ, Welch MJ, Bergmann SR. Assessment of regional myocardial and renal blood flow with copper-PTSM and positron emission tomography. Circulation 1990; 82: 990–7.

10. Beanlands RS, Muzik O, Mintun M, et al. The kinetics of copper-62-PTSM in the normal human heart. J Nucl Med 1992; 33: 684–90.

11. Herrero P, Hartman JJ, Green MA, et al. Regional myocardial perfusion assessed with generator-produced copper-62-PTSM and PET. J Nucl Med 1996; 37: 1294–300.

12. Herrero P, Markham J, Weinheimer CJ, et al. Quantification of regional myocardial perfusion with generator-produced 62Cu-PTSM and positron emission tomography. Circulation 1993; 87: 173–83.

13. Yu M, Guaraldi MT, Mistry M, et al. BMS-747158-02: a novel PET myocardial perfusion imaging agent. J Nucl Cardiol 2007; 14: 789–98.

14. Nekolla SG, Reder S, Saraste A, et al. Evaluation of the novel myocardial perfusion positron-emission tomography tracer 18F-BMS-747158-02: comparison to 13N-ammonia and validation with microspheres in a pig model. Circulation 2009; 119: 2333–42.

15. Sherif HM, Nekolla SG, Saraste A, et al. Simplified quantification of myocardial flow reserve with flurpiridaz F 18: validation with microspheres in a pig model. J Nucl Med 2011; 52: 617–24.

16. Gallagher BM, Ansari A, Atkins H, et al. Radiopharmaceuticals XXVII. 18F-labeled 2-deoxy-2-fluoro-d-glucose as a radiopharmaceutical for measuring regional myocardial glucose metabolism in vivo: tissue distribution and imaging studies in animals. J Nucl Med 1977; 18: 990–6.

17. Chow BJ, Beanlands RS, Lee A, et al. Treadmill exercise produces larger perfusion defects than dipyridamole stress N-13 ammonia positron emission tomography. J Am Coll Cardiol 2006; 47: 411–6.

18. Stabin MG. Radiopharmaceuticals for nuclear cardiology: radiation dosimetry, uncertainties, and risk. J Nucl Med 2008; 49: 1555–63.

19. Senthamizhchelvan S, Bravo PE, Esaias C, et al. Human biodistribution and radiation dosimetry of 82Rb. J Nucl Med 2010; 51: 1592–9.

20. Senthamizhchelvan S, Bravo PE, Lodge MA, et al. Radiation dosimetry of 82Rb in humans under pharmacologic stress. J Nucl Med 2011; 52: 485–91.

21. Go RT, Marwick TH, MacIntyre WJ, et al. A prospective comparison of rubidium-82 PET and thallium-201 SPECT myocardial perfusion imaging utilizing a single dipyridamole stress in the diagnosis of coronary artery disease [see comments]. J Nucl Med 1990; 31: 1899–905.

22. Stewart RE, Schwaiger M, Molina E, et al. Comparison of rubidium-82 positron emission tomography and thallium-201 SPECT imaging for detection of coronary artery disease. Am J Cardiol 1991; 67: 1303–10.

23. Bateman TM, Heller GV, McGhie AI, et al. Diagnostic accuracy of rest/stress ECG-gated Rb-82 myocardial perfusion PET: comparison with ECG-gated Tc-99m sestamibi SPECT. J Nucl Cardiol 2006; 13: 24–33.

24. Berman DS, Kang X, Slomka PJ, et al. Underestimation of extent of ischemia by gated SPECT myocardial perfusion imaging in patients with left main coronary artery disease. J Nucl Cardiol 2007; 14: 521–8.

25. Dorbala S, Vangala D, Sampson U, et al. Value of vasodilator left ventricular ejection fraction reserve in evaluating the magnitude of myocardium at risk and the extent of angiographic coronary artery disease: a 82Rb PET/CT study. J Nucl Med 2007; 48: 349–58.

26. Parkash R, deKemp RA, Ruddy Td T, et al. Potential utility of rubidium 82 PET quantification in patients with 3-vessel coronary artery disease. J Nucl Cardiol 2004; 11: 440–9.

27. Di Carli MF, Hachamovitch R. New technology for noninvasive evaluation of coronary artery disease. Circulation 2007; 115: 1464–80.

28. Di Carli MF, Dorbala S, Curillova Z, et al. Relationship between CT coronary angiography and stress perfusion imaging in patients with suspected ischemic heart disease assessed by integrated PET-CT imaging. J Nucl Cardiol 2007; 14: 799–809.

29. Kajander S, Joutsiniemi E, Saraste M, et al. Cardiac positron emission tomography/computed tomography imaging accurately detects anatomically and functionally significant coronary artery disease. Circulation 2010; 122: 603–13.

30. Naya M, Murthy VL, Blankstein R, et al. Quantitative relationship between the extent and morphology of coronary atherosclerotic plaque and downstream myocardial perfusion. J Am Coll Cardiol 2011; 58: 1807–16.

31. Sangiorgi G, Rumberger JA, Severson A, et al. Arterial calcification and not lumen stenosis is highly correlated with atherosclerotic plaque burden in humans: a histologic study of 723 coronary artery segments using nondecalcifying methodology. J Am Coll Cardiol 1998; 31: 126–33.

32. Schenker MP, Dorbala S, Hong EC, et al. Interrelation of coronary calcification, myocardial ischemia, and outcomes in patients with intermediate likelihood of coronary artery disease: a combined positron emission tomography/computed tomography study. Circulation 2008; 117: 1693–700.

33. Marwick TH, Shan K, Patel S, Go RT, Lauer MS. Incremental value of rubidium-82 positron emission tomography for prognostic assessment of known or suspected coronary artery disease. Am J Cardiol 1997; 80: 865–70.

34. Yoshinaga K, Chow BJ, Williams K, et al. What is the prognostic value of myocardial perfusion imaging using rubidium-82 positron emission tomography? J Am Coll Cardiol 2006; 48: 1029–39.

35. Dorbala S, Hachamovitch R, Curillova Z, et al. Incremental prognostic value of gated Rb-82 positron emission tomography myocardial perfusion imaging over clinical variables and rest LVEF. JACC Cardiovasc Imaging 2009; 2: 846–54.

36. Lertsburapa K, Ahlberg AW, Bateman TM, et al. Independent and incremental prognostic value of left ventricular ejection fraction determined by stress gated rubidium 82 PET imaging in patients with known or suspected coronary artery disease. J Nucl Cardiol 2008; 15: 745–53.

37. Cecchi F, Olivotto I, Gistri R, et al. Coronary microvascular dysfunction and prognosis in hypertrophic cardiomyopathy. N Engl J Med 2003; 349: 1027–35.

38. Neglia D, Michelassi C, Trivieri MG, et al. Prognostic role of myocardial blood flow impairment in idiopathic left ventricular dysfunction. Circulation 2002; 105: 186–93.

39. Dorbala S, Hassan A, Heinonen T, Schelbert HR, Di Carli MF. Coronary vasodilator reserve and Framingham risk scores in subjects at risk for coronary artery disease. J Nucl Cardiol 2006; 13: 761–7.

40. Murthy VL, Naya M, Foster CR, et al. Improved cardiac risk assessment with noninvasive measures of coronary flow reserve. Circulation 2011; 124: 2215–24.

41. Hachamovitch R, Hayes SW, Friedman JD, Cohen I, Berman DS. Comparison of the short-term survival benefit associated with revascularization compared with medical therapy in patients with no prior coronary artery disease undergoing stress myocardial perfusion single photon emission computed tomography. Circulation 2003; 107: 2900–7.

42. Tonino PA, De Bruyne B, Pijls NH, et al. Fractional flow reserve versus angiography for guiding percutaneous coronary intervention. N Engl J Med 2009; 360: 213–24.

43. Bech GJ, De Bruyne B, Pijls NH, et al. Fractional flow reserve to determine the appropriateness of angioplasty in moderate coronary stenosis: a randomized trial. Circulation 2001; 103: 2928–34.

44. Chamuleau SAJ, Meuwissen M, Koch KT, et al. Usefulness of fractional flow reserve for risk stratification of patients with multivessel coronary artery disease and an intermediate stenosis. Am J Cardiol 2002; 89: 377–80.

45. Shaw LJ, Hachamovitch R, Berman DS, et al. The economic consequences of available diagnostic and prognostic strategies for the evaluation of stable angina patients: an observational assessment of the value of precatheterization ischemia. Economics of Noninvasive Diagnosis (END) Multicenter Study Group. J Am Coll Cardiol 1999; 33: 661–9.

46. Shreibati JB, Baker LC, Hlatky MA. Association of coronary CT angiography or stress testing with subsequent utilization and spending among Medicare beneficiaries. JAMA 2011; 306: 2128–36.

47. Hacker M, Jakobs T, Matthiesen F, et al. Comparison of spiral multidetector CT angiography and myocardial perfusion imaging in the noninvasive detection of functionally relevant coronary artery lesions: first clinical experiences. J Nucl Med 2005; 46: 1294–300.

48. Schuijf JD, Wijns W, Jukema JW, et al. Relationship between noninvasive coronary angiography with multi-slice computed tomography and myocardial perfusion imaging. J Am Coll Cardiol 2006; 48: 2508–14.

49. Gaemperli O, Schepis T, Kalff V, et al. Validation of a new cardiac image fusion software for three-dimensional integration of myocardial perfusion SPECT and stand-alone 64-slice CT angiography. Eur J Nucl Med Mol Imaging 2007; 34: 1097–106.

50. Gaemperli O, Schepis T, Valenta I, et al. Cardiac image fusion from stand-alone SPECT and CT: clinical experience. J Nucl Med 2007; 48: 696–703.

51. Rispler S, Roguin A, Keidar Z, et al. Integrated SPECT/CT for the assessment of hemodynamically significant coronary artery lesions. J Am Coll Cardiol 2006; 47: 115A.

52. Malkerneker D, Brenner R, Martin WH, et al. CT-based attenuation correction versus prone imaging to decrease equivocal interpretations of rest/stress Tc-99m tetrofosmin SPECT MPI. J Nucl Cardiol 2007; 14: 314–23.

53. Hacker M, Jakobs T, Hack N, et al. Combined use of 64-slice computed tomography angiography and gated myocardial perfusion SPECT for the detection of functionally relevant coronary artery stenoses. First results in a clinical setting concerning patients with stable angina. Nuklearmedizin 2007; 46: 29–35.

54. Opie LH. The Heart. Physiology and Metabolism. 2nd edn. New York: Raven Press, 1991.

55. Young LH, Coven DL, Russell RR 3rd. Cellular and molecular regulation of cardiac glucose transport. J Nucl Cardiol 2000; 7: 267–76.

56. Opie LH. Effects of regional ischemia on metabolism of glucose and fatty acids. Circ Res 1976; 38(Suppl I): 152–74.

57. Liedtke AJ. Alterations of carbohydrate and lipid metabolism in the acutely ischemic heart. Prog Cardiovasc Dis 1981; 23: 321–36.

58. Camici P, Araujo LI, Spinks T, et al. Increase uptake of 18F-fluorodeoxyglucose in postischemic myocardium of patients with exercise-induced angina. Circulation 1986; 74: 81–8.

59. Tillisch J, Brunken R, Marshall R, et al. Reversibility of cardiac wall-motion abnormalities predicted by positron tomography. N Engl J Med 1986; 314: 884–8.

60. Phelps ME, Hoffman EJ, Selin C, et al. Investigation of [18F] 2-fluoro-2-deoxyglucose for the measure of myocardial glucose metabolism. J Nucl Med 1978; 19: 1311–9.

61. Di Carli MF. Advances in positron emission tomography. J Nucl Cardiol 2004; 11: 719–32.

62. Di Carli MF. Predicting improved function after myocardial revascularization. Curr Opin Cardiol 1998; 13: 415–24.

63. Beanlands RS, Ruddy TD, deKemp RA, et al. Positron emission tomography and recovery following revascularization (PARR-1): the importance of scar and the development of a prediction rule for the degree of recovery of left ventricular function. J Am Coll Cardiol 2002; 40: 1735–43.

64. Ragosta M, Beller GA, Watson DD, Kaul S, Gimple LW. Quantitative planar rest-redistribution 201Tl imaging in detection of myocardial viability and prediction of improvement in left ventricular function after coronary bypass surgery in patients with severely depressed left ventricular function. Circulation 1993; 87: 1630–41.

65. Perrone-Filardi P, Pace L, Prastaro M, et al. Dobutamine echocardiography predicts improvement of hypoperfused dysfunctional myocardium after revascularization in patients with coronary artery disease. Circulation 1995; 91: 2556–65.

66. Kim RJ, Wu E, Rafael A, et al. The use of contrast-enhanced magnetic resonance imaging to identify reversible myocardial dysfunction. N Engl J Med 2000; 343: 1445–53.

67. Di Carli MF, Asgarzadie F, Schelbert HR, et al. Quantitative relation between myocardial viability and improvement in heart failure symptoms after revascularization in patients with ischemic cardiomyopathy. Circulation 1995; 92: 3436–44.

68. Rohatgi R, Epstein S, Henriquez J, et al. Utility of positron emission tomography in predicting cardiac events and survival in patients with coronary artery disease and severe left ventricular dysfunction. Am J Cardiol 2001; 87: 1096–9; A1096.

69. Marwick TH, Zuchowski C, Lauer MS, et al. Functional status and quality of life in patients with heart failure undergoing coronary bypass surgery after assessment of myocardial viability. J Am Coll Cardiol 1999; 33: 750–8.

70. Senior R, Kaul S, Raval U, Lahiri A. Impact of revascularization and myocardial viability determined by nitrate-enhanced Tc-99m sestamibi and Tl-201 imaging on mortality and functional outcome in ischemic cardiomyopathy. J Nucl Cardiol 2002; 9: 454–62.

71. Bax JJ, Poldermans D, Elhendy A, et al. Improvement of left ventricular ejection fraction, heart failure symptoms and prognosis after revascularization in patients with chronic coronary artery disease and viable myocardium detected by dobutamine stress echocardiography. J Am Coll Cardiol 1999; 34: 163–9.

72. Allman K, Shaw LJ, Hachamovitch R, Udelson JE. Myocardial viability testing and impact of revascularization on prognosis in patients with coronary artery disease and left ventricular dysfunction: a meta-analysis. J Am Coll Cardiol 2002; in press.

73. Udelson JE, Bonow RO, Dilsizian V. The historical and conceptual evolution of radionuclide assessment of myocardial viability. J Nucl Cardiol 2004; 11: 318–34.

74. Beanlands RS, Nichol G, Huszti E, et al. F-18-fluorodeoxyglucose positron emission tomography imaging-assisted management of patients with severe left ventricular dysfunction and suspected coronary disease: a randomized, controlled trial (PARR-2). J Am Coll Cardiol 2007; 50: 2002–12.

75. Bonow RO, Maurer G, Lee KL, et al. Myocardial viability and survival in ischemic left ventricular dysfunction. N Engl J Med 2011; 364: 1617–25.

76. Cleland JG, Pennell DJ, Ray SG, et al. Myocardial viability as a determinant of the ejection fraction response to carvedilol in patients with heart failure (CHRISTMAS trial): randomised controlled trial. Lancet 2003; 362: 14–21.

77. Sampson UK, Dorbala S, Limaye A, Kwong R, Di Carli MF. Diagnostic accuracy of rubidium-82 myocardial perfusion imaging with hybrid positron emission tomography/computed tomography in the detection of coronary artery disease. J Am Coll Cardiol 2007; 49: 1052–8.

78. Marwick TH, Nemec JJ, Stewart WJ, Salcedo EE. Diagnosis of coronary artery disease using exercise echocardiography and positron emission tomography: comparison and analysis of discrepant results. J Am Soc Echocardiogr 1992; 5: 231–8.

79. Grover-McKay M, Ratib O, Schwaiger M, et al. Detection of coronary artery disease with positron emission tomography and rubidium 82. Am Heart J 1992; 123: 646–52.

80. Demer LL, Gould KL, Goldstein RA, et al. Assessment of coronary artery disease severity by positron emission tomography. Comparison with quantitative arteriography in 193 patients. Circulation 1989; 79: 825–35.

81. Tamaki N, Yonekura Y, Senda M, et al. Value and limitation of stress thallium-201 single photon emission computed tomography: comparison with nitrogen-13 ammonia positron tomography. J Nucl Med 1988; 29: 1181–8.

82. Gould KL, Goldstein RA, Mullani NA, et al. Noninvasive assessment of coronary stenoses by myocardial perfusion imaging during pharmacologic coronary vasodilation. VIII. Clinical feasibility of positron cardiac imaging without a cyclotron using generator-produced rubidium-82. J Am Coll Cardiol 1986; 7: 775–89.

83. Herzog BA, Husmann L, Valenta I, et al. Long-term prognostic value of 13N-ammonia myocardial perfusion positron emission tomography added value of coronary flow reserve. J Am Coll Cardiol 2009; 54: 150–6.

84. Slart RH, Zeebregts CJ, Hillege HL, et al. Myocardial perfusion reserve after a PET-driven revascularization procedure: a strong prognostic factor. J Nucl Med 2011; 52: 873–9.

85. Fukushima K, Javadi MS, Higuchi T, et al. Prediction of short-term cardiovascular events using quantification of global myocardial flow reserve in patients referred for clinical 82Rb PET perfusion imaging. J Nucl Med 2011; 52: 726–32.

86. Ziadi MC, Dekemp RA, Williams KA, et al. Impaired myocardial flow reserve on rubidium-82 positron emission tomography imaging predicts adverse outcomes in patients assessed for myocardial ischemia. J Am Coll Cardiol 2011; 58: 740–8.

87. Carrel T, Jenni R, Haubold-Reuter S, et al. Improvement in severely reduced left ventricular function after surgical revascularization in patients with preoperative myocardial infarction. Eur J Cardiothorac Surg 1992; 6: 479–84.

88. Vanoverschelde JL, Wijns W, Depre C, et al. Mechanisms of chronic regional postischemic dysfunction in humans. New insights from the study of noninfarcted collateral-dependent myocardium. Circulation 1993; 87: 1513–23.

89. Maes A, Borgers M, Flameng W, et al. Assessment of myocardial viability in chronic coronary artery disease using technetium-99m sestamibi SPECT. J Am Coll Cardiol 1997; 29: 62–8.

90. Grandin C, Wijns W, Melin JA, et al. Delineation of myocardial viability with PET. J Nucl Med 1995; 36: 1543–52.

91. Schwarz ER, Schaper J, vom Dahl J, et al. Myocyte degeneration and cell death in hibernating human myocardium. J Am Coll Cardiol 1996; 27: 1577–85.

92. Wolpers HG, Burchert W, van den Hoff J, et al. Assessment of myocardial viability by use of 11C-acetate and positron emission tomography. Threshold criteria of reversible dysfunction. Circulation 1997; 95: 1417–24.

93. vom Dahl J, Altehoefer C, Sheehan FH, et al. Effect of myocardial viability assessed by technetium-99m-sestamibi SPECT and fluorine-18-FDG PET on clinical outcome in coronary artery disease. J Nucl Med 1997; 38: 742–8.

94. Di Carli MF, Dorbala S, Meserve J, et al. Clinical Myocardial Perfusion PET/CT. J Nucl Med 2007; 48: 783–93.

11 From conventional to three-dimensional coronary angiography: Potential clinical implications
Chrysafios Girasis

OUTLINE

Coronary angiography is still considered as a cornerstone in the diagnosis of coronary artery disease (CAD), despite its inherent limitations. Quantitative coronary angiography (QCA) is an accurate and reproducible way to quantify the extent of coronary stenoses, as opposed to highly variable visual estimates. Conventional single-vessel analysis is inadequate for bifurcation lesions; dedicated QCA algorithms have been developed and validated instead. The validity of two-dimensional (2D) angiography is limited by foreshortening, variable magnification, and vessel overlap; 3D angiographic reconstruction eliminates these shortcomings providing reliable results in real time. Rotational coronary angiography can minimize contrast use, radiation exposure, and procedure time without jeopardizing its diagnostic accuracy. Angiographic measurements can be used on-line to guide coronary interventions, whereas off-line they serve as surrogate endpoints for clinical events in angiographic trials. It is expected that recent advances in coronary angiography will improve its correlation with functional indices and invasive imaging modalities; the potential to improve clinical outcome remains to be proven.

INTRODUCTION

Since its inception in 1958 (1), invasive coronary angiography has been considered essential in the diagnostic evaluation of CAD and the guidance of percutaneous coronary interventions (PCIs). Ongoing advances in interventional cardiology have prompted the development of high-resolution digital angiographic systems; by performing a series of intra-coronary contrast injections in carefully selected angiographic projections, it is possible to acquire a wealth of information from the entire coronary artery tree (2).

Visual assessment has been the intuitive way to interpret the coronary angiogram; even to date this "eyeballing" technique is commonly employed to determine coronary stenosis severity. Nevertheless, visual estimates have been proven to be rather inaccurate and highly variable even among experienced interventional cardiologists, usually resulting in the overestimation of severe stenoses and *vice versa* (3–8). Having evolved from the era of digital calipers into highly sophisticated software algorithms, QCA provides an objective and reproducible approach for the analysis of contrast-filled coronary arteries (9–12). However, conventional angiographic analysis is limited by the 2D representation of 3D coronary anatomy (13). Owing to flat-panel detectors and increased computational power of contemporary workstations, a spatially accurate 3D reconstruction of the vessel lumen can be made available in real time for single-vessel and bifurcation lesions (14–17). Angiographic measurements can be used on-line in order to size and deploy intracoronary devices, whereas off-line they can help us evaluate the efficacy of coronary interventions as well as the progression of coronary atherosclerosis (18). A standardized operating procedure is of evident importance at every individual step during angiographic analysis (9,19).

2D QUANTITATIVE CORONARY ANALYSIS

Acquisition and Calibration

A first requirement for reliable angiographic analysis is the acquisition of high-quality images. Projections with the least possible vessel foreshortening should be selected, whereas overlap with adjacent vessel branches and/or non-coronary structures (sternal wires, pacemaker leads, metallic markers) should be avoided. Intracoronary injection of nitrates prior to contrast injection for controlling vasomotor tone, and use of 100% low-osmolar contrast at 37°C should be standardized; radiographic settings should be optimized and kept constant throughout acquisition. Correct selection and engagement of angiographic catheters, proper patient positioning and table height, optimal breath hold by the patient, use of wedge filters, adequate duration of contrast injection are all of paramount importance (20) and are detailed in textbooks and relevant references (21).

Calibration of 2D projection images has to be performed before we start with actual image analysis; the following options are available:

1. Automatic calibration: Automatic calibration is based on the acquisition geometry of the angiographic projections; in order to compute a valid calibration factor, the target vessel segment has to be placed at the angiographic system isocenter (i.e. center of rotation). Nevertheless, the automatically derived pixel size can be valid on only one plane (the isocenter plane) (17). The course of coronary vessels does not usually lie on a single plane inside the human thorax; hence analysis of different vessel segments on the same 2D angiographic image is subject to errors from variable magnification (13). Naturally, the same phenomenon applies to catheter calibration as well.

2. Calibration is performed using an object of known dimensions as a scaling device, conventionally the angiographic catheter. The system's edge-detection algorithm is applied to the non-tapered catheter tip resulting in automatic detection of its outer contour, whereby the system assumes a cylindrical shape of the catheter (22). However, this calibration method has several limitations. Digital images acquired in earlier technology angiographic systems suffered from the so-called pin-cushion (geometric) distortion; that is a selectively increased magnification of objects viewed in the periphery of the angiographic field, commonly the location of the angiographic catheter. This resulted in an erroneously small calibration factor, thus an underestimation of luminal dimensions (23). This distortion is not present in the flat-panel detectors; however, even so, catheter calibration is susceptible to error due to different intra-thoracic locations of catheter and target vessel segment (out-of-plane magnification). The magnitude and direction of error are dependent on the coronary artery and the angiographic projection (24). The angiographic catheter true size is known to deviate from the nominal dimensions. Furthermore, catheter radio-opacity and thereby its outer contour detection is dependent on its composition and wall thickness (25); variability from this source is more pronounced with nylon catheters (up to 10% overestimation) (22). Whereas in validation studies a precision micrometer can be used to measure the exact size of the catheter tip, this approach is not practical in clinical cases. Finally, contour detection varies considerably with contrast filling of the catheters; that is why it has been suggested, that the non-tapered, saline-flushed tip of the catheter is used as a calibration object (26); however, there is no unanimous policy on this issue.

3. Manual calibration: The pixel size has already been derived, usually based on a geometric calibration of an object of known dimensions such as a centimeter grid, and is entered into the system manually by the analyst; this option usually applies to validation studies, in an attempt to enhance accuracy and minimize the intra- and inter-observer variability (27).

Single-Vessel Analysis

From each acquired cine-run that clearly displays the target vessel segment, we usually select an image in the second or third heart cycle after contrast administration to ensure homogeneous contrast filling. Furthermore, end-diastolic frames are usually selected for analysis, in order to avoid motion blur and minimize variability from frame selection (Focus Box 11.1) (28,29).

The analyst defines the target vessel segment by indicating proximal and distal delimiter points at easily identifiable

---

Focus Box 11.1 Standard Operation Procedure for Quantitative Coronary Angiography Analysis

- Good visualization of target vessel segment (no overlap, minimal foreshortening)
- Homogeneous contrast filling (end-diastolic images, frame in second or third heart cycle after contrast administration)
- Automatic or catheter calibration (automatic preferable, although not error-free)
- Analysis of target vessel segments between adjacent bifurcations (bifurcation to bifurcation)
- Minimal user interaction
- Analysis in at least two orthogonal views fulfilling these criteria
- For serial angiographic studies, acquisitions in identical projections are essential

---

landmarks, such as major coronary bifurcations, in order to limit operator selection bias. A path-line is then automatically calculated between these delimiting points based on a wave propagation algorithm. Alternatively, if the automatic path-line does not correspond to the vessel's course, this can be indicated by the analyst using the computer mouse. Subsequently, detection of luminal contours is performed based on an edge-detection algorithm, which consists in a two-step iteration. In the first step, tentative vessel contours are computed based on the brightness profiles along scan-lines perpendicular to the vessel path-line. In the second step, a so-called minimum cost algorithm searches for an optimal path along the entire vessel segment using the tentative vessel contours as a model; based on some connectivity criterion the final vessel contours are computed. If necessary, the analyst can edit the initially detected contours in various ways, ultimately by manually redrawing them (usually in part); nevertheless, minimal user-interaction is preferred (11,30).

Minimal Lumen Diameter/Area (MLD/MLA)

From the final luminal contours, the diameter function is determined by computing the shortest distances between the left and right contour positions. The obstruction site and length is determined from the diameter function on the basis of curvature analysis; MLD is taken as the absolute shortest distance between the two-vessel contours (11). However, most coronary lesions are known to have an elliptical shape; MLA values extrapolated from a single or even two orthogonal MLD measurements can be at gross variance with intravascular ultrasound (IVUS) derived values. This discrepancy is aggravated after balloon angioplasty, which results in hazy, irregular lumen contours (31–33). Video-densitometry would be expected to quantify the stenosis and the changes conferred by angioplasty more accurately, being independent of lumen morphology. This method is based on the Beer-Lambert law, which states that the logarithmic attenuation of an X-ray beam through a vessel is proportional to the thickness of the contrast medium inside that vessel (34). Although this method is theoretically appealing, in vitro and in vivo validation studies have demonstrated higher accuracy and precision for edge-detection in the detection of larger vessel lumens (26,35). Video-densitometry is limited by the effects of spectral hardening and scatter of the X-ray beam, veiling glare, background noise, vessel foreshortening, and overlap; inhomogeneous contrast filling of the vessel as a result of blood turbulence or intra-luminal dissection makes things worse (26). Notably, restoration of a near-circular vessel lumen configuration and sealing of dissections after stent implantation improves the performance of both edge-detection and video-densitometry (32).

On the other hand, edge-detection of small objects is historically known to be affected by blurring due to the limitations of the X-ray systems and noise (27). Notwithstanding the introduction of flat-panel detectors and increased software sophistication, these phenomena are still present as evidenced by the overestimation of lumen diameters <1.00 mm in recent validation studies (12,36). Several approaches have been reported to improve the accuracy of small diameters for single-vessel analysis. Recently, an algorithm has been validated, where video-densitometric information is dynamically integrated in the process of lumen detection, in order to reduce the overestimation of small diameters resulting from stand-alone edge-detection. This new approach benefits from the relative strengths of both techniques (video-densitometry is better for small lumens whereas edge-detection is better for larger lumens), by dynamically combining them (37). In any event, cross-sectional area measurements from either edge-detection or video-densitometry based on a single projection should be interpreted with caution (38). Acquisition and evaluation of the target vessel segment in as many angiographic projections as possible (at least two orthogonal views) is strongly recommended (Fig. 11.1); in serial angiographic studies, time-related changes should be evaluated in identical angiographic projections.

Reference Vessel Diameter (RVD)/Percent Diameter Stenosis (DS)

In order to determine the reference size of a target vessel segment, the analyst can select either a "user-defined" or an "interpolated" reference (9,11,39). The former is usually the average of the mean diameters of apparently normal segments proximally and distally to the target lesion, resulting in a horizontal RVD function. A single reference point can also be selected, under the assumption that healthy vessel segments between adjacent bifurcations are not expected to taper. In the latter method, the reference diameter function is determined by a regression technique (interpolation) based on the entire analyzed vessel segment, wherein stenotic or ectatic coronary segments are not taken into account. This technique, proprietary to each software package, results in a straight tapering line which approximates the perceived normal or disease-free arterial contour over the obstruction site.

Applying the user-defined method, one can have a constant reference throughout the intervention and follow-up studies, however, with the inherent bias of user selection; in excessively long or tapered vessel segments the validity of this approach is even more limited. On the other hand, the interpolated reference method requires minimal user interaction; however, in diffusely diseased vessel segments without a healthy reference point/segment the RVD function can be grossly underestimated (Fig. 11.2). Moreover, since the RVD is usually reported at the site of the MLD, migration of the MLD within the target vessel segment in successive studies will result in diverse RVD values (39).

The DS value is derived at the location of the MLD according to the following equation DS = $(1 - MLD/RVD) \times 100\%$. The integral of the distances between the luminal and the reference contours over the obstructive region of the coronary artery is defined as "plaque area."

Lesion Curvature – Angulation

The curvature of a given vessel segment is defined as the infinitesimal rate of change in the tangent to the vessel centerline. The curvature value is calculated in cm^{-1} as the inverse radius of the perfect circle drawn through three centerline points defined at the beginning, the center and the end of the analyzed vessel segment (Fig. 11.3) (40). The angulation of a vessel segment located in a coronary bend is defined as the angle in degrees that the tip of a guidewire would need to have in order to reach the distal part of the bend. Angulation is calculated as the angle created by the intersection of centerline tangent vectors for the proximal and distal parts of the analyzed vessel segment. Increased coronary angulation is known to predispose to atheroma formation and is associated with higher rates of acute procedural complications (usually due to dissections) (41), as well as increased restenosis, mostly due to stent strut fractures. Determination of such parameters can quantify the changes in vessel geometry after stent implantation and the conformability of the stents used (40).

Clinical Applications and Potential Limitations

QCA has been long used in the study of pharmacologically induced coronary vasomotion. Essential to this study is the minimization of variability in data acquisition and analysis, as already detailed. The mean lumen diameter for the target vessel segment is computed in serial acquisitions of the same single projection at baseline and after methylergonovine or acetylcholine administration; this allows quantification of the reactivity of the arterial wall to provocative stimuli and determination of the degree of endothelial dysfunction (42).

In order to determine the functional significance of a coronary stenosis, QCA software can provide estimates for the anticipated pressure drop for certain levels of coronary flow. However, there is a large discrepancy between estimated and actually measured trans-stenotic pressure gradients due to limited applicability of proposed fluid-dynamic equations especially at high flows; estimates assume non-pulsatile flow in rigid and straight tubes (18,43). In the absence of fractional flow reserve (FFR) measurements, interventional cardiologists extrapolate the functional significance of a coronary stenosis based on respective DS values. On one hand, DS estimates as high as 90% or even higher,

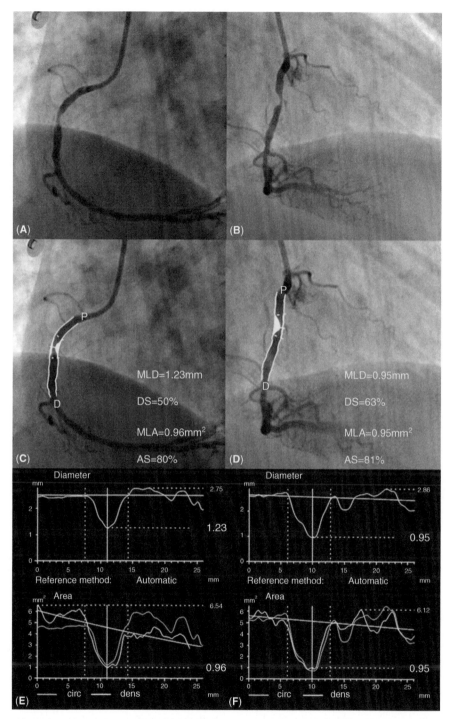

Figure 11.1 Edge-detection versus videodensitometry. Orthogonal views (**A, B**) of the right coronary artery show an eccentric lesion in the proximal vessel. (**C, D**) Quantitative coronary angiography analysis in 2D images; MLD/DS vary considerably between images, whereas MLA/AS is remarkably consistent. (**E, F**) Diameter and area graphs for respective images. Diameters are derived from edge-detection; there are two area curves, one based on edge detection, one on videodensitometry. *Abbreviations*: AS, area stenosis; DS, diameter stenosis; MLA, minimal lumen area; MLD, minimal lumen diameter.

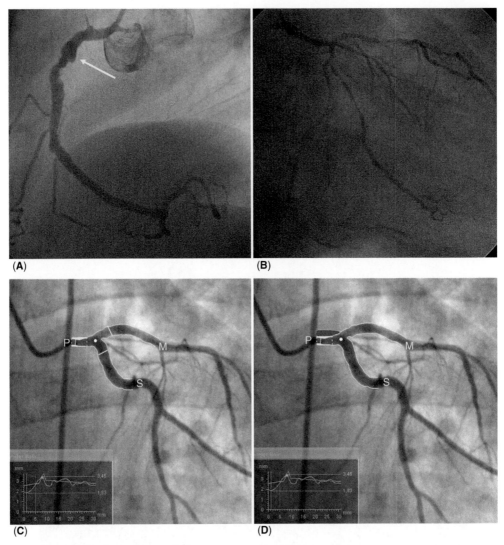

Figure 11.2 Pitfalls of quantitative coronary angiography analysis. Reference vessel diameter can be severely over-, or under-estimated in ectatic (A) or diffusely diseased (B) vessels respectively. In a diffusely diseased proximal vessel segment, there is no clear reference (C); in the left main, a more credible reference size can be defined by the user, based on the law of Finet assuming that the distal bifurcation branches are not diffusely diseased themselves (D).

common in visual assessment, are physiologically impossible. Even assuming an RVD of 3.0–3.5 mm, MLD would correspond to 0.35 mm, barely the width of a guidewire; residual lumens smaller than 0.5–0.6 are prone to intra-luminal thrombosis and occlusion, thereby not bound to be open for visual inspection (26,31,43). On the other hand, even the more credible QCA derived DS values are relative measurements limited by the assumption of a healthy reference vessel segment. It is known that in the early stages of atherosclerotic lesion formation, the vessel undergoes an outward expansion, concealing the presence of disease. At the stage that plaque begins to encroach on the lumen, it has already taken up 40% of the remodeled vessel cross-sectional area (44). Thus, assumed healthy reference segments are not necessarily disease-free, thereby limiting the

reliability of QCA derived RVD, DS, plaque area, and volume measurements (18).

In the end, MLD, being the only absolute unambiguous measurement, has been found to correlate more closely with FFR measurements for the simple reason that changes in MLD will affect the pressure gradient by a power of four. A cut-off value of 1.45–1.54 mm identifies with high sensitivity and specificity both the onset of angina and a steep increase in trans-stenotic gradients (45,46); this range of values is by fortunate coincidence where edge-detection algorithms perform the best.

Following this reasoning, MLD is more suitable than any other relative measurement to evaluate the efficacy of intra-coronary devices and the progression/regression of atherosclerosis over time. Angiographic surrogate endpoints derived

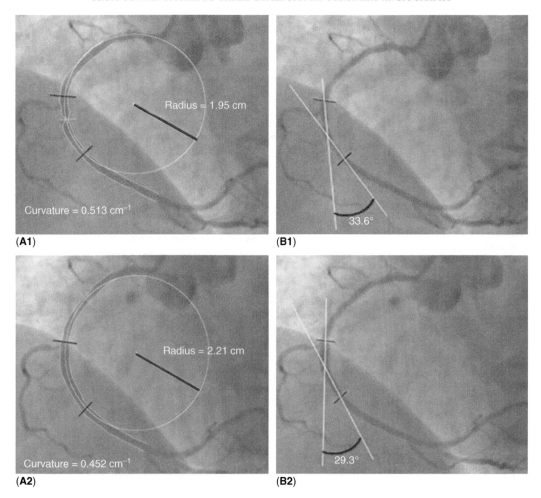

Figure 11.3 Curvature (**A**) and angulation (**B**) analysis is shown before (**A1-B1**) and after stent implantation (**A2-B2**). Curvature is calculated in cm^{-1} as the inverse radius of a circle drawn through three centerline points at the beginning, the center and the end of the analyzed vessel segment. Angulation is defined by the tangents of the centerline at the beginning and end of the target vessel segment.

from MLD are employed for this purpose; the acute lumen gain is calculated as the difference in measurements between post- and pre-procedural analysis, whereas the late lumen loss is the difference in MLD between follow-up and post-procedural angiography. Higher reproducibility in MLD measurements as achieved with last generation QCA software allows a downward re-definition of restenosis (a late loss of ≤0.4 mm) and thereby a reduction of sample size in serial angiographic studies (47). However, late lumen loss is calculated without taking into account the possible axial relocation of the MLD in the target vessel segment between post-procedure and follow-up QCA analysis, thereby limiting its correlation with the restenotic process as evidenced by IVUS (Focus Box 11.2) (48–50).

BIFURCATION ANALYSIS
In accordance with the European Bifurcation Club, a bifurcation lesion is defined as "a coronary artery narrowing adjacent to, and/or involving the origin of a significant side-branch (SB)";

significant is defined as a SB that the operator does not want to lose (51). Currently, bifurcation lesions are classified according to Medina (52). The proximal main vessel (PMV), the distal main vessel (DMV), and the SB are visually adjudicated for the presence of significant stenosis; every vessel segment, following the same order, is assigned an integer of 1 when DS exceeds 50%, and an integer of 0 when DS<50%. Lesions with Medina class (1,1,1), (1,0,1), and (0,1,1), where both the main vessel and the SB show significant stenosis, are designated as "true" bifurcation lesions.

However, inaccuracy and variability of visual DS estimates are even more pronounced in bifurcation lesions compared with single-vessel segments (53). This probably represents an additive effect between the shortcomings of visual assessment and the particularities in bifurcation lesion interpretation. The vessel segments distal to the bifurcation carina taper in size, their reference diameter being dictated by laws of fractal geometry, such as Murray's Law ($[PMV]^3 = [DMV]^3 + [SB]^3$) or the more simplified law of Finet (54), wherein PMV = 0.678*(DMV + SB). However, the intuitive way, in which even experienced operators interpret stenosis severity at or close to the ostium of distal bifurcation branches, is by referring to the PMV segment, thus resulting in overestimated DS values. Conversely, lesions in the PMV may be underestimated.

These phenomena are also reflected in the way single-vessel QCA analysis has been applied in the bifurcation lesions (Fig. 11.4). Manual extension of vessel contours from the SB/DMV into the PMV and vice versa is an arbitrary and tedious procedure (55); not unexpectedly this results in DS measurements that correlate poorly with FFR values of ostial SB stenoses (56). To make up for these shortcomings, dedicated bifurcation QCA algorithms have been developed, wherein the RVD function is separately determined for PMV, DMV, and SB (57,58). The bifurcation region itself is treated in a different way compared with single-vessel segments; luminal diameters, MLD, and RVD function for this region are derived with methodology specific to individual software developers. Results are reported over a number of segments including the stented areas, the peri-stent areas and the ostia of SB and DMV. This segmentation facilitates the accurate localization of MLD in serial angiographic studies, thereby providing more reliable late lumen loss measurements. This way we can increase our understanding of the mechanisms that lead to post-intervention failure and restenosis, especially at the SB ostium (39).

In order to determine the actual impact of different definitions on the accuracy and precision of QCA measures, validation studies have been performed using precision manufactured bifurcation phantoms; their design reflected the anatomic variation and the fractal nature of coronary bifurcations as derived from the relevant literature (59). In the latest edition of the Cardiovascular Angiography Analysis System (CAAS, Pie Medical Imaging, Maastricht, The Netherlands) 2D bifurcation QCA software, accuracy and precision (mean difference ± SD) for MLD was 0.01 ± 0.08 mm, for RVD -0.03 ± 0.05 mm and for DS $-0.48 \pm 3.66\%$ (in anteroposterior views) (37); respective measures for QAngio XA (Medis medical imaging systems, Leiden, The Netherlands) were 0.02 ± 0.10 mm, -0.01 ± 0.04 mm and $-0.60 \pm 4.23\%$ (60). Reproducibility was very high for both 2D software algorithms, whereas the effect of modest gantry rotation on measurements was limited; it should be emphasized that results over the entire bifurcation are obtained during a single analysis. The superiority of the dedicated 2D bifurcation software over conventional QCA was confirmed by a study showing an improved correlation with invasive functional testing in real coronary cases (61). This correlation is expected to improve further through the integration of dedicated bifurcation QCA algorithms with a spatially accurate 3D reconstruction of bifurcation lesions. Naturally, definitive conclusions on the anatomical and functional relevance of QCA-derived measures in bifurcation lesions will be drawn from ongoing major randomized trials in the field, such as EXCEL and TRYTON.

Bifurcation Angle

Next to the diameter-derived measures the bifurcation angle (BA) is another important piece of information that can be derived from QCA analysis of bifurcation lesions; however, definitions and measurement methods are still at variance. The European Bifurcation Club has adopted a definition, according to which proximal and distal BA are delineated between the PMV and the SB, and between the DMV and the SB, respectively (Fig. 11.5) (51). Regarding BA quantification, until recently a binary approach was adopted; bifurcations used to be divided in T-shaped (BA≥70°) and Y-shaped ones (BA<70°) according to visual assessment or calculations using digital calipers (62). The T-shaped bifurcations were associated with unfavorable SB access and increased procedural complexity (63). Automated algorithms for BA calculation have been implemented in 2D and 3D QCA software (14,57,64); meticulous quantification requires adherence to the following acquisition and documentation guidelines: (*i*) A coronary bifurcation is a 3D structure; if 3D reconstruction is not available, the 2D angiographic view in which foreshortening of the three vessel segments is minimal provides a reliable approximation of the BA true size. (*ii*) The temporary insertion of an angioplasty guidewire into the SB is sufficient for the BA to be considerably modified; operators tend to use this very maneuver in order to facilitate access to the SB (62). Therefore, BA calculations are better performed either pre- or post-procedure without guidewires in place. (*iii*) There is a significant systolic-diastolic variation for BA, distal values increasing in diastole (65); hence to be consistent, similar phases of the heart cycle should be analyzed.

BA has gained attention due to growing evidence that it can affect immediate procedural success and long-term outcome (66). Bench studies have shown that in the context of Crush stenting, a steep proximal angle and consequently a larger distal

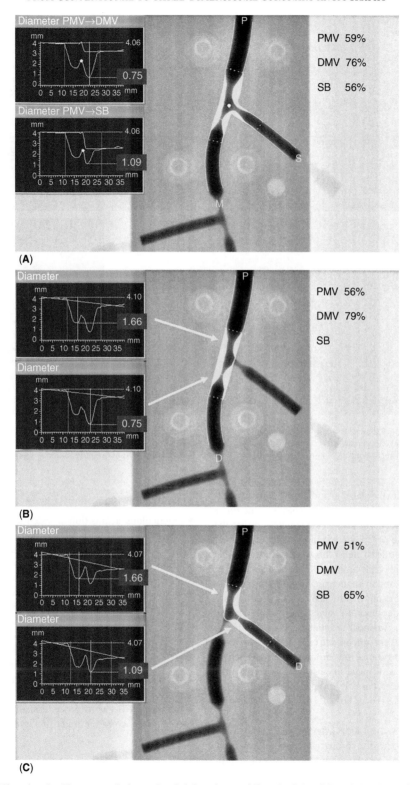

Figure 11.4 Dedicated bifurcation algorithms versus single-vessel analysis in a phantom bifurcation lesion. (**A**) Analysis with a dedicated algorithm provides results for all three vessel segments. Single-vessel analysis along the main vessel (**B**) and from the PMV into the SB (**C**) results in under-estimation for PMV and over-estimation for distal branch lesion; the greater the discrepancy in vessel branch size the greater the inaccuracy. P, M, and S stand for PMV, DMV, and SB. *Abbreviations*: DMV, distal main vessel; PMV, proximal main vessel; SB, side branch.

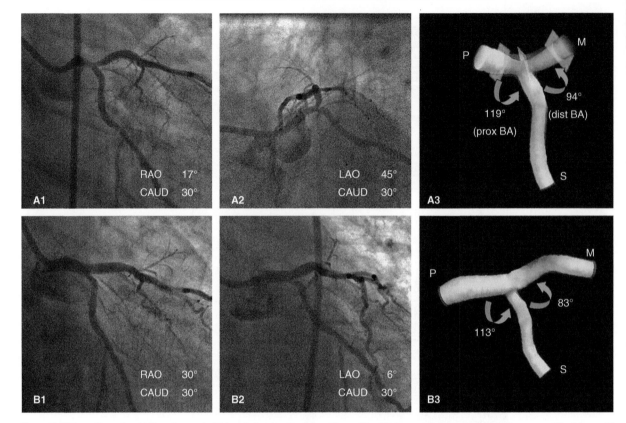

Figure 11.5 Three-dimensional bifurcation angle (BA) analysis using CardiOp software. Two 2D images of a left main bifurcation are combined into a 3D reconstruction before (**A**) and after percutaneous coronary intervention (**B**). Distal BA is decreased post-procedure. P, M, and S stand for PMV, DMV, and SB. *Abbreviations*: CAUD, caudal angulation; DMV, distal main vessel; PMV, proximal main vessel; RAO/LAO, right/left anterior oblique rotation; SB, side branch.

angle results in less optimal expansion and apposition of the SB stent, especially at the site of the ostium (67,68). On the other hand, theoretical considerations lead to the conclusion that the outcome of either Crush or Culotte technique will be adversely influenced by a narrower distal angle; this would be attributable to a more probable carina shift limiting the diameter of the SB ostium with Crush (69) and to an increased stent cell size necessary to span an oblique ostium with Culotte (70). In the long-term, it appears that wider distal BA values might incur a worse outcome especially with two-stent techniques (66,71,72). High- and low-shear stress areas are supposed to exist in close proximity in steeply angulated bifurcations, thus promoting platelet activation and stasis; an excess of metal in such an area would only aggravate these phenomena, possibly leading to increased rates of thrombosis and restenosis (Focus Box 11.3).

3D RECONSTRUCTION AND QUANTITATIVE ANALYSIS

Expert recommended views for coronary arteries do not apply to all patients due to anatomic variation; notwithstanding individual operator skill to mentally reconstruct coronary anatomy from a number of suboptimal projection images, this procedure is prone to substantial error (73). Vessel overlap and tortuosity

Focus Box 11.3 Bifurcation Analysis

- Meticulous acquisition is essential; there is one single optimal projection.
- Medina classification (visual assessment)
- Single-vessel analysis in bifurcations overestimates side branch and underestimates proximal main vessel lesions
- Dedicated bifurcation quantitative coronary angiography software algorithms are accurate, precise, and reproducible; correlation with fractional flow reserve values is improved
- Steep bifurcation angle (BA) between main vessel and side-branch increases procedural complexity
- BA modification after percutaneous coronary intervention is dependent on technique (number of stents used in the bifurcation)
- BA can predict acute procedural and long-term outcomes (generally worse for larger BA, at least when ≥2 stents are used)

interfere with angiographic analysis and can mask obstructive coronary lesions. Furthermore, out-of-plane magnification and foreshortening, often not fully appreciated, result in inaccurate

Focus Box 11.4 Pitfalls of 2D Analysis (Merits of 3D quantitative coronary angiography)

- Vessel overlap
- Vessel tortuosity
- Vessel foreshortening
- Lesion eccentricity
- Out-of-plane magnification/errors from catheter calibration (full automatic calibration)
- Bifurcation angle underestimation/side-branch take-off obscured (optimal projection determination)

estimates for vessel size and lesion length and thus erroneous stent sizing and deployment. Selection of a stent that is too short will result in incomplete coverage of the lesion and possibly in the need for a second stent inflating procedural cost; conversely, an excessively long stent will result in geographic miss, potential SB jailing and increased restenosis rates (15,17,74). On the other hand, the clinical implications of over- or under-sized stents would be edge dissections or even vessel perforations for the former, with malapposition and stent thrombosis as potential complications of the latter (Focus Box 11.4) (75).

In the last 10–15 years several algorithms for 3D reconstruction and subsequent QCA analysis have been developed (14–17). Most of them do not create a true volumetric reconstruction of the vessel lumen, which still is computationally demanding and cannot be made available online (see section on *rotational angiography*), but rather a 3D model, which is based on the reconstruction of the vessel centerline.

Such a reconstruction requires at least two 2D angiographic images separated by a viewing angle ≥30°; images acquired by a biplane, monoplane or a rotational angiographic system can be combined. The accuracy of the 3D model heavily relies on digital flat-panel detectors being free from "pincushion" distortion as well as on the acquisition geometry of the 2D projection images, which is stored in the DICOM headers of the angiographic system. However, this information alone is not sufficient to obtain an accurate 3D reconstruction because of the isocenter offset of the angiographic system. The isocenter offset is the spatial difference between the isocenters of the frontal and lateral C-arms in a biplane gantry and can be affected by gravity; even in a monoplane system rotating the gantry to a different acquisition angle could cause a significant shift of more than 20 mm to its isocenter. The spatial correspondence between 2D derived centerlines is re-established by identifying 1–3 reference points, which represent corresponding anatomical landmarks (e.g. bifurcation points) in the 2D images; this procedure also corrects for the respiration induced heart motion (17,64).

Notwithstanding subtle differences between available algorithms, a standard operator procedure for a 3D reconstruction of a coronary lesion consists in the following steps:

1. Angiographic images of the target vessel segment (possibly a bifurcation) showing minimal foreshortening and overlap are selected. For images acquired

on a monoplane system, electrocardiographic-gating can ensure proper time alignment of analyzed image frames.

2. If necessary, catheter calibration is performed in one of the images (14). However, full automatic calibration is the default (and only) choice in most algorithms (17,64).

3. The target vessel segment is identified and automatic contour detection is performed. The same procedure is repeated in the next selected image(s); the region of interest is automatically indicated by the epipolar lines, thereby assisting the analyst in correctly placing the delimiter points.

4. Reference points are identified; automatically determined common image points are verified or relocated, as appropriate (17,64,74).

5. The 3D model is created by fitting the contour information derived from the 2D images to the 3D vessel centerline. An image of the reconstructed vessel is provided together with quantitative data on vessel diameter/area, stenosis severity, length and BA, when applicable (Fig. 11.6).

The performance of commercially available 3D QCA software in single-vessel segments has been reported in a number of validation studies. Length measurements were shown to have very high accuracy and precision compared with objects of known dimensions (14,16,17), whereas correlation was excellent with IVUS (76,77), multi-slice computed tomography (MSCT) (76) and 3D reconstructions based on fusion of biplane angiography and IVUS (ANGUS) (78). Regarding luminal diameter and area measurements, the highest in-vitro accuracy and precision was reported for 3D CAAS, specifically 0.01 ± 0.09 mm for MLD and 0.02 ± 0.14 mm^2 for MLA (15); respective in-vivo measures were 0.37 ± 0.37 mm and 0.45 ± 1.49 mm^2 when compared with ANGUS reconstructions (78). Equally important, using CardiOp-B 3D QCA software (Paieon Medical, Ltd., Rosh Ha'ayin, Israel), MLA and percent area stenosis were shown to have higher power for predicting significantly reduced FFR values, when compared with parameters derived from 2D analysis (79). Finally, experience with 3D bifurcation reconstructions has been reported comparing results with 2D analysis (80,81); however, accuracy and precision of 3D bifurcation QCA measurements has not been established compared with a gold standard; validation is currently under way.

A relative merit of most 3D modeling algorithms is the determination of the optimal viewing angle, which is especially important for bifurcation lesions (82,83). Absence of vessel-overlap, minimal foreshortening and widest possible opening of the bifurcation can be found together in one single best view, if at all. It follows that in any other projection, certain parts of the anatomy, usually the ostia of the daughter branches, are obscured due to overlap. Three-dimensional QCA algorithms can retrieve missing information even from a combination of suboptimal views (64); nevertheless, a reconstruction including the optimal

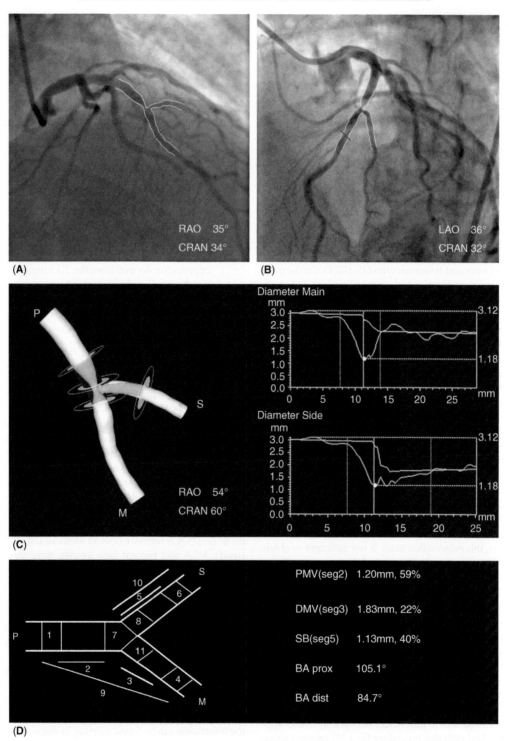

Figure 11.6 Three-dimensional reconstruction and quantitative coronary angiography bifurcation analysis with a dedicated algorithm (Cardiovascular Angiography Analysis System software). (**A, B**) 2D images of an left anterior descending artery-diagonal bifurcation lesion; red cross marks a common image point. (**C**) 3D reconstructed bifurcation shown in the optimal projection (lesion in blue) together with diameter graphs (simplified) (**D**). *Left*: 11-segment model schematic. *Right*: MLD and DS results for PMV, DMV and SB together with BA values. *Abbreviations*: BA, bifurcation angle; DMV, distal main vessel; DS, diameter stenosis; MLD, minimal lumen diameter; PMV, proximal main vessel; SB, side branch.

2D projection is expected to be even more robust (82). Furthermore, the optimal working view could facilitate stent positioning keeping radiation and contrast usage to a minimum. However, limitations imposed by patients' anatomy (vessel overlap) or proximity between the gantry and the patient/table may make it difficult to acquire the optimal view exactly as suggested (Focus Box 11.5).

ROTATIONAL ANGIOGRAPHY

Similar to the analysis of individual lesions, the overall screening adequacy of a routine angiographic study is dependent on a limited number of subjectively selected fixed-view images; anatomic features such as eccentric lesions, tortuous vessels, and/or BAs may not be appreciated, if the optimal projection is not acquired (84). Rotational angiography provides a standardized approach to acquire significantly more information from the entire coronary tree, at the same time minimizing acquisition time, contrast usage, and radiation exposure (85–88). New gantries have been developed that allow rapid isocentric rotations of the imaging camera; acquisitions over a long trajectory (arcs up to 200°) with pre-defined cranial or caudal orientation can be completed within few seconds. Moreover, dual-motion coronary angiography allows rotation in several axes rather than in a simple arc, offering a multiple-angle

perspective within a single, continuous, slightly longer (7.2 sec) contrast injection (88,89). Information obtained from rotational acquisitions can then be used for tomographic reconstructions of the coronary vessels similar to the ones provided by conventional CT-scans (Dyna-CT) (Fig. 11.7) (90); as opposed to 3D modeling algorithms, no user interaction is required (84). Currently, the major limitation of this method is the decreased temporal resolution of rotational angiography (~5 sec per half gantry rotation as opposed to around 180 ms per half rotation on a modern MSCT scanner); dedicated algorithms are being developed to minimize the effect of coronary motion thereby improving the quality of reconstruction (Focus Box 11.6) (91–93).

QUALITATIVE ASSESSMENT OF CORONARY LESION MORPHOLOGY

Coronary angiography cannot evaluate coronary plaque composition and therefore is unable to distinguish between stable and high-risk vulnerable plaques; solely based on the extent of obstruction, one will fail to predict the location and timing of a future symptomatic plaque rupture (94). However, prognostic information regarding the immediate and long-term outcome after PCI can be inferred from the study of flow characteristics and lesion morphology patterns.

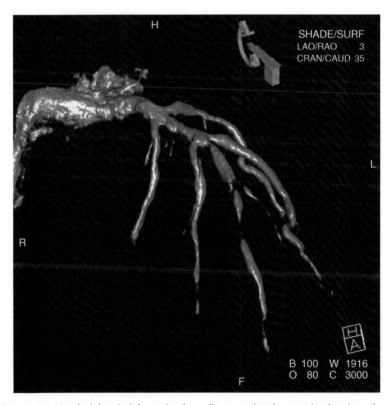

Figure 11.7 Volumetric 3D reconstruction of a left main-left anterior descending artery based on rotational angiography with motion compensation. Reconstructed vessel is shown in a cranial orientation.

Focus Box 11.5 Acquisition Guidelines Aiming at a 3D Reconstruction (Including Bifurcations)

- Use a flat-panel detector system, if available
- Use biplane gantry, if available
- Record the electrocardiogram; it is essential for temporal alignment of images acquired on a monoplane system
- Obtain angiograms during breath hold
- Do not shift/move the patient/table during the recording of a single projection
- Each angiogram has to be preceded by intra-coronary injection of nitrates
- Acquire at least two different projection images, separated by at least 30° in viewing angle
- Try to acquire the optimal projection for a given bifurcation; side-branch ostium should be clearly visible with the least possible overlap. Alternatively, try to acquire the optimal projection suggested after a 3D reconstruction
- Acquire angiograms before the insertion of guidewires
- At the end of the procedure, do not forget to repeat the same angiographic views (at least two) without guidewires in place

---

Focus Box 11.6 3D Models Versus 3D Volumetric Reconstructions

Centerline based	Volumetric reconstruction
Monoplane, biplane or rotational acquisition	Rotational angiography
At least two (up to four) 2D projection images	Multiple views (rotation arcs up to 200 deg); preselected cranial-caudal angulation; dual axis rotation feasible
Available in real time	Time consuming (requires at least 3 min, usually considerably longer)
Requires some user-interaction	No user interaction needed
Need for visual skill for initial acquisitions; indicates optimal projection	Automated or semi-automated procedure
Trial and error	Minimization of contrast usage and radiation exposure
Correction for isocenter offset	Need for motion compensation

Coronary artery flow has been classified according to the Thrombolysis In Myocardial Infarction (TIMI) grading scale; this classification was initially devised to grade coronary reperfusion in patients with acute myocardial infarction and has now become the standard method for semi-quantitative evaluation of coronary flow in clinical trials. TIMI grade 3 corresponds to brisk antegrade flow (also by comparison to non-culprit vessels) and heralds best clinical outcomes, whereas TIMI grade 0 and 1 indicate minimal perfusion or none at all (95). Angiographic contrast run-off can be further quantified with the TIMI frame count, namely the number of cineframes required

for contrast to reach a predetermined distal landmark, standardized for each coronary artery. Delayed flow corresponds to more than a doubling of normal frame counts and has been associated with increased mortality rates (96).

Qualitative assessment of coronary morphology was first employed in 1985 to explain the pathogenesis of unstable angina (97). Subsequently, a number of morphological lesion characteristics, including but not limited to lesion length, eccentricity, angulation, irregularity, calcification, thrombus, and coronary occlusion, have been associated with increased rates of acute complications after PCI (98,99). The classification established by the American College of Cardiology/American Heart Association (ACC/AHA) integrated several adverse angiographic characteristics in lesion types of increasing complexity (Types A, B1, B2, and C), in order to assist the selection of patients suitable for PCI and to stratify procedural risk independent of clinical presentation (Table 11.1) (100,101). This classification retained its long-term prognostic value, when lesions were reclassified into simple (A plus B1) and complex ones (B2 plus C) (102).

Including many of the adverse lesion characteristics, the SYNTAX score grades the angiographic complexity of CAD referred to above at a patient level (103). In the SYNTAX trial, it proved effective in predicting clinical outcomes after elective PCI procedures in patients with three-vessel and/or left main CAD (104,105). Furthermore, the score's predictive ability for a number of clinical outcomes has subsequently been confirmed in patient cohorts with a varying extent of CAD undergoing both elective and emergent PCI procedures (106). The calculation of the SYNTAX score is lesion based; all coronary lesions with a visually assessed percent DS ≥50%, in vessels ≥1.5 mm are scored using the SYNTAX score algorithm, which is available online (www.syntaxscore.com). The algorithm takes into account the functional impact and the stenosis severity of the lesion; occlusive lesions are weighed more heavily than non-occlusive ones. All other adverse lesion characteristics considered in the SYNTAX score have an additive and not multiplicative value. Finally, the total SYNTAX score is derived from the summation of all individual lesion scorings (103).

Visual assessment for stenosis severity and vessel size coupled with variable adjudication of coronary bifurcations and adverse lesion characteristics such as thrombus and diffuse disease may limit the reproducibility of the SYNTAX score (107). Motion compensated 3D reconstruction of rotational angiograms and subsequent quantification could potentially render a more objective score (Focus Box 11.7).

PERSONAL PERSPECTIVE

The major challenge for QCA is to achieve integration into the daily interventional routine and to be considered essential in device sizing and deployment. The primary role of angiography in the guidance of PCI has increasingly been contested by invasive imaging modalities such as IVUS and optical coherence tomography (OCT) and by invasive functional testing. However, while the information from these techniques has potential added

TABLE 11.1 American College of Cardiology/American Heart Association Lesion Classification System in the Percutaneous Coronary Intervention Stent Era

Type A High success – low risk	Type B[a] Moderate success – moderate risk	Type C Low success – high risk
Discrete (length<10 mm)	Tubular (length 10–20 mm)	Diffuse (length>20 mm)
Concentric	Eccentric[b]	
Readily accessible	Moderate tortuosity of proximal segment[c]	Excessive tortuosity of proximal segment[c]
Non-angulated vessel segment (<45°)	Moderately angulated vessel segment (>45°, <90°)	Extremely angulated vessel segment (>90°)
Smooth contour	Irregular contour[d]	
Little or no calcification	Moderate or heavy calcification[e]	
Less than totally occlusive	Total occlusion[f] <3 months old	Total occlusion >3 months old and/or bridging collaterals
Not ostial in location	Ostial in location[g]	
No side-branch (RVD≥1.5 mm) involvement	True bifurcation lesions	Inability to protect major side-branch
Absence of thrombus	Some thrombus present[h]	
		Degenerated vein grafts with friable lesions[i]

[a]Lesions with one type B characteristic are classified as B1, lesions with ≥2 Type B characteristics are classified as B2.
[b]One of the luminal edges is located in the outer one-quarter of the apparent normal lumen.
[c]Moderate = up to two bends of 45° to 90° proximal to target lesion; excessive = one or more bends of 90° or more, or three or more bends of 45° to 90°.
[d]One or more of: ulceration, intimal flap, aneurysm, saw-tooth pattern.
[e](Multiple) persisting opacifications of the apparent coronary vessel wall at the site of the lesion.
[f]Thrombolysis in myocardial infarction 0/1 intra-luminal flow.
[g]Lesion starts within 3 mm of the vessel origin.
[h]Discrete intra-luminal filling defect, surrounded on three sides by contrast medium, seen just distal or within the coronary stenosis; alternatively, visible embolization of intra-luminal material downstream.
[i]lumen irregularity or ectasia covering >50% of the graft length.
Abbreviations: PCI, percutaneous coronary intervention; RVD, reference vessel diameter.

Focus Box 11.7 Qualitative Assessment of Coronary Lesion Morphology

- Coronary angiography cannot provide information on vessel wall composition
- Delayed antegrade coronary artery flow (less than thrombolysis in myocardial infarction 3 flow or respective frame count) is associated with adverse clinical outcomes
- A number of adverse lesion characteristics has been identified (Table 1)
- American College of Cardiology/American Heart Association lesion type classification (Types A, B1, B2, and C) retains its prognostic value in the stent era
- SYNTAX score is a lesion based angiographic score; it grades angiographic complexity at a patient level; it can risk-stratify patients with a varying extent of coronary artery disease undergoing both elective and emergent percutaneous coronary intervention procedures

value, IVUS, OCT, and/or FFR measurements are not invariably available or applicable. Moreover, the additional cost is currently a major issue. On the other hand, QCA can provide reliable information in real time from already acquired projection images at no extra cost beyond the initial purchase (one-off) of the software license. Admittedly, coronary angiography cannot provide information on vessel wall composition, nor can angiographic

measures such as MLD or DS account for all anatomic and hemodynamic components reflected in FFR values. Nevertheless, recent advances in angiographic analysis have not yet been integrated in current PCI strategies; prospective long-term outcome and cost-effectiveness trials are necessary to determine the clinical relevance of QCA-derived measures including the impact of local geometry (BA, curvature) that cannot be derived from other invasive imaging modalities.

Conceptually, a fusion of angiography with other imaging modalities into a 4-D "roadmap" could facilitate diagnosis and treatment in challenging lesions. Information derived from IVUS, OCT, and MSCT helps us understand the local pathology; however, none of these modalities is available in real time during stent implantation. Therefore, the operator has to mentally map the region of interest from analyzed image frames onto the fluoroscopy screen; in the absence of easily identifiable landmarks, such as a large SB, this process could result in geographical miss, vessel dissections, and/or perforations. Regarding invasive imaging, co-registration algorithms are now available accurately aligning 3D angiographic centerlines with IVUS/OCT pullbacks on a point-to-point basis (108); thereby vessel dimensions and plaque information can also be assessed at every corresponding position. On the other hand, co-registration of cardiac CT data with coronary angiography is also feasible quantifying calcified plaque and suggesting a reference vessel path in chronic total occlusions; IVUS-like images of the occluded vessel can be obtained helping the operator to tailor his/her strategy in this demanding lesion dataset (109). Further steps have yet to be taken for the actual fusion of imaging techniques.

REFERENCES

1. Sones FM Jr, Shirey EK. Cine coronary arteriography. Mod Concepts Cardiovasc Dis 1962; 31: 735–8.
2. Bruschke AV, Sheldon WC, Shirey EK, Proudfit WL. A half century of selective coronary arteriography. J Am Coll Cardiol 2009; 54: 2139–44.
3. Detre KM, Wright E, Murphy ML, Takaro T. Observer agreement in evaluating coronary angiograms. Circulation 1975; 52: 979–86.
4. Zir LM, Miller SW, Dinsmore RE, Gilbert JP, Harthorne JW. Interobserver variability in coronary angiography. Circulation 1976; 53: 627–32.
5. DeRouen TA, Murray JA, Owen W. Variability in the analysis of coronary arteriograms. Circulation 1977; 55: 324–8.
6. Beauman GJ, Vogel RA. Accuracy of individual and panel visual interpretations of coronary arteriograms: implications for clinical decisions. J Am Coll Cardiol 1990; 16: 108–13.
7. Fleming RM, Kirkeeide RL, Smalling RW, Gould KL. Patterns in visual interpretation of coronary arteriograms as detected by quantitative coronary arteriography. J Am Coll Cardiol 1991; 18: 945–51.
8. Bertrand ME, Lablanche JM, Bauters C, Leroy F, Mac Fadden E. Discordant results of visual and quantitative estimates of stenosis severity before and after coronary angioplasty. Cathet Cardiovasc Diagn 1993; 28: 1–6.
9. Reiber JH, Serruys PW, Kooijman CJ, et al. Assessment of short-, medium-, and long-term variations in arterial dimensions from computer-assisted quantitation of coronary cineangiograms. Circulation 1985; 71: 280–8.
10. Reiber JH, van der Zwet PM, Koning G, et al. Accuracy and precision of quantitative digital coronary arteriography: observer-, short-, and medium-term variabilities. Cathet Cardiovasc Diagn 1993; 28: 187–98.
11. Gronenschild E, Janssen J, Tijdens F. CAAS. II: a second generation system for off-line and on-line quantitative coronary angiography. Cathet Cardiovasc Diagn 1994; 33: 61–75.
12. Tuinenburg JC, Koning G, Seppenwoolde Y, Reiber JH. Is there an effect of flat-panel-based imaging systems on quantitative coronary and vascular angiography? Catheter Cardiovasc Interv 2006; 68: 561–6.
13. Green NE, Chen SY, Messenger JC, Groves BM, Carroll JD. Three-dimensional vascular angiography. Curr Probl Cardiol 2004; 29: 104–42.
14. Gradaus R, Mathies K, Breithardt G, Bocker D. Clinical assessment of a new real time 3D quantitative coronary angiography system: evaluation in stented vessel segments. Catheter Cardiovasc Interv 2006; 68: 44–9.
15. Ramcharitar S, Daeman J, Patterson M, et al. First direct in vivo comparison of two commercially available three-dimensional quantitative coronary angiography systems. Catheter Cardiovasc Interv 2008; 71: 44–50.
16. Agostoni P, Biondi-Zoccai G, Van Langenhove G, et al. Comparison of assessment of native coronary arteries by standard versus three-dimensional coronary angiography. Am J Cardiol 2008; 102: 272–9.
17. Tu S, Koning G, Jukema W, Reiber JH. Assessment of obstruction length and optimal viewing angle from biplane X-ray angiograms. Int J Cardiovasc Imaging 2010; 26: 5–17.
18. de Feyter PJ, Serruys PW, Davies MJ, et al. Quantitative coronary angiography to measure progression and regression of coronary atherosclerosis. Value, limitations, and implications for clinical trials. Circulation 1991; 84: 412–23.
19. Herrington DM, Siebes M, Sokol DK, Siu CO, Walford GD. Variability in measures of coronary lumen dimensions using quantitative coronary angiography. J Am Coll Cardiol 1993; 22: 1068–74.
20. Di Mario C, Sutaria N. Coronary angiography in the angioplasty era: projections with a meaning. Heart 2005; 91: 968–76.
21. Seiler C, Di Mario C. Invasive Imaging and Haemodynamics. In: Camm A, Luescher T, Serruys PW, eds. The ESC Textbook of Cardiovascular Medicine. Oxford, UK: Blackwell Publishing, 2006: 159–87.
22. Reiber JH, Kooijman CJ, den Boer A, Serruys PW. Assessment of dimensions and image quality of coronary contrast catheters from cineangiograms. Cathet Cardiovasc Diagn 1985; 11: 521–31.
23. Haase J, Di Mario C, Slager CJ, et al. In-vivo validation of on-line and off-line geometric coronary measurements using insertion of stenosis phantoms in porcine coronary arteries. Cathet Cardiovasc Diagn 1992; 27: 16–27.
24. Wunderlich W, Roehrig B, Fischer F, et al. The impact of vessel and catheter position on the measurement accuracy in catheter-based quantitative coronary angiography. Int J Card Imaging 1998; 14: 217–27.
25. Fortin DF, Spero LA, Cusma JT, et al. Pitfalls in the determination of absolute dimensions using angiographic catheters as calibration devices in quantitative angiography. Am J Cardiol 1991; 68: 1176–82.
26. Di Mario C, Haase J, den Boer A, Reiber JH, Serruys PW. Edge detection versus densitometry in the quantitative assessment of stenosis phantoms: an in vivo comparison in porcine coronary arteries. Am Heart J 1992; 124: 1181–9.
27. Keane D, Haase J, Slager CJ, et al. Comparative validation of quantitative coronary angiography systems. Results and implications from a multicenter study using a standardized approach. Circulation 1995; 91: 2174–83.
28. Reiber JH, van Eldik-Helleman P, Visser-Akkerman N, Kooijman CJ, Serruys PW. Variabilities in measurement of coronary arterial dimensions resulting from variations in cineframe selection. Cathet Cardiovasc Diagn 1988; 14: 221–8.
29. Fischell TA, Maheshwari A, Mirza RA, et al. Impact of frame selection on quantitative coronary angiographic analysis after coronary stenting. Catheter Cardiovasc Interv 2005; 64: 460–7.
30. Reiber JH, Kooijman CJ, Slager CJ, et al. Coronary artery dimensions from cineangiograms methodology and validation of a computer-assisted analysis procedure. IEEE Trans Med Imaging 1984; 3: 131–41.
31. Serruys PW, Reiber JH, Wijns W, et al. Assessment of percutaneous transluminal coronary angioplasty by quantitative coronary angiography: diameter versus densitometric area measurements. Am J Cardiol 1984; 54: 482–8.
32. Strauss BH, Juilliere Y, Rensing BJ, Reiber JH, Serruys PW. Edge detection versus densitometry for assessing coronary stenting quantitatively. Am J Cardiol 1991; 67: 484–90.
33. Ozaki Y, Violaris AG, Kobayashi T, et al. Comparison of coronary luminal quantification obtained from intracoronary ultrasound and both geometric and videodensitometric quantitative

angiography before and after balloon angioplasty and directional atherectomy. Circulation 1997; 96: 491–9.

34. Hermiller JB, Cusma JT, Spero LA, et al. Quantitative and qualitative coronary angiographic analysis: review of methods, utility, and limitations. Cathet Cardiovasc Diagn 1992; 25: 110–31.

35. Haase J, Escaned J, van Swijndregt EM, et al. Experimental validation of geometric and densitometric coronary measurements on the new generation Cardiovascular Angiography Analysis System (CAAS II). Cathet Cardiovasc Diagn 1993; 30: 104–14.

36. Girasis C, Schuurbiers JC, Onuma Y, et al. Two-dimensional quantitative coronary angiographic models for bifurcation segmental analysis: in vitro validation of CAAS against precision manufactured plexiglas phantoms. Catheter Cardiovasc Interv 2011; 77: 830–9.

37. Girasis C, Schuurbiers JC, Onuma Y, et al. Advances in two-dimensional quantitative coronary angiographic assessment of bifurcation lesions: improved small lumen diameter detection and automatic reference vessel diameter derivation. EuroIntervention 2011; In revision.

38. Escaned J, Foley DP, Haase J, et al. Quantitative angiography during coronary angioplasty with a single angiographic view: a comparison of automated edge detection and videodensitometric techniques. Am Heart J 1993; 126: 1326–33.

39. Lansky A, Tuinenburg J, Costa M, et al. Quantitative angiographic methods for bifurcation lesions: a consensus statement from the European Bifurcation Group. Catheter Cardiovasc Interv 2009; 73: 258–66.

40. Gomez-Lara J, Garcia-Garcia HM, Onuma Y, et al. A comparison of the conformability of everolimus-eluting bioresorbable vascular scaffolds to metal platform coronary stents. JACC Cardiovasc Interv 2010; 3: 1190–8.

41. Ellis SG, Topol EJ. Results of percutaneous transluminal coronary angioplasty of high-risk angulated stenoses. Am J Cardiol 1990; 66: 932–7.

42. Serruys PW, Ormiston JA, Onuma Y, et al. A bioabsorbable everolimus-eluting coronary stent system (ABSORB): 2-year outcomes and results from multiple imaging methods. Lancet 2009; 373: 897–910.

43. Rensing BJ, Hermans WR, Deckers JW, et al. Lumen narrowing after percutaneous transluminal coronary balloon angioplasty follows a near gaussian distribution: a quantitative angiographic study in 1,445 successfully dilated lesions. J Am Coll Cardiol 1992; 19: 939–45.

44. Glagov S, Weisenberg E, Zarins CK, Stankunavicius R, Kolettis GJ. Compensatory enlargement of human atherosclerotic coronary arteries. N Engl J Med 1987; 316: 1371–5.

45. Wijns W, Serruys PW, Reiber JH, et al. Quantitative angiography of the left anterior descending coronary artery: correlations with pressure gradient and results of exercise thallium scintigraphy. Circulation 1985; 71: 273–9.

46. Rensing BJ, Hermans WR, Deckers JW, de Feyter PJ, Serruys PW. Which angiographic variable best describes functional status 6 months after successful single-vessel coronary balloon angioplasty? J Am Coll Cardiol 1993; 21: 317–24.

47. Pocock SJ, Lansky AJ, Mehran R, et al. Angiographic surrogate end points in drug-eluting stent trials: a systematic evaluation based on individual patient data from 11 randomized, controlled trials. J Am Coll Cardiol 2008; 51: 23–32.

48. Sabate M, Costa MA, Kozuma K, et al. Methodological and clinical implications of the relocation of the minimal luminal diameter

after intracoronary radiation therapy. Dose Finding Study Group. J Am Coll Cardiol 2000; 36: 1536–41.

49. Escolar E, Mintz GS, Popma J, et al. Meta-analysis of angiographic versus intravascular ultrasound parameters of drug-eluting stent efficacy (from TAXUS IV, V, and VI). Am J Cardiol 2007; 100: 621–6.

50. Semeraro O, Agostoni P, Verheye S, et al. Re-examining minimal luminal diameter relocation and quantitative coronary angiography–intravascular ultrasound correlations in stented saphenous vein grafts: methodological insights from the randomised RRISC trial. EuroIntervention 2009; 4: 633–40.

51. Louvard Y, Thomas M, Dzavik V, et al. Classification of coronary artery bifurcation lesions and treatments: time for a consensus! Catheter Cardiovasc Interv. 2008; 71: 175–83.

52. Medina A, Suarez de Lezo J. Pan M. [A new classification of coronary bifurcation lesions]. Rev Esp Cardiol 2006; 59: 183.

53. Girasis C, Onuma Y, Schuurbiers JC, et al. Validity and variability in visual assessment of stenosis severity in phantom bifurcation lesions: a survey in experts during the Fifth Meeting of the European Bifurcation Club. Catheter Cardiovasc Interv 2012; 79: 361–8. doi: 10.1002/ccd.23213

54. Finet G, Gilard M, Perrenot B, et al. Fractal geometry of arterial coronary bifurcations: a quantitative coronary angiography and intravascular ultrasound analysis. EuroIntervention 2008; 3: 490–8.

55. Goktekin O, Kaplan S, Dimopoulos K, et al. A new quantitative analysis system for the evaluation of coronary bifurcation lesions: comparison with current conventional methods. Catheter Cardiovasc Interv 2007; 69: 172–80.

56. Koo BK, Kang HJ, Youn TJ, et al. Physiologic assessment of jailed side branch lesions using fractional flow reserve. J Am Coll Cardiol 2005; 46: 633–7.

57. Ramcharitar S, Onuma Y, Aben JP, et al. A novel dedicated quantitative coronary analysis methodology for bifurcation lesions. EuroIntervention 2008; 3: 553–7.

58. Tuinenburg JC, Koning G, Rares A, et al. Dedicated bifurcation analysis: basic principles. Int J Cardiovasc Imaging 27: 167–74.

59. Girasis C, Schuurbiers JC, Onuma Y, Serruys PW, Wentzel JJ. Novel bifurcation phantoms for validation of quantitative coronary angiography algorithms. Catheter Cardiovasc Interv 2011; 77: 790–7.

60. Girasis C, Serruys PW. Dedicated Software for Bifurcation QCA. Pie Medical (CAAS 5.9) and MEDIS (QAngio XA 7.2.34.0): Validation on Phantom analysis. 6th meeting of the European Bifurcation Club. Budapest.

61. Sarno G, Garg S, Onuma Y, et al. Bifurcation lesions: Functional assessment by fractional flow reserve vs. anatomical assessment using conventional and dedicated bifurcation quantitative coronary angiogram. Catheter Cardiovasc Interv 2010; 76: 817–23.

62. Lefevre T, Louvard Y, Morice MC, et al. Stenting of bifurcation lesions: classification, treatments, and results. Catheter Cardiovasc Interv 2000; 49: 274–83.

63. Louvard Y, Lefevre T, Morice MC. Percutaneous coronary intervention for bifurcation coronary disease. Heart 2004; 90: 713–22.

64. Onuma Y, Girasis C, Aben JP, et al. A novel dedicated 3Dimensional quantitative coronary analysis methodology for bifurcation lesions. EuroIntervention 2011; 7: 629–35.

65. Girasis C, Serruys PW, Onuma Y, et al. 3Dimensional bifurcation angle analysis in patients with left main disease: a substudy of the SYNTAX trial (SYNergy Between Percutaneous Coronary Intervention with TAXus and Cardiac Surgery). JACC Cardiovasc Interv 2010; 3: 41–8.

66. Dzavik V, Kharbanda R, Ivanov J, et al. Predictors of long-term outcome after crush stenting of coronary bifurcation lesions: importance of the bifurcation angle. Am Heart J 2006; 152: 762–9.

67. Ormiston JA, Currie E, Webster MW, et al. Drug-eluting stents for coronary bifurcations: insights into the crush technique. Catheter Cardiovasc Interv 2004; 63: 332–6.

68. Murasato Y. Impact of three-dimensional characteristics of the left main coronary artery bifurcation on outcome of crush stenting. Catheter Cardiovasc Interv 2007; 69: 248–56.

69. Vassilev D, Gil RJ. Relative dependence of diameters of branches in coronary bifurcations after stent implantation in main vessel–importance of carina position. Kardiol Pol 2008; 66: 371–8; discussion 379.

70. Ormiston JA, Webster MW, El Jack S, et al. Drug-eluting stents for coronary bifurcations: bench testing of provisional side-branch strategies. Catheter Cardiovasc Interv 2006; 67: 49–55.

71. Adriaenssens T, Byrne RA, Dibra A, et al. Culotte stenting technique in coronary bifurcation disease: angiographic follow-up using dedicated quantitative coronary angiographic analysis and 12-month clinical outcomes. Eur Heart J 2008; 29: 2868–76.

72. Serruys PW. SYNTAX Left Main: 3-year outcome and techniques. 6th meeting of the European Bifurcation Club. Budapest, 2010.

73. Green NE, Chen SY, Hansgen AR, et al. Angiographic views used for percutaneous coronary interventions: a three-dimensional analysis of physician-determined vs. computer-generated views. Catheter Cardiovasc Interv 2005; 64: 451–9.

74. Gollapudi RR, Valencia R, Lee SS, et al. Utility of three-dimensional reconstruction of coronary angiography to guide percutaneous coronary intervention. Catheter Cardiovasc Interv 2007; 69: 479–82.

75. Gomez-Lara J, Diletti R, Brugaletta S, et al. Angiographic maximal luminal diameter and appropriate deployment of the everolimus-eluting bioresorbable vascular scaffold as assessed by optical coherence tomography: an ABSORB cohort B trial sub-study. EuroIntervention 2011; In press.

76. Bruining N, Tanimoto S, Otsuka M, et al. Quantitative multi-modality imaging analysis of a bioabsorbable poly-L-lactic acid stent design in the acute phase: a comparison between 2- and 3D-QCA, QCU and QMSCT-CA. EuroIntervention 2008; 4: 285–91.

77. Tu S, Huang Z, Koning G, Cui K, Reiber JH. A novel three-dimensional quantitative coronary angiography system: In-vivo comparison with intravascular ultrasound for assessing arterial segment length. Catheter Cardiovasc Interv 2010; 76: 291–8.

78. Schuurbiers JC, Lopez NG, Ligthart J, et al. In vivo validation of CAAS QCA-3D coronary reconstruction using fusion of angiography and intravascular ultrasound (ANGUS). Catheter Cardiovasc Interv 2009; 73: 620–6.

79. Yong AS, Ng AC, Brieger D, et al. Three-dimensional and two-dimensional quantitative coronary angiography, and their prediction of reduced fractional flow reserve. Eur Heart J 2010; 32: 345–53.

80. Dvir D, Assali A, Lev EI, et al. Percutaneous interventions in unprotected left main lesions: novel three-dimensional imaging and quantitative analysis before and after intervention. Cardiovasc Revasc Med 2010; 11: 236–40.

81. Galassi AR, Tomasello SD, Capodanno D, et al. A novel 3d reconstruction system for the assessment of bifurcation lesions treated by the mini-crush technique. J Interv Cardiol 2010; 23: 46–53.

82. Schlundt C, Kreft JG, Fuchs F, et al. Three-dimensional on-line reconstruction of coronary bifurcated lesions to optimize side-branch stenting. Catheter Cardiovasc Interv 2006; 68: 249–53.

83. Tu S, Hao P, Koning G, et al. In vivo assessment of optimal viewing angles from X-ray coronary angiography. EuroIntervention 2011; 7: 112–20.

84. Neubauer AM, Garcia JA, Messenger JC, et al. Clinical feasibility of a fully automated 3D reconstruction of rotational coronary X-ray angiograms. Circ Cardiovasc Interv 2010; 3: 71–9.

85. Maddux JT, Wink O, Messenger JC, et al. Randomized study of the safety and clinical utility of rotational angiography versus standard angiography in the diagnosis of coronary artery disease. Catheter Cardiovasc Interv 2004; 62: 167–74.

86. Akhtar M, Vakharia KT, Mishell J, et al. Randomized study of the safety and clinical utility of rotational vs. standard coronary angiography using a flat-panel detector. Catheter Cardiovasc Interv 2005; 66: 43–9.

87. Garcia JA, Agostoni P, Green NE, et al. Rotational vs. standard coronary angiography: an image content analysis. Catheter Cardiovasc Interv 2009; 73: 753–61.

88. Klein AJ, Garcia JA, Hudson PA, et al. Safety and efficacy of dual-axis rotational coronary angiography vs. standard coronary angiography. Catheter Cardiovasc Interv 2011; 77: 820–7.

89. Garcia JA, Chen SY, Messenger JC, et al. Initial clinical experience of selective coronary angiography using one prolonged injection and a 180 degrees rotational trajectory. Catheter Cardiovasc Interv 2007; 70: 190–6.

90. Rittger H, Rieber J, Sinha AM, Schmidt M, Brachmann J. Feasibility of a new C-arm Angiography (DYNA-CT) based three-dimensional Coronary Reconstruction Algorithm. Am J Cardiol 2009; 104: 164D–5D.

91. Hansis E, Schafer D, Dossel O, Grass M. Projection-based motion compensation for gated coronary artery reconstruction from rotational x-ray angiograms. Phys Med Biol 2008; 53: 3807–20.

92. Schoonenberg G, Florent R, Lelong P, et al. Projection-based motion compensation and reconstruction of coronary segments and cardiac implantable devices using rotational X-ray angiography. Med Image Anal 2009; 13: 785–92.

93. Rohkohl C, Lauritsch G, Biller L, et al. Interventional 4D motion estimation and reconstruction of cardiac vasculature without motion periodicity assumption. Med Image Anal 2010; 14: 687–94.

94. Stone GW, Maehara A, Lansky AJ, et al. A prospective natural-history study of coronary atherosclerosis. N Engl J Med 2011; 364: 226–35.

95. Anderson JL, Karagounis LA, Becker LC, Sorensen SG, Menlove RL. TIMI perfusion grade 3 but not grade 2 results in improved outcome after thrombolysis for myocardial infarction. Ventriculographic, enzymatic, and electrocardiographic evidence from the TEAM-3 Study. Circulation 1993; 87: 1829–39.

96. Gibson CM, Murphy SA, Rizzo MJ, et al. Relationship between TIMI frame count and clinical outcomes after thrombolytic administration. Thrombolysis In Myocardial Infarction (TIMI) Study Group. Circulation 1999; 99: 1945–50.

97. Ambrose JA, Winters SL, Stern A, et al. Angiographic morphology and the pathogenesis of unstable angina pectoris. J Am Coll Cardiol 1985; 5: 609–16.

98. Ellis SG, Vandormael MG, Cowley MJ, et al. Coronary morphologic and clinical determinants of procedural outcome with angioplasty for multivessel coronary disease. Implications for patient selection. Multivessel Angioplasty Prognosis Study Group. Circulation 1990; 82: 1193–202.

99. Ellis SG, Guetta V, Miller D, Whitlow PL, Topol EJ. Relation between lesion characteristics and risk with percutaneous intervention in

the stent and glycoprotein IIb/IIIa era: an analysis of results from 10,907 lesions and proposal for new classification scheme. Circulation 1999; 100: 1971–6.

100. Ryan TJ, Faxon DP, Gunnar RM, et al. Guidelines for percutaneous transluminal coronary angioplasty. A report of the American College of Cardiology/American Heart Association Task Force on Assessment of Diagnostic and Therapeutic Cardiovascular Procedures (Subcommittee on Percutaneous Transluminal Coronary Angioplasty). Circulation 1988; 78: 486–502.

101. Smith SC Jr, Dove JT, Jacobs AK, et al. ACC/AHA guidelines for percutaneous coronary intervention (revision of the 1993 PTCA guidelines)-executive summary: a report of the American College of Cardiology/American Heart Association task force on practice guidelines (Committee to revise the 1993 guidelines for percutaneous transluminal coronary angioplasty) endorsed by the Society for Cardiac Angiography and Interventions. Circulation 2001; 103: 3019–41.

102. Kastrati A, Schomig A, Elezi S, et al. Prognostic value of the modified american college of Cardiology/American heart association stenosis morphology classification for long-term angiographic and clinical outcome after coronary stent placement. Circulation 1999; 100: 1285–90.

103. Sianos G, Morel MA, Kappetein AP, et al. The SYNTAX Score: an angiographic tool grading the complexity of coronary artery disease. EuroIntervention 2005; 1: 219–27.

104. Serruys PW, Morice MC, Kappetein AP, et al. Percutaneous coronary intervention versus coronary-artery bypass grafting for severe coronary artery disease. N Engl J Med 2009; 360: 961–72.

105. Serruys PW, Onuma Y, Garg S, et al. Assessment of the SYNTAX score in the Syntax study. EuroIntervention 2009; 5: 50–6.

106. Garg S, Sarno G, Girasis C, et al. A patient-level pooled analysis assessing the impact of the SYNTAX (synergy between percutaneous coronary intervention with taxus and cardiac surgery) score on 1-year clinical outcomes in 6,508 patients enrolled in contemporary coronary stent trials. JACC Cardiovasc Interv 2011; 4: 645–53.

107. Garg S, Girasis C, Sarno G, et al. The SYNTAX score revisited: a reassessment of the SYNTAX score reproducibility. Catheter Cardiovasc Interv 2010; 75: 946–52.

108. Tu S, Holm NR, Koning G, Huang Z, Reiber JH. Fusion of 3D QCA and IVUS/OCT. Int J Cardiovasc Imaging 2011; 27: 197–207.

109. Roguin A, Abadi S, Engel A, Beyar R. Novel method for real-time hybrid cardiac CT and coronary angiography image registration: visualising beyond luminology, proof-of-concept. EuroIntervention 2009; 4: 648–53.

12   Fractional flow reserve: Role in guiding clinical decision making

Aaron Peace, Stylianos A. Pyxaras, and Bernard De Bruyne

OUTLINE

Coronary angiography is a "lumen-o-gram" and therefore, may not provide reliable information on the potential of an angiographically visible stenosis to be responsible for ischemia. Many patients do not have a comprehensive non-invasive functional testing prior to planned angiography. Further, while these tests help demonstrate whether ischemia is present, all have limitations in that they are relatively subjective, have lower than desired sensitivities and specificities, are often unable to localize ischemia and may be associated with high radiation exposure. The ideal test is one that can be done rapidly and simply and provide accurate, objective and reproducible result in a cost effective fashion. Fractional Flow Reserve usually abbreviated to FFR has all these. In this chapter we provide a step-by-step guide to obtaining and interpreting FFR measurements highlighting potential pitfalls and providing Tips and Tricks to facilitate easy incorporation of this validated but still underused technique into the catheterization laboratory.

INTRODUCTION

Coronary angiography is still considered by many who do not have access to techniques such as intravascular ultrasound (IVUS) to be the gold standard diagnostic investigation to establish whether or not a patient has significant coronary atherosclerosis. Although it is a highly effective tool to detect the presence of atheromatosis, in reality it only provides us with 2D pictorial information. Essentially, the coronary angiogram is a "lumen-o-gram" and, therefore, provides only little information on the functional relevance of an angiographically visible stenosis. In other words, the simple question that coronary angiography fails to answer is whether or not a given atherosclerotic lesion(s) is/are ischemic. We need to know this fundamental piece of information since ischemia is prognostically important (1,2).

In the vast majority of cardiology departments worldwide, functional evaluation is done before angiography using non-invasive tests such as exercise stress testing on a treadmill or bicycle, exercise stress echocardiography, dobutamine stress echocardiography (DSE), myocardial sestamibi scanning (MIBI), or positron emission tomography (PET) scanning. Surprisingly, comprehensive non-invasive functional testing is only performed in around 45% of cases, even in cases of stable coronary artery disease (CAD) (3).

While these tests can help to demonstrate whether ischemia is present, each of these modalities has limitations. In all of the tests mentioned above there is an element of subjectivity that is highly operator dependent. Although DSE and MIBI scanning (which itself involves high radiation exposure) have better sensitivities and specificities than mere exercise stress testing, these are still lower than desired. The spatial resolution of all of these non-invasive tests is not ideal in that treadmill testing tells us about ischemia to a "per patient" accuracy whereas DSE, MIBI, and PET give accuracy to at best "per vessel." The ideal test is one that achieves "per segment" accuracy. With such a test the operator learns about the functional significance of a stenosis to within a few millimeters. In summary, the above tests can be poor localizers to where the ischemia is or is not occurring.

For the cardiologist, the ideal test is one that can be done rapidly, simply, accurately (with a high spatial resolution), objectively, and provide reproducible results. The "icing on the cake" is that the diagnostic test is cost-effective and provides reliable results that ultimately guide decision making in order to achieve optimal therapy for the patient.

This brings us on to the measurement of fractional flow reserve (FFR), which possesses all of the above-mentioned features. Recognition of the clinical value of using FFR is evident from the recent myocardial revascularization guidelines that have elevated the use of FFR to a Class IA recommendation in the functional assessment of stenosis in patients with stable CAD (4).

With regard to the technical aspects of performing FFR, we will discuss some broad concepts to help fully understand the principles behind FFR. Before embarking upon how to actually use FFR to guide clinical decision making, it is important to discuss how important one's "mind set" is before establishing FFR as a routine tool in the cardiac catheterization laboratory.

Succeeding in Measuring FFR in the Catheterization Laboratory

The phrase "practice makes perfect" applies to the measurement of FFR. Once the decision has been made to use FFR, it is advisable to get everyone "on board" to facilitate its success. To achieve this, it is important to educate all staff, in particular the nursing staff. If there is obvious enthusiasm among any members of the nursing staff, then they should be identified and asked to "champion FFR." This strategy will facilitate the routine use of FFR in the laboratory.

It has been said that "protocol is everything" and in this case it is vital because the success of your program hinges on establishing a protocol that will be followed religiously by everyone in the catheterization laboratory every time FFR is measured. For the operator themselves, it is advisable to begin by becoming confident in using the technology. To achieve this, it is advisable to start by measuring FFR in lesions where the stenosis is clearly significant by visual estimation. By measuring this type of lesion the operator quickly learns to trust the FFR measurement, as it confirms their visual estimation in the first place. In turn, this approach will also build the trust of the allied staff and so the use of the pressure wire to measure visually estimated intermediate lesions will establish itself.

The next step toward success is to be consistent in how the patient is managed once you have measured FFR. Despite what you or anyone else might think, the pressure measurement never lies as long as the same protocol is rigidly adhered to. Remember that FFR provides us with an objective measure of the functional relevance of a stenosis as opposed to its more subjective visual estimation.

The final step in ensuring that FFR becomes a routine diagnostic tool and an adjunct to coronary angiography is to have a low threshold for using the pressure wire. In other words, if you are not sure whether a lesion is hemodynamically important or not, then measure it and remove the doubt.

Definition of FFR

The mathematical derivation of FFR is quite complicated. FFR is essentially the ratio of two flows, that is, the ratio of hyperemic myocardial blood flow in the presence of a stenosis to hyperemic myocardial blood flow in the hypothetical case where the same artery is normal. Previous studies have shown that the two flows can be derived from two pressures as long as they are both obtained during maximal hyperemia. The bottom line is

that FFR = P_d/P_a where P_d is the pressure measured at the distal end of the coronary beyond a stenosis and P_a is the aortic pressure (Fig. 12.1) (5,6).

Unique Characteristics of FFR

FFR Is Not Influenced by Systemic Hemodynamics

In the catheterization laboratory, systemic pressure, heart rate, and left ventricular contractility are prone to change. In contrast to many other indices measured in the catheterization laboratory, changes in systemic hemodynamics do not influence the value of FFR in a given coronary stenosis (7). This is due not only to the fact that aortic and distal coronary pressures are measured simultaneously, but also to the extraordinary capability of the microvasculature to repeatedly vasodilate to exactly the same extent. In addition, FFR measurements are extremely reproducible. FFR has also been shown to be independent of gender and risk factors such as hypertension and diabetes (8). These characteristics contribute to the accuracy of the method and to the acceptance of its value for decision making.

FFR Takes into Account the Contribution of Collaterals

Whether myocardial flow is provided antegradely by the epicardial artery or retrogradely through collaterals does not really matter for the myofilaments. Distal coronary pressure during maximal hyperemia reflects both antegrade and retrograde flows according to their respective contributions. This is true for the stenoses supplied by collaterals and for

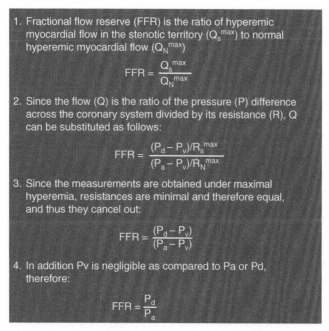

1. Fractional flow reserve (FFR) is the ratio of hyperemic myocardial flow in the stenotic territory (Q_s^{max}) to normal hyperemic myocardial flow (Q_N^{max})

$$FFR = \frac{Q_s^{max}}{Q_N^{max}}$$

2. Since the flow (Q) is the ratio of the pressure (P) difference across the coronary system divided by its resistance (R), Q can be substituted as follows:

$$FFR = \frac{(P_d - P_v)/R_s^{max}}{(P_a - P_v)/R_N^{max}}$$

3. Since the measurements are obtained under maximal hyperemia, resistances are minimal and therefore equal, and thus they cancel out:

$$FFR = \frac{(P_d - P_v)}{(P_a - P_v)}$$

4. In addition Pv is negligible as compared to Pa or Pd, therefore:

$$FFR = \frac{P_d}{P_a}$$

Figure 12.1 Simplified mathematical derivation of FFR. *Abbreviations*: P_a, aortic pressure; P_d, distal coronary pressure; P_v, venous pressure; Q_s^{max}, hyperemic myocardial blood flow in the stenotic territory; Q_N^{max}, hyperemic myocardial blood flow in the normal territory; R_s^{max}, hyperemic myocardial resistance in the stenotic territory; R_N^{max}, hyperemic myocardial resistance in the normal territory.

stenosed arteries providing collaterals to another more critically diseased vessel.

FFR Specifically Relates the Severity of the Stenosis to the Mass of Tissue to be Perfused

The larger the myocardial mass subtended by a vessel, the larger the hyperemic flow, and in turn, the larger the gradient and the lower the FFR. This explains why a stenosis with a minimal cross-sectional area of 4 mm² has a totally different hemodynamic significance in the proximal left anterior descending artery (LAD) versus the second marginal branch.

Understanding the principles discussed in sections above is important, particularly in the scenario of measuring FFR in an intermediate lesion seen in a vessel (e.g., mid-LAD) that is supplying collaterals to an occluded vessel [e.g., occluded right coronary artery (RCA)]. As mentioned above, the larger the myocardial territory supplied by a vessel, the larger the hyperemic flow, and in turn, the larger the gradient and the lower the FFR. At first, the lesion in the mid-LAD may appear to be ischemic with an FFR of 0.73; however, this may be overestimated since the LAD is supplying both its own territory and that of the occluded RCA.

Once the RCA is successfully re-opened, the size of the myocardial territory that the LAD then supplies is smaller, which means reduced hyperemic flow, a lower gradient, and a higher FFR value. In certain circumstances, the FFR value in the LAD increases to such an extent that the intermediate lesion which was deemed significant before opening of the RCA is now above the ischemic threshold and therefore not significant; for example, if the FFR of the mid-LAD increases from 0.73 to 0.84, it indicates that the mid-LAD is actually not flow limiting. This is a fundamental principle to remember since the RCA, in this case, has changed the LAD from being ischemic as first thought to being non-ischemic because the original FFR was overestimated.

Basic Concepts of FFR

Anatomical Issues

There are several anatomical issues that must be dealt with before delving into the coronary physiology of FFR. The endothelium is privy to a highly complex environment consisting of hemodynamic shear stresses and interactions with various blood cells, most notably platelets. In addition, the endothelium is affected by a multitude of vasoactive substances that in turn alter its function and integrity, thereby affecting the flow dynamics within the artery. All these processes are in a very fine equilibrium which changes in case of a vascular endothelial injury. When such a disruption occurs, the balance between endothelial relaxants (e.g., nitric oxide) and endothelial constricting agents (e.g., endothelin) results in disturbances in the coronary blood flow.

When considering the basic concepts of FFR it is vital to remind ourselves that a clear correlation exists between the cross-sectional area of a coronary artery at each point along its length and the amount of myocardial territory that it supplies. This is a very important issue when considering the potential prognostic significance of a stenosis in the proximal part of a large artery such as the LAD compared with smaller coronary arteries such as a diagonal or marginal side branch.

Physiological Issues

Pressure, Flow, and Resistance

The key elements of circulatory function are flow, pressure, and resistance (Fig. 12.1).

The 'Holy Grail' of vascular physiology is to have a technique that allows for accurate measurement of both absolute coronary flow and absolute resistance. However, some would argue that a clinical application that allows the measurement of absolute coronary flow and resistance is of relatively limited value since these parameters may, at best, only have a modest impact on changes in clinical management. In addition, there is no uniformly normal value for flow and resistance along the epicardial arteries. Flow (Q), pressure (P), and resistance (R) are mathematically related by the equation:

$$Q = \Delta P / R$$

Flow and resistance are dependent upon the size of the territory that is being perfused. In other words, both flow and resistance are dependent upon the myocardial mass to be perfused. Thus, there is no clear normal value that can be assigned to coronary flow or indeed resistance. It is important to understand that under normal conditions coronary pressure is equal to aortic pressure along the whole length of an epicardial vessel. This principle also applies during maximal hyperemia, which is defined as the point at which minimal microvascular resistance has been achieved.

The Epicardial and Microvascular Compartments and Their Role in Coronary Autoregulation

Myocardial blood flow is regulated by several elements such as neuro-humoral, endothelial, endocrine and paracrine, metabolic, and physical factors. Not surprisingly, none of these factors operate in isolation, and indeed the regulation of blood flow involves a complex interaction between many if not all of the processes mentioned above.

To make things easier, the coronary circulation should be considered a two-compartment model. The first compartment consists of epicardial vessels, referred to as "conductance vessels" because they do not provide any resistance to blood flow. The second compartment consists of arteries <400 μm or "resistive vessels." It is these vessels that primarily control myocardial blood flow, as they are able to vasodilate under physiological and pharmacological stress. At coronary angiography, they are not clearly delineated but appear as a myocardial blush of contrast medium. During exercise or any other form of increased oxygen demand, the resistance of the microvasculature decreases allowing for an increased blood flow. Similarly, when a stenosis is present in an epicardial artery, the increased epicardial resistance is compensated for by an equivalent decrease in the microvascular resistance. This results in a maintained total resistance to blood flow and a preserved resting flow, with residual—albeit reduced—coronary flow reserve. When an epicardial stenosis progresses further, its relative contribution to the total resistance increases. At the other extreme, when the stenosis becomes "critical," the compensation capacity of the microvascular circulation is exhausted. Any additional increase in the epicardial resistance will result in an increase in the total resistance and in a decrease in the myocardial flow.

The Flow–Function Relationship
In normal circumstances, about 5% of the cardiac output is devoted to myocardial blood flow. As the heart is constantly working, its resting myocardial oxygen demand is high; so high that the amount of oxygen that is being pulled out is close to maximum, which is much higher than in other organs. For example, oxygen saturation in the coronary sinus venous blood is close to 20%. This is in stark contrast to, for instance, the renal vein where oxygen saturations are more than four times higher at around 85%. Since there is very little scope for the myocardium to extract any additional oxygen, the coronary circulation is forced to compensate by fine-tuning the myocardial blood flow. Moreover, as soon as the myocardial blood flow decreases to <90% of its normal resting levels, myocardial function starts to decrease. It is obvious that the control of myocardial blood flow must be remarkably tight to avoid wall motion abnormalities. Conversely, this also implies that when the myocardial wall motion is normal, its resting perfusion must be normal.

TECHNICAL ASPECTS OF MEASURING FFR
The Practicalities of Measuring FFR
It is probably fair to say that the introduction of a new technology such as pressure wires into a catheterization laboratory is met with some trepidation by the staff. However, this fear is quickly dispelled on discovering how easy it is to install, use, and interpret results from the pressure wire. Conveniently, only three pieces of equipment are necessary to measure FFR: a catheter, a pressure wire, and a hyperemic stimulus.

The Equipment
Catheters
Although guide catheters are routinely used to measure FFR, one could argue that it is feasible to use diagnostic catheters. However, a guide catheter has several advantages over a standard diagnostic catheter: less friction in the guide facilitates better wire manipulation and therefore less potential to influence the pressure measurement due to the larger internal luminal diameter. Also, the guide allows for the possibility of ad-hoc percutaneous coronary intervention (PCI) should the decision be made to proceed using the pressure wire as a PCI wire.

Wires
There are two commercially available wires used to measure FFR, the Certus PressureWire™ (St. Jude Medical, St. Pauls, MN; Radi Medical Systems, Uppsala, Sweden) and PrimeWire Prestige™ (Volcano Inc, Rancho Cordova, California, USA). In keeping with the wireless era we live in, the Certus PressureWire is also

available as a wireless system known as the Aeris™ Wireless FFR measurement system. The advantage of the Aeris system is that it can be directly linked to your hemodynamic monitoring software without the need for an interface.

The wire sensor itself is situated 3 cm proximal to the tip, at the intersection between the non-opaque and opaque segments of the wire. Proximal to the sensor is a hydrophilic segment of wire which improves handling. Proximal to the hydrophilic segment is a polymer (PTFE) coated segment of wire which extends all the way back to the start of the wire. The distal end of the pressure wire measures 0.014 inches in diameter, similar to that of most standard angioplasty wires. Historically, these pressure wires were quite cumbersome as they were difficult to manipulate, although the new generation of pressure wires are virtually equivalent to your standard PCI wire. This makes crossing stent struts to assess side branches more achievable than ever before.

Vasodilators
To correctly measure FFR we need to maximally vasodilate the epicardial vessels and the microcirculation. To do this, the epicardial vessels are first dilated using isosorbide dinitrate at a dose of nitroglycerin 200 μg. Then the microcirculation is maximally vasodilated using one of several agents including intracoronary (IC) or intravenous (IV) adenosine (by far the most commonly used agent), IC papaverine, or sodium nitroprusside (Focus Box 12.2)

Equalization (Focus Box 12.3)
It cannot be emphasized enough as to how important it is to understand the process of equalization and how to do it correctly. Before equalization the fluid-filled transducer for aortic pressure and the microchip transducer on the pressure wire must be calibrated. Once this is done, the wire can be passed into the proximal part of the vessel that is to be assessed.

Once the pressure sensor is correctly positioned at 1–2 mm outside of the tip of the guide catheter, equalization can take place. Sometimes, after positioning the sensor the aortic pressure and wire pressures can differ. This is usually explained by incorrect positioning of the aortic pressure transducer in relation to the patient's sternum. Ideally, the aortic transducer should be positioned 5–7 cm below the patient's sternum.

Focus Box 12.1 Essential Checklist before Measuring FFR

1. Explain what you are going to do, in particular emphasize the fact that adenosine will cause some discomfort and possibly breathlessness
2. Heparin at an equivalent to that given for PCI (recommended 100 U/kg UFH or as per your catheterization laboratory)
3. If you have not already done so, administer IC nitrates

Abbreviations: PCI, percutaneous coronary intervention; UFH, unfractionated heparin; IC, intracoronary.

Focus Box 12.2 Agents to Obtain Maximal Hyperemia

Agent	Recommended dose	Speed of onset and duration (min)	Potential adverse effects
Adenosine IC	At least 50 μg bolus IC	0.5–1	Bradycardia, heart block, bronchospasm, chest tightness
Adenosine IV	140 μg/kg/min infusion IV	1–2	Bradycardia, heart block, bronchospasm, chest tightness
Papaverine	12 mg bolus IC	2	Ventricular fibrillation
Sodium nitroprusside	0.6 μg/kg bolus IC	1	Hypotension

Abbreviations: IC, intracoronary; IV, intravenous.

Focus Box 12.3 Equalization

1. Before positioning the wire, again check that heparin and nitrates have been administered
2. Now position the sensor just distal to the end of the catheter (Fig. 12.2)
3. For ostial disease, equalize the pressure wire in the aorta

After correctly positioning the wire, the equalize button should be pressed to allow the two pressure traces to superimpose on one another so that the ratio of P_d/P_a is 1.00.

Many operators question whether the introducer needle should be left in the Y-connector or whether it should be removed. This does not really matter as long as the measurement of P_d is done in the same way as when equalization was performed. Thus, if the needle was inside the Y-connector during equalization, then it should be left there when maximal hyperemia is being induced. The same applies if the needle was out during equalization. In that case, it should be removed after positioning the sensor beyond the lesion but before inducing hyperemia. It is worth mentioning that large-caliber introducer needles should be avoided as these allow leakage, which can lead to a slightly less accurate reading (Fig. 12.2).

In the case of ostial disease, the simplest technique is to position the wire in the ascending aorta and then equalize. Once this is done, retract the wire, fix the torquer adjacent to the Y-connector to prevent the wire diving into the coronary with the next injection of contrast, and then engage the ostium. Then advance the wire beyond the lesion, but before inducing hyperemia be sure to disengage the guide catheter from the ostium so that the reading is accurate.

Crossing the Lesion and Positioning of the Pressure Wire

Once equalization has been done correctly, advance the wire through the stenosis. Based on personal experience, we recommend positioning the wire sensor just beyond where a surgeon is likely to anastomose a graft such as an internal mammary artery in the case of the LAD. Again, the same principle applies when measuring the left circumflex, or the RCA. Although not entirely necessary in all cases, it is probably good practice in every case to carefully disengage the guide

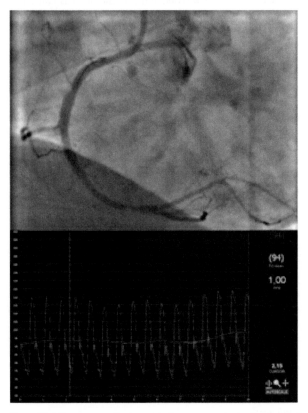

Figure 12.2 Pressure equalization with the pressure wire in the proximal right coronary artery.

catheter from the ostium of the coronary immediately after the vasodilator has been administered to avoid inappropriate dampening from the catheter. This is usually achieved by opening the Y-connector and simultaneously pushing the pressure wire forward while pulling the guide catheter out of the coronary ostium.

Hyperemia

The key aspect to successfully measuring FFR is to achieve maximal hyperemia, meaning that maximal vasodilation has been obtained in both the microvascular circulation and the epicardial vessels.

First, the epicardial vessels must be maximally vasodilated using IC nitrate. The aim of IC nitrates is to not only lower epicardial resistance to as low a value as possible but to also help avoid coronary vasospasm from wire manipulation in the vessels. After correctly following the steps described above, hyperemia of the microcirculation can be achieved using various agents, the most common being IC or IV adenosine.

Apart from this, several other vasodilators can be used such as IC papaverine or sodium nitroprusside (Focus Box 12.3). It is vital to give heparin equivalent to that given for PCI, which may vary from one laboratory to another; therefore, local protocols should be developed and applied accordingly.

Adenosine is the preferred choice to induce maximal hyperemia and can be administered either by the IV or IC route. Both methods achieve the same endpoint, although there are pros and cons to each. IC administration is faster because it requires less setup time and can be delivered more quickly than IV administration, giving a virtually instant hyperemic response. However, some laboratories are so accustomed to giving IV adenosine that they are equally proficient in both techniques. The advantage of the IV route is that maximal hyperemia can be achieved and a steady state is obtained which persists for a longer time than when IC adenosine is given. A prolonged steady state if tolerated by the patient allows for a more detailed assessment of long diffuse segments of disease or sequential lesions. Another setting where the IV route is more advantageous than the IC route is in the evaluation of ostial disease. Ideally, if IV adenosine is used, it should be delivered through a large-caliber vein such as the brachio-cephalic or femoral vein. The maximal effect of adenosine through this route is normally achieved in approximately one minute.

There are several clues that the effect of adenosine is beginning. First, there is often a transient increase in systolic pressure followed by an increase in the trans-stenotic gradient. Second, the patient begins to feel some tightness in their chest or even breathlessness. It is important to pre-warn the patient that this may happen as this feeling can be very unpleasant. If the patient does not experience such a sensation, then the operator must check whether adenosine has reached the heart or, yours, whether adequate amounts were given. In this case, all lines should be carefully checked. Failing that IC adenosine can be given after ensuring that the catheter is selectively engaged in the coronary ostium.

In the case of IC adenosine, the effect is very fast, in about 10 seconds. It is not uncommon to see complete or second-degree heart block but this is virtually always transient. As the duration of action is only around 20 seconds, the assessment of long diffuse segments of disease or sequential lesions can be difficult and at times inaccurate.

Interpretation of the FFR Value (Fig. 12.3)

Confusion still remains over which threshold should be applied, 0.75 or 0.8, to identify ischemia. Simply put, if vessels are ≥2.5 mm apply a threshold of 0.80. A value above 0.80 means the lesion in question is not causing ischemia.

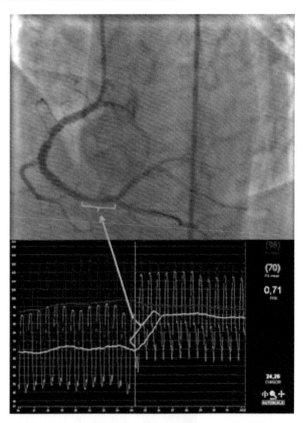

Figure 12.3 In this case, a fractional flow reserve (FFR) value of 0.71 is documented during maximal IV adenosine-induced hyperemia (ischemic lesion). Note the "jump" in the FFR registered values during the passage of the pressure wire through the lesion.

Interpretation of the Pullback

Ideally, a recorded pullback should be done in every case to ascertain whether the coronary disease is focal, sequential, or diffuse. The exact position of the sensor in the coronary tree can be monitored using fluoroscopy, and documented angiographically (Fig. 12.4). Pulling back the sensor under maximal hyperemia (usually IV adenosine) provides the operator with an instantaneous assessment of the abnormal resistance of the arterial segment located between the guide catheter and the sensor. While other functional tests achieve a "per patient" accuracy (exercise ECG) or, at best, a "per vessel" accuracy (myocardial perfusion imaging), FFR achieves a "per segment" accuracy with a spatial resolution of a few millimetres (Focus Box 12.4) (Fig. 12.4).

TIPS AND TRICKS

There are several tips and tricks that can be useful when measuring FFR. For clarity, we have created a table of these tips and tricks that describes, in a stepwise fashion, the optimal technique to measure FFR, which is outlined in Focus Box 12.5 and in Video clip 12.1.

Focus Box 12.4 The Simple Guide to Measuring FFR

1. After all the equipments have been calibrated, advance the wire until the sensor is positioned just at the tip of the guide catheter
2. Now equalize the P_a and P_d pressures so that the ratio is 1.00. If the ratio of the pressure signals is already 1.00, then proceed without equalization
3. Now cross the lesion to be measured by advancing the pressure wire sensor distal to the lesion
4. If the lesion is ostial, then it is important to disengage the guide catheter from it to avoid damping of the signal
5. Once the wire has been appropriately positioned, then induce hyperemia
6. Perform a pullback to localize the most important lesion
7. Ensure that when the sensor comes back to the tip of the catheter the ratio of $P_d/P_a = 1.00$ and that drifting is not an issue

Abbreviations: P_a, aortic pressure; P_d, distal pressure.

PITFALLS AND COMPLICATIONS

There are very few settings in which FFR presents problems; these issues are outlined in Focus Box 12.6.

COST-EFFECTIVENESS

One of the major aspects of any diagnostic tool is whether it is cost-effective. While there are several studies which suggest that the use of FFR to guide revascularization strategies is a cost-saving exercise, more recent evidence from the FAME (Fractional Flow Reserve Versus Angiography for Multivessel Evaluation) cohort provided conclusive evidence that the use of FFR saves healthcare resources when compared with an angio-guided PCI strategy. Not only were the healthcare costs lower at the time of the index procedure in the FFR-guided group ($13,182 ± 9667 vs. $14,878 ± 9509; $p < 0.0001$) but the same was also true at 1-year follow-up ($14,315 ± 11,109 vs. $16,700 ± 11,868; $p < 0.0001$).

FFR IN CLINICAL PRACTICE

Interventional cardiologists are increasingly faced with patients presenting with complex coronary diseases such as multi-vessel disease, bifurcation disease, left main disease, or stenoses in

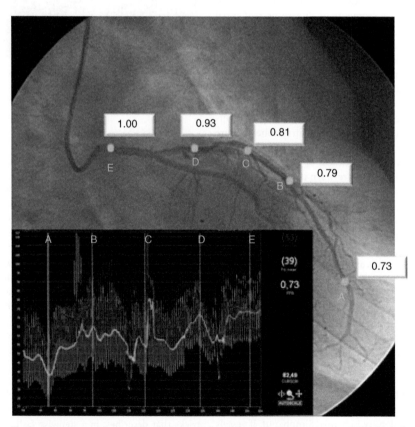

Figure 12.4 Recorded pullback of the pressure wire in a diffusely diseased left anterior descending coronary artery (LAD) during maximal IV adenosine-induced hyperemia. Note that different FFR value "jumps" correspond to different angiographic lesions. The sum of these lesions results in ischemia distally (A and B) that gradually "fades away" in the more proximal segments of the LAD (C and D).

Focus Box 12.5 Useful Tips and Tricks when Measuring FFR

	Tips
Handling the wire	Be gentle with the wire as the sensor can be damaged relatively easily
Introducer needles	It is preferable to use the smallest caliber needle. If the needle is in the Y-connector during equalization leave it in during hyperemia
IV adenosine	If the patient does not feel symptoms when giving IV adenosine, then check the infusion lines. Increasing the dose does not work
IC adenosine	Switch to IC adenosine if IV adenosine does not appear to be having any effect. Always check that it is travelling down the coronary by flushing with 3–4 ml of contrast. Repeat the measurement
Whipping	When the guide wire sensor hits the coronary wall, an increase in the pressure signal can be seen. Pull back (or advance) the wire a few millimeters
Ventricularization	This can occur when the tip of the guide catheter is hitting the wall of the coronary and results in a pressure drop during hyperemia. Simply push the wire while pulling the catheter thereby disengaging the catheter so that the morphology of the two traces are the same
Guide catheter with side holes	The guiding pressure will reflect a pressure 'somewhere in between' the coronary and the aortic pressure (side holes and end-hole). Intracoronary administration of drugs is unreliable. One should avoid using a side-hole catheter for FFR measurements
Disconnection and reconnection of the wire	When the pressure wire has been disconnected, it is advisable to wipe the end of the wire with a wet gauze and to dry it with a dry gauze before reconnecting to avoid loss of the signal

calcified or tortuous vessels in elderly patients. In this section, the utility of FFR in various clinical scenarios will be discussed.

FFR in Diffuse Disease

Histopathology studies and, more recently, IVUS have shown that atherosclerosis is diffuse in nature and that a discrete stenosis in an otherwise normal artery is actually rare. The concept of a focal lesion is mainly an angiographic description but it does not reflect pathology. Until recently, it was believed that when no focal narrowing of >50% was seen at the angiogram no abnormal resistance was present in the epicardial artery. It was therefore assumed that the distal pressure was normal and that "diffuse mild disease without focal stenosis" could not cause myocardial ischemia. This paradigm has recently been shifted: the presence of diffuse disease is often associated with a progressive decrease in coronary pressure (9) and flow (10), and this cannot be predicted from the angiogram. In contrast, this decline in pressure correlates with the total atherosclerotic burden (11). In approximately 10% of patients this abnormal epicardial resistance may be responsible for reversible myocardial ischemia. In these patients chest pain is often considered noncoronary because no single focal stenosis is found, and the myocardial perfusion imaging is wrongly considered false positive ("false false positive") (12). Such diffuse disease and its hemodynamic impact should always be kept in mind when performing functional measurements. In a large multicenter registry of 750 patients FFR was obtained after technically successful stenting. A post-PCI FFR value <0.9 was still present in almost one-third of the patients and was associated with a poor clinical outcome (13). The only way to demonstrate the hemodynamic impact of diffuse disease is by performing a careful pull-back manoeuvre of the pressure sensor under steady-state maximal hyperemia.

FFR After Myocardial Infarction

After a myocardial infarction, previously viable tissue is partially replaced by scar tissue. Therefore, the total mass of the functional myocardium supplied by a given stenosis in an infarct-related artery will tend to decrease (14). By definition, hyperemic flow and thus hyperemic gradient will both decrease as well. Assuming that the morphology of the stenosis remains identical, FFR must therefore increase. This does not mean that FFR underestimates lesion severity after myocardial infarction. It simply illustrates the relationship that exists between flow, pressure gradient, and myocardial mass and, conversely, illustrates that the mere morphology of a stenotic segment does not necessarily reflect its functional importance. Recent data confirm that the hyperemic myocardial resistance in viable myocardium within the infarcted area remains normal (15). This further supports the application of the established FFR cut-off value in the setting of partially infarcted territories. Earlier data had suggested that microvascular function was abnormal in non-infarcted regions that are remote from a recent myocardial infarction (16,17). However, more recent work taking into account distal coronary pressure indicates that hyperemic resistance is normal in these remote segments (18). These data support the use of FFR to evaluate stenoses in patients with recent myocardial infarction when the lesions are in a territory other than the infarcted region.

FFR in Sequential Stenoses

When several stenoses are present in the same artery, the concept and the clinical value of FFR is still valid to assess the effect of all stenoses together. Yet, it is important to realize that when several discrete stenoses are present in the same coronary artery, each of them will influence hyperemic flow and therefore the pressure gradient across the other stenoses. The influence of the distal lesion on the proximal lesion is more

Focus Box 12.6 Potential Pitfalls of FFR

	Pitfalls	How to avoid
Incorrect height of pressure transducer	The guiding catheter pressure transducer is >5–10 cm from the estimated location of the aortic root	The transducer must be placed at the same height, resulting in the absence of any difference in pressures.
Use of a guidewire introducer	The space around the wire within the introducer may leak and decrease P_a by 0–5 mmHg if it is too large caliber	This type of introducer must be removed prior to all measurements
Damping of pressure by guiding catheter	A large (>7F) guiding catheter can blunt maximum blood flow through the artery, resulting in a lower gradient and an overestimated FFR value	Pull back the guiding catheter carefully from the ostium, leaving the pressure wire in the distal vessel Use an intravenous instead of an intracoronary hyperemic stimulus
Guiding catheters with side holes	Pressure signal influenced by both coronary and aortic pressure	Pull back the catheter outside the coronary ostium before the FFR measurements
Signal drift during procedure	Gradient between the proximal and the distal pressure signal with almost identical pressure curves	Pull the sensor back to the guiding catheter and recheck the calibration Make the pullback under maximum hyperemia
Reversed or paradoxical gradient	P_d exceeds P_a	Physiologic phenomenon; generally these differences are small and do not confound the interpretation of data or clinical decision making
Proportionality between P_a and P_d	Changes in systemic blood pressure during maximum hyperemia are accompanied by proportional changes in DP_{max}	Physiologic phenomenon; FFR is not affected
Inadequate or submaximum hyperemia	If maximum hyperemia is not completely achieved, the actual severity of the lesion will be underestimated and patients may be undertreated	Check carefully the composition and dosage of the drug used Check that all stopcocks of the manifold are in the right position and that there is no leakage; a higher dosage of the respective drug or another hyperemic stimulus (IV instead of IC) should be tried
Left ventricular hypertrophy	The natural physiologic reserve capacity of the myocardial vascular bed will be affected when LVH develops; because growth of the vascular bed is not proportional to the increase in muscle mass	Higher FFR values (>0.80) may not exclude ischemia; attention is needed in the interpretation of the results
Exercise-induced vasoconstriction	Paradoxical vasoconstriction at the site of an otherwise non-significant lesion may be induced only by exercise and not by pharmacologically induced hyperemia in the catheterization laboratory	Attention is needed in the interpretation of the results
Microvascular disease	Microvascular disease cannot be detected by coronary pressure measurement	Integrate software module which includes CFR, IMR, or absolute flow measurements
Myocardial infarction	Only a small gradient or high FFR might be observed despite a severe anatomic stenosis	Combination of coronary flow velocity and pressure measurements
Whipping	When the guide wire sensor hits the coronary wall, an artifact can be seen in the form of a brief but pronounced increase (spike) in the pressure signal measured by the wire	Pull back (or advance) the wire a few millimeters
Accordion effect	Folds in the vessel wall induce stenosis due to the presence of the wire	When the wire is pulled back, the folds immediately disappear

Abbreviations: CFR, coronary flow reserve; FFR, fractional flow reserve; IMR, index of microvascular resistance; LVH, left ventricular hypertrophy; P_a, aortic pressure; P_d, distal pressure; DP_{max}, maximum pressure difference.

important than the reverse. The FFR can theoretically be calculated for each stenosis individually (19,20). However, this is neither practical nor easy to perform and therefore of little use in the catheterization laboratory. Practically, similar to diffuse disease, a pull-back maneuver under maximal hyperemia is the only way to determine the exact location and the physiological significance of sequential stenoses.

FFR in Multivessel Disease

A complete functional percutaneous revascularization strategy for patients with multivessel disease consists of stenting all the functionally significant lesions, that is, those that induce ischemia, while treating with optimal medical therapy the lesions that do not induce ischemia. The latter in fact are better deferred with good long-term clinical outcome. The DEFER study showed that the incidence of death and non-fatal myocardial infarction at 5 years was not significantly different between patients deferred on the basis of non-functionally significant lesion assessment and patients undergoing PCI in spite of negative FFR (3.3% vs. 7.9%; p = 0.21) (21,22). In addition, the percentage of patients free from angina at follow-up was not different between the two groups of patients. These findings have also been confirmed in the setting of left main disease. In a registry of 213 patients with angiographically equivocal left main coronary artery stenosis, the 5-year survival of patients deferred on the basis of FFR > 0.80 and treated with optimal medical therapy was favourable, and comparable with that of patients with FFR < 0.80 treated with coronary bypass surgery (89.8% vs. 85.4%; p = 0.48). In other words, patients with non-hemodynamically significant stenoses do not derive any additional benefit when undergoing revascularization.

In contrast, revascularization of ischemia-inducing lesions is associated with improvement of symptoms and better clinical outcomes (2,23). In patients with multivessel disease, a complete functional revascularization strategy guided by FFR measurement was compared with a complete anatomical revascularization strategy guided by angiography in the FAME trial (24). Patients assigned to the angio-guided PCI underwent stenting of all indicated lesions, whereas patients assigned to FFR-guided PCI underwent stenting of indicated lesions only if the FFR was ≤0.80. Compared with the angio-guided strategy, the FFR-guided strategy was associated with a significant reduction of major adverse cardiac events at 1 year (13.2% vs. 18.3%, p = 0.02). This beneficial effect was also preserved at 2 years, with a significantly lower rate of myocardial infarction (6.1% vs. 9.9%; p = 0.03) and of the combined endpoint of death and myocardial infarction (8.4% vs. 12.9%; p = 0.02) (25). Importantly, the FFR-guided strategy was found to not only improve clinical outcome but also significantly reduce costs (26).

The beneficial effect of the FFR-guided strategy was also achieved thanks to a functional redefinition of coronary atherosclerosis severity: among those patients (n = 115) with angiographic three-vessel disease, only 14% had functional three-vessel disease, while 43% had functional two-vessel disease and 34% had functional single-vessel disease. In 9% of the cases no functionally severe stenosis could be detected (27). Changing the diagnosis from three-vessel to two- or one-vessel disease could have a huge impact on clinical decision making. According to the guidelines and/or local revascularization strategy, patients with three-vessel disease who are referred for surgery were indeed downgraded on the basis of the functional severity of the stenosis by FFR. In extreme cases, the patient may be reclassified to single-vessel disease based on the FFR assessment and may end up with a single stent. Avoidance of complex coronary intervention or coronary artery bypass graft through FFR-guided reclassification is a very attractive scenario for the patient and the health service when we consider the potential risk exposure to the patient and the potential cost savings involved.

FFR in Bifurcation Disease

Atherosclerosis frequently occurs at branch points of coronary vessels and for many cardiologists the management of bifurcation disease remains a challenge. Recent evidence suggests that in the majority of cases provisional stenting is a more effective strategy than a "two-stent strategy" when treating bifurcations (28). Regardless of the strategy chosen, it is frequently the case that the ostium of the side branch is compromised either through plaque shift or carina shift. Trying to decide whether to treat or not to treat the side branch is not a straightforward task and visual estimation, quantitative coronary analysis, and IVUS have not been found to be reliable in determining the functional relevance. While many authors propose dilating the jailed side branch following plaque shift using final kissing balloons, the recently published NORDIC III study suggests that a final kissing balloon strategy is unnecessary as no clinical benefit was seen using this strategy for up to 6 months (29).

However, one possible explanation for this could be that in the side branches where a final kissing balloon was used the stenosis was not functionally significant in the first place. In addition, when we consider the data from Koolen et al. (30), showing that, on average, approximately 32% of the jailed side branches are functionally significant, and apply it to the NORDIC III data, it could be argued that this study did not find a difference from the final kissing balloons because it was not powered to answer this. One might speculate that had the strategy to dilate the side branch been based on the detection of inducible ischemia using FFR, the conclusion may have differed.

FFR in Left Main Stem Disease

Left main coronary artery (LMCA) lesions are sometimes difficult to appreciate angiographically for several reasons: (i) the catheter obscures the angiographic image; (ii) coexistent atherosclerosis makes it difficult to estimate the stenosis; (iii) the mixing effect of blood and contrast at the ostium affects image quality; (iv) the LMCA can be remarkably short. In extreme cases, even an angiographically mild to moderate LMCA stenosis can provoke such a reflex action that patients may undergo surgical revascularization for a lesion that is functionally irrelevant. The implications of this are far reaching since the patient may be subjected to sternotomy and bypass grafting. Moreover, this strategy may be in vain since grafts anastomosed to a vessel with a functionally hemodynamically non-significant stenosis are more likely to occlude (30).

One of the many things we have learned from FFR is that the threshold to measure FFR in the left main or the proximal LAD should indeed be low since it supplies such a large myocardial mass. When speaking of the safety of FFR to evaluate left main stem disease we have several small studies supporting this practice and one more recent study in 223 patients (31). In each case, FFR was measured and if the value was ≤0.80 the patient was referred for surgery whereas if the patient had an FFR > 0.80 the patient was prescribed optimal medical therapy alone. The results of this study showed that the survival rates were comparable (89.8% vs. 85.4%, p = 0.48) as were event-free survival estimates (74.2% vs. 82.8%, p = 0.50) after a 5-year follow-up. Incidentally, up to 23% of the patients with LMCA stenosis in this study deemed as angiographically non-significant had FFR values <0.80. In other words, a significant proportion of left main stem disease patients were denied revascularization incorrectly. These data support the use of FFR in left main disease.

PERSONAL PERSPECTIVE

Despite the growing body of evidence supporting a revascularization strategy aimed at targeting the ischemic substrate, the data from the Courage trial raised several issues with regard to the merits of invasive revascularization strategies compared with a policy of aggressive medical optimal management of patients, particularly those with stable angina (32). The Courage study, in fact, demonstrated that there was no difference in the primary endpoint of death and myocardial infarction between a strategy of PCI plus optimal medical therapy and optimal medical therapy alone. Not surprisingly, these findings were met with criticisms questioning the real applicability of the Courage data to the real world of clinical practice. The fact that only a small number of patients were included, compared with the ones initially screened, and the very high rate of non-invasive functional assessment (uncommon in clinical practice) raised the suspicion of a highly selected patient population (1). In addition, it is very possible that non-functionally significant coronary lesions have been stented just on the basis of their angiographic appearance, which actually should have been left alone.

Following on from the FAME trial and based on the results of the Courage trial, the FAME II trial was designed and is underway. The purpose of the FAME II trial is simple in that it aims to compare the clinical outcomes, safety, and cost-effectiveness of FFR-guided PCI plus optimal medical therapy versus optimal medical therapy alone in patients with stable CAD, including those that may necessitate complex PCI. This study will address the question as to which patient and which lesion subsets will benefit most from percutaneous coronary revascularization and optimal medical therapy.

In conclusion, there are still several question marks over the relative merits of PCI in the management of complex coronary disease; however, one thing that seems clear is that as clinicians we cannot continue to guide complex intervention solely on the basis of visual estimation. We can speculate that if an FFR-guided approach had been applied in several recent studies to guide the mode of revascularization, the results may well have been different.

FFR measurement represents a valuable tool that enables the interventional cardiologist to base his decision making on the functional severity of the stenosis and, therefore, tailor the treatment to those lesions and those vessels responsible for the patient's symptoms.

VIDEO CLIP

Video clip 12.1 Measurement of funtional flow reserve in ostial lesions.

REFERENCES

1. Shaw LJ, Berman DS, Maron DJ, et al. Optimal medical therapy with or without percutaneous coronary intervention to reduce ischemic burden: results from the Clinical Outcomes Utilizing Revascularization and Aggressive Drug Evaluation (COURAGE) trial nuclear substudy. Circulation 2008; 117: 1283–91.
2. Erne P, Schoenenberger AW, Burckhardt D, et al. Effects of percutaneous coronary interventions in silent ischemia after myocardial infarction. JAMA 2007; 297: 1985–91.
3. Lin GA, Dudley RA, Lucas FL, et al. Frequency of stress testing to document ischemia prior to elective percutaneous coronary intervention. JAMA 2008; 300: 1765–73.
4. Wijns W, Kolh P, Danchin N, et al. The Task Force on Myocardial Revascularization of the European Society of Cardiology (ESC) and the European Association for Cardio-Thoracic Surgery (EACTS). Guidelines on myocardial revascularization. Eur Heart J 2010; 31: 2501–55.
5. Pijls NH, van Son JA, Kirkeeide RL, De Bruyne B, Gould KL. Experimental basis of determining maximum coronary, myocardial, and collateral blood flow by pressure measurements for assessing functional stenosis severity before and after percutaneous transluminal coronary angioplasty. Circulation 1993; 87: 1354–67.
6. De Bruyne B, Baudhuin T, Melin JA, et al. Coronary flow reserve calculated from pressure measurements in humans. Validation with positron emission tomography. Circulation 1994; 89: 1013–22.
7. De Bruyne B, Bartunek J, Sys SU, et al. Simultaneous coronary pressure and flow velocity measurements in humans. Feasibility, reproducibility, and hemodynamic dependence of coronary flow velocity reserve, hyperemic flow versus pressure slope index, and fractional flow reserve. Circulation 1996; 94: 1842–9.
8. Murtagh B, Higano S, Lennon R, et al. Role of incremental doses of intracoronary adenosine for fractional flow reserve assessment. Am Heart J 2003; 146: 99–105.
9. De Bruyne B, Hersbach F, Pijls NH, et al. Abnormal epicardial coronary resistance in patients with diffuse atherosclerosis but "Normal" coronary angiography. Circulation 2001; 104: 2401–6.
10. Gould KL, Nakagawa Y, Nakagawa K, et al. Frequency and clinical implications of fluid dynamically significant diffuse coronary artery disease manifest as graded, longitudinal, base-to-apex myocardial perfusion abnormalities by noninvasive positron emission tomography. Circulation 2000; 101: 1931–9.
11. Fearon WF, Nakamura M, Lee DP, et al. Simultaneous assessment of fractional and coronary flow reserves in cardiac transplant recipients: Physiologic Investigation for Transplant Arteriopathy (PITA Study). Circulation 2003; 108: 1605–10.
12. Aarnoudse WH, Botman KJ, Pijls NH. False-negative myocardial scintigraphy in balanced three-vessel disease, revealed by coronary pressure measurement. Int J Cardiovasc Intervent 2003; 5: 67–71.
13. Pijls NH, Klauss V, Siebert U, et al. Coronary pressure measurement after stenting predicts adverse events at follow-up: a multicenter registry. Circulation 2002; 105: 2950–4.
14. De Bruyne B, Pijls NH, Bartunek J, et al. Fractional flow reserve in patients with prior myocardial infarction. Circulation 2001; 104: 157–62.
15. Marques KM, Knaapen P, Boellaard R, et al. Microvascular function in viable myocardium after chronic infarction does not influence fractional flow reserve measurements. J Nucl Med 2007; 48: 1987–92.

16. Uren NG, Crake T, Lefroy DC, et al. Reduced coronary vasodilator function in infarcted and normal myocardium after myocardial infarction. N Engl J Med 1994; 331: 222–7.

17. Claeys MJ, Vrints CJ, Bosmans J, et al. Coronary flow reserve during coronary angioplasty in patients with a recent myocardial infarction: relation to stenosis and myocardial viability. J Am Coll Cardiol 1996; 28: 1712–9.

18. Marques KM, Knaapen P, Boellaard R, et al. Hyperaemic microvascular resistance is not increased in viable myocardium after chronic myocardial infarction. Eur Heart J 2007; 28: 2320–5.

19. De Bruyne B, Pijls NH, Heyndrickx GR, et al. Pressure-derived fractional flow reserve to assess serial epicardial stenoses: theoretical basis and animal validation. Circulation 2000; 101: 1840–7.

20. Pijls NH, De Bruyne B, Bech GJ, et al. Coronary pressure measurement to assess the hemodynamic significance of serial stenoses within one coronary artery: validation in humans. Circulation 2000; 102: 2371–7.

21. Pijls NH, van Schaardenburgh P, Manoharan G, et al. Percutaneous coronary intervention of functionally nonsignificant stenosis: 5-year follow-up of the DEFER Study. J Am Coll Cardiol 2007; 49: 2105–11.

22. Pijls NH, De Bruyne B, Peels K, et al. Measurement of fractional flow reserve to assess the functional severity of coronary-artery stenoses. N Engl J Med 1996; 334: 1703–8.

23. Davies RF, Goldberg AD, Forman S, et al. Asymptomatic Cardiac Ischemia Pilot (ACIP) study two-year follow-up: outcomes of patients randomized to initial strategies of medical therapy versus revascularization. Circulation 1997; 95: 2037–43.

24. Tonino PA, De Bruyne B, Pijls NH, et al. Fractional flow reserve versus angiography for guiding percutaneous coronary intervention. N Engl J Med 2009; 360: 213–24.

25. Pijls NH, Fearon WF, Tonino PA, et al. Fractional flow reserve versus angiography for guiding percutaneous coronary intervention in patients with multivessel coronary artery disease: 2-year follow-up of the FAME (Fractional Flow Reserve Versus Angiography for Multivessel Evaluation) study. J Am Coll Cardiol 2010; 56: 177–84.

26. Fearon WF, Bornschein B, Tonino PA, et al. Economic evaluation of fractional flow reserve-guided percutaneous coronary intervention in patients with multivessel disease. Circulation 2010; 122: 2545–50.

27. Tonino PA, Fearon WF, De Bruyne B, et al. Angiographic versus functional severity of coronary artery stenoses in the FAME study fractional flow reserve versus angiography in multivessel evaluation. J Am Coll Cardiol 2010; 55: 2816–21.

28. Hildick-Smith D, de Belder AJ, Cooter N, et al. Randomized trial of simple versus complex drug-eluting stenting for bifurcation lesions: the British Bifurcation Coronary Study: Old, New, and Evolving Strategies. Circulation 2010; 121: 1235–43.

29. Niemela M, Kervinen K, Erglis A, et al. Randomized comparison of final kissing balloon dilatation versus no final kissing balloon dilatation in patients with coronary bifurcation lesions treated with main vessel stenting: the Nordic-Baltic Bifurcation Study III. Circulation 2011; 123: 79–86.

30. Botman CJ, Schonberger J, Koolen S, et al. Does stenosis severity of native vessels influence bypass graft patency? A prospective fractional flow reserve-guided study. Ann Thorac Surg 2007; 83: 2093–7.

31. Hamilos M, Muller O, Cuisset T, et al. Long-term clinical outcome after fractional flow reserve-guided treatment in patients with angiographically equivocal left main coronary artery stenosis. Circulation 2009; 120: 1505–12.

32. Boden WE, O'Rourke RA, Teo KK, et al. Optimal medical therapy with or without PCI for stable coronary disease. N Engl J Med 2007; 356: 1503–16.

13   Intravascular ultrasound: Role in patient diagnosis and management

Kenji Sakamoto, Yasuhiro Honda, and Peter J. Fitzgerald

OUTLINE

In recent decades, intravascular ultrasound (IVUS) has evolved as a valuable adjunct to angiography, providing valuable clinical insights by direct visualization of atherosclerosis and other pathologic conditions within the vessel wall. Because the ultrasound signal is able to penetrate below the wall of the artery, the entire cross section, including the complete thickness of the plaque, can be imaged in real time. This offers the opportunity to gather diagnostic information about the process of atherosclerosis and directly observe the effects of various interventions on the plaque and arterial wall. Moreover, IVUS has proven to be a practically useful tool in the evaluation and optimal guidance of interventional vascular medicine. While devices for the treatment of coronary artery disease have seen great progress, for example, the latest generation of drug-eluting stents, IVUS continues to play a vital role as operators are faced with more difficult anatomical and technical challenges in the treatment of complex lesions. In this chapter, we detail the current use of IVUS in the clinical setting with evidence-based data provided by precise analysis of IVUS images.

INTRODUCTION

By the late 1980s, the first images of human vessels were recorded by Yock and colleagues (1). Since then, intravascular ultrasound (IVUS) has become a pivotal catheter-based imaging technology that can provide scientific insights into vascular biology and practical guidance for percutaneous coronary interventions (PCIs) in clinical settings. The detailed anatomic information obtained with IVUS has proven extremely helpful in clinical practice. IVUS before intervention can help to determine the need for treatment and the optimal treatment strategy; IVUS is also invaluable in evaluating the results of stent implantation and in determining the need for adjunct intervention to optimize the result. In addition, IVUS can provide very sensitive imaging endpoints for the evaluation of new drugs and devices to facilitate smaller sample sizes and shorter study durations thereby shortening the approval process for novel technological advances. IVUS is particularly suitable because of its easy availability and its relatively high image resolution that provides accurate and reproducible measurements. The ability of IVUS to detect mild silent atherosclerosis that can be a precursor of future coronary events is superior to that of coronary angiography. Recently, intravascular optical coherence tomography (OCT) has been introduced into the clinical arena, offering higher image resolution at the expense of penetration depth in the tissue. However, the capability for interactive on-line guidance owing to the visibility of the image

Focus Box 13.1

IVUS has evolved as a pivotal imaging technology to directly visualize atherosclerosis and other pathologic conditions within the vessel wall in vivo.

transducer position on fluoroscopy, the deeper penetration that allows imaging of the entire vessel wall, and the fact that additional contrast for repeated imaging is unnecessary are the specific advantages of IVUS.

IMAGING SYSTEMS AND PROCEDURES

IVUS imaging systems use reflected sound waves to visualize the vessel wall structure in a two-dimensional format, analogous to a histological cross-section. This technology enables in vivo acquisition of detailed information that cannot be accurately provided by angiography: this includes vessel diameter, lesion length, and the amount and distribution of plaque. In general, higher frequencies of ultrasound limit the scanning depth but improve the axial resolution, with current IVUS catheters having center frequencies ranging from 20 to 45 MHz. There are two different designs of IVUS transducer systems: the solid-state dynamic aperture system (the electronically switched multi-element array system) and the mechanically rotating single-transducer system. Image quality is generally better in the mechanically rotating single-transducer system, but a guide wire artifact and occasional non-uniform rotational distortion (NURD) are limitations specific to this system (Fig. 13.1). A stationary outer sheath of the mechanical catheters allows the transducer to be moved through a segment of interest in a precise and controlled manner (Video clip 13.1A–D).

For patient use, both require preprocedural administration of intravenous heparin (5,000–10,000 U or equivalent anticoagulation) along with intracoronary nitroglycerin (100–300 µg). Standard interventional techniques and equipment are used for imaging catheter delivery, and image acquisition is performed by retracting the transducer from the distal segment to the region of interest. During imaging, the most frequent acute complication is transient coronary spasm (up to 3%) (2). Although major complications are rare (dissection, thrombosis, or abrupt closure in <0.5%), careful catheter manipulation is mandatory, similar to other interventional procedures. Regarding possible endothelial injury and disease progression as a chronic complication of intracoronary instrumentation, a study of transplant patients confirmed no acceleration of coronary artery disease associated with repeated IVUS examinations (3).

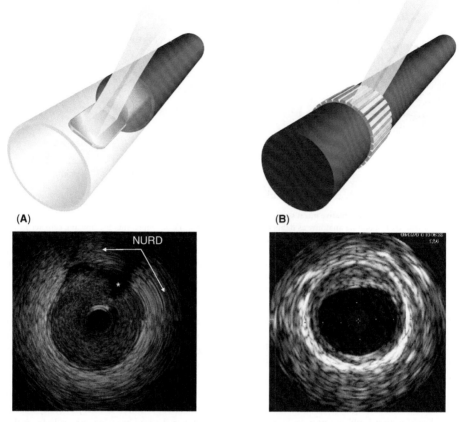

Figure 13.1 Basic diagrams of the two imaging catheter designs with representative ultrasound images. The mechanically rotating single-transducer system (**A**) can offer higher image resolution due to the higher center frequency and the larger effective aperture of the transducer element. On the other hand, the solid-state dynamic aperture system (**B**) is free from guide wire artifact (* in image **A**) and non-uniform rotational image distortion that can occasionally be seen with the mechanical system.

PRINCIPLES OF IMAGE INTERPRETATION

The interpretation of coronary IVUS images is possible because the layers of a diseased arterial wall can be identified separately. The media of the coronary artery is characterized by a darker band compared with the intima and adventitia (Fig. 13.2). The relative echolucency of the media because of less collagen and elastin contents than in the neighboring layers gives rise to a three-layered appearance (bright-dark-bright). "Blooming," a spillover effect, can be seen since the intimal layer reflects ultrasound more strongly than the media. This results in a slight overestimation of the thickness of the intima and a corresponding underestimation of the medial thickness. Conversely, the fibrous plaque may lead to overestimation of the medial thickness owing to ultrasound signal attenuation behind the plaque. In patients with significant plaque burden, thinning of the media underlying the plaque can occur. As a result, the media is often indistinct or undetectable in some part of the IVUS cross-section, and this problem can be exacerbated by the blooming phenomenon. Even in these cases, however, the media/adventitial boundary (at the level of the external elastic membrane [EEM]) can be accurately rendered, because a step-up in echoreflectivity

occurs at this boundary and no blooming appears. For this reason, current IVUS studies measure and report the plaque-plus-media area as a surrogate measure for plaque area alone.

The determination of the position of the imaging plane within the artery is one important aspect of image interpretation. For example, the IVUS beam penetrates beyond the coronary artery, providing images of perivascular structures, including the cardiac veins, myocardium, and pericardium. These structures provide useful landmarks regarding the position of the imaging plane because they have a characteristic appearance when viewed from various positions within the arterial tree. The branching patterns of the arteries are also distinctive and help identify the position of the transducer. During pullback in the left anterior descending coronary artery (LAD) from the distal to the proximal segments, for example, the septal perforators appear to bud away from the LAD much more abruptly than the diagonals. The pericardium, which can be seen in the distal portion of the coronary artery, contains fibrous material that generates a radial acoustic shadow (Fig. 13.3) (Video clip 13.2). The geographic relationship between the pericardium and the right ventricular branch of the right coronary artery is similar to the relationship

153

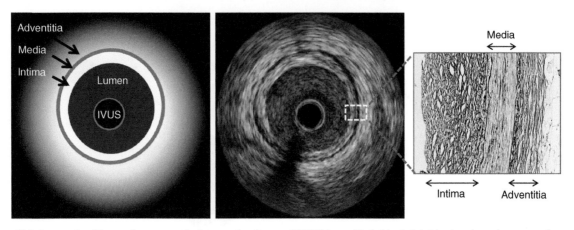

Figure 13.2 Cross-sectional format of a representative intravascular ultrasound (IVUS) image. The bright-dark-bright, three-layered appearance is seen on the ultrasound image (*left*) with corresponding anatomy as defined (*middle* and *right*). "IVUS" represents the imaging catheter in the vessel lumen. The media has lower ultrasound reflectance owing to less collagen and elastin compared with neighboring layers. The outer boundary of the media (external elastic membrane) can be rendered more accurately than the inner boundary (internal elastic membrane), because of a step-up in echoreflectivity at the media/adventitial boundary precluding the effect of ultrasound blooming or attenuation. The adventitial and peri-adventitial tissues are similar enough in echoreflectivity that a clear outer adventitial border cannot be defined.

Focus Box 13.2

Fundamental knowledge of ultrasound and coronary anatomy is essential for accurate image interpretation and orientation in the coronary tree.

between the pericardium and the diagonal branch of the LAD (branched from the direction that is 90° counterclockwise from the pericardium—however, anatomic variation may occur). Longitudinal image orientation facilitates accurate stent implantation in the aspects of optimal stent edge positioning, while cross-sectional image orientation is important particularly for guide wire orientation in the treatment of chronic total occlusion (CTO) lesions. In off-line IVUS analysis, accurate orientation in both longitudinal and short axes is essential, in order to be able to compare images at the same site obtained at different time points.

IVUS MEASUREMENTS FOR QUANTITATIVE ASSESSMENT

Using an intrinsic distance calibration, electronic caliper (diameter) and tracing (area) measurements can be performed at the tightest cross-section as well as at reference segments located proximal and distal to the lesion. The maximum and minimum diameters (i.e., the major and minor axes of an elliptical cross-section) are the most widely used dimensions. The ratio of maximum to minimum diameter defines a measure of symmetry. Area measurements are performed with computer planimetry and lumen area is determined by tracing the leading edge of the blood/intima border, whereas vessel (or EEM) area is defined as the area enclosed by the outermost interface between the media and the adventitia. Plaque area (or plaque-plus-media area) is calculated as the difference between the vessel and lumen areas. The ratio of plaque area to vessel area is termed percent plaque area, plaque burden, or percent cross-sectional narrowing. Area measurements can be added to calculate volumes using the modified Simpson's rule, which involves the use of motorized pullback.

TISSUE CHARACTERIZATION FOR QUALITATIVE ASSESSMENT

Regions of calcification are very brightly echoreflective and create a dense shadow more peripherally from the catheter, a phenomenon known as acoustic shadowing. Shadowing prevents determination of the true thickness of a calcific deposit and precludes visualization of structures in the tissue beyond the calcium. Calcification also causes an appearance of multiple ghost images of the leading calcium interface, spaced at regular radial intervals, known as ultrasound reverberation. Like calcium, densely fibrotic tissue appears bright on the ultrasound scan. Fatty plaque is less echogenic than fibrous plaque. The brightness of the adventitia can be used as a gauge to discriminate between predominantly fatty and fibrous plaque (an area of plaque that appears darker than the adventitia is considered fatty). In an image of extremely good quality, the presence of a lipid pool can be inferred from the appearance of a dark region within the plaque. In thrombus-containing lesions, an accurate diagnosis of thrombus may often be difficult because various compositions and changes over time can be associated with the thrombus. Injection of contrast or saline may disperse the stagnant flow, clear the lumen (Video clip 13.3), and allow differentiation between blood stasis and thrombus. Mobility, lobulation, pedunculated appearance, speckled or scintillating sign, and blood flow in cleft or microchannels are entities thought to suggest thrombus (Video clip 13.4A,B).

Since the visual interpretation of conventional grayscale IVUS images is limited in the detection and quantification of specific plaque components, computer-assisted analysis of raw

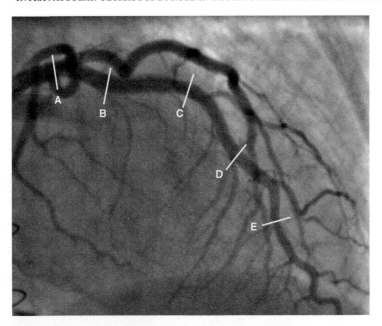

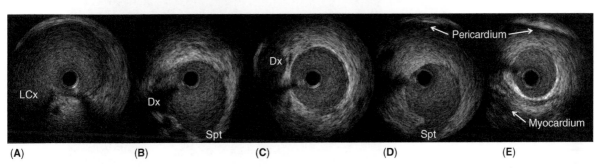

Figure 13.3 Image orientation of intravascular ultrasound images. In the pullback imaging sequence from the distal to the proximal portion of the left anterior descending artery (LAD), the left circumflex artery (LCx) emerges on the same side as the diagonal branches (Dx) (A and B). The septal branches (Spt) typically emerge on the side of the myocardium (the opposite side of the pericardium), while the diagonal branches emerge roughly orthogonal (90° counterclockwise) to the pericardium (B, D, and E). The angle between the septal and diagonal branches can increase to as much as 180° depending on the portion of the LAD. The diagonals first appear in the periphery of the image and gradually come closer to the LAD (C), while the septals appear to bud away from the LAD abruptly. The mid- and the distal portions of the LAD often lie deeper in the interventricular sulcus than the proximal LAD such that myocardium can be observed at this level on the opposite side of the pericardium (E).

radiofrequency (RF) signals in the reflected ultrasound beam has recently been developed. Virtual Histology™ (VH) IVUS (Volcano Corporation, Rancho Cordova, CA) is recognized as the first commercialized RF analysis technology. A classification tree algorithm developed from ex vivo human coronary data sets generates color-mapped images of the vessel wall with a distinct color for each category: fibrous, necrotic, calcific, and fibro-fatty. Another mathematical technique used in RF ultrasound backscatter analysis is the integrated backscatter (IB) IVUS (YD Corporation, Nara, Japan). This method utilizes IB values calculated as the average power of the backscattered ultrasound signal from a sample tissue volume. The IB-IVUS system then constructs color-coded tissue maps, providing a quantitative visual readout for four types of plaque composition: calcification, fibrosis, dense fibrosis, and lipid

pool. More recently, iMap™ (Boston Scientific Inc, Natick, MA) has been commercialized as the latest tissue characterization method that is compatible with the 40-MHz mechanical IVUS imaging system. iMap allows identification and quantification of four different types of atherosclerotic components (fibrotic, necrotic, lipidic, and calcified tissues) based on the degree of spectral similarity between the backscattered signal and a reference library of spectra from preserved histological data. A confidence level assessment is carried out and displayed for each tissue type (Fig. 13.4).

ASSESSMENT OF PLAQUE DISTRIBUTION AND INSTABILITY
Contrast coronary arteriography is limited in its ability to assess the extent or distribution of atherosclerosis or to identify changes within the vessel wall. One of the causes for this

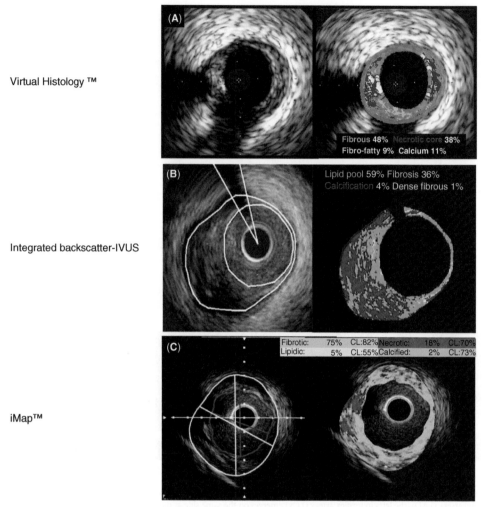

Virtual Histology ™

Integrated backscatter-IVUS

iMap™

Figure 13.4 Plaque characterization by radiofrequency intravascular ultrasound (IVUS) signal analyses. (**A**) Virtual Histology™ employs spectral radiofrequency analyses with a classification tree algorithm developed from ex vivo coronary datasets, showing a distinct color for each of the fibrous, fibro-fatty, necrotic core, and calcific components (*right*). (**B**) Integrated backscatter-IVUS utilizes integrated backscatter values calculated as the average power of the backscattered ultrasound signal from a sample tissue volume, to differentiate the following tissue types: fibrosis, dense fibrous, lipid pool, and calcification. (**C**) iMap™ identifies four different types of plaque components (fibrotic, lipidic, necrotic, and calcified tissue) based on the degree of spectral similarity between the backscattered signal and a reference library of spectra from known tissue types. This allows a confidence level assessment of each plaque component.

Focus Box 13.3

To complement the limitation of grayscale IVUS in precise tissue characterization, several radiofrequency signal analysis techniques have been introduced for the quantitative assessment of plaque components in clinical settings.

discrepancy is the phenomenon of vessel remodeling (Fig. 13.5), a process which is in fact bidirectional, with some segments showing positive remodeling (or expansion) and others showing negative remodeling (or constriction). In IVUS studies, a remodeling index (the ratio of vessel area at

the lesion site to that at the reference site) as a continuous variable is often used in addition to the categorical classifications. The assessment of remodeling is clinically important not only for optimal therapeutic device sizing but also for risk stratification regarding plaque rupture or evaluating procedural and long-term outcomes of an intervention. Vulnerable lesions responsible for acute coronary syndromes have usually undergone extensive positive remodeling with large plaque burden and less calcification. Histopathologic studies support these clinical IVUS observations by demonstrating that these lesion subsets frequently represent large, lipid-rich plaques with increased inflammatory cell infiltrates. Furthermore, multiple clinical studies have shown that pre-interventional positive

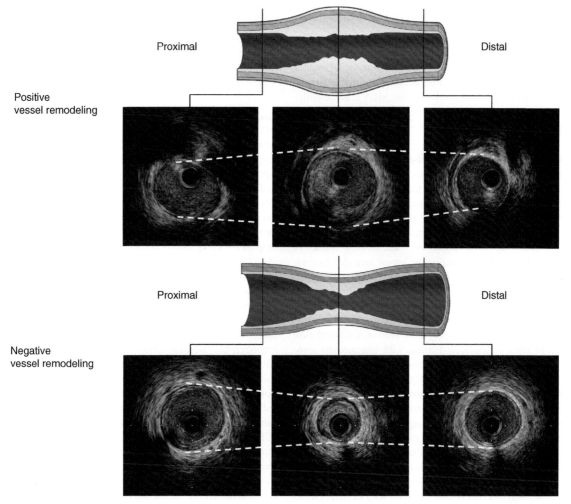

Figure 13.5 Intravascular ultrasound images showing remodeling. *Upper:* Positive remodeling (or vessel expansion), where there is localized enlargement of the vessel in the area of plaque accumulation. *Lower:* Negative remodeling (or vessel shrinkage), where the lesion has a smaller media-to-media diameter than the adjacent, less diseased sites.

remodeling or large plaque burden assessed by IVUS predicts unfavorable acute or long-term outcomes following coronary interventions (4).

While the characteristics of the ruptured plaque after the event (eccentric plaque, positive remodeling, and hypoechoic plaque) have already been reported, there is increasing interest in the ability of IVUS to predict future coronary events. One of the largest natural history studies is the Providing Regional Observations to Study Predictors of Events in the Coronary Tree (PROSPECT) trial that employed three-vessel imaging with VH-IVUS in 697 acute coronary syndrome patients (5). Multivariate analysis identified three baseline IVUS characteristics that independently predicted events: (i) plaque burden >70% (hazard ratio [HR] = 5.03); (ii) VH-determined thin-cap fibroatheroma (TCFA) (HR = 3.35); and (iii) minimal luminal area <4.0 mm² (HR = 3.21). Major adverse cardiac

> **Focus Box 13.4**
>
> Positive vessel remodeling, large plaque burden, and VH-determined TCFA, all of which cannot be identified using angiography, are the IVUS-specific predictive factors for unfavorable future events.

events occurred in 18% of lesions that had all three of these characteristics and in <1% of lesions with none of them.

INTERVENTIONAL APPLICATIONS OF IVUS

Assessment of Functional Significance in Intermediate Lesions

Intermediate coronary lesions identified by angiography (40–70% angiographic stenosis) represent a challenge for revascularization decision-making. Several IVUS or physiologic studies have

Focus Box 13.5

IVUS-determined minimum lumen area (MLA) reasonably correlates with results from physiologic assessments for functional significance of intermediate coronary stenosis. Despite the limited specificity to identify ischemia-inducible stenoses, the negative predictive value of the MLA is sufficiently high to defer the intervention in lesions with an MLA larger than the cut-off.

Focus Box 13.6

Pre-interventional IVUS assessment of plaque composition and distribution can help clarify the risk of peri-procedural complications and determine the optimal procedural strategy.

suggested that a considerable number of intermediate lesions referred for elective interventions are in fact hemodynamically insignificant and can be successfully managed with medical treatment alone. In addition to the increased health care costs, unnecessary interventions can expose the patient to increased stent-related risks and the need for prolonged antiplatelet therapy when drug-eluting stents (DESs) are used. In early studies of proximal coronary lesions, minimum lumen area (MLA) measured by IVUS demonstrated reasonable correlations with results from physiologic assessments. The ischemic MLA threshold was identified as 3.0–4.0 mm^2 for major epicardial coronary arteries, and 5.5–6.0 mm^2 for the left main coronary artery, based on physiologic assessment with coronary flow reserve, fractional flow reserve, or stress scintigraphy. Patients with intermediate coronary lesions in whom intervention was deferred based on IVUS findings (MLA > 4.0 mm^2) had a target lesion revascularization rate of only 2.8% with a composite event rate of 4.4% (6). More recent studies expanded the study population into a wide variety of lesions and indicated that the diagnostic accuracies and the optimal cut-off values of the MLA can vary depending on the location or the amount of myocardium supplied by the target segment (7). Nevertheless, the consistently high negative predictive values of the MLA in these studies suggest that interventions can still be safely deferred at least in lesions with an MLA greater than the proposed cut-offs.

Preinterventional Plaque Type Assessment

Preinterventional IVUS imaging is useful in determining the appropriate interventional strategy. In particular, it is important to identify the calcified plaque since the presence, degree, and location of calcium within the target vessel can substantially affect the delivery and subsequent deployment of coronary stents. One important advantage of on-line IVUS guidance is its ability to assess the extent and distance from the lumen of calcium deposits within a plaque. For example, lesions with extensive superficial calcium may require rotational atherectomy prior to stenting. Conversely, apparently significant calcification identified by fluoroscopy may subsequently be found by IVUS to be distributed in a deep portion of the vessel wall or to have a lower degree of calcification (calcium arc <180°). In these cases, standalone stenting is generally adequate to achieve lumen expansion large enough for DESs, particularly given the significant neointimal suppression at follow-up.

Preinterventional evaluation of plaque composition may also predict the occurrence of distal emboli during balloon dilatation or stenting that can result in the "slow-flow" or "no-reflow" phenomenon leading to peri-procedural myocardial infarction (8,9). In grayscale IVUS, predictive findings include large plaque burden with signal attenuation (unrelated to calcification), a large low-echoic region suggesting a lipid pool, and a thrombus-containing plaque. Recent studies with IB-IVUS or VH also demonstrated that the amount of lipid or necrotic core at preintervention was related to findings suggesting distal emboli. Identification of high-risk plaques may help in selecting lesions suitable for distal protection devices (Fig. 13.6).

Precise Selection of Device Size and Length

Vessel size and lesion length are often underestimated by angiography due to the technical limitations as described previously. For example, several IVUS studies have shown that angiographic "normal" reference segments for interventions have 35–51% of plaque burden when assessed by IVUS. Precise measurements of vessel size and lesion length can guide the optimal sizing of devices to be employed. A direct approach to balloon sizing, based on IVUS images, was first systematically pursued by the Clinical Outcomes with Ultrasound Trial (CLOUT) investigators (10), who reasoned that aggressive balloon sizing might be safely accomplished using the "true" vessel size and plaque characteristics as determined by IVUS. In this prospective, non-randomized study, balloon sizes were chosen to equal the average of the lumen and media-to-media diameters at the reference segment for cases with no extensive calcification. This led to an average 0.5-mm "oversizing" of the balloon compared with sizing based on standard angiographic criteria, and resulted in a significant decrease in post-procedure residual stenosis (from 28% to 18%) with no increase in clinically significant complications. In a contemporary DES trial of complex lesions, known as the Angiography Versus IVUS Optimization (AVIO) study, the size of the post-dilatation balloon was selected based on the average of the media-to-media diameters at multiple sites within the stented segment. The precise vessel size measurement is also critically important for size selection of self-expanding or fully biodegradable stents because undersizing of these devices is not amendable once deployed in the lesion.

Assessment of true lesion length by IVUS dictates the exact length of stent necessary to appropriately scaffold a lesion. Several IVUS studies of DESs have identified greater reference plaque burden as an independent predictor of subsequent stent edge restenosis or thrombosis. The Impact of Stent Deployment Techniques on Clinical Outcomes of Patient Treated with the CYPHER Stent (STLLR) trial also demonstrated that geographic miss

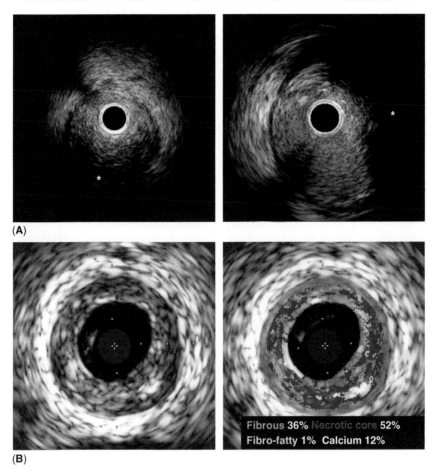

(A)

(B)

Fibrous 36% Necrotic core 52%
Fibro-fatty 1% Calcium 12%

Figure 13.6 Preinterventional intravascular ultrasound (IVUS) evaluation demonstrating high-risk plaques possibly prone to distal embolization during interventions. (**A**) Two examples of lesions with large plaque burden and ultrasound signal attenuation (*). The signal attenuation, observed despite absence of calcium, may suggest thrombus, lipid or necrotic core, and/or microcalcification within the plaque. (**B**) An example of a lesion with a large amount of necrotic core suggested by Virtual Histology IVUS: a conventional grayscale image (*left*) and a color-mapped presentation of the plaque components (*right*).

(defined as the length of the injured or stenotic segment not fully covered by the DES) had a significant negative impact on both clinical efficacy and safety at 1 year following sirolimus-eluting stent implantation (11). Therefore, complete coverage of the reference disease is currently recommended. Importantly, however, longer stent length has also been reported to be independently associated with DES restenosis and thrombosis. On-line IVUS guidance can facilitate the determination of appropriate stent length for anchoring the stent ends in relatively plaque-free vessel segments while minimizing the stent length for complete lesion coverage. One practical approach has recently been proposed in a single-center registry, where unique stepwise IVUS criteria (plaque burden <50% as the primary target zone) determined the optimal landing zone for sirolimus-eluting stents (12).

Optimization of Stent Expansion

There is compelling clinical evidence that procedure-related factors are important contributors to the development of both

restenosis and thrombosis after stent implantation, regardless of the stent type. In particular, the most consistent risk factor is stent underexpansion, the incidence of which has been reported to be 60–80% of current DES failures. In the bare metal stent (BMS) era, the predicted risk of restenosis was reported to decrease 19% for every 1-mm^2 increase in minimum stent area (MSA) (13). In the Can Routine Ultrasound Improve Stent Expansion (CRUISE) trial, IVUS guidance by operator preferences increased MSA from 6.25 to 7.14 mm^2, leading to a 44% relative reduction in target vessel revascularization at 9 months compared with angiographic guidance alone (14). In the Angiography Versus IVUS-Directed Stent Placement (AVID) trial, IVUS-guided stent implantation resulted in larger acute dimensions compared with angiography alone (7.54 vs. 6.94 mm²), with no increase in complications, and lower 12-month target lesion revascularization rates for complex lesion subsets (15). A number of studies have also suggested a link between suboptimal stent expansion detected by IVUS and stent thrombosis (16).

In the DES era, the relationship between post-implantation MSA and in-stent restenosis can further be enhanced when variability of the biologic response (neointimal proliferation) is reduced. In the SIRIUS trial, significant positive correlation was observed between baseline MSA and 8-month MLA with a stronger correlation with a higher regression coefficient in sirolimus-eluting stents than control BMS (17). In another clinical IVUS study of native coronary lesions treated with sirolimus-eluting stents, the only independent predictors of angiographic restenosis were post-procedural final MSA <5.5 mm² and IVUS-measured stent length >40 mm (odds ratio = 0.586 and 1.029, respectively) (18). In a series of restenotic BMS lesions treated with sirolimus-eluting stents, 82% of recurrent lesions had an MSA <5.0 mm² versus 26% of non-recurrent lesions (p = 0.003) (19).

As consistently observed in other stent studies, a pooled analysis of paclitaxel-eluting stent trials also identified baseline MSA as the independent predictor of subsequent in-stent restenosis in both paclitaxel-eluting stents and control BMS (20). Interestingly, while the overall antiproliferative effect of paclitaxel-eluting stents resulted in a smaller optimal threshold of MSA, the c-statistic and odds ratio in predicting 9-month restenosis were virtually identical for the two types of stents. This discrepancy can occur since the diagnostic accuracy of MSA for follow-up lumen patency is a function of lesion-to-lesion variability in neointimal hyperplasia rather than the average power of neointimal suppression. In general, the relative benefit of further obtaining larger MSA to ensure a greater "safety margin" for an unexpected amount of neointima (the so-called the bigger-is-better theory) can significantly vary among DESs, depending on the variability of subsequent neointimal proliferation. Given the wide variety of clinical backgrounds, patient risk factors, lesion morphologies, and disease complexities that we routinely face in our clinical practice, it is unlikely that one single pre-specified MSA endpoint could be effectively applied to all target lesions. Nevertheless, the ability of IVUS to assess the results of stent implantation more precisely than angiography can significantly contribute to our clinical judgment for individual patients. The utility of IVUS to ensure adequate stent expansion cannot be overemphasized, particularly if there are clinical risk factors for DES failure (e.g., diabetes, renal failure).

Assessment of Acute Complications

IVUS can identify several stent deployment issues. Incomplete expansion occurs when a portion of the stent is inadequately expanded compared with the distal and proximal reference dimensions, especially when dense fibrocalcific plaque is present.

Focus Box 13.8

Regardless of the stent type, IVUS-measured minimum stent area at post-implantation is a strong and independent parameter to predict subsequent events including both thrombosis and in-stent restenosis.

Incomplete apposition occurs when part of the stent structure is not fully in contact with the vessel wall. After stent implantation, tears at the edge of the stent (marginal tears or pocket flaps) can occur, which may be recognized as haziness by angiography. The stent edge tears have been attributed to the shear forces created at the junction between the metal edge of the stent and the adjacent, more compliant tissue, or to the effect of balloon expansion beyond the edge of the stent.

In fact, when investigated by IVUS, angiographic hazy lesions can represent a spectrum of during- and post-intervention anatomic morphologies, including calcium, dissection, thrombus, hematoma, spasm, and excessive plaque burden with extreme remodeling at the reference segment (Video clip 13.5). The etiology of persistent haziness can be precisely defined by IVUS owing to its higher sensitivity than contrast angiography for detecting the abnormal entities in the vessel wall (Video clip 13.6A,B). In addition, IVUS can also demonstrate the precise location and severity of those findings. For example, the location of the dissection can be important for risk of extension. Dissections on the free wall (same side as the pericardium) may have a higher likelihood of propagating through to the vessel wall compared with dissections on the mural wall, where the surrounding muscle constrains further propagation. Other criteria of vulnerable dissection are large, moving flaps, and extensive medial tears occupying greater than 50% of the vessel circumference (onion skin-like appearance). Identification of these patients at high risk of abrupt closure, who require preventive treatment such as (additional) stent implantation, is often possible and augments the angiographic findings. Practical IVUS checkpoints in the cardiac catheterization laboratory are shown in Table 13.1.

IVUS is also helpful in evaluating the involvement of side branches during the treatment of bifurcation lesions, which can have a significant impact on treatment strategy. Significant narrowing or occlusion of a side branch may occur during balloon dilatation and stenting of the parent artery, due to the "snowplow effect" of a plaque from the main vessel, a carina shift toward the side branch orifice, or their combination. It is important to note that contrast angiography sometimes shows false ostial narrowing of a side branch following parent artery stenting. Potential causes include spasm, flow disturbance, or dye streaming due to jailing of the branch, all of which can be differentiated by IVUS from true ostial plaque encroachment that may require further intervention.

Assessment of Chronic Complications

The primary mechanism of restenosis can be accurately identified by IVUS, which significantly affects the treatment strategy

Table 13.1 Practical IVUS Checklist for PCI in the Cardiac Catheterization Laboratory

Purpose	Location	Check point	Parameter	Details
Before PCI				
Assess lesion severity	Target	Lumen size	Minimum Lumen Area (MLA)	Minimum lumen CSA
		Plaque amount	% Plaque CSA	Plaque CSA/EEM CSA
Assess lesion morphology	Target	Eccentricity	Plaque eccentricity index	(Max-Min) Plaque CSA/Max P CSA
	Target and reference	Remodeling	Remodeling index	Lesion EEM CSA/Reference EEM CSA, Positive >1.0–1.05; negative <0.95–1.0
	Target	Plaque composition		Soft, fibrous, calcific, mixed, thrombus
		Calcification		Size (the arcs), location (superficial, deep, mixed)
		Plaque distribution		Diffuse or focal
		Relation to the branch		Plaque encroachment of side branch orifice
Device sizing	Target	Lumen and vessel size	Lumen and EEM CSA	
		Lesion length	% Plaque CSA	Plaque CSA/EEM CSA <50%
	Reference	Disease amount		
		Lumen and vessel size	Lumen and EEM CSA	
Safe delivery	Proximal vessel	Occult stenosis	MLA	Minimum lumen CSA
		Calcification		Size (the arcs), location (superficial, deep, mixed)
During and after PCI				
Assess stent expansion	Stented site	Stent expansion	%Stent expansion	Min stent CSA/Predefined reference area
		ISA		Size and location (body or edge)
		Stent eccentricity	Stent eccentricity index	(Max-Min) stent diameter/Max stent diameter or Min stent diameter/Max stent diameter
Assess complications	Stented site	Prolapse		Longitudinal length and extent of luminal encroachment
		Relation to the branch		Presence of jailed side branch
	Stented and reference sites	Hematoma		Location β (intra- or extravascular), longitudinal length and extent of luminal encroachment
	Reference	Edge dissection		Size and severity (intimal or medial)

Abbreviations: CSA, cross-sectional area; EEM, external elastic membrane; ISA, incomplete stent apposition; IVUS, intravascular ultrasound; MLA, minimum lumen area; MSA, minimum stent area; PCI, percutaneous coronary intervention.

Focus Box 13.9

IVUS can clarify the etiology of angiographic ambiguity observed during intervention and helps determine the appropriate strategy to treat complications.

---

in patients with restenotic lesions. An IVUS study of in-stent restenosis (ISR) lesions following BMS demonstrated that 20% of lesions had an MSA <5.0 mm² and an additional 4.5% had other mechanical problems that contributed to restenosis. In most of these cases, stent underexpansion or other mechanical problems were not suspected angiographically at the time of reintervention. For this type of ISR, mechanical optimization is the first priority, and IVUS can be helpful to differentiate mechanical issues from exaggerated neointimal proliferation that may truly require DES implantation within the original restenotic stent.

For DES treatment of ISR, early clinical studies suggested a hypothesis that full DES coverage of the original stent might be important for the prevention of recurrent restenosis. This aggressive optimization strategy, however, can be associated with several clinical issues, and thus may not be feasible in every case. In a retrospective IVUS study of BMS restenosis treated with sirolimus-eluting stents, 77% of the uncovered BMS segments maintained adequate lumen patency at follow-up (21). Therefore, as long as the original BMS is well expanded and has a segment with sufficient lumen area, conservative coverage with DES can be a clinical option (the so-called spot stenting strategy). Another study from the TAXUS trials evaluated 9-month IVUS results of patients who did not require revascularization at the time of 9-month angiography. At 3 years, revascularization was required in 4.9% of paclitaxel-eluting stents and 6.7% of BMS. Multivariate analysis identified MLA at 9 months as a significant predictor of later revascularization for both stent types (22).

Several IVUS studies have demonstrated that late-acquired incomplete stent apposition (LISA) is frequently observed in lesions of late DES thrombosis (Fig. 13.7) (Video clip 13.7). A literature-based meta-analysis also suggested a significantly higher risk of late or very late DES thrombosis in patients with incomplete stent apposition at follow-up (OR 6.51, P = 0.02) (23). The main mechanism of LISA after DES is often focal, positive vessel remodeling, whereas plaque regression or thrombus resolution is the predominant mechanism for LISA after BMS (24). In LISA with positive vessel remodeling, incompletely apposed struts are seen primarily in eccentric plaques, and gaps develop mainly on the disease-free side of the vessel wall. Thus, the combination of mechanical vessel injury during stent implantation and biologic vessel injury with pharmacological agents or polymers in the setting of little underlying plaque may predispose the vessel wall to chronic, pathologic dilation. It remains controversial, however, whether this morphologic abnormality independently contributes to the occurrence of stent thrombosis (Video clip 13.8).

Other IVUS-detected conditions that may be of importance in DESs include non-uniform stent strut distribution and stent fractures after implantation (Fig. 13.7) (Video clip 13.7). Theoretically, both abnormalities can reduce the local drug dose delivered to the arterial wall and affect the mechanical scaffolding of the treated lesion segment. By IVUS, strut fracture is defined as longitudinal strut discontinuity and can be categorized based upon its morphological characteristics: (i) strut separation, (ii) strut subluxation, or (iii) strut intussusceptions (25). Angiographic or IVUS studies have reported the incidence of DES fracture as 0.8–7.7%, wherein ISR or stent thrombosis occurred in 22–88% of cases (26). The exact incidence and clinical implications of strut fractures remain to be investigated in large clinical studies.

Focus Box 13.10

IVUS assessment is useful to evaluate the vessel response and stent morphology in the chronic phase, facilitating the understanding of new stent devices and the decision to implement additional treatment strategies in individual patients if required.

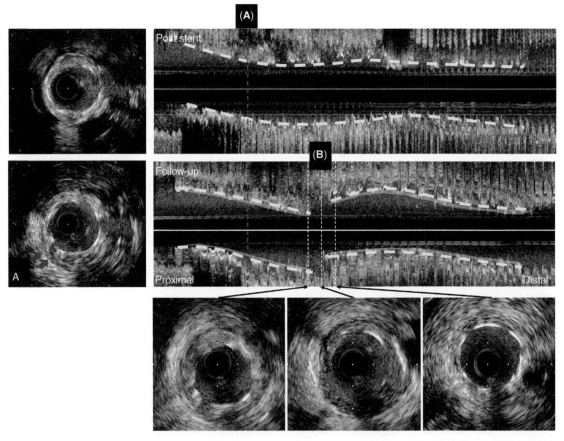

Figure 13.7 Intravascular ultrasound (IVUS)-detected problems 8 months after drug-eluting stent deployment. The longitudinal presentations show post-stent (*upper*) and 8-month follow-up (*lower*) results. At follow-up, newly acquired incomplete stent apposition (*arrows*, 5 to 8 o'clock) is observed at the proximal in-stent segment (**A**) where stent struts were well apposed to the vessel wall at baseline (cross-sectional images on the *left*). The gap developed on the relatively disease-free side of the vessel wall, accompanied by a focal vessel expansion at follow-up. At the mid-in-stent segment (**B**), newly acquired stent strut discontinuity is observed at follow-up. On the cross-sectional IVUS image (*bottom, middle*), no stent struts can be detected at 2 to 10 o'clock, while the proximal (*bottom, left*) and distal (*bottom, right*) adjacent segments shows a complete, circumferential distribution of stent struts.

Impact of IVUS Guidance in Stent Implantations

In the BMS era, multiple studies have indicated the long-term benefits of IVUS in stent implantation, whereas controversial results were also reported in some IVUS-guided stent trials. This may be partly due to differing procedural endpoints for IVUS-guided stenting as well as various adjunctive treatment strategies that were used in these trials in response to suboptimal results. Overall, a meta-analysis of nine clinical studies (2972 patients) demonstrated that IVUS-guided stenting significantly lowers 6-month angiographic restenosis (OR 0.75, P = 0.01) and target vessel revascularizations (OR 0.62, P = 0.00003), with a neutral effect on death and non-fatal myocardial infarction compared with angiographic optimization (27).

The impact of IVUS guidance during DES implantation on long-term clinical outcomes has also been assessed in several large studies. In a single-center study of IVUS-guided DES implantation versus a propensity score matched control population with angiographic guidance alone, a higher rate of definite stent thrombosis was seen in the angiography-guided group at both 30 days (0.5 vs. 1.4%, P = 0.046) and 12 months (0.7 vs. 2.0%, P = 0.014) (28). In addition, a trend was seen in favor of IVUS guidance for 12-month target lesion revascularization (5.1 vs. 7.2%, P = 0.07). Recent results of the Revascularization for Unprotected Left Main Coronary Artery Stenosis: Comparison of Percutaneous Coronary Angioplasty versus Surgical Revascularization (MAIN-COMPARE) registry showed a significantly lower 3-year mortality in the IVUS-guidance group as compared with the conventional angiography-guidance group (4.7% vs. 16.0%, log-rank P = 0.048) in patients treated with DES (29). A single-center registry of IVUS-guided DES implantation for the treatment of bifurcation lesions has also reported a significantly reduced 4-year mortality compared with angiography-guided stenting (HR 0.24, Cox model P = 0.03) (30). As previously described, the AVIO study was recently conducted to establish modern, universal criteria for IVUS optimization of DES implantation in complex coronary lesions. This study proposed the target stent area be determined according to the size of a post-dilation, non-compliant balloon chosen on the basis of IVUS measurements. Post-procedure minimum lumen diameter, as the primary endpoint of this study, was significantly larger in the IVUS-guided group, particularly when optimal IVUS criteria were met, with no increase in complications as compared with the angiography-guided group (target IVUS criteria met: 2.86 mm, target IVUS criteria not met: 2.6 mm, angiography alone: 2.51 mm).

FUTURE DIRECTIONS AND PERSONAL PERSPECTIVE

Currently, examination of clinical IVUS utility in third-generation stents (e.g., bioabsorbable vascular scaffolds) is

---

Focus Box 13.11

The usefulness of IVUS-guided intervention compared with angiographic optimization has been shown in the studies of the left main coronary lesions, bifurcation lesions, and complex lesions.

---

under way. The vascular response to these new generation stent implantations represents another important field to investigate with coronary imaging devices. Regarding technologic developments of imaging devices, an interesting approach would be to combine IVUS with a therapeutic device. In 2010, one angioplasty balloon catheter to integrate IVUS imaging (Vibe™ RX, Volcano Corporation, Rancho Cordova, CA) gained CE-mark clearance in Europe. This device is designed to provide precise IVUS-guided balloon dilatation with immediate confirmation of interventional results without additional catheters or catheter exchanges. Another interesting area is "forward-looking" IVUS (FLIVUS) technology that examines the vessel wall distal to the imaging catheter thereby having the potential to visualize the true and false lumens or penetration in CTO lesions. Currently, integration of an RF ablation feature into the FLIVUS catheter is also being explored for the CTO application. The potential synergy of different technologies may include a combination of diagnostic modalities also. LipiScan™ IVUS coronary imaging system (InfraReDx, Burlington, MA) that recently received FDA approval combines grayscale IVUS with NIR spectroscopy to visualize coronary lesions with simultaneous detection and localization of the lipid-rich plaque (Fig. 13.8A). Integration of IVUS and OCT into one imaging catheter is also under development to combine the advantages of the two imaging technologies. Finally, the next-generation higher-frequency IVUS catheter is under preclinical testing. Theoretically, an increase of center frequency from 40 MHz to 50 MHz corresponds to a 25% improvement in the axial resolution (Fig. 13.8B). Although some of these new technologies are yet to mature, the advances in diagnostic modalities will enhance our understanding of coronary pathophysiology and further enhance new treatment strategies to benefit our patients.

Focus Box 13.12

Ongoing technical developments of IVUS technology are exploring greater operator convenience, synergistic combination with therapeutic or other diagnostic modalities, and improved image quality with higher resolution.

ACKNOWLEDGMENT

The authors acknowledge Heidi N. Bonneau, RN, MS, CCA, for her review and editing advice.

VIDEO CLIPS

Video clip 13.1 Movies of common IVUS image artifacts during pullback. (A) Non-uniform rotational distortion (NURD) results in a wedge-shaped, smeared appearance in the image (between 9 and 12 o'clock in this example). (B) A "halo" or a series of bright rings immediately around the mechanical IVUS catheter are often due to air bubbles (between the transducer and the outer sheath) that need to be flushed out. (C) Radiofrequency noise appears as alternating radial spokes or random white dots in the outer aspect of the image due to interference from another electrical device. (D) Side lobe artefacts may lead to incorrect interpretation of the IVUS images. In this case, stent struts appear to be protruding into the lumen.

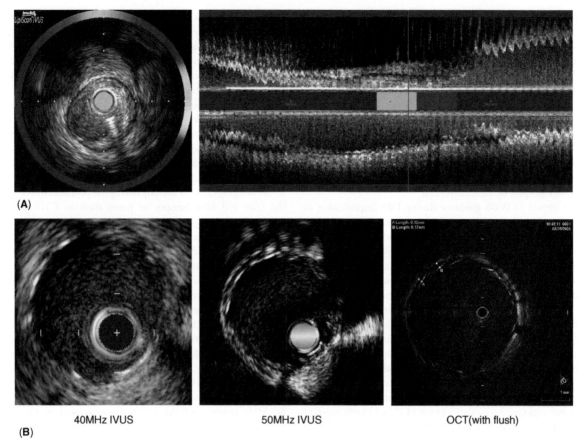

(A)

(B)   40MHz IVUS   50MHz IVUS   OCT(with flush)

Figure 13.8 Two examples of new intravascular ultrasound (IVUS) technologies. (A) Synergy of two different diagnostic modalities: grayscale IVUS with NIR spectroscopy (LipiScan™ IVUS Coronary Imaging System). Compared with the conventional grayscale presentation (*left*), the combined imaging catheter offers simultaneous detection and localization of the lipid-rich plaque (*middle* and *right*) superimposed on the anatomical information. (B) High-frequency IVUS for improved image quality. Compared with the conventional 40-MHz image (*left*), a new IVUS system with a center frequency of 50 MHz (Silicon Valley Medical Instrument, Inc., Fremont, CA) offers greater axial image resolution, allowing the detection of fine incomplete stent apposition (*right*).

Video clip 13.2 Movie showing image orientation in IVUS, from distal to proximal (movie of Figure 13.3).

Video clip 13.3 Recording showing contrast injection during IVUS. Injection of contrast allows interspersing of stagnant blood flow, clarifying the differentiation between blood stasis and the lumen wall.

Video clip 13.4 An example of an acute thrombus. After the severe stenotic lesion in the left anterior descending artery (LAD) was crossed with a guide wire, advancing the second guide wire into the diagonal branch took a long time. (A) An angiogram immediately after ST elevation in the EKG monitor shows significant filling defects along the proximal LAD. (B) IVUS pullback from distal to proximal shows a large amount of thrombus accumulation around the IVUS catheter.

Video clip 13.5 An example of a hematoma. The formation of an extensive hematoma within the vessel wall (behind the stent struts) is observed along the stent.

Video clip 13.6 An example of an angiographically ambiguous lesion. (A) An angiogram of the left coronary artery shows haziness localized in the ostium of the left anterior descending artery. (B) An IVUS image from distal to proximal shows a large neointimal flap at the proximal edge of the stent (2–8 o'clock).

Video clip 13.7 An 8-month follow-up IVUS image after drug-eluting stent deployment (movie of Figure 13.7). At the mid-in-stent segment, stent strut discontinuity (fracture) is observed with abnormal paucity of stent struts at 2–10 o'clock. During pullback from distal to proximal, the cross-sectional stent image jumps to the lower left on the IVUS image at the fracture site (subluxation). At the proximal in-stent segment, incomplete stent apposition at 5–8 o'clock is observed.

Video clip 13.8 An example IVUS image of the left anterior descending artery, from distal to proximal, with very late stent thrombosis (VLST) after drug-eluting stent implantation. Considerable vessel enlargement is observed at the proximal stent segment. Incomplete stent apposition is observed at multiple sites.

REFERENCES

1. Yock PG, Linker DT, Angelsen BA. Two-dimensional intravascular ultrasound: technical development and initial clinical experience. J Am Soc Echocardiogr 1989; 2: 296–304.
2. Hausmann D, Erbel R, Alibelli-Chemarin MJ, et al. The safety of intracoronary ultrasound. A multicenter survey of 2207 examinations. Circulation 1995; 91: 623–30.

3. Ramasubbu K, Schoenhagen P, Balghith MA, et al. Repeated intravascular ultrasound imaging in cardiac transplant recipients does not accelerate transplant coronary artery disease. J Am Coll Cardiol 2003; 41: 1739–43.

4. Okura H, Hayase M, Shimodozono S, et al. Impact of pre-interventional arterial remodeling on subsequent vessel behavior after balloon angioplasty: a serial intravascular ultrasound study. J Am Coll Cardiol 2001; 38: 2001–5.

5. Stone GW, Maehara A, Lansky AJ, et al. A prospective natural-history study of coronary atherosclerosis. N Engl J Med 2011; 364: 226–35.

6. Abizaid AS, Mintz GS, Mehran R, et al. Long-term follow-up after percutaneous transluminal coronary angioplasty was not performed based on intravascular ultrasound findings: importance of lumen dimensions. Circulation 1999; 100: 256–61.

7. Koo BK, Yang HM, Doh JH, et al. Optimal intravascular ultrasound criteria and their accuracy for defining the functional significance of intermediate coronary stenoses of different locations. JACC Cardiovasc Intervent 2011; 4: 803–11.

8. Endo M, Hibi K, Shimizu T, et al. Impact of ultrasound attenuation and plaque rupture as detected by intravascular ultrasound on the incidence of no-reflow phenomenon after percutaneous coronary intervention in ST-segment elevation myocardial infarction. JACC Cardiovasc Intervent 2010; 3: 540–9.

9. Kawaguchi R, Oshima S, Jingu M, et al. Usefulness of virtual histology intravascular ultrasound to predict distal embolization for ST-segment elevation myocardial infarction. J Am Coll Cardiol 2007; 50: 1641–6.

10. Stone GW, Hodgson JM, St Goar FG, et al. Improved procedural results of coronary angioplasty with intravascular ultrasound-guided balloon sizing: the CLOUT Pilot Trial. Clinical Outcomes With Ultrasound Trial (CLOUT) Investigators. Circulation 1997; 95: 2044–52.

11. Costa MA, Angiolillo DJ, Tannenbaum M, et al. Impact of stent deployment procedural factors on long-term effectiveness and safety of sirolimus-eluting stents (final results of the multicenter prospective STLLR trial). Am J Cardiol 2008; 101: 1704–11.

12. Morino Y, Tamiya S, Masuda N, et al. Intravascular ultrasound criteria for determination of optimal longitudinal positioning of sirolimus-eluting stents. Circ J 2010; 74: 1609–16.

13. Kasaoka S, Tobis JM, Akiyama T, et al. Angiographic and intravascular ultrasound predictors of in-stent restenosis. J Am Coll Cardiol 1998; 32: 1630–5.

14. Fitzgerald PJ, Oshima A, Hayase M, et al. Final results of the Can Routine Ultrasound Influence Stent Expansion (CRUISE) study. Circulation 2000; 102: 523–30.

15. Russo RJ, Silva PD, Teirstein PS, et al. A randomized controlled trial of angiography versus intravascular ultrasound-directed bare-metal coronary stent placement (the AVID Trial). Circ Cardiovasc Interv 2009; 2: 113–23.

16. Uren NG, Schwarzacher SP, Metz JA, et al. Predictors and outcomes of stent thrombosis: an intravascular ultrasound registry. Eur Heart J 2002; 23: 124–32.

17. Sonoda S, Morino Y, Ako J, et al. Impact of final stent dimensions on long-term results following sirolimus-eluting stent implantation: serial intravascular ultrasound analysis from the sirius trial. J Am Coll Cardiol 2004; 43: 1959–63.

18. Hong MK, Mintz GS, Lee CW, et al. Intravascular ultrasound predictors of angiographic restenosis after sirolimus-eluting stent implantation. Eur Heart J 2006; 27: 1305–10.

19. Fujii K, Mintz GS, Kobayashi Y, et al. Contribution of stent under-expansion to recurrence after sirolimus-eluting stent implantation for in-stent restenosis. Circulation 2004; 109: 1085–8.

20. Doi H, Maehara A, Mintz GS, et al. Impact of post-intervention minimal stent area on 9-month follow-up patency of paclitaxel-eluting stents: an integrated intravascular ultrasound analysis from the TAXUS IV, V, and VI and TAXUS ATLAS Workhorse, Long Lesion, and Direct Stent Trials. JACC Cardiovasc intervent 2009; 2: 1269–75.

21. Sakurai R, Ako J, Hassan AH, et al. Neointimal progression and luminal narrowing in sirolimus-eluting stent treatment for bare metal in-stent restenosis: a quantitative intravascular ultrasound analysis. Am Heart J 2007; 154: 361–5.

22. Doi H, Maehara A, Mintz GS, et al. Impact of in-stent minimal lumen area at 9 months poststent implantation on 3-year target lesion revascularization-free survival: a serial intravascular ultrasound analysis from the TAXUS IV, V, and VI trials. Circulation Cardiovasc Intervent 2008; 1: 111–8.

23. Hassan AK, Bergheanu SC, Stijnen T, et al. Late stent malapposition risk is higher after drug-eluting stent compared with bare-metal stent implantation and associates with late stent thrombosis. Eur Heart J 2010; 31: 1172–80.

24. Ako J, Morino Y, Honda Y, et al. Late incomplete stent apposition after sirolimus-eluting stent implantation: a serial intravascular ultrasound analysis. J Am Coll Cardiol 2005; 46: 1002–5.

25. Honda Y. Drug-eluting stents. Insights from invasive imaging technologies. Circ J 2009; 73: 1371–80.

26. Doi H, Maehara A, Mintz GS, et al. Classification and potential mechanisms of intravascular ultrasound patterns of stent fracture. Am J Cardiol 2009; 103: 818–23.

27. Casella G, Klauss V, Ottani F, et al. Impact of intravascular ultrasound-guided stenting on long-term clinical outcome: a meta-analysis of available studies comparing intravascular ultrasound-guided and angiographically guided stenting. Catheter Cardiovasc Interv 2003; 59: 314–21.

28. Roy P, Steinberg DH, Sushinsky SJ, et al. The potential clinical utility of intravascular ultrasound guidance in patients undergoing percutaneous coronary intervention with drug-eluting stents. Eur Heart J 2008; 29:1851–7.

29. Park SJ, Kim YH, Park DW, et al. Impact of intravascular uvltrasound guidance on long-term mortality in stenting for unprotected left main coronary artery stenosis. Circ Cardiovasc Interv 2009; 2: 167–77.

30. Kim SH, Kim YH, Kang SJ, et al. Long-term outcomes of intravascular ultrasound-guided stenting in coronary bifurcation lesions. Am J Cardiol 2010; 106: 612–8.

14 Photoacoustic imaging of coronary arteries: Current status and potential clinical applications

Krista Jansen, Gijs van Soest, and Ton van der Steen

OUTLINE

Plaque composition is a major determinant of the risk of future clinical events, of which plaque rupture is the most common. Intravascular photoacoustic imaging (IVPA) has the potential to fully characterize lesion vulnerability by imaging both plaque structure and composition. It is a natural extension of intravascular ultrasound (IVUS) that adds tissue type specificity to the images. Like near-infrared reflection spectroscopy (NIRS), it utilizes differences in the optical absorption spectra of different tissues to differentiate plaque components that are associated with vulnerability from those associated with stability. IVPA has a distinct advantage over NIRS in that it is an imaging modality; it uses the acoustic time-of-flight to create depth resolution as in IVUS.

In this chapter, we discuss the development of IVPA and its current status. We focus on the small diameter catheter that we have developed for combined IVUS/IVPA imaging and the ex vivo demonstration of lipid-specific imaging in human coronary plaques. We also discuss the future steps required for the application of this technique in clinical practice.

INTRODUCTION

The rupture of vulnerable atherosclerotic plaques is a major contributor to acute cardiovascular events and sudden cardiac deaths (1), which result in 17 million deaths annually worldwide (World Health Organization 2005). The vulnerability of an atherosclerotic plaque—its susceptibility to rupture—is known to be related to the composition of the plaque, the distribution of mechanical stress within it, and the presence and extent of associated inflammation (2–4). One of the most common types of vulnerable plaques is the thin-cap fibroatheroma. These lesions are characterized by a thin fibrous cap, weakened by the presence of macrophages, covering a lipid-rich necrotic core (2). Rupture of the cap due to high mechanical stress will release the thrombogenic contents of the necrotic core into the bloodstream. The subsequent formation of a platelet-rich thrombus may result in occlusion, either at the location of the rupture or upstream from the lesion site. If this occlusion takes place in a coronary artery, the result may be unstable angina or a myocardial infarction. An occlusion in the carotid artery results in a stroke. The key to plaque vulnerability is still elusive, even though recent advances in intravascular imaging technology have enabled the collection of a wealth of data on unstable atherosclerosis in all its stages of development (5), both in clinical and in ex vivo settings. Plaque type and morphology are relevant for planning percutaneous coronary intervention, and have a significant effect on long-term clinical outcome (6).

The current intravascular standard to assess coronary atherosclerotic disease and guide interventional procedures is intravascular ultrasound (IVUS). This modality produces images based on the reflected amplitude of ultrasound pulses, providing information on both lumen geometry and the structure of the vascular wall with a resolution of approximately 100 μm and an imaging depth of 7 mm. The sensitivity and specificity of IVUS grayscale for plaque composition is limited (7). IVUS radiofrequency data analysis techniques for tissue characterization have been developed as an extension to grayscale imaging (8). Recently, our laboratory collaborated with InfraReDx Inc. to develop a hybrid near-infrared spectroscopy (NIRS)/IVUS catheter that combines morphological imaging and lipid detection (9–11). This technology identifies the lipid-containing sectors of the IVUS image in order to detect lipid-core plaques. A major limitation of NIRS is that it is not an imaging modality: it has no depth resolution. NIRS can identify the presence but not the amount or the location, relative to the lumen, of the lipid content. Intravascular optical coherence tomography (IVOCT) is another modality based on the echo delay of light backscattered from the tissue. IVOCT provides high resolution images (15 μm) but with limited depth penetration (1–2 mm) (12). OCT tissue characterization is currently a topic of intense research (13).

Intravascular photoacoustics (IVPA) has demonstrated the ability to directly image tissue components in the vessel wall. Its potential for the detection of lipids has been demonstrated, and there is potential to extend the technology to identify other factors, such as dense macrophage infiltration, associated with plaque vulnerability. The same catheter can be used simultaneously to image the arterial wall architecture by IVUS.

PRINCIPLE OF PHOTOACOUSTICS

In photoacoustic imaging, the tissue is irradiated by short laser pulses for a duration of several nanoseconds. Absorption of laser radiation in the tissue transfers the optical energy to the tissue, which, under conditions of stress confinement and thermal confinement (the pulse is shorter than both the stress relaxation and the thermal diffusion times), causes a pressure rise, ΔP, in the irradiated volume (14):

$$\Delta P = \frac{c_0^2 \beta}{C_p} \mu_a F(z) = \Gamma \mu_a F(z). \tag{1}$$

where c_0 (m/s) is the sound velocity in the tissue, β (K^{-1}) is the thermal coefficient of volume expansion, C_p (J/kg·K) is the heat capacity at constant pressure, μ_a (m^{-1}) is the absorption

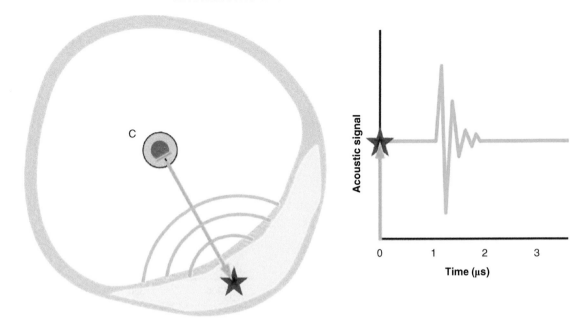

Figure 14.1 Sketch of the IVPA principle. A laser pulse (green) is sent from the catheter C to the vessel wall containing a plaque (yellow). The light excites an acoustic wave (blue curves) through optical absorption and the associated thermoelastic expansion (red star). The graph on the right shows a time trace of the acoustic signal after the laser fires at time $t = 0$.

coefficient of the tissue, and $F(z)$ is the laser fluence (J/m^2). The dimensionless Grüneisen parameter Γ represents the thermoacoustic efficiency (14). This pressure rise is the result of a brief thermoelastic expansion following the absorption of light in the tissue. It propagates as a broadband ultrasonic wave which travels through the tissue. This pressure wave can be detected with an ultrasound transducer. In IVPA, the same ultrasound transducer that is used in IVUS can be employed. The principle of IVPA is shown in Figure 14.1.

As can be seen from Eq. 1, the signal strength in photoacoustics depends on the absorption coefficient, μ_a, of the tissue being irradiated. This absorption coefficient varies with the excitation wavelength which is in turn dictated by the chemical absorption spectrum of the tissue constituents. Different biological tissues can be identified by their distinct optical absorption spectra (Fig. 14.2). In photoacoustic imaging, these absorption spectra can be used as chemical fingerprints. The photoacoustic excitation wavelengths can be selected to give maximum absorption contrast between the relevant vessel wall and plaque components, such as collagen, calcified tissue, and lipid material (15,16), and so image plaque composition.

DEVELOPMENT OF IVPA

The first spectroscopic measurements to discriminate between atheromatous plaque and healthy arterial tissue focused on the visible wavelength range (410–680 nm). Prince et al. (17) showed preferential optical attenuation in atheroma in the spectral range 420–530 nm by performing spectrophotometric measurements on human cadaveric atherosclerotic aorta. Al Dhahir et al. (18)

Focus Box 14.1

IVPA provides direct imaging of tissue type and thus adds chemical specificity to IVUS and OCT imaging

---

Focus Box 14.2

IVPA imaging adds depth resolution to NIRS

---

performed the first in vitro time-resolved photoacoustic experiments to measure optical attenuation using a pulsed dye laser and confirmed the preferential attenuation in atheroma over the 440–500 nm wavelength range. Using an excimer laser at 308 nm, Crazzolara et al. (19) showed that the photoacoustic signature of calcified plaques is different to that of normal arterial tissue based on in vitro time-resolved photoacoustic measurements.

Beard and Mills (20) used time-resolved photoacoustic spectroscopy to characterize post mortem human aorta for the purpose of discriminating between normal and atheromatous areas (soft yellow plaques) of arterial tissue. They illuminated the tissue with nanosecond laser pulses at 436, 461, and 532 nm and used a PVDF membrane hydrophone to detect the thermoelastic waves. At 436 nm, they found a wide variation in the photoacoustic signature, but at 461 nm they found a significant and reproducible difference between the photoacoustic response of atheroma and normal tissue due to the increased optical absorption in atheroma. Lower absorption at 532 nm enabled light penetration over the full thickness of the tissue, providing a means of determining the structure and thickness

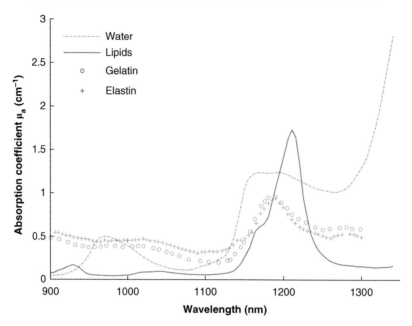

Figure 14.2 Absorption coefficient spectra of water (37°C), fatty acid mixture (lipids) (40°C), gelatin (25°C), and elastin of eye lens (25°C) determined by Tsai et al. (34), for standardized samples.

of the tissue sample. They suggested that pulsed photoacoustic spectroscopy at 461 and 532 nm may find application in characterizing arterial tissue in situ by providing information about both the composition and the thickness of the vessel wall.

Discrimination between normal and atheromatous areas of arterial tissue based on photoacoustic absorption in the visible range (410–680 nm) has an important drawback: at these wavelengths blood (hemoglobin) absorption is also very high. Therefore, a wider range of excitation wavelengths (740–1800 nm) was investigated in experiments conducted by several groups, starting in 2005.

Sethuraman et al. (21) performed the first catheter-based IVPA imaging with external light delivery. They imaged atherosclerotic rabbit arteries ex vivo using a commercial IVUS catheter (Atlantis SR Plus, Boston Scientific Inc.) with external illumination to evaluate the ability of IVPA imaging to detect the presence of inflammation in the plaque. Their results suggested that it may be possible to utilize the difference in the magnitude of the photoacoustic response from free lipids, macrophage foam cells, blood, and the rest of the arterial wall to identify fibrocellular inflammatory plaques.

The same group performed multi-spectral IVPA imaging of ex vivo samples of normal and atherosclerotic rabbit aorta at several wavelengths within the 680–900 nm range (22). They found different spectral slopes in the IVPA image in regions identified as lipid-rich, collagen type I, and collagen type III. Wang et al. (23) imaged lipids in atherosclerotic rabbit aorta using a bench-top setup with external illumination near 1200 nm. This study demonstrated that spectroscopic IVPA imaging in the 1200–1230 nm wavelength range can

Focus Box 14.3

Current status of IVPA: successful combined IVPA/IVUS imaging of the lipid content of a human atherosclerotic plaque ex vivo

successfully identify lipid-rich regions in the atherosclerotic rabbit aorta.

All the experiments discussed above were done in saline-filled experimental settings. Allen and Beard (24) were the first to exploit the low blood absorption in the 900–1300 nm wavelength range and the peak in the lipid absorption curve around 1200 nm to discriminate between lipid-rich and normal vascular tissue. They successfully imaged human aorta samples through blood.

Recently, we reported the first IVPA imaging of human atherosclerotic coronary arteries ex vivo (25). Specific imaging of lipids was shown by spectroscopic imaging over the wavelength range 715–1400 nm, making use of the peak in the lipid absorption spectrum around 1200 nm. In contrast to earlier work, an actual prototype IVPA catheter, with intravascular illumination of tissue, was used to image the arteries. These experiments provide proof of principle for IVPA imaging of plaque composition.

Lipids have a distinct absorption structure near 1200 nm, which was used to differentiate them from other tissue components in the studies cited above. Meanwhile, it was suggested that IVPA imaging may be able to identify other tissue types. Wang et al. (26) proposed that IVPA imaging could identify the presence and the location of macrophage-rich atherosclerotic plaques using gold nanoparticles as a contrast agent. They used IVPA in atherosclerotic rabbit aorta injected with macrophages loaded with gold nanoparticles in a bench-top experimental setting using an external light source. They detected that the signal from the macrophages was enhanced by aggregated gold nanoparticles by illuminating the sample around 700 nm. Aggregated gold nanoparticles, metabolized by the macrophages, do absorb at this wavelength, while (extracellular) single gold nanoparticles do not, providing a usable contrast mechanism.

IVPA CATHETER DEVELOPMENT

Practical in vivo implementation of IVPA required the development of a dedicated catheter device, for which various designs have been proposed. The first IVPA probes were developed in the context of laser angioplasty, and therefore were forward looking. The devices were aimed at the intravascular detection of athero-sclerotic plaques and were meant to provide device guidance during laser angioplasty procedures. These included a miniature all-optical intravascular photoacoustic probe (27) with a transparent Fabry–Perot ultrasound sensor at the end of an optical fiber to detect the thermoelastic waves. A hybrid scheme using a piezoelectric transducer for detection has also been described (28).

Later designs of IVPA probes shifted focus to sideways imaging of the arterial wall to provide information about its composition and structure. In 1997, Pérennès et al. (29) proposed the design of a miniature, all-optical sideward looking IVPA probe consisting of a transparent polymer film, acting as a low finesse Fabry–Perot interferometer, glued to a glass prism which in turn was mounted on the end of an optical fiber. To demonstrate the feasibility of the proposed design, they mounted the same Fabry–Perot polymer film sensor on the end of a 1 mm diameter optical fiber in a forward looking configuration and tested it on a liquid absorber with an absorption coefficient in the same range as the effective attenuation coefficient of arterial tissue (50–100 cm^{-1}). They also showed that it was sufficiently sensitive to detect pho-toacoustic signatures in post mortem arterial tissue (27). All these designs still lacked pulse-echo imaging capability.

This shortcoming was overcome by Karpiouk et al. (30), who developed two prototype catheters that combined an optical fiber for light delivery with a commercially available IVUS imaging catheter (Atlantis™ SR plus, Boston Scientific, Inc.) for both pulse-echo ultrasound imaging and detection of photo-acoustic signals. To deflect the light toward the vessel wall, one design used an angle-polished fiber ("side-fire fiber"); in the other design a silver coated glass mirror redirected the light. The catheters were tested on vessel mimicking phantoms and images were obtained by rotating the phantoms.

In a more recent paper, Karpiouk et al. (31) presented an advanced rotating design of the integrated IVPA/IVUS imaging catheter based on a 40-MHz single-element ultrasound trans-ducer and a 600-µm diameter core single optical fiber. The light was redirected using the side-fire fiber approach. Using this catheter, they demonstrated combined IVPA/IVUS imaging through blood.

Hsieh et al. (32) fabricated an integrated scan-head design for combined IVPA/IVUS imaging. The catheter consisted of a multimode optical fiber coupled to a cone-shaped mirror for illumination and a polymer microring resonator with a wide detection bandwidth to detect low-frequency photoacoustic signals for IVPA imaging and high-frequency ultrasound for IVUS imaging. A homemade, single-element, ring-shaped transducer was used for sideward ultrasound transmission. The outer diameter of the device was 3 mm. Future designs will be miniaturized by using a small-diameter optical fiber and fabri-cating a small-element ring transducer.

Since the diameters of the sideward looking catheters used in the above-mentioned studies were too large to allow use in human coronary arteries, they have only been tested on phan-toms, rabbit aortas, and on human arteries that were opened up to allow raster scanning of the luminal surface. Recently, we achieved a vital step towards miniaturization of IVPA devices by building a hybrid IVPA/IVUS catheter with an outer diameter of 1.25 mm. We imaged intact human coronary arteries ex vivo (25), within 24 hours post mortem. The catheter consisted of a 400-µm diameter core optical fiber (Pioneer Optics, Bloom-field, CT) and a lead-zirconium-titanate (PZT) ultrasound transducer with a diameter of 1.0 mm (custom built by TUDelft; design by DuMED, Rotterdam) (33). A schematic illustration and a photograph of the catheter tip are shown in Figure 14.3A and B, respectively. The tip of the fiber was positioned at an angle of 34° and covered with a glued-on quartz cap to preserve an air-glass interface deflecting the beam by total reflection. The transducer had a center frequency of 30 MHz and a 6-dB frac-tional bandwidth of 65%. The fiber and the transducer were mounted in an assembly with an outer diameter of 1.25 mm (Fig. 14.3B). The fiber tip and transducer center were separated by approximately 1 mm. The angle between the optical and the acoustical beams was 22°; the beams overlapped between 0.5 and 4.5 mm from the transducer.

We demonstrated the imaging performance of the catheter using a vessel phantom with metal wires as point absorbers and quantified its imaging characteristics by taking measurements at isolated point targets. The axial and lateral point spread function widths were 110 and 550 µm, respectively, for IVPA imaging and 89 and 420 µm, respectively, for IVUS imaging. The signal-to-noise ratios were 50 dB (photoacoustics, unaver-aged) and 54 dB (ultrasound, 10 times averaged).

IMAGING OF HUMAN CORONARY ATHEROSCLEROSIS

Using the catheter described above, we imaged fresh human cor-onary arteries, showing different stages of disease, ex vivo (25). The arteries were obtained from the Department of Pathology of the Erasmus MC at autopsy and imaged within 24 hours post mortem. Consent was obtained from the relatives and the proto-col was sanctioned by the Medical Ethics Committee of the Eras-mus MC. The specimens were mounted on two cannulas in a tank containing saline solution. Large side branches were closed and arteries were pressurized to 100 mmHg to maintain an open lumen. The arteries were screened by an IVUS pullback (Boston

Scientific iLab, Atlantis SR Pro catheters) and sites of interest were marked with suture needles. Markers were located with IVPA and cross-sectional scans were made at sites of interest.

A diagram of the experimental setup is shown in Figure 14.3A. A tunable laser provided the excitation light (pulse width 5 ns, repetition rate 10 Hz, pulse energy 1.2 mJ at catheter tip) for photoacoustic imaging. Pulse-echo imaging was performed using an arbitrary waveform generator (30 MHz; 10 V peak-to-peak; 100%

bandwidth). Images were obtained by rotation of the catheter in 1° steps using a motorized rotor. At every position, IVPA and IVUS image lines were acquired, ensuring image co-registration. All IVUS and IVPA signals obtained were band-pass filtered, amplified, and digitized. No averaging was applied for IVPA imaging; IVUS traces were averaged 10-fold. Acquisition of one IVPA/IVUS image took 36 s. The dynamic range of all IVUS and IVPA images shown in Figures 14.4 and 14.6 is 40 dB.

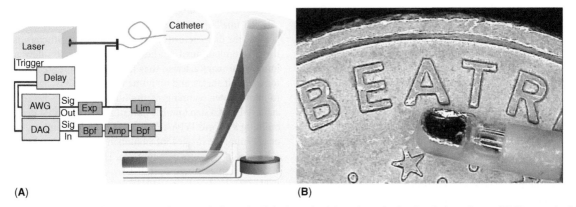

(A)   **(B)**

Figure 14.3 (**A**) Diagram of the experimental setup, including a detailed schematic of the catheter tip showing the beam layout. (**B**) Photograph of the catheter tip on the edge of a 10 eurocent coin. *Abbreviations*: Amp, amplifier; AWG, arbitrary wave generator; bpf, band-pass filter; DAQ, data acquisition; Exp, expander; Lim, limiter.

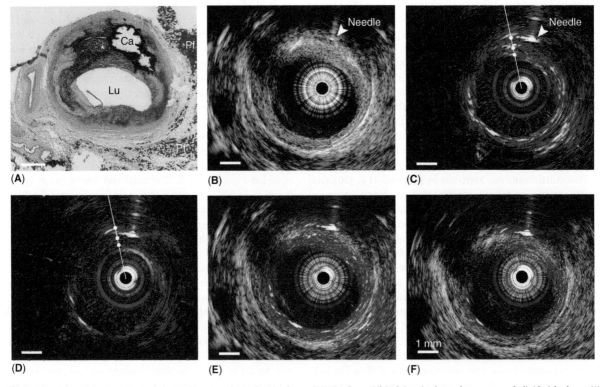

Figure 14.4 IVPA/IVUS imaging of an advanced human atherosclerotic plaque. (**A**) Histology: Oil Red O stain shows the presence of a lipid-rich plaque (*) as well as a calcified area (Ca). (**B**) IVUS image; IVPA images at (**C**) 1210 nm (high lipid absorption) and (**D**) 1230 nm (low lipid absorption). Arrowheads indicate the needle used for marking. Full spectral scans were made along the white line in (**C**) and (**D**). The spectra at the locations marked by the white dots are shown in Figure 14.5. (**E**) and (**F**) show combined IVPA/IVUS images at 1210 and 1230 nm, respectively. *Abbreviations*: Lu: lumen, Pf: peri-adventitial fat.

LIPID DETECTION

We obtained a co-registered IVPA/IVUS image in an advanced lesion (left anterior descending artery, male aged 56 years). The results arc shown in Figure 14.4. The histology shows circumferential intimal thickening with a large eccentric lipid-rich lesion, as well as a calcified area and regions of peri-adventitial fat. The IVUS data confirms this morphology. The IVPA image at 1210 nm exhibits a bright signal along the intimal border, and also from deeper tissue layers in the eccentric plaque and the peri-adventitial fat in the bottom right corner. At 1230 nm the signal in these regions is markedly lower, in accordance with the absorption spectrum of lipids in this wavelength range. Collocated with the enhanced 1210 nm IVPA signal a positive Oil Red O stain is observed, particularly in the plaque, indicating the presence of lipids. Variation in the laser pulse energy and tissue-scattering properties is negligible over the wavelength range 1210–1230 nm.

Photoacoustic spectra were acquired along image lines sampling the plaque tissue. The resulting data sets are two-dimensional matrices of wavelength versus depth. In Figure 14.5, spectra are shown at three locations, two inside the lipid-rich plaque region and one just outside. The absorption spectra of lipids and connective tissue (34) are included for reference. The two spectra located in the plaque clearly match the lipid reference, while the third lacks the pronounced peak.

Spectroscopic imaging is demonstrated on a second specimen (left main stem, female aged 43 years). The results are shown in Figure 14.6. The IVUS part of these combined IVPA/IVUS images shows mild fibrous intimal thickening.

Comparison of the images shows the presence of lipids outside the vessel wall. This peri-adventitial fat is part of the normal anatomy. The average IVPA signal strength in this region, acquired from IVPA images at various wavelengths between 1180 and 1230 nm, closely tracks the lipid absorption peak shape (Fig. 14.7).

POTENTIAL APPLICATIONS AND LIMITATIONS

IVPA is an experimental technique that is currently being used and undergoing further refinement in ex vivo experiments. It is in a very early stage of its development. Although it has demonstrated the ability to fill an important niche, many facets of real-time clinical imaging still need to be resolved. Several important aspects of the optimal image acquisition sequence, laser sources, details of catheter design, etc., are currently being investigated. The road to in vivo IVPA imaging will present some specific challenges as discussed.

In order to obtain an optimal photoacoustic signal strength, it is desirable to deliver as much light to the vessel wall as is possible within the physical boundaries of the instrument, and within the safety limits. Blood is a strongly scattering tissue, which can markedly reduce the light intensity at the vessel wall, even at wavelengths in the near infrared region. It appears likely that IVPA imaging will require flushing of the blood from the artery, even in a clinical setting. The details of the flush procedure and the flush media will have to be determined.

Blood clearing is standard practice in IVOCT imaging. IVPA does not depend on the coherence of the light, so complete

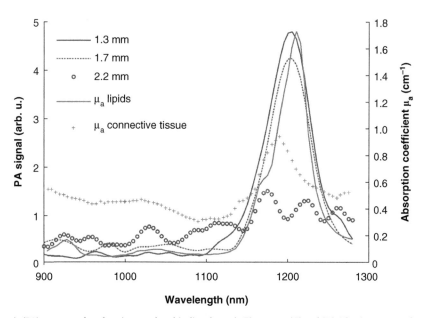

Figure 14.5 Photoacoustic (PA) spectra at three locations on the white line shown in Figure 14.4 (**C**) and (**D**). The sites at 1.4 and 1.7 mm distance from the catheter are located within the lipid-rich plaque. The corresponding PA spectra show strong resemblance to the lipid absorption reference. The site at 2.2 mm is located just outside the plaque area.

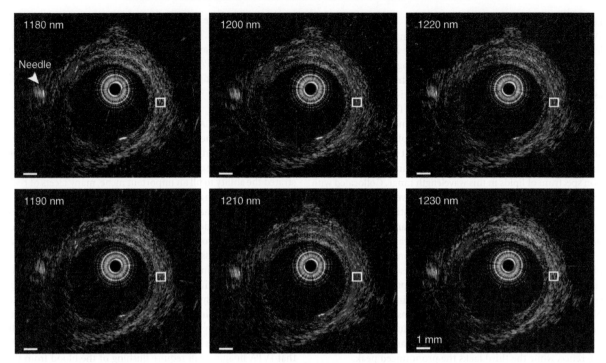

Figure 14.6 Combined IVPA/IVUS image at 1180, 1190, 1200, 1210, 1220, and 1230 nm of a healthy human coronary artery. The white squares indicate the area in which the IVPA signal strength is averaged and compared with the lipid absorption spectrum of Tsai et al. (34) (Fig. 14.7).

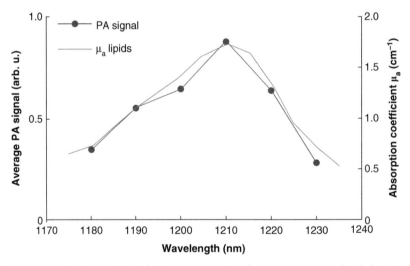

Figure 14.7 Average IVPA signal strength in the area indicated in Figure 14.6, obtained from the images at wavelengths between 1180 and 1230 nm, closely tracks the peak in the reference lipid absorption spectrum. *Source*: From Ref. 34.

clearing of the artery under investigation may not be necessary. On the other hand, the ultrasonic properties of the flush media used for OCT (iodixanol, a coronary angiography contrast agent, trade name Visipaque™) are not precisely known, so investigation of alternatives may be needed.

The development of a fast laser source at the desired wavelengths is necessary. The currently available light sources for IVPA at near infrared wavelengths, with sufficient pulse power, have a repetition rate of only 10 Hz. This low pulse frequency prevents in vivo imaging. Particularly if flushing is used, the optimal imaging sequence will be modeled on that of Fourier domain OCT: high frame rate, high pullback speed, short pullback time of <10 s. To meet these requirements, and to reduce motion artifacts to an acceptable level, an illumination source

REFERENCES

1. Falk E, Shah PK, Fuster V. Coronary Plaque Disruption. Circulation 1995; 1995; 92: 657–71.
2. Schaar JA, Muller JE, Falk E, et al. Terminology for high-risk and vulnerable coronary artery plaques. Eur Heart J 2004; 25: 1077–82.
3. Virmani R, Kolodgie FD, Burke AP, Farb A, Schwartz SM. Lessons from sudden coronary death - A comprehensive morphological classification scheme for atherosclerotic lesions. Arterioscler Thromb Vasc Biol 2000; 20: 1262–75.
4. Richardson PD, Davies MJ, Born GV. Influence of plaque configuration and stress distribution on fissuring of coronary atherosclerotic plaques. Lancet 1989; 334: 941–4.
5. Waxman S, Ishibashi F, Muller JE. Detection and treatment of vulnerable plaques and vulnerable patients - Novel approaches to prevention of coronary events. Circulation 2006; 114: 2390–411.
6. Kolodgie FD, Burke AP, Farb A, et al. The thin-cap fibroatheroma: a type of vulnerable plaque - The major precursor lesion to acute coronary syndromes. Curr Opin Cardiol 2001; 16: 285–92.
7. de Korte CL, van der Steen AFW, Cespedes EI, et al. Characterization of plaque components and vulnerability with intravascular ultrasound elastography. Phys Med Biol 2000; 45: 1465–75.
8. Nair A, Kuban BD, Tuzcu EM, et al. Coronary plaque classification with intravascular ultrasound radiofrequency data analysis. Circulation 2002; 106: 2200–6.
9. Garg S, Serruys PW, van der Ent M, et al. First use in patients of a combined near infra-red spectroscopy and intra-vascular ultrasound catheter to identify composition and structure of coronary plaque. EuroIntervention 2010; 5: 755–6.
10. Gardner CM, Tan H, Hull EL, et al. Detection of lipid core coronary plaques in autopsy specimens with a novel catheter-based near-infrared spectroscopy system. Jacc 2008; 1: 638–48.
11. Moreno PR, Lodder RA, Purushothaman KR, et al. Detection of lipid pool, Thin fibrous cap, and inflammatory cells in human aortic atherosclerotic plaques by near-infrared spectroscopy. Circulation 2002; 105: 923–7.
12. Tearney GJ, Waxman S, Shishkov M, et al. Three-dimensional coronary artery microscopy by intracoronary optical frequency domain imaging. J Am Coll Cardiol Img 2008; November 1, 2008; 1: 752–61.
13. van Soest G, Goderie T, Regar E, et al. Atherosclerotic tissue characterization in vivo by optical coherence tomography attenuation imaging. J Biomed Opt 2010; 15: 011105–9.
14. Oraevsky AA, Karabutov AA. Optoacoustic tomography. In: Vo-Dinh T, ed. Biomedical Photonics Handbook. Boca Raton, FL: CRC Press, 2003: 34–1.
15. Van Veen RLP, Sterenborg HJCM, Pifferi A, Torricelli A, Cubeddu R. Determination of VIS- NIR absorption coefficients of mammalian fat, with time- and spatially resolved diffuse reflectance and transmission spectroscopy. OSA Biomed Opt Topical Meeting; 2004.
16. Tromberg BJ, Shah N, Lanning R, et al. Non-invasive in vivo characterization of breast tumors using photon migration spectroscopy. Neoplasia 2000; 2: 26–40.
17. Prince MR, Deutsch TF, Mathews-Roth MM, et al. Preferential light absorption in atheromas in vitro. Implications for laser angioplasty. J Clin Invest 1986; 78: 295–302.
18. Al Dhahir RK, Dyer PE, Zhu Z. Photoacoustic studies and selective ablation of vascular tissue using a pulsed dye laser. Appl Phys B-Photophysics Laser Chem 1990; 51: 81–5.
19. Crazzolara H, Vonmuench W, Rose C, et al. Analysis of the acoustic response of vascular tissue irradiated by an ultraviolet-laser pulse. J Appl Phys 1991; 70: 1847–9.

Focus Box 14.4

The best of two worlds: IVPA combines optical contrast with ultrasound imaging depth

Focus Box 14.5

Multimodality imaging: combined IVPA/IVUS to provide information on plaque composition (IVPA) and morphology (IVUS)

with a repetition rate of the order of 10 kHz would be needed. These lasers will be developed in the near future.

The smallest IVPA catheter diameter manufactured to date is 1.25 mm. Current IVUS catheters have an outer diameter of less than 1 mm, including the protective sheath in which they rotate. Future developments will reduce the IVPA catheter diameter to 1 mm or less for successful application in clinical practice.

PERSONAL PERSPECTIVE

IVPA is a very promising technique that is currently in the experimental stage: several experimental IVPA/IVUS catheters have been developed and successful combined IVPA/IVUS imaging of the lipid content of a human atherosclerotic plaque ex vivo has recently been demonstrated.

IVPA can differentiate between plaque components by using the differences in the optical absorption spectra of different tissues, like NIRS. However, it has an important advantage over NIRS in terms of depth resolution. This makes it possible to know the exact spatial location of the identified components. Thus, it can distinguish lipid located within a plaque, which is pathological, from peri-adventitial lipid, which is a part of the normal vessel wall structure. IVPA provides optical contrast with ultrasound imaging depth. If used in combination with IVUS, IVPA can provide information on plaque composition that complements the morphological information provided by IVUS. In the future, useful combinations with other imaging modalities might be considered, such as an IVPA/OCT combination.

IVPA can potentially become a very powerful tool in exploring the vulnerable plaque and in the monitoring of responses to different forms of intervention (genetic, pharmacologic, lifestyle changes). It could be used as an imaging endpoint in clinical studies to show changes in the lipid content of atherosclerotic plaques (35,36). The use of IVPA during percutaneous coronary intervention could potentially minimize the risk of incomplete stent coverage of lipid-rich plaques and the associated risks for the patient. The occurrence of incomplete stent coverage of lipid-rich plaques, despite adequate coverage of the angiographic stenosis, demonstrates the limitations of standard angiography to delineate the borders of the plaque. Incomplete stent coverage can potentially cause lipid-rich plaque disruption during stent placement, which can result in distal embolization (37). Incomplete stent coverage is also suspected to be associated with plaque progression leading to stent failure due to edge restenosis (38).

20. Beard PC, Mills TN. Characterization of post mortem arterial tissue using time-resolved photoacoustic spectroscopy at 436, 461 and 532 nm. Phys Med Biol 1997; 42: 177–98.

21. Sethuraman S, Amirian JH, Litovsky SH, Smalling RW, Emelianov SY. Ex vivo characterization of atherosclerosis using intravascular photoacoustic imaging. Opt Express 2007; Dec 10;15: 16657–66.

22. Sethuraman S, Amirian JH, Litovsky SH, Smalling RW, Emelianov SY. Spectroscopic intravascular photoacoustic imaging to differentiate atherosclerotic plaques. Opt Express 2008; 16: 3362–7.

23. Wang B, Su JL, Amirian J, et al. Detection of lipid in atherosclerotic vessels using ultrasound-guided spectroscopic intravascular photoacoustic imaging. Opt Express 2010; 18: 4889–97.

24. Allen TJ, Beard PC. Photoacoustic characterisation of vascular tissue at NIR wavelengths. Photons Plus Ultrasound: Imaging and Sensing. San Jose, CA, USA: SPIE, 2009; 71770A–9.

25. Jansen K, van der Steen AF, van Beusekom HM, Oosterhuis JW, van Soest G. Intravascular photoacoustic imaging of human coronary atherosclerosis. Opt Lett 2011; 36: 597–9.

26. Wang B, Yantsen E, Larson T, et al. Plasmonic intravascular photoacoustic imaging for detection of macrophages in atherosclerotic plaques. Nano Lett 2009; 9: 2212–17.

27. Beard PC, Mills TN. Evaluation of an optical fibre probe for in vivo measurement of the photoacoustic response of tissues. Adv Fluoresc Sensing Technol II 1995; 2388: 446–57.

28. Chen QX, Davies A, Dewhurst RJ, Payne PA. Photo-acoustic probe for intra-arterial imaging and therapy. Electron Lett 1993; 29: 1632–3.

29. Pérennès F, Beard PC, Mills TN. Intravascular photoacoustic-photothermal imaging of the arterial wall using a miniature optical fibre probe. In Horizons de l'Optique. Orsay Cedex, France: Société Française d'Optique, 1997: A13.

30. Karpiouk AB, Wang B, Emelianov SY. Development of a catheter for combined intravascular ultrasound and photoacoustic imaging. Rev Sci Instruments 2010; Jan; 81: 014901–1–7.

31. Karpiouk AB, Wang B, Emelianov SY. Integrated catheter for intravascular ultrasound and photoacoustic imaging. Photons Plus Ultrasound Imaging Sensing 2010; 7564: 756408–1–6.

32. Hsieh BY, Chen SL, Ling T, Guo LJ, Li PC. Integrated intravascular ultrasound and photoacoustic imaging scan head. Opt Lett 2010; Sep 1; 35: 2892–4.

33. Jansen K, Springeling G, Lancée C, et al. An Intravascular Photoacoustic Imaging Catheter. Ultrasonics Symposium (IUS), 2010 IEEE International 2010: 378–81.

34. Tsai CL, Chen JC, Wang WJ. Near-infrared absorption property of biological soft tissue constituents. J Med Biol Eng 2001; 21: 7–14.

35. Serruys PW, Garcia-Garcia HM, Buszman P, et al. Effects of the direct lipoprotein-associated phospholipase A(2) inhibitor darapladib on human coronary atherosclerotic plaque. Circulation 2008; 118: 1172–82.

36. Van Mieghem CA, McFadden EP, de Feyter PJ, et al. Noninvasive detection of subclinical coronary atherosclerosis coupled with assessment of changes in plaque characteristics using novel invasive imaging modalities: the Integrated Biomarker and Imaging Study (IBIS). J Am Coll Cardiol 2006; 47: 1134–42.

37. Schultz CJ, Serruys PW, van der Ent M, et al. First-in-man clinical use of combined near-infrared spectroscopy and intravascular ultrasound: a potential key to predict distal embolization and no-reflow? J Am Coll Cardiol 2010; 56: 314.

38. Waxman S, Freilich MI, Suter MJ, et al. A case of lipid core plaque progression and rupture at the edge of a coronary stent: Elucidating the mechanisms of drug-eluting stent failure. Circ Cardiovasc Interv 2010; 3: 193–6.

15 Plaque imaging with optical coherence tomography: Current status and potential clinical implications

Francesco Prati, Eleonora Ficarra, Vito Ramazzotti, and Mario Albertucci

OUTLINE

Optical Coherence Tomography (OCT) is a light-based imaging technique, provides resolution in the range of 10–15 microns, an order of magnitude greater than IVUS thus allowing unparalleled in vivo detail on the structure of the vessel wall. FD-OCT technology provides rapid imaging of long vessel segments without the need for vessel occlusion. Despite its limited penetration depth, OCT could provides novel insights into the atherosclerotic process. During coronary interventions the high resolution, the thinner profile of the probe, and the high speed of the pull-back of OCT offers a wealth of information, despite the incomplete definition of plaque burden, whose clinical utility needs validation. OCT has a high enough resolution to study vessel healing after coronary stent implantation and provide insights into modes of stent failure.

Integration of OCT with other complementary imaging modalities will provide an excellent tool to study atherosclerotic coronary disease and optimize treatment.

INTRODUCTION: PHYSICAL PRINCIPLES OF OCT

Optical coherence tomography (OCT) is an imaging modality that uses light instead of sound and offers significantly improved resolution as compared with intravascular ultrasound (IVUS) (1–8). In fact, the resolution of OCT is about 10 times higher than that of IVUS, being in the range of 10–15 μm, as a result of the very short wavelength of the imaging light (1,5). Cross-sectional images are generated by measuring the echo time delay and the intensity of light that is reflected or backscattered from internal structures in the tissue (1–5). As the speed of light does not allow direct measurement of the echo time delay, interferometric techniques have been developed to analyze the reflected light signal.

There are two main technologies that can be used to obtain OCT images: time domain (TD) and frequency domain (FD) (5–7). TD is the older technology and its use is now confined to countries where the latter technology, FD-OCT, has not been approved yet. The LightLab Dragonfly™ FD-OCT catheter is so far the only one in the market, but in the near future two other systems from Volcano and Terumo, which have functions similar to the Dragonfly, will also be available. TD-OCT is obtained with the M3 LightLab OCT wire (Imagewire™), having an outer diameter of 0.019 inch, and containing a 0.006 inch fiber-optic imaging core (<0.4 mm in diameter). The TD-OCT imagewire has a distal radiopaque spring tip, similar to conventional guide wires.

Like the TD-OCT catheter, the FD-OCT catheter (Dragonfly; LightLab Imaging, Westford, MA, USA) also uses a single-mode

Focus Box 15.1

OCT is a light-based imaging modality whose resolution (10–15 μm) is an order of magnitude greater than IVUS

Adoption in clinical practice has been limited by catheter size and the need to interrupt blood flow

Current technology allows image acquisition over a few seconds, with a rapid exchange system, and vessel occlusion is no longer required

The ability of light to penetrate tissue limits resolution to between 0.5 and 2 mm

optical fiber, which is enclosed in a hollow metal torque wire that rotates at a speed of 100 revolutions per second. The catheter is designed for rapid-exchange delivery and is compatible with a conventional 0.014 inch angioplasty guide wire inserted in a short monorail lumen at the tip, a solution similar to the one adopted for mechanical IVUS catheters. The main advantage of FD-OCT is that the technology enables rapid imaging of the coronary artery, with the capability to scan long coronary segments in few seconds at a pull-back speed that can reach a maximum of 25 mm/sec, using a single, non-occlusive catheter (5–7).

FD-OCT has an improved lateral resolution, reduced motion artifacts, and an increased scan diameter up to 11 mm, features that have significantly improved both the quality and the ease of use of OCT in the catheterization laboratory (5–7).

The penetration depth of OCT is between 0.5 and 2 mm in most tissue types and remains the main limitation of the technique, because optical scattering losses and tissue attenuation limit light penetration and focusing in vascular tissues (8,9). However, a slight improvement in the penetration depth of FD-OCT compared with TD-OCT can be observed in most tissues.

Image Acquisition

As TD-OCT will be soon replaced by FD-OCT, we will focus only on aspects of OCT acquisition obtained with the latter system. The description of acquisition will refer to the St Jude Dragonfly™ FD-OCT catheter, which at present is the only one in the market.

The main obstacle to the adoption of OCT imaging in clinical practice is that OCT cannot image through a blood field, as infrared light cannot penetrate red blood cells. Therefore, unlike IVUS, OCT requires clearing or flushing of the blood from the lumen. This drawback particularly affected TD-OCT acquisition as the moderate pull-back speed of this first-generation OCT required complex technical solutions to overcome the problem (5,9).

The technique of acquisition by FD-OCT has been optimized using the concept developed specifically for the non-occlusive modality of TD-OCT acquisition (10–12). Contrast solution, due to its viscosity, can displace blood cells for a sufficient period of time so as to be able to record OCT images in a certain coronary segment. Obviously, the fact that FD-OCT images can be obtained at speeds up to 25 mm/sec enables the acquisition of long coronary segments in a very short time. The size of the OCT image is first calibrated by adjusting the z-offset, the zero-point setting of the system. In FD-OCT systems, the calibration procedure can be done in a completely automated manner. To maintain accurate measurements, the z-offset must be readjusted prior to off-line analysis and monitored throughout the pullback (12).

The OCT probe is first positioned over a regular guide wire, distal to the region of interest. Identification of the pull-back starting point is a simple task as a dedicated marker identifies the exact position of the OCT lens, located 10 mm proximal to the marker itself.

The acquisition of a rapid OCT image sequence with fast pull-back can be automatically commenced by injecting a bolus of solution through the guiding catheter, with the acquisition speed set at between 5 and 20 mm/sec. The infusion rate of contrast is usually set at 3–4 ml/sec for the left coronary artery and 2–3 ml/sec for the right coronary, but can be modified based on the vessel run-off and size. When the OCT catheter is positioned and blood clearance is visually obtained distally to the catheter through the contrast injection, the acquisition of a rapid OCT image sequence with fast pullback can be automatically or manually commenced by injecting a bolus of solution through the guiding catheter, with the acquisition speed set at between 5 and 25 mm/sec (11).

The automated contrast injection is the modality of acquisition preferred by the majority of operators (11).

SAFETY AND EFFECTIVENESS
Previous experiences with TD-OCT technology, both occlusive and non-occlusive, show OCT acquisition to be safe and effective (5,13). OCT provides excellent differentiation between the lumen and the arterial wall, facilitating the determination of lumen areas and volumes and the depiction of stent struts with high accuracy (14). Furthermore, early studies of quantitative measurements of the lumen, stent, and neointimal areas reveal a high reproducibility, primarily driven by the high resolution of the technology (15).

Preliminary data on the safety of the use of FD-OCT technology are even more promising. A preliminary study on 14 patients (7) and a more recent one on 90 subjects with coronary artery disease (CAD) did not report complications: in fact, no ischemic ECG changes or arrhythmias developed during the short injection period. This is due to the marked simplification of the acquisition procedures and the consequent reduction in the required contrast volume (7,12). These preliminary data also indicate that FD-OCT is highly effective, as it can study longer segments with clear images compared with TD-OCT (7,12). As

with TD-OCT, the image quality in FD-OCT depends on the use of an accurate acquisition technique and proper guiding catheter engagement is needed to optimize directional contrast flushing.

NORMAL CORONARY MORPHOLOGY
In normal vessels and at the sites of thin plaques, with thicknesses not exceeding 1.2 mm, the *coronary artery wall* appears as a three-layer structure in OCT images. Unlike IVUS, OCT can clearly distinguish the intimal layer from the medial layer of the coronary arterial wall and measure its thickness (range 125–350 µm, mean 200 µm) (16,17). The media appears as a dark band, delimited by the internal elastic lamina (IEL) and external elastic lamina (EEL). However, the assessment of a normal intima is beyond the resolution of OCT because its thickness is only approximately 4 µm, which corresponds to a small subendothelial collagen layer and a single layer of endothelial cells that are flattened in normal vessels of children and youths.

The limited penetration of OCT does not allow the study of vessel remodelling in a consistent manner, which is well addressed by IVUS. This phenomenon involves the thinning of the media in the quadrants of plaque accumulation as a result of asymmetric expansion of the vessel wall.

Nearly all coronary arteries of adults show some grade of *intimal thickness* with increase in age. However, the identification of pathologic neointimal growth is limited by the lack of an established cut-off value. Despite this limitation, OCT, compared with IVUS (17–19), detects even the earliest stages of intimal thickening, which is depicted as a bright, homogeneous thin rim of tissue having a texture similar to that of fibrous plaque components. A comparative study between OCT and integrated backscatter IVUS (IB-IVUS) showed that both methods detect intimal hyperplasia with high specificity (100% vs. 99%) but OCT is more sensitive (86% vs. 67%) (16).

ASSESSMENT OF ATHEROSCLEROSIS
As already mentioned, OCT studies plaque components at a very high resolution; however, this comes at a cost of limited penetration that makes the assessment of deeper structures difficult. Jang and colleagues provided one of the first comparisons between OCT and IVUS. The former provided a more precise measurement of the thickness of the fibrous cap, and improved the study of structures located behind superficial macrocalcification (5). Furthermore, OCT was able to identify tissue components such as intimal hyperplasia and lipid-rich plaques with high accuracy (5).

Focus Box 15.2

Unlike IVUS, OCT can clearly distinguish the intima from the media

Although entirely normal intima (with a thickness of 4 µm) cannot be seen on OCT, angiographically normal adult coronary vessels have a three-layer appearance on OCT reflecting "normal" intimal thickening

Limited penetration does not allow for assessment of vessel remodeling with OCT

It is well known that angiography has poor sensitivity in the detection of calcific deposits, especially when they have a radial extension less than 180° (19). On the other hand, IVUS can identify calcium with a high degree of accuracy although the shadowing effect caused by calcific deposits does not permit the measurement of their thickness. Infrared light penetrates calcium better, but calcific components with a thickness greater than 1–1.3 mm can prove impossible to penetrate. Calcium deposits located in deep intraplaque regions may be missed by OCT. However, this is rather uncommon as calcium deposits are often subendothelial.

Unlike angiography or IVUS, OCT holds promises in identifying thrombi, measuring their dimensions, and guiding their removal (11,20).

Qualitative Descriptions

Calcifications appear as well-delineated, low backscattering heterogeneous regions (5,21).

Superficial microcalcifications, considered to be a distinctive feature of plaque vulnerability, are revealed as small superficial calcific deposits (22).

Fibrous plaques consist of homogeneous high backscattering areas (5,21). *Necrotic lipid pools* are less well-delineated than calcifications and exhibit lower signal density and more heterogeneous backscattering than fibrous plaques. Lipid pools most often appear as diffusely bordered, signal-poor regions with overlying signal-rich bands, corresponding to fibrous caps (5,21). Importantly, OCT can also identify the early stages of atherosclerosis. An experimental study carried out in rabbit carotid arteries showed that OCT has a high sensitivity and specificity (80% and 95%, respectively) in detecting Stary III lesions, which correspond to intimal xanthomas (23).

Thrombi are identified as masses protruding into the vessel lumen discontinuous from the surface of the vessel wall. Red thrombi consist mainly of red blood cells; the corresponding OCT images are characterized as high backscattering protrusions with signal-free shadowing. White thrombi consist mainly of platelets and white blood cells and are characterized by signal-rich, low backscattering billowing projections protruding into the lumen (21).

Despite the high resolution of OCT, in some circumstances non-protruding red thrombi can be misinterpreted as necrotic lipid pools. This may occur due to the similar OCT signal pattern of the two plaque components (24).

Thrombi are frequently found within *culprit lesions* of patients with *acute coronary syndromes* (ACS) (10,21). A fresh

or large thrombus may hamper the visualization of plaque features such as ulceration beneath the thrombus itself.

Quantitative Descriptions

It has to be stressed that identification and quantification of atherosclerotic plaque components by OCT depends on the penetration depth of the incident light beam into the vessel wall. The depth of penetration is greatest for fibrous tissue and least for thrombi with calcium whereas lipid tissue have intermediate values (Fig. 15.1).

OCT can measure the arc of superficial calcium deposits (in degrees) with a protractor centered in the middle of the lumen (5,21). By applying a semi-quantitative grading, calcium can be classified according to the number of quadrants it subtends (1, 2, 3, or 4). Superficial microcalcifications are small calcific deposits that subtend an angle less than 90° and are separated from the lumen by a rim of tissue less than 100 μm thick (5,21). As the penetration of OCT through superficial *necrotic lipid pools* is less than that through calcified and fibrous tissues, in the majority of lesions the thickness of lipid pools cannot be measured (5,21). However, OCT enables measurements of the *thickness of the fibrous cap*, which delimits superficial lipid pools. The thickness of the fibrous cap can be obtained either as a single measurement at the cross-section where it is considered minimal (25,26) or as the average of multiple (three or more) measurements (20). The arc (in degrees) and the longitudinal extent of a superficial necrotic lipid pool can be measured analogous to the semi-quantitative grading of calcium (5,20,21).

OCT has the potential to identify *inflammatory cells* such as clusters of lymphocytes and macrophages. Streaks of macrophages or foam cells appear as bands of high reflectivity in OCT images. When they are located in a plaque with a lipid pool, macrophage streaks appear within the fibrous cap covering the lipid pool. However, the interface between the fibrous cap and the lipid pool produces a bright OCT appearance that can be difficult to distinguish from tightly packed foam cells (27,28).

Previous studies have shown that the application of OCT algorithms can identify inflammatory cells with high specificity and sensitivity. Off-line use of these dedicated algorithms may be instrumental in identifying and possibly quantifying plaque inflammation.

PATHOPHYSIOLOGY OF ACS

Acute plaque ulceration or rupture can be detected by OCT as a ruptured fibrous cup that connects the lumen with the lipid pool. These ulcerated or ruptured plaques may occur with or without a superimposed thrombus. When signs of ulceration are present without evidence of thrombus, the lesion cannot be defined as a "culprit" with certainty, unless clinical criteria provide some evidence that the lesion is responsible for the acute events. Use of thrombolysis, IIb-IIIa GP inhibitors, or other anti-thrombotic drugs facilitate clot degradation and in some circumstances may lead to complete disappearance.

Identification of *erosion* as a mechanism of plaque instability is a challenge even for a technique with a resolution below 20 μm. Thrombosis with an apparently normal endothelial

---

Focus Box 15.3

Areas of calcification appear as well-defined, low backscattering heterogenous regions

Fibrous plaques appear as homogenous, high backscattering regions

Lipid pools appear as diffusely bordered, signal-poor regions with overlying signal-rich bands (fibrous caps)

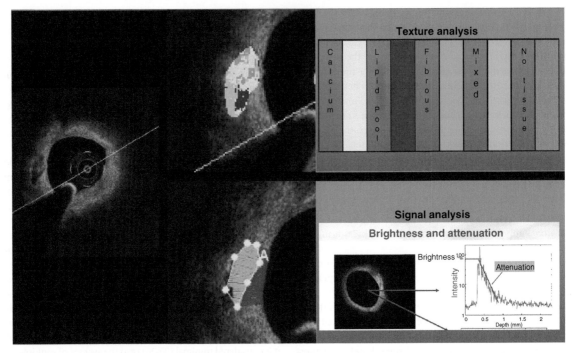

Figure 15.1 The figure shows the ability of optical coherence tomography (OCT) to detect plaque components. The panel on the *left* shows an OCT cross-section obtained at a plaque site with mixed composition. The panel on the *right* shows the corresponding texture and signal analysis with color coding.

lining underneath may be indicative of erosion. Validation studies that combine OCT with techniques that provide a functional assessment of the endothelium may be able to give us more information on vessel thrombosis induced by erosion.

Localization of Plaques with High-Risk Morphology

OCT studies confirmed the histological notion that ruptured plaques are mainly located in the proximal segments (proximal 30 mm) (29). An in vivo three-vessel OCT study in patients with stable angina and ACS showed that 76% of the thin cap fibrous atheromas (TCFAs) in the left anterior descending (LAD) artery were located in the most proximal 30 mm, while in the other arteries TCFAs were evenly distributed throughout the entire coronary length (30). In the same study, the clustering of the TCFAs was similar in culprit segments as compared with non-culprit segments (30).

Pathological studies carried out in patients who died due to ACS identified the morphology of vulnerable plaques (5,31). Consistent with previous observations, OCT studies confirmed that culprit plaques of patients with ACS have greater lipid content, thinner fibrous cap thickness, and greater macrophage concentration as compared with non-culprit plaques (9,32,33). Also patients with acute myocardial infarction had a greater incidence of thrombus and TCFA in the non-culprit lesion (34).

Moreover, morphological differences are not restricted to patients with or without ACS, but are also evident between different presentations of ACS. According to Tanaka et al., plaque rupture in exertion-onset ACS is associated with greater fibrous

cap thickness and is more often located at the shoulder of the plaque (35).

The Link Between Plaque Morphology and Inflammation

Plaque composition at OCT was found to be related to the presence of systemic inflammation. Raffel et al. showed an inverse relationship between the thickness of the fibrous cap thickness and its infiltration by macrophages in culprit lesions of ACS (28). Furthermore, this finding was related to the white blood cell count as a systemic marker of inflammation (28). In another study, the authors identified a cut-off of hs-CRP of 1.66mg/L as the only significant independent predictor of TCFA (36). In the same study, inflammatory markers such as interleukin 18, tumor necrosis factor α, and white blood cell count showed a significant inverse linear correlation with fibrous cap thickness. Also inflammatory markers tended to increase with increasing plaque lipid content (36).

Plaque Morphology, Vulnerability, and Progression

IVUS currently plays an important role in the identification of plaque volume changes in response to specific treatments aimed at promoting plaque regression or limiting progression (19). OCT may become, in the near future, a viable technique to address plaque changes as it can discriminate among the different plaque components.

Preliminary data indicate that statin therapy can modify plaque composition. In fact patients on statin therapy have a reduced incidence of plaque rupture as compared with the control group (37). In a prospective study with 3-month follow-up

OCT examination, statin therapy increased the thickness of the fibrous cap in culprit lesions of patients with stable angina. This, however, occurred only in the presence of a thin fibrous cap at baseline assessment (38).

However, robust validation studies are needed to verify whether OCT is capable of measuring serial changes in plaque components indicative of vulnerability such as fibrous cap thickness or lipid pool extension. It is possible that in the future OCT will have a role in assessing the risk of myocardial infarction.

Also, due to its ability to address plaque components, OCT can be used to establish an association between plaque morphology and clinical characteristics. Surprisingly, plaque composition is similar among diabetics and non-diabetics (39).

Comparison with Other Invasive Imaging Methods for Assessment of Plaque Vulnerability

One of the future challenges in the field of interventional cardiology is the characterization of the vulnerable plaque and how best to manage. A number of IVUS studies based on grayscale assessment or signal radiofrequency analysis of IVUS backscatter have attempted to characterize the appearance of vulnerable plaques, containing superficial necrotic-lipid cores. Recently, the PROSPECT trial showed for the first time that IVUS characteristics or coronary plaques can predict the risk of a plaque-related adverse cardiac event at 3 years. Angiographically mild lesions with certain morphologic features on grayscale and virtual histology (VH) IVUS, such as lesion severity, as detected by lumen area measurement, plaque burden, and thin cap fibrous atheroma, conferred a 3-year higher risk of cardiac events (40). OCT, due to its high accuracy in the detection of superficial plaque components, can directly measure fibrous cap thickness and has the potential to detect plaques at risk of rupture with greater accuracy. However, the limited penetration of OCT may pose some problems in the identification of lesion components and, as a consequence, in the recognition of plaque vulnerability. For this reason, the utility of a combined approach based on the use of OCT and VH IVUS has been proposed (41,42).

Angioscopy has great potential in the identification of superficial tissue components. However, the complexity of the technique and the difficulty in obtaining quantitative information are two factors that limited the widespread use of angioscopy, confining its use in Japan. In vivo comparative studies between OCT and angioscopy showed that the plaque color observed at angioscopy is strongly associated with the thickness of the fibrous cap, whereas correlation with the size of the lipid core is lower (43).

The combined use of IVUS and thermography represents a solution to merge morphological and functional characteristics. In fact, ruptured plaques with expansive remodeling are associated with increased local inflammatory activation, as demonstrated by increased temperature difference (44). Furthermore, the development of algorithms capable of detecting plaque deformation or calculating shear stress using OCT (45) provides an excellent combination of morphological and functional imaging using a single catheter.

CURRENT CLINICAL APPLICATIONS: ADVANTAGES AND DISADVANTAGES OF OCT AS COMPARED WITH IVUS

Angiographically Normal Coronary Arteries

Normal angiograms or angiograms with minimal irregularities are found in around 10–15% of patients undergoing coronary angiography for suspected CAD (19). Like IVUS, OCT can confirm the absence of significant atherosclerosis or indicate the degree of subclinical atherosclerotic lesion formation. This may be of relevance in modulating the aggressiveness of medical therapeutic strategies for primary prevention.

Evaluation of Intermediate Stenoses and Ambiguous Lesions

Suboptimal angiographic visualization impairs the accurate assessment of stenosis severity. This may happen in the presence of intermediate lesions of uncertain severity, very short lesions, pre- or post-aneurysmal lesions, ostial or left main stem stenoses, disease at branching sites, sites with focal spasm, or angiographically hazy lesions. OCT has the potential to become a routine clinical tool to guide interventional procedures as it provides accurate luminal measurements of lesion severity due to a better delineation of the lumen-wall interface, as compared with IVUS.

Like IVUS, OCT can quantify lesion severity more accurately than quantitative coronary angiography. The OCT measured minimal lumen area (MLA) of 2.4–3.0 mm² is considered the significant cut-off threshold for a clinically significant flow-limiting stenosis in appropriately sized (>3 mm) vessels excluding the left main coronary artery (46). Further validation studies are needed in this area. Comparison of the MLA with reference lumen areas is an alternative method for assessment of the degree of stenosis.

In particular, OCT is indicated for the assessment of angiographically hazy lesions and focal vessel spasm. In angiographically hazy lesions, OCT often detects ruptured plaques with thrombus attached to the site of rupture of the fibrous cap over a partially emptied lipid pool (Figs. 15.2 and 15.3). Under these circumstances, the decision to proceed with treatment may be more influenced by these morphologic observations than by absolute measurements of the lumen area.

Furthermore, the relatively small size of the OCT imaging catheters, compared with IVUS catheters, may reduce the incidence of catheter wedging and coronary spasm (12).

The main limitation of OCT lies in its inability to measure plaque burden when the thickness exceeds 1.3–1.5 mm. This drawback may affect the role of OCT in guiding interventional procedures as well as in the assessment of overall plaque burden and the presence or extent of positive remodeling.

A technical drawback of both TD-OCT and FD-OCT in this application is that plaque located at the ostium of the left or right coronary arteries cannot be accurately imaged (5). Unlike IVUS, OCT assessment requires the displacement of blood with contrast or other clear fluids (e.g., dextran or ringer lactate). This requires the firm engagement of the coronary ostium with a guiding catheter. As infrared light cannot penetrate the

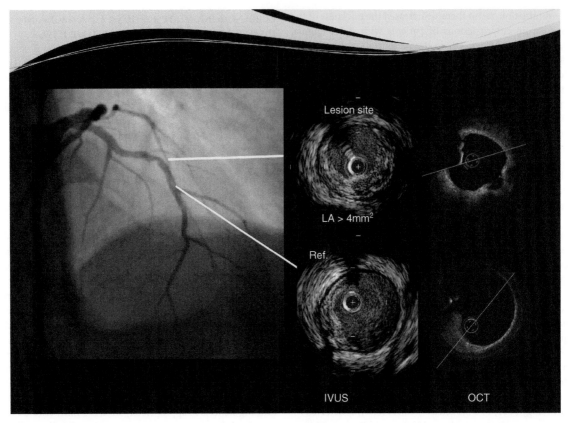

Figure 15.2 Application of OCT in a patient with ACS due to left anterior descending disease (*right panel*). IVUS (*middle panel*) shows a superficial soft plaque without indicating the presence of plaque rupture. OCT (*right panel*) confirms the presence of a plaque rupture without thrombus.

partially metallic structure of guide catheters, the structures beneath cannot be visualized by OCT.

Previous studies using IVUS to guide interventional procedures in the presence of ambiguous and intermediate angiographic lesions reported a modification of the overall revascularization strategy in 40% of patients, with aborted planned revascularizations in a high percentage of patients and a trend toward improved clinical outcome (47). As for IVUS, preliminary data indicate that OCT may alter the operator's intended treatment plan, avoiding unnecessary interventional procedures or modifying the strategy in some cases (12).

Comparison with IVUS

Assessment of target lesions by IVUS is frequently a demanding task. In spite of the miniaturization of ultrasound catheters, IVUS probes tend to occlude the lumen in tight lesions during the time required to acquire pull-back images at a relatively low pull-back speed of 1 mm/sec and consequently the symptoms and signs of myocardial ischemia may develop. Moreover, blood stagnation can complicate image interpretation. As FD-OCT probes have a slightly thinner profile than IVUS probes, pull-back imaging can be done at very high speeds (normally 20 mm/sec) and a significant fraction of severely diseased target

lesions can be imaged without causing luminal obstruction, thus rendering symptomatic ischemia less likely. If the probe causes luminal obstruction, however, blood cannot be cleared and OCT imaging becomes impossible beyond or at the level of the most severe stenosis. Furthermore, the fact that vessel flushing is required to displace blood may further impair image acquisition. Therefore, in subocclusive lesions it may be a better strategy to perform OCT after gentle predilatation.

POST-INTERVENTION ASSESSMENT
The Advantage of an IVUS-Guided Approach of Stent Deployment

Many studies have addressed the ability of IVUS guidance to reduce restenosis and thrombosis. Results have been conflicting but meta-analyses indicate a potential advantage, particularly in complex lesions (48). In particular, left main stenting benefits from an IVUS-guided approach that results in a significant decrease in mortality when compared with simple angiographic guidance. Intravascular imaging modalities also have a role in tackling the occurrence of thrombosis, as suggested by recent IVUS data obtained in a large propensity-score matched population after drug-eluting stent (DES) positioning (49). In the presence of a DES, a threshold of the absolute minimal lumen cross-sectional

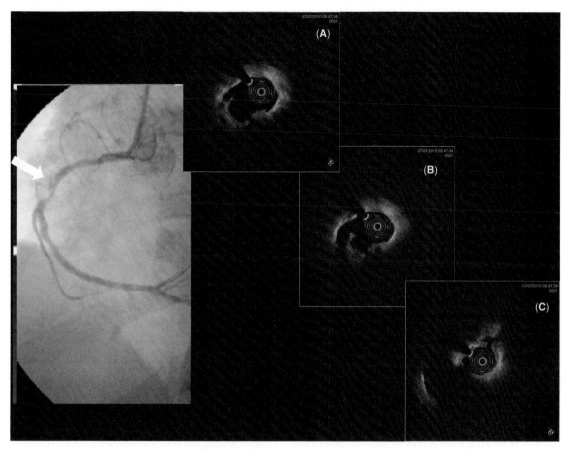

Figure 15.3 Example of plaque ulceration. Angiography shows a tight lesion in the middle portion (*arrow in the left panel*). OCT depicts the pathophysiology of the acute event. The fissuration of the plaque rupture is shown in panels A and B, while panel C shows the large lipid pool located beneath.

area within the stent of at least 5.0–5.5 mm² has been advocated as the target minimum stent area necessary to prevent failure (48).

The Potential of OCT for Stent Guidance
Most of the IVUS-guided criteria for stent expansion used in the era of bare metal stenting are based on a comparison with the lumen area in the reference segments (48). The optimal resolution of OCT further facilitates the assessment of optimal stent expansion, by comparing minimal stent area and reference areas (Fig. 15.4).

Unlike IVUS, OCT has sufficient resolution to perform a per-strut analysis, revealing mild levels of malapposition, small intra-stent thrombi formations, and minor degrees of dissection at the stent edges (50).

In the presence of stent underexpansion or haziness within the stent or at the stent edges, which may be due to plaque prolapse or edge dissection, OCT can precisely identify and quantify the factors responsible for the angiographic appearances.

The role of malapposition as a possible cause of stent thrombosis is still unclear. Potentially, acute and late-acquired malapposition can contribute to stent thrombosis, hampering the process of re-endothelialization and neointima formation,

thereby leading to platelet adhesion and subsequent thrombotic stent occlusion. However, to date, IVUS data suggest that stent malapposition does not increase the risk of major adverse cardiac events. A possible explanation is that IVUS may miss important findings, identifying only gross malapposition without enabling a per-strut analysis.

OCT is capable of detecting very small thrombi depositions on stent struts, a common finding in patients with ACS after stenting of the culprit lesions (12). Although the clinical significance of this finding is still unknown, we can speculate that the presence of thrombus after stenting increases the risk for acute and subacute stent thrombosis.

Advantages and Pitfalls of OCT for Guidance of Coronary Interventions
The need for serial OCT acquisitions to guide the selection of balloons and stents and to correct underexpansion means repeated contrast injections that may significantly increase the total amount of procedural contrast. The main drawbacks of OCT are its inability, unlike IVUS, to outline the vessel architecture and measure the external elastic membrane and the longitudinal extent of plaque burden in lesions whose depth

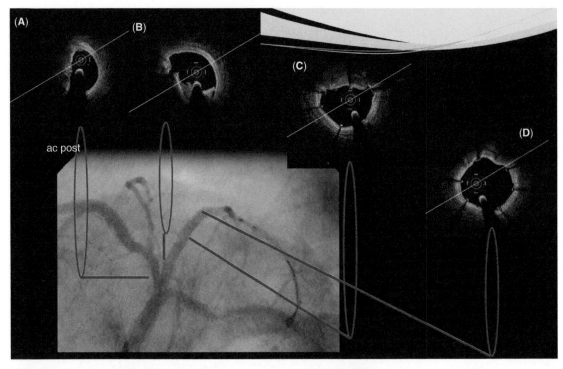

Figure 15.4 Suboptimal stent deployment despite an apparently good angiographic result. OCT shows edge dissection (B), residual proximal lumen narrowing (A), stent underexpansion and asymmetry (C), and stent site with appropriate expansion (D).

exceeds 1.0–1.5 mm. These drawbacks may have some clinical implications, as the accepted criterion for identification of reference segments by IVUS is a plaque burden less than 40%. This definition derives from the IVUS finding that a plaque burden greater than 40% at the stent margin represents a risk factor for late restenosis and thrombosis (48). IVUS proved to be a valid technical solution to select the appropriate stent size and length in diffusely diseased vessels, in an attempt to position stent edges at sites with a mild plaque burden, potentially reducing edge restenosis. On the other hand, pre-intervention use of OCT in this anatomical context may be questionable.

In presence of extensive calcification on angiography, OCT is able to accurately address the measurement of the extent and depth of superficial calcium; this may guide the selection of lesions more likely to benefit from the use of rotational atherectomy.

After stenting, OCT can identify the presence of dissection at the stent margins capable of reducing flow and thrombotic formations encroaching on the lumen or reducing the lumen area either in the stented segments or at reference sites. All these features can affect the clinical outcome.

OCT may also be useful in the treatment of late in-stent restenosis because the strong reflective power of the stent struts allows their detection through thick layers of hyperplasia, thus permitting optimal sizing of high pressure balloons to correct underexpansion and cutting balloons to deeply score up to the level of the previously implanted stent the intimal hyperplasia, when restenosis is mainly due to excessive proliferation (50).

Stent Follow-Up

Delayed healing and poor endothelialization are common findings in pathologic specimens of vessels treated with DES and recent post-mortem studies demonstrated that late stent thrombosis was highly associated with the ratio of uncovered/total stent struts (51).

OCT is potentially capable of circumventing many of these limitations and assessing the in-vivo tissue response following stent implantation (Figs. 15.5 and 15.6).

OCT anecdotal studies in patients with stent thrombosis revealed a high incidence of uncovered struts. Also, ongoing registries on stent thrombosis confirm the presence of a high incidence of uncovered struts.

At present, OCT represents an established method to verify the presence of stent coverage despite the fact that it is unable to identify the endothelium (1). In a subanalysis of the ODESSA trial, 20 of the 250 stented segments with no detectable neointima by IVUS were found to have neointimal coverage ranging from 67% to 100% by OCT (52).

Follow-up OCT data revealed that the majority of stent struts of first- and second-generation DES, including those with biodegradable polymers, are covered with thin neointima (50,52). Recent data revealed that incomplete stent apposition and the absence of OCT tissue coverage are more frequently detected by OCT in patients presenting with ACS. This finding is probably due to the presence of thrombus, a mileu that facilitates stent strut malapposition and hampers the process of vessel healing. Furthermore, in

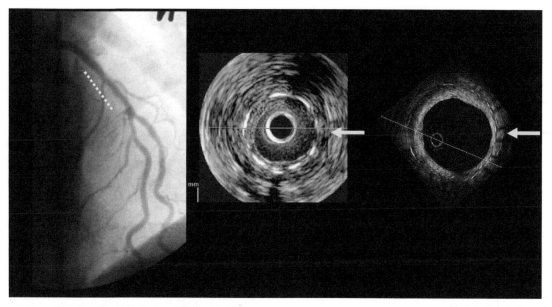

Figure 15.5 Example of OCT detection of complete drug-eluting stent coverage at 1-year follow-up. IVUS is able to identify stent coverage at 3 o'clock (*arrow in the middle panel*). OCT (*right panel*) shows complete coverage throughout the stent circumference.

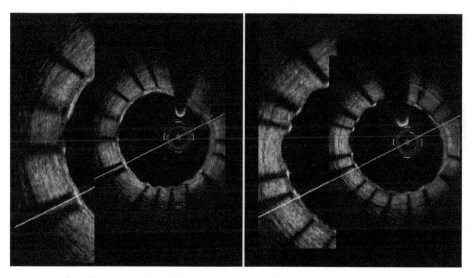

Figure 15.6 Representative OCT images of covered (*left*) and uncovered (*right*) stent struts.

patients with ST elevation myocardial infarction, the use of DES as opposed to BMS was found to increase the risk of incomplete strut apposition and uncovered struts (53). It is difficult to offer any recommendation at this stage for the use of OCT for late follow-up in individual patients, but anecdotal cases of OCT application to rule out the need for prolongation of dual antiplatelet treatment in patients requiring surgery that cannot be deferred have been reported. At present, the main application is the comparison of different stent platforms, based on the assumption that a more uniform strut coverage will improve the late outcome.

FUTURE OCT DEVELOPMENTS

Currently, standard OCT interpretation is limited to the evaluation of grayscale images generated by infrared light reflections at tissue interfaces. Identification of individual plaque components by OCT requires experience and sometimes it is not easy to distinguish calcific from lipidic elements.

The application of post-processing color-coding software that apply algorithms to analyse either spectral OCT backscattered data or other optical tissue properties should improve the characterization of atherosclerotic coronary plaques and provide a more objective assessment (54).

Macrophages show high reflectivity in OCT images and can be observed as streaks displaying a high backscatter. However, OCT identification is challenging. Macrophages are mainly located within the fibrous cap covering the lipid pool; the interface between the fibrous cap and the lipid pool produces a bright OCT appearance that can be difficult to distinguish from tightly packed foam cells (5). For this reason, dedicated software capable of identifying these inflammatory cells by improving the signal to noise ratio should be applied.

Three-dimensional (3D) reconstruction of OCT images of vessel segments may facilitate histopathologic OCT studies by providing a true view of the coronary architecture. 3D reconstruction also holds promise for facilitating OCT guidance of complex procedures, particularly for the treatment of bifurcation lesions. A 3D view can clarify the angle between a side branch and the main vessel, aiding decisions on the choice of the optimal treatment strategy. After stent positioning, 3D reconstruction can be used to address the exact location of stent struts at the site of the bifurcation.

Lastly, a catheter that enables the combination of two imaging modalities, offering complementary information, would represent a further step forward. In this respect, some research centers are experimenting with the combination of OCT with IVUS and infrared spectroscopy: the latter is a novel technique that enables the chemical definition of plaque components.

ACKNOWLEDGMENT
We acknowledge the CLI Foundation for supporting the present manuscript.

REFERENCES
1. Huang D, Swanson EA, Lin CP, et al. Optical coherence tomography. Science 1991; 254: 1178–81.
2. Brezinski ME, Tearney GJ, Bouma BE, et al. Optical coherence tomography for optical biopsy properties and demonstration of vascular pathology. Circulation 1996; 93: 1206–13.
3. Fujimoto JG, Schmitt JM. Principles of OCT. In: Regar E, van Leeuwen TG, Serruys P, eds. Optical Coherence Tomography in Cardiovascular Research. London: Informa Healthcare, 2006: 19–33.
4. Jang IK, Bouma BE, Kang DH, et al. Visualization of coronary atherosclerotic plaques in patients using Optical Coherence Tomography: comparison with intravascular ultrasound. J Am Coll Cardiol 2002; 39: 604–9.
5. Prati F, Regar E, Mintz GS, et al. for the Expert's OCT Review Document. Expert review document on methodology and clinical applications of OCT. Physical principles, methodology of image acquisition and clinical application for assessment of coronary arteries and atherosclerosis. Eur Heart J 2010; 31: 401–15.
6. Tearney GJ, Waxman S, Shishkov M, et al. Three-dimensional coronary artery microscopy by intracoronary Optical Frequency Domain Imaging. J Am Coll Cardiol Img 2008; 1: 752–61.
7. Takarada S, Imanishi T, Liu Y, et al. Advantage of next-generation frequency-domain optical coherence tomography compared with conventional time-domain system in the assessment of coronary lesion. Catheter Cardiovasc Interv 2010; 75: 202–6.
8. Jang IK, Tearney GJ, MacNeill B, et al. In vivo characterization of coronary atherosclerotic plaque by use of Optical Coherence Tomography. Circulation 2005; 111: 1551–5.
9. Regar E, Prati F, Serruys PW. Intracoronary OCT applications. In: Regar E, van Leeuwen TG, Serruys P, eds. Optical Coherence Tomography in Cardiovascular Research. London: Informa Healthcare, 2006: 53–64.
10. Prati F, Cera M, Ramazzotti V, et al. From bench to bed side: a novel technique to acquire OCT images. Circ J 2008; 72: 839–43.
11. Prati F, Cera M, Ramazzotti V, et al. Safety and feasibility of a new non-occlusive technique for facilitated intracoronary optical coherence tomography (OCT) acquisition in various clinical and anatomical scenarios. EuroInterv 2007; 3: 365–70.
12. Imola F, Mallus MT, Ramazzotti V, et al. Safety and feasibility of frequency domain Optical Coherence Tomography to guide decision making in percutaneous coronary intervention. EuroInterv 2010; 6: 575–81.
13. Barlis P, Gonzalo N, Di Mario C, et al. A multicentre evaluation of the safety of intracoronary optical coherence tomography. EuroInterv 2009; 5: 90–5.
14. Tanigawa J, Barlis P, Di Mario C. Intravascular optical coherence tomography: optimization of image acquisition and quantitative assessment of stent strut apposition. EuroInterv 2007; 3: 128–36.
15. Capodanno D, Prati F, Pawlowsky T, et al. Comparison of optical coherence tomography and intravascular ultrasound for the assessment of in-stent tissue coverage after stent implantation. EuroInterv 2009; 5: 538–43.
16. Kawasaki M, Bouma BE, Bressner J, et al. Diagnostic accuracy of optical coherence tomography and integrated backscatter intravascular ultrasound images for tissue characterization of human coronary plaques. J Am Coll Cardiol 2006; 48: 81–8.
17. Kume T, Akasaka T, Kawamoto T, et al. Assessment of coronary intima-media thickness by Optical Coherence Tomography. Comparison with intravascular ultrasound. Circ J 2005; 8: 903–7.
18. Rieber J, Meissner O, Babaryka G, et al. Diagnostic accuracy of optical coherence tomography and intravascular ultrasound for the detection and characterization of atherosclerotic plaque composition in ex-vivo coronary specimens: a comparison with histology. Coron Artery Dis 2006; 17: 425–33.
19. Mintz GS, Nissen SE, Anderson WD, et al. ACC Clinical Expert Consensus Document on Standards for the acquisition, measurement and reporting of intravascular ultrasound studies: a report of the American College of Cardiology Task Force on Clinical Expert Consensus Documents (Committee to Develop a Clinical Expert Consensus Document on Standards for Acquisition, Measurement and Reporting of Intravascular Ultrasound Studies (IVUS]. J Am Coll Cardiol 2001; 37: 1478–92.
20. Prati F, Capodanno D, Pawlowski T, et al. Local versus standard intracoronary infusion of abciximab in patients with acute coronary syndromes. J Am Coll Cardiol Intv 2010; 3: 928–34.
21. Kubo T, Imanishi T, Takarada S, et al. Assessment of culprit lesion morphology in acute myocardial infarction: ability of Optical Coherence Tomography compared with intravascular ultrasound and coronary angioscopy. J Am Coll Cardiol 2007; 50: 933–9.
22. Cilingiroglu M, Oh JH, Sugunan B, et al. Detection of vulnerable plaque in a murine model of atherosclerosis with optical coherence tomography. Catheter Cardiovasc Interv 2006; 67: 915–23.
23. Zimarino M, Prati F, Stabile E, et al. Optical coherence tomography accurately identifies intermediate atherosclerosis lesions. An

in-vivo evaluation in the rabbit carotid artery. Atherosclerosis 2007; 193: 94–101.

24. Takano M, Jang IK, Inami S, et al. In vivo comparison of Optical Coherence Tomography and angioscopy for the evaluation of coronary plaque characteristics. Am J Cardiol 2008; 101: 471–8.

25. Kume T, Akasaka T, Kawamoto T, et al. Measurements of the thickness of the fibrous cap by optical coherence tomography. Am Heart J 2006; 152: 755, e1–755. e4.

26. Barlis P, Serruys PW, Gonzalo N, et al. Assessment of culprit and remote coronary narrowings using Optical Coherence Tomography with long-term outcomes. Am J Cardiol 2008; 102: 391–5.

27. Tearney GJ, Yabushita H, Houser SL, et al. Quantification of macrophage content in atherosclerotic plaques by optical coherence tomography. Circulation 2003; 107: 113–9.

28. Raffel OC, Tearney GJ, Gauthier DD, et al. Relationship between a systemic inflammatory marker, plaque inflammation, and plaque characteristics determined by intravascular optical coherence tomography. Arterioscler Thromb Vasc Biol 2007; 27: 1820–7.

29. Wang JC, Normand SL, Mauri L, Kuntz RE. Coronary artery spatial distribution of acute myocardial infarction occlusions. Circulation 2004; 110: 278–84.

30. Fujii K, Kawasaki D, Masutani M, et al. OCT assessment of thin-cap fibroatheroma distribution in native coronary arteries. J Am Coll Cardiol Img 2010; 3: 168–75.

31. Virmani R, Burke AP, Farb A, Kolodgie FD. Pathology of the vulnerable plaque. J Am Coll Cardiol 2006; 47: C13–8.

32. Fujii K, Masutani M, Okumura T, et al. Frequency and predictor of coronary thin-cap fibroatheroma in patients with acute myocardial infarction and stable angina pectoris a 3-vessel optical coherence tomography study. J Am Coll Cardiol 2008; 52: 787–8.

33. MacNeill BD, Jang IK, Bouma BE, et al. Focal and multi-focal plaque macrophage distributions in patients with acute and stable presentations of coronary artery disease. J Am Coll Cardiol 2004; 44: 972–9.

34. Kubo T, Imanishi T, Kashiwagi M, et al. Multiple coronary lesion instability in patients with acute myocardial infarction as determined by optical coherence tomography. Am J Cardiol 2010; 105: 318–22.

35. Tanaka A, Imanishi T, Kitabata H, et al. Morphology of exertion-triggered plaque rupture in patients with acute coronary syndrome: an optical coherence tomography study. Circulation 2008; 118: 2368–73.

36. Li QX, Fu QQ, Shi SW, et al. Relationship between plasma inflammatory markers and plaque fibrous cap thickness determined by intravascular optical coherence tomography. Heart 2010; 96: 196–201.

37. Chia S, Raffel OC, Takano M, et al. Comparison of coronary plaque characteristics between diabetic and non-diabetic subjects: an in vivo optical coherence tomography study. Diabetes Res Clin Pract 2008; 81: 155–60.

38. Takarada S, Imanishi T, Kubo T, et al. Effect of statin therapy on coronary fibrous-cap thickness in patients with acute coronary syndrome: assessment by optical coherence tomography study. Atherosclerosis 2009; 202: 491–7.

39. Peterson CL, Schmitt JM. Design of an OCT imaging system for intravascular applications. In: Regar E, van Leeuwen TG, Serruys P, eds. Optical Coherence Tomography in Cardiovascular Research. London: Informa Healthcare, 2006: 35–42.

40. Stone GW, Maehara A, Lansky AJ, et al.; for the PROSPECT Investigators. A prospective natural-history study of coronary atherosclerosis. N Engl J Med 2011; 364: 226–35.

41. Manfrini O, Mont E, Leone O, et al. Sources of error and interpretation of plaque morphology by optical coherence tomography. Am J Cardiol 2007; 99: 1350.

42. Sawada T, Shite J, Garcia-Garcia HM, et al. Feasibility of combined use of intravascular ultrasound radiofrequency data analysis and optical coherence tomography for detecting thin-cap fibroatheroma. Eur Heart J 2008; 29: 1136–46.

43. Gonzalo N, Garcia-Garcia HM, Regar E, et al. In vivo assessment of high-risk coronary plaques at bifurcations with combined intravascular ultrasound and optical coherence tomography. J Am Coll Cardiol Img 2009; 2: 473–82.

44. Toutouzas K, Synetos A, Stefanadis E, et al. Correlation between morphologic characteristics and local temperature differences in culprit lesions of patients with symptomatic coronary artery disease. J Am Coll Cardiol 2007; 49: 2264–71.

45. Rogowska J, Patel NA, Fujimoto JG, Brezinski ME. Optical coherence tomographic elastography technique for measuring deformation and strain of atherosclerotic tissues. Heart 2004; 90: 556–62.

46. Kang Y, Mintz GS. IVUS vs. FFR for the assessment of intermediate lesions. Circ Card Interv In press.

47. Abizaid AS, Mintz GS, Mehran R, et al. Long-term follow-up after percutaneous transluminal coronary angioplasty was not performed based on intravascular ultrasound findings: importance of lumen dimensions. Circulation 1999; 100: 256–61.

48. Mintz GS, Weissman NJ. Intravascular ultrasound in the drug-eluting stent era. J Am Coll Cardiol 2006; 48: 421–9.

49. Roy P, Steinberg DH, Sushinsky SJ, et al. The potential clinical utility of intravascular ultrasound guidance in patients undergoing percutaneous coronary intervention with drug-eluting stents. Eur Heart J 2008; 29: 1851–7.

50. Bezerra HG, Costa MA, Guagliumi G, Rollins AM, Simon DI. Intracoronary optical coherence tomography: a comprehensive review clinical and research applications. J Am Coll Cardiol Interv 2009; 2: 1035–46.

51. Finn AV, Joner M, Nakazawa G, et al. Pathological correlates of late drug-eluting stent thrombosis: strut coverage as a marker of endothelialization. Circulation 2007; 115: 2435–41.

52. Guagliumi G, Sirbu V, Bezerra H, et al. Strut coverage and vessel wall response to zotarolimus eluting and bare metal stents implanted in patients with ST segment elevation myocardial infarction: the OCTAMI (Optical coherence tomography in acute myocardial infarction) study. J Am Coll Cardiol Interv 2010; 3: 680–7.

53. Gonzalo N, Barlis P, Serruys PW, et al. Incomplete stent apposition and delayed tissue coverage are more frequent in drug-eluting stents implanted during primary percutaneous coronary intervention for ST-segment elevation myocardial infarction than in drug eluting stents implanted for stable/unstable angina. J Am Coll Cardiol Interv 2009; 2: 445–52.

54. Nair A, Kuban BD, Tuzcu EM, et al. Coronary plaque classification with intravascular ultrasound radiofrequency data analysis. Circulation 2002; 106: 2200–6.

16 Thermal assessment of the human coronary atherosclerotic plaque: Current status and potential clinical implications

Konstantinos Toutouzas, Maria Drakopoulou, Archontoula Michelongona, Eleftherios Tsiamis, and Christodoulos Stefanadis

INTRODUCTION

Although enormous progress has been made in the prevention and treatment of cardiovascular disease, it remains the leading cause of death worldwide (1). Despite advances in current imaging modalities, the ability to identify patients who are at high risk for a future acute coronary event is still limited mainly because these events may occur as the first manifestation of coronary atherosclerosis in previously apparently asymptomatic individuals with non–flow-limiting plaques (2).

The concept of the 'vulnerable' plaque has emerged in recent years to describe quiescent atherosclerotic plaques that are prone to rupture and cause an acute coronary event (3). Advances in the identification of vulnerable plaque are of great importance in the quest to prevent myocardial infarction (AMI) and sudden cardiac death. Several histological characteristics of vulnerable plaques have been identified: (*i*) a thin fibrous cap, (*ii*) a large lipid pool, and (*iii*) the presence of activated macrophages near the fibrous cap (4). The first prospective trial of the natural history of atherosclerosis using multimodality imaging to characterize the coronary tree [Providing Regional Observations to Study Predictors of Events Coronary Tree Trial (PROSPECT)] showed that most non-culprit plaques, which may cause a future event have a large plaque burden, a large lipid core, and a small lumen area (5).

Our understanding of the pathophysiology of vulnerable plaque has led to the recognition that an intense inflammatory response, as manifested by local invasion of macrophages and lymphocytes and activation of matrix metalloproteinases, plays a pivotal role in degrading the supporting collagen and promoting plaque fragility. However, although inflammation seems to be an integral part of vulnerable plaque development and progression, leading eventually to plaque instability, its impact has not been studied in prospective studies (6).

Local heat production has long been recognized as one of the principal signs of inflammation. In atherosclerotic plaques, the high metabolic rate of the inflammatory cell infiltrate, increased neoangiogenesis, and ineffective thermogenesis are mechanisms that result in enhanced heat production, which can be detected by temperature recordings (7). Given that inflammation has a central role in atherosclerosis, intracoronary thermography has been introduced as a novel technique for the identification of the local inflammatory activation of vulnerable plaques (8). The increased heat production from unstable plaques has been confirmed in several ex vivo human studies, experimental models, and clinical studies.

The feasibility of intracoronary thermography for the assessment of thermal heterogeneity in vivo has been validated in multiple animal studies (9–12). Although there are significant differences in the technological characteristics of the device design, the reported studies have provided important pathophysiological insights in the development of the unstable plaque. Naghavi et al. developed a contact-based 'thermobasket' catheter for measuring in vivo the temperature at several points on the vessel wall in the presence of blood flow (10,13). The system was tested in a canine and a rabbit model of atherosclerosis. In inbred cholesterol-fed dogs with femoral atherosclerosis, marked thermal heterogeneity was found on the surface of atherosclerotic regions, but not in disease-free regions (Fig. 16.1). This device showed satisfactory results in terms of accuracy, reproducibility, and safety.

TECHNICAL ASPECTS

Different types of intracoronary thermography catheters have been designed (Fig. 16.2). The intracoronary thermography catheter utilized in a series of clinical studies is a thermistor-based sensor that consists of two lumens (Epiphany; Medispes S. W., Zug, Switzerland) (14–21). The first lumen runs through the distal 20 cm of the device and is used for insertion of a 0.014-inch guidewire that serves as a monorail system. The thermistor is positioned at the distal part of the thermography catheter of the second lumen. The technical characteristics of this particular polyamide thermistor include (*i*) temperature accuracy of 0.05°C; (*ii*) time constant of 300 ms; (*iii*) spatial resolution of 0.5 mm; and (*iv*) linear correlation of resistance versus temperature over the range of 33–43°C. This catheter is 3 Fr, 3.5 Fr, or 4 Fr in diameter, depending on the size of the vessel.

Another system of intracoronary thermography is the ThermoCoil system that consists of a 0.014-inch guidewire, a pullback handle, and a data acquisition system (22). The temperature sensor is located at the tip of the wire and has a resolution of 0.08°C. The tip of the wire is pre-bent in an angled curve 10 mm proximal to the tip, which brings the tip into contact with the vessel wall. The signals are converted to temperature readings and displayed in real time as a digital readout and in graphical form.

Other clinical studies have been also performed with a 3.5 F thermography catheter that has a self-expanding basket with five nitinol arms and a thermocouple on each arm (Volcano Therapeutics Inc., Rancho Cordova, CA) (23,24). This catheter of 0.05°C sensitivity has two radio-opaque markers and a

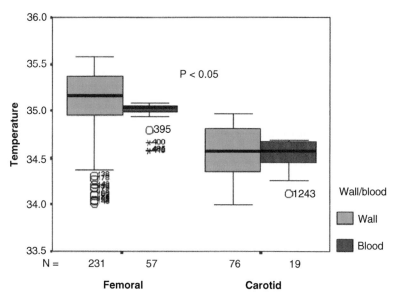

Figure 16.1 The thermography basket catheter showed higher absolute temperatures as well as temperature heterogeneity on atherosclerotic lesions compared to lesion-free segments.

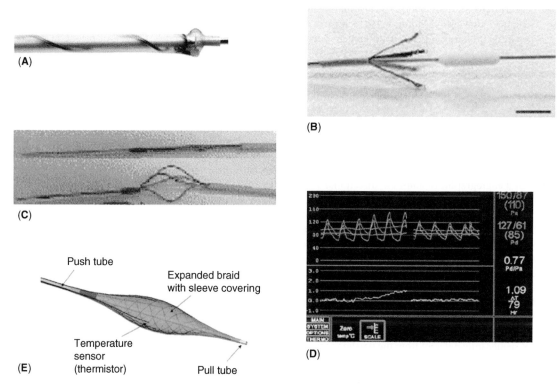

Figure 16.2 (**A**) Epiphany thermography system (Epiphany, Medispes S.W., Zug, Switzerland). A monorail system containing two lumens with a temperature accuracy 0.05°C and the time constant 300 ms. (**B**) Thermocore thermography system with a functional probe containing four thermistors with an accuracy of 0.01°C. Epiphany coronary thermography system. (**C**) Volcano non-occluding thermography catheter (Volcano Therapeutics, Orange County, California) with a self-expanding basket, five nitinol arms at its tip, with one thermocouple on each arm and another one on the central wire, allowing for real-time, cross-sectional thermal mapping of the arterial wall. (**D**) Radi PressureWire® (Radi Medical Systems, Inc., Uppsala, Sweden): a 0.014-inch wire that contains a high-sensitivity thermistor of 0.1°C. (**E**) Accumed Systems, Inc. (Ann Arbor, MI, US): A blood-flow-occluding feature with a temperature-sensing structure at its distal end and a proximal end including a manually operated expansion control.

thermocouple in the center of the shaft to allow monitoring of core blood temperature.

More recently, clinical studies have been performed with the 0.014-inch Radi wire (Medical Systems, Uppsala, Sweden) equipped with a high-sensitivity thermistor (sensitivity 0.1°C) (25,26).

CLINICAL STUDIES

The first clinical study with intracoronary thermography (Epiphany Medispes system) performed by Stefanadis et al. in 1999 demonstrated that the temperature difference between atherosclerotic plaques and adjacent healthy segments increased progressively from control subjects through the ACS spectrum, with patients with AMI recording the highest values (18). Temperature was constant within the arteries of the control subjects, whereas most atherosclerotic plaques showed a higher temperature compared with the healthy vessel wall. Plaque temperature heterogeneity was present in 20%, 40%, and 67% of the patients with stable angina, unstable angina, and AMI, respectively, and did not correlate with the degree of stenosis. Thermal heterogeneity was absent in the control group. Another study including 55 patients showed increased plaque temperature for an extended period after AMI, indicating that the inflammatory process is sustained after plaque rupture (19). Schmermund et al. recorded intracoronary temperature differences ranging from 0.14°C to 0.36°C. Focal temperature heterogeneity was observed in 50% of patients with unstable angina and in 27% of patients with stable angina. Although this study showed a difference between the two groups, there was still a considerable overlap (23). Wainstein et al. used a different thermography catheter (ThermoCoil Guidewire). Thirteen patients presenting with either acute or chronic coronary syndromes as indications for percutaneous coronary intervention (PCI) were evaluated by intracoronary thermography, intravascular ultrasound, and angiography. In addition, directional atherectomy was performed in two patients and tissue was analyzed by histology. Intra-arterial temperature differences between 0.1°C and 0.3°C were noted in four subjects. Intravascular ultrasound findings and atherectomy tissue histology suggested a correlation between plaque vulnerability and elevated temperature (22).

Worthley et al., using the 0.014-inch Radi PressureWire XT (Radi Medical Systems, Uppsala, Sweden), found a mean temperature difference of 0.02 ± 0.01°C at the culprit lesion of patients with ACS, which was below the resolution of the thermistor and not significantly different from the baseline temperature difference of 0.00°C ± 0.01°C (26). In a recent article, Cuisset et al. used the same system and assessed intracoronary pressure and temperature variations in 18 patients with AMI. In this study, when the sensor was advanced across the lesion, an increase in the temperature signal (average, 0.059 ± 0.028°C) was uniformly observed in all patients. However, the increase in the temperature signal was proportional to the pressure drop across the stenosis ($R = 0.72$, $p < 0.001$) (25). This study

suggested that thermistor-based sensors may not be suitable for assessing in vivo coronary thermal heterogeneity, and that the data obtained so far in patients with acute coronary syndrome (ACS) may be affected by pressure and flow artefacts. These studies, however, may have been limited by the fact that the Radi wire is not designed for measuring the coronary plaque temperature, but rather for measuring the blood temperature within the lumen and its thermistor is not always in contact with the arterial wall (26). However, the correct interpretation of intravascular thermographic measurements might require knowledge of the flow and morphological characteristics of the atherosclerotic plaque that are not readily available at this stage. Takumi et al. assessed the hypothesis that the site where the highest temperature is detected, as measured by thermal wire, coincides with the culprit plaque, detected by intravascular ultrasound, in patients with AMI (27). This study of 45 consecutive patients presenting with anterior AMI demonstrated that the site where the maximal temperature measured by the pressure/temperature guidewire (Pressure Wire RADI 5; Radi Medical Systems, Uppsala, Sweden) was observed distallyl to the angiographic site of occlusion in patients with total vessel occlusion. In the same study, the site where the maximal temperature was observed as opposed to the site of angiographic occlusion coincided with the ruptured 'culprit' plaque as assessed by intravascular ultrasound (Fig. 16.3). Thus, thermography identified accurately the culprit plaque in patients with AMI and coronary total occlusion, which did not always correspond with the angiographic findings (perhaps related to retrograde propagation of thrombus).

LIMITATIONS

In light of the complex pathophysiological background of coronary atherosclerosis and inflammation, intracoronary thermography has provided important information regarding the mechanisms involved (Table 16.1). However, although coronary thermography is a safe and feasible method for the functional evaluation of atherosclerotic plaques, it has certain technical limitations. There is a discrepancy in temperature differences between ex vivo and in vivo measurements raising concern over the accuracy of the method. This discrepancy has been attributed to the (i) 'cooling effect' of coronary blood flow, and (ii) inability of the sensors to reliably remain in contact with the arterial vessel wall, thus underestimating plaque heat production in clinical practice.

To assess the possible influence of coronary blood flow, temperature measurements have been performed during complete interruption of flow (28). During vessel occlusion, the observed temperature was elevated in patients with stable angina as well as those with ACS, suggesting that coronary flow has a cooling effect on thermal heterogeneity, which may lead to underestimation of local heat production. Specifically, complete obstruction of blood flow has been shown to increase the degree of detected temperature heterogeneity by 60–76% (29). However, other studies have shown that normal physiological flow conditions reduce temperature heterogeneity only by

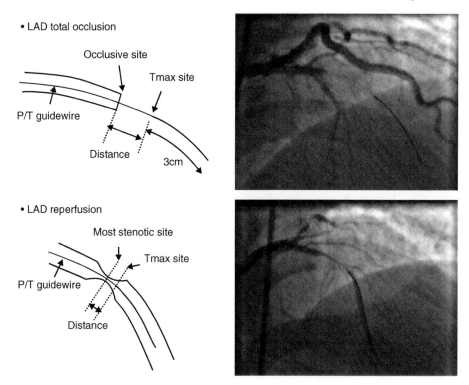

Figure 16.3 Methods to measure the distance between the maximal temperature (Tmax) site by the pressure/temperature (P/T) guidewire and the occlusive site by angiography in patients with an occluded left anterior descending coronary artery (LAD) (*top panel*), and that between the Tmax site and the most stenotic site in patients with LAD reperfusion (*bottom panel*).

Table 16.1 Human in Vivo Thermography Studies

Author	Year	Main finding	Type of catheter
Stefanadis et al. (18)	1999	Temperature differences between atherosclerotic plaque and healthy vessel wall increased through the clinical spectrum	Epiphany catheter: Single-channel, thermistor-based
Stefanadis et al. (39)	2000	Positive correlation of C-reactive protein and serum amyloid A with the temperature difference of the plaque	Epiphany catheter: Single-channel, thermistor-based
Stefanadis et al. (17)	2001	Increased local temperature in atherosclerotic plaques is strong predictor of an unfavorable clinical outcome in patients with CAD undergoing percutaneous interventions	Epiphany catheter: Single-channel, thermistor-based
Stefanadis et al. (16)	2002	Statin intake showed a favorable effect on heat release from atherosclerotic plaques	Epiphany catheter: Single-channel, thermistor-based
Webster et al. (37)	2002	Increased thermal heterogeneity detected in atherosclerotic plaques. No correlation with C-reactive protein was found	RADI PressureWire high-sensitivity thermistor
Stefanadis et al. (29)	2003	Thermal heterogeneity was underestimated in atherosclerotic plaques due to the 'cooling effect' of coronary blood flow	Epiphany catheter: Single-channel, thermistor-based
Stefanadis et al. (28)	2003	In vivo atherosclerotic plaque temperature recording was feasible with the new balloon-thermography catheter. A higher temperature difference was found after complete interruption of blood flow by inflation of the balloon	A balloon-thermography catheter designed for temperature measurements during coronary flow interruption. The thermistor probe is positioned at the distal segment of the catheter with a balloon at the opposite site. By inflation of the balloon, coronary flow is interrupted

(Continued)

Table 16.1 Human in Vivo Thermography Studies (*Continued*)

Author	Year	Main finding	Type of catheter
Schmermund et al. (23)	2003	Increased thermal heterogeneity of atherosclerotic plaques in patients with stable or unstable angina	Volcano catheter: Self-expanding basket with five nitinol arms, one on each arm and one on the central wire
Stefanadis et al. (44)	2004	Coronary sinus temperature was increased in patients with CAD and was found to be a prognostic factor for mid-term clinical outcome	A 7Fr thermographic catheter possessing a steering arm at the proximal part of the catheter and a thermistor probe at the catheter tip. Manipulation of the steering arm proximally enables the distal end of the catheter to be curved (0° to 180°)
Toutouzas et al. (19)	2004	Increased plaque temperature was observed for an extended period after myocardial infarction. Statin intake showed a beneficial effect on plaque temperature after myocardial infarction	Epiphany catheter: Single-channel, thermistor-based
Dudek et al. (24)	2005	Thermography was unable to differentiate between lesions at risk, despite the selection of lesions that seemed most likely to show significant differences distinct to differentiate	Volcano catheter
Toutouzas et al. (41)	2005	Systemic inflammation correlated with coronary sinus temperature independent of the extent of CAD	A 7Fr thermographic catheter possessing a steering arm at the proximal part of the catheter and a thermistor probe at the catheter tip. Manipulation of the steering arm proximally enables the distal end of the catheter to be curved (0° to 180°)
Toutouzas et al. (36)	2005	Patients with diabetes mellitus had an increased temperature difference compared to patients without diabetes. Statin intake showed a beneficial effect on plaque temperature	Epiphany catheter: Single-channel, thermistor-based
Toutouzas et al. (38)	2006	The temperature gradient at non-culprit lesions progressively increased with the lowest values in patients with stable angina and the highest in patients with ACS	Epiphany catheter: Single-channel, thermistor-based
Rzeszutko et al. (45)	2006	Intracoronary thermography was safe and feasible. It was unable to differentiate between lesions at risk, despite a selection of lesions that should appear most distinct to differentiate	Volcano catheter
Worthley et al. (26)	2006	No significant temperature increase in patients with ACS, compared to baseline temperature	RADI PressureWire high-sensitivity thermistor
Wainstein et al. (22)	2007	Intracoronary thermography detected vulnerable plaques, as assessed by intravascular ultrasound and on histology performed on atherectomy specimens	ThermoCoil guidewire
Toutouzas et al. (40)	2007	Local inflammatory activation in non-culprit lesions correlated with systemic inflammation. Statins showed a beneficial effect on non-culprit lesion heat production	Epiphany catheter: Single-channel, thermistor-based
Toutouzas et al. (21)	2007	Culprit lesions with plaque rupture and positive arterial remodeling had increased thermal heterogeneity	Epiphany catheter: Single-channel, thermistor-based
Takumi et al. (27)	2007	Thermography accurately identified the culprit lesion in patients with AMI and coronary total occlusion	RADI PressureWire high-sensitivity thermistor
Cuisset et al. (25)	2009	The temperature increase across the lesion correlated with the pressure drop across the stenosis ($R = 0.72$, $p < 0.001$)	RADI PressureWire high-sensitivity thermistor

8–13% compared to surface temperature measured in the absence of flow (11). An in vitro model of a focal, eccentric, heat-generating lesion demonstrated that a guidewire-based system (Themocoil System) can detect changes in surface temperature. However, temperature measurements increased linearly with source temperature and decreased with increases in flow by an exponent of –0.33 ($p < 0.001$ for both). This study showed that both flow rates and heat source properties can significantly influence the measurement and interpretation of thermographic data (30). Similarly, another mathematical simulation of a model of a coronary artery segment also containing a heat source predicted that measured temperature is strongly affected by blood flow, cap thickness, source geometry, and maximal flow velocity. Specifically, maximal temperature differences at the lumen wall decreased when the source volume increased and blood flow was acting as a coolant to the lumen wall (31). Additionally, when cap thickness increased, maximal temperatures decreased, and the influence of flow increased. In vitro investigations in a model of 'hot' plaque showed that the sensor of the RadiWire could detect changes in the temperature of the wall of 0.58°C as long as the distance from the wall was less than 0.5 mm and the flow less than 60 ml/min. For flow values larger than 60 ml/min, the pressure wire could not detect any significant increase in temperature when crossing the 'hot spot'. An inverse correlation was observed between the flow and the observed temperature changes (25). Rzeszutko et al. performed intracoronary thermography in 40 patients with ACS using a thermography catheter containing five thermocouples measuring vessel wall temperature and one thermocouple measuring blood temperature (accuracy 0.05°C). The temperature gradient between blood temperature and the maximum wall temperature was measured. In 40% of patients, the temperature gradient was found to be >0.10°C. There was a significant difference in ΔT between culprit and adjacent non-culprit segments when blood flow was interrupted during thermography. However, this difference was marginally non-significant when the flow was preserved. The most important observation from this pilot study appears to be the impact of blood flow on the thermography readings. In patients with transient blood flow interruption lower temperatures (cooling) were recorded in proximal reference segments. There was a significant inverse correlation between plaque temperature and the presence of blood flow at the beginning of the thermographic evaluation. This effect of blood flow on vessel wall temperature has been investigated in vitro and in vivo, as well as by mathematical modeling (31).

To eliminate these shortcomings and the inability of sensors to achieve contact with the arterial wall in intermediate lesions, other catheter designs have been introduced. Verheye et al. observed more pronounced temperature differences when blood flow was stopped by balloon occlusion in rabbit aorta (11). Belardi et al. presented preliminary results with a basket-catheter with multiple thermistors that can also measure atheromatic plaque temperature during complete interruption of coronary blood flow (32). All these devices need to be investigated in a large number of patients in order to draw conclusions regarding their safety and prognostic value. Another limitation is the inability of the proposed devices to scan the long segments of coronary arteries; hence, they can only perform spot measurements at pre-selected sites. Thus, early local inflammatory activation cannot be detected in intermediate lesions and a prospective study to investigate the prognostic role of local inflammatory activation cannot be performed. Moreover, a cut-off value of temperature in order to characterize a plaque as 'inflamed' is not feasible, and thus the clinical application of intracoronary thermography is problematic.

All these shortcomings prohibit the performance of large prospective clinical trials with intravascular thermography. Therefore, research should be focused on alternative pathways,

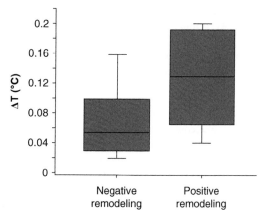

Figure 16.4 Difference in atherosclerotic plaque temperature from background temperature (ΔT) between patients with negative remodeling and those with positive remodeling.

such as the combination of intracoronary thermography with an imaging method, e.g., intravascular ultrasound (IVUS) or optical coherence tomography (OCT). IVUS has been widely used for detection of the morphologic characteristics of the vulnerable plaque (8). Distinct morphologic characteristics, including positive arterial wall remodeling, and an increased number of rupture sites have been detected in plaques of patients with ACS. In a study by IVUS, a strong and positive correlation was found between the coronary remodelling index (defined as the ratio of the external elastic membrane area at the lesion, to that at the proximal site) and the temperature difference between the atherosclerotic plaque and healthy vascular wall (21). Specifically, patients with ACS had a greater remodeling index than those with stable angina and increased atherosclerotic plaque temperature. Moreover, patients with positive remodeling had higher thermal heterogeneity than those with negative remodeling (Fig. 16.4). In patients with negative remodeling no difference was found in thermal heterogeneity between ACS and stable angina. Patients with plaque rupture had an increased temperature difference compared to patients without rupture as determined by IVUS. This study showed that culprit lesions with ruptured plaque and positive arterial remodeling have increased thermal heterogeneity, although in certain patients a discrepancy was observed between morphologic and functional characteristics. These results confirm that a combination of morphologic and functional examination may offer additional diagnostic information.

The OCT generates real-time tomographic images from backscattered reflections of infrared light (2,33). The greatest advantage of this method is its resolution that is significantly higher than ultrasound-based approaches. This improvement, however, comes at the expense of poorer penetration through blood and tissue (1–3 mm). The potential feasibility of OCT for in vivo vulnerable plaque macrophage quantification has been demonstrated in recent studies (34). In recent preliminary studies, assessment of culprit lesions in patients with ACS has been performed both by intracoronary thermography and OCT (20,35). Plaques with increased thermal heterogeneity had thinner fibrous caps compared to plaques without increased temperature. Moreover, the presence of intraluminal thrombus was not related to plaque temperature.

CLINICAL EFFECTIVENESS

Intracoronary thermography, with the above-mentioned limitations overcome, could have a role in the assessment of specific groups of patients, as well as in risk stratification and treatment evaluation in patients with coronary artery disease (CAD).

In patients with diabetes mellitus, inflammation is particularly pronounced and atherosclerotic lesions have denser inflammatory cell infiltrates than patients without diabetes. In a study including 45 patients with diabetes mellitus and 63 controls without diabetes, patients with diabetes mellitus had a greater temperature difference compared to patients without diabetes (14,20,36). Moreover, patients with diabetes mellitus suffering from ACS or stable angina showed increased local inflammatory involvement compared to patients without diabetes mellitus. This finding is in accordance with previous observations that patients with diabetes mellitus have more severe inflammation in their coronary atherosclerotic plaques, suggesting that diabetes mellitus has a strong impact on plaque destabilization by inflammatory activation. The increased local inflammatory activation in patients with diabetes mellitus is a possible explanation for the failure of trials to lower cardiovascular events in patients with diabetes mellitus, even in patients with intensive treatment to control blood glucose levels. The combination of strict control of glucose levels with stabilization of local inflammatory involvement could potentially reduce the cardiovascular mortality in this high-risk group of patients.

Another emerging application of thermography is in the prognostic assessment of patients with CAD. The impact of intracoronary thermography on risk stratification of patients undergoing percutaneous coronary intervention (PCI) has been also investigated. In a study population including 86 patients after successful PCI with bare metal stents at the culprit lesion, the relationship between the temperature difference between the atherosclerotic plaque and the healthy vessel wall with event-free survival was been studied (17). The patients that were enrolled had stable angina (34.5%), unstable angina (34.5%), or AMI (30%). Temperature difference increased progressively from stable angina to AMI. After a median clinical follow-up period of 17.88 ± 7.16 months, thermal heterogeneity was greater in patients with adverse cardiac events than in patients without events ($p < 0.0001$). In addition, temperature difference was found to be a strong predictor of adverse cardiac events during the follow-up period (OR = 2.14, p = 0.043). However, the impact of local inflammatory activation on (i) restenosis in the era of drug-eluting stents and (ii) on the progression of non-culprit lesions remains to be determined in large prospective studies.

With respect to treatment evaluation, intracoronary thermography has been demonstrated effective in evaluating the effect of diet and medications on atherosclerotic plaque thermal heterogeneity (16). Statins are the only drugs in cardiovascular medicine with proven anti-inflammatory action in atherosclerotic plaques. Therefore, the potential of statins to prevent rupture of atherosclerotic plaques has been the focus of intense research effort.

Statins have well-recognized anti-inflammatory effects and can reduce the number of macrophages while increasing the collagen content and the thickness of the fibrous cap of atherosclerotic plaques (as assessed by OCT), hence stabilizing the plaque (4). The possible stabilizing effect of statins on hot plaques has been investigated in several studies. In a study of 72 patients (37 patients receiving statins for more than 4 weeks and 35 not receiving statins), thermal heterogeneity of the culprit lesion was lower in patients on treatment, independent of their clinical syndrome (16). The effect of statin on temperature was independent of both the serum cholesterol level at hospital admission and clinical presentation. Furthermore, statin therapy had a more marked beneficial effect in patients with diabetes mellitus. In this study, patients with diabetes mellitus treated with statins had a decreased temperature difference compared with untreated patients, suggesting that statins have a favorable effect in patients with diabetes mellitus and CAD (14,36). The effect of statin therapy on non-culprit lesion thermal heterogeneity has been investigated in 71 patients undergoing PCI (40 patients treated with statin and 31 untreated patients). This study demonstrated that thermal heterogeneity was decreased both in patients with ACS and in those with stable angina receiving statins (21). These findings indicate that aggressive treatment with statins may be essential for the stabilization of the vulnerable atherosclerotic plaque in patients with CAD. This is likely secondary to the proven anti-inflammatory 'pleiotropic' vascular effects of statins. Intracoronary thermography remains the only method demonstrating the effect of statin treatment on in vivo local inflammatory status.

Thermography provided new insights supporting the concept of diffuse destabilization of coronary atherosclerotic plaques: although only a single lesion may be responsible for clinical symptoms, ACSs were associated with diffuse thermal heterogeneity. It is increasingly recognized that the mechanisms leading to an acute coronary event involve the complete coronary tree and can be regarded as a pan-coronary process. In a study that recruited 20 patients (6 with unstable angina and 14 with stable angina), the investigators after choosing a cut-off temperature value $\geq 0.1°C$ identified 10 patients without temperature heterogeneity, 4 with a single hot spot, 3 with 2 hot spots, and 3 with 3 hot spots (37). Thermal heterogeneity of non-culprit lesions was investigated in a study of 40 patients with ACS by a multisensor thermography basket catheter (Volcano Therapeutics, Rancho Cordova, CA, USA). The temperature difference, defined as the maximum temperature difference between blood and any thermal couple, was measured. This study showed increased temperature difference in non-culprit segments, although the difference remained lower than that observed at culprit lesions. The temperature difference was inversely correlated with blood flow during thermal mapping. Thus, the presence of blood flow led to a significant decrease in the recorded temperature difference between culprit and non-culprit segments (24). However, in another study that included 42 patients (23 with stable angina and 19 with ACS), thermal heterogeneity in non-culprit intermediate lesions was found to be similar to that in culprit lesions (38). In the same study, patients with ACS had increased thermal heterogeneity in both culprit and non-culprit lesions compared to patients with stable angina supporting a pan-coronary inflammatory activation. In another study with 71 patients with ACS or stable angina undergoing PCI in the culprit lesion, thermography of the intermediate non-culprit lesion showed increased thermal heterogeneity (40). In patients with ACS compared to those with stable angina, patients higher temperature differences were noted compared to patients with stable angina in non-culprit lesions. Several studies have demonstrated a correlation between systemic inflammation determined by elevated levels of serum biomarkers, such as C-reactive protein, and local plaque temperature. The correlation of systemic inflammatory markers with potential plaque vulnerability has been investigated in 60 patients with CAD (20 with stable angina, 20 with unstable angina, and 20 with AMI) and 20 sex- and age-matched controls without CAD. In this study, there was a strong correlation between C-reactive protein and serum amyloid A levels and observed differences in temperature (39). This study demonstrated that systemic inflammatory activation as assessed by the levels of C-reactive protein correlates with local inflammatory activity of non-culprit intermediate lesions (40). A linear correlation was detected between temperature differences of non-culprit lesions and CRP values in the total study population, and in patients with ACS and stable angina alone ($R = 0.46$, p b0.001, $R = 0.39$, p = 0.01, $R = 0.42$, p = 0.01, respectively) (22). An apparently higher mean C-reactive protein level has been demonstrated in patients with higher temperature heterogeneity compared to those without elevated temperature (14.0 vs. 6.2 mg/L) (25). Some other studies, however, such as that by Webster et al., failed to show such a relationship, as most patients had normal CRP levels possibly resulting from a higher use of statins and anti-inflammatory medications (37).

On the basis of these findings, blood temperature differences between the coronary sinus and the right atrium were measured in patients with symptomatic CAD, thus evaluating whether diffuse coronary inflammation increases blood temperature during its passage through the coronary tree to the coronary sinus. Thermography was performed by a catheter possessing a steering arm that passes through the lumen of the catheter and is attached to its tip. The catheter has a thermistor probe at the center of the tip with a sensitivity of 0.05°C and a time constant of 300 msec. Temperature difference between the coronary sinus and the right atrium was greater in patients with ACS and with stable angina compared to patients without angiographically significant CAD. Though patients with ACS had greater thermal heterogeneity compared to stable angina patients, the difference did not reach statistical significance. The levels of C-reactive protein were well correlated with thermal heterogeneity ($R = 0.35$,

$p < 0.01$) (41). This study showed that systemic inflammation correlates with coronary sinus blood temperature suggesting thus that an inflammatory process is potentially the underlying mechanism for increased heat production from the myocardium. Moreover, coronary sinus blood temperature was found to be greater than right atrial blood temperature in patients with angiographically significant lesions, independent of the site of the lesion, compared to subjects without CAD. These findings provide further support for the hypothesis that an extensive inflammatory process within the coronary arterial tree may contribute to the pathogenesis of ACS in patients with CAD.

POTENTIAL COMPLICATIONS

Although intracoronary thermography is a valuable technique to evaluate the vulnerability of a coronary plaque, its invasive nature may, albeit rarely, result in severe complications. It should be specified though, that these complications, such as renal dysfunction, are due to the coronary angiography and not intracoronary thermography itself. However, it cannot be excluded that the catheters themselves might, on rare occasions, cause coronary dissection.

PERSONAL PERSPECTIVE: EVOLVING INDICATIONS

The invasive approach of intravascular thermography excludes the application of this modality in primary prevention. The non-invasive assessment of 'hot' plaques in coronary arteries and peripheral arteries (e.g., carotids), however, would be ideal for the primary prevention of adverse cardiovascular events. A promising method is the microwave radiometry (RTM-01-RES system), a new method already applied in oncology for the non-invasive temperature measurement. The system includes a personal computer and a printer. The device is connected to a PC through a serial port. Results of RTM-diagnosis are shown in the monitor of the computer or printed out as a thermogram and temperature field superimposed on the projection of an investigated organ. Microwave radiometry detects natural electromagnetic radiation from internal tissues at microwave frequencies, and as the intensity of the radiation is proportional to the temperature of tissue, microwave radiometry can provide accurate temperature measurements (Table 16.2). Theoretically, thermal scanning by microwave radiometry can be performed in all arterial segments in a depth of 1–7 cm from the skin.

This proposal of thermal mapping in arterial segments has been successfully investigated in an experimental hypercholesterolemic model. In specific, 24 New Zealand rabbits were randomized to either a normal ($n = 12$) or cholesterol-rich (0.3%) diet ($n = 12$) for 6 months. Thereafter, temperature measurements of the abdominal aortas were performed (i) invasively with intravascular catheter-based thermography and (ii) noninvasively with microwave radiometry. All animals were euthanized after the procedure and aortas were extracted for histological and immunohistochemical analysis. Both techniques detected that temperature differences of atherosclerotic aortic segments were significantly higher compared to temperature differences of the controls ($p < 0.001$) (Fig. 16.5). In all segments,

Table 16.2 Technical Characteristics of the RTM-01-RES System

Items	Specifications
Thermal abnormality (i.e., a lower or higher temperature) is detected at a depth of, cm	3–7 (depending on water content tissue type)
Accuracy of measuring the averaged internal temperature, when a temperature is 32–38°C, °C	± 0,2
Time required for measuring internal temperature at a point, seconds	10
Antenna diameter, mm	39
Accuracy of measuring the skin temperature, °C	± 0,2
Time required for measuring skin temperature at a point, when the temperature is 32–38 °C, seconds	1
Device mass, kg	4
Power supply	220 ± 22 V, 1 phase, 50–60 Hz
Power consumption, Watt	20

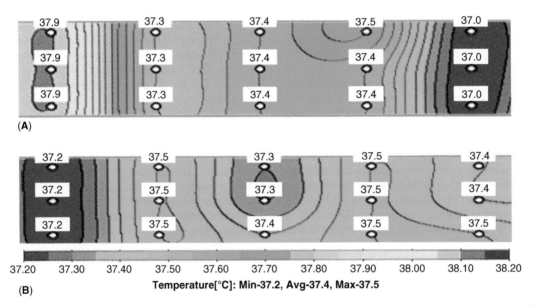

Figure 16.5 Thermal mapping of the abdominal aorta of the rabbits with the use of the microwave radiometry. (A) A representative temperature difference of 0.9°C measured at the aorta o a hypercholesterolemic rabbit. (B) A representative temperature field of the aorta of a control rabbit showing equally distributed temperatures with ΔT of 0.3°C. Each temperature corresponds to a specific color and the scale is depicted in the bottom of the temperature fields.

temperature differences detected by the two methods, correlated positively ($p < 0.001$, $R = 0.94$). Histological analysis of the atherosclerotic aortic segments showed that mean plaque thickness was 352.1 ± 152.2 μm. Temperature heterogeneity of atherosclerotic segments assessed by both methods had good correlation with plaque thickness assessed by histology (MR: $R = 0.60$, $p < 0.001$, IVT: $R = 0.41$, $p = 0.004$). Moreover, segments with higher thermal heterogeneity measured by both methods had also higher inflammatory cell (density lymphocytes and mast cells) (Fig. 16.6) (42).

The method is also currently under clinical evaluation in human carotid arteries. A recent study of a group of 60 patients (30 patients with atherosclerosis in one or both carotid arteries and 30 subjects with normal carotid arteries matched by sex and age), showed that thermal heterogeneity detected by microwave thermography along the atherosclerotic carotid arteries was significantly higher compared to that detected in controls (1.32 ± 0.55°C vs. 0.39 ± 0.18°C, $p < 0.001$). All patients were also evaluated by ultrasound echo-color Doppler (US-ECD) study of both carotid arteries and subsequent association of thermographic and ultrasound findings were performed. Among carotid arteries with atherosclerosis, fatty plaques (43.3%) had higher ΔT compared to mixed (23.3%) and calcified (33.3%) ones (1.78 ± 0.54°C vs. 1.09 ± 0.17°C vs. 0.88 ± 0.16°C, accordingly, $p < 0.01$ for all comparisons). Plaques with an ulcerated surface (23.33%) had higher ΔT compared to plaques with irregular (30%) and regular surfaces (23.3%) (2.07 ± 0.59°C vs. 1.32 ± 0.21°C vs. 0.94 ± 0.18°C, accordingly, $p < 0.01$ for all comparisons). Heterogenous plaques (70%) had higher ΔT compared to homogenous (30%) (1.52 ± 0.53°C vs. 0.83 ± 0.13°C, $p < 0.01$) (43). Further clinical evaluation is needed to validate the clinical application of this promising method.

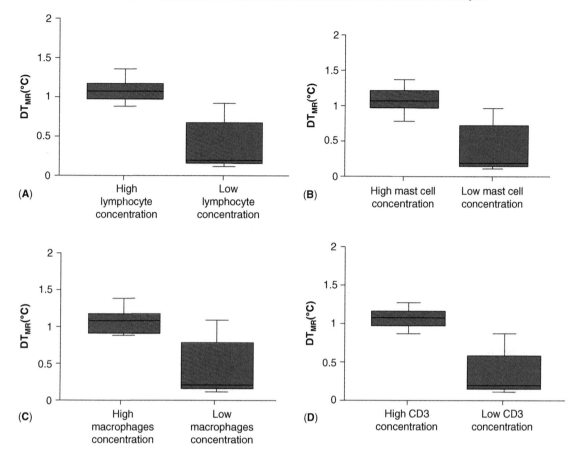

Figure 16.6 Temperature differences by microwave radiometry (ΔT MR (°C)) in segments with intense versus low expression of inflammatory indexes. (A) Intense versus low expression of lymphocyte concentration. (B) Intense versus low expression of mast cell concentration. (C) Intense versus low expression of macrophage concentration (CD68). (D) Intense versus low expression of CD3.

Focus Box 16.1

- Inflammation plays a crucial role not only in initiation and propagation, but also in development of acute complications of atherosclerosis
- Temperature heterogeneity assessed by intracoronary thermography devices along the inner surface of a coronary artery may be a surrogate marker of impending plaque rupture and has been associated with an increased likelihood of future coronary events
- The potential development of a combination technique including intracoronary thermography and IVUS or OCT will hopefully lead to the (*i*) early and (*ii*) accurate detection of inflamed plaques
- Although intracoronary thermography provided important information regarding the functional characteristics of the vulnerable plaque, its clinical application has several shortcomings, and most of them are due to its invasive character
- The new non-invasive technique of microwave radiometry reveals itself as a promising method for the in vivo measurement of thermal heterogeneity indicating plaque inflammation

REFERENCES

1. World Health Organization. Cardiovascular diseases. Fact sheet N°317. [Available from: http://www.who.int/mediacentre/factsheets/fs317/en/2011] [Assessed January 2011].
2. Honda Y, Fitzgerald PJ. Frontiers in intravascular imaging technologies. Circulation 2008; 117: 2024–37.
3. Naghavi M, Falk E, Hecht HS, et al. From vulnerable plaque to vulnerable patient–Part III. Executive summary of the Screening for Heart Attack Prevention and Education (SHAPE) Task Force report. Am J Cardiol 2006; 98: 2H–15H.
4. Naghavi M, Libby P, Falk E, et al. From vulnerable plaque to vulnerable patient: a call for new definitions and risk assessment strategies: part I. Circulation 2003; 108: 1664–72.
5. Stone GW, Maehara A, Lansky AJ, et al. A prospective natural-history study of coronary atherosclerosis. N Engl J Med 2011; 364: 226–35.
6. Libby P, Ridker PM, Hansson GK. Inflammation in atherosclerosis: from pathophysiology to practice. J Am Coll Cardiol 2009; 54: 2129–38.
7. Lilledahl MB, Larsen EL, Svaasand LO. An analytic and numerical study of intravascular thermography of vulnerable plaque. Phys Med Biol 2007; 52: 961–79.
8. Hamdan A, Assali A, Fuchs S, Battler A, Kornowski R. Imaging of vulnerable coronary artery plaques. Catheter Cardiovasc Interv 2007; 70: 65–74.

9. Verheye S, De Meyer GR, Van Langenhove G, Knaapen MW, Kockx MM. In vivo temperature heterogeneity of atherosclerotic plaques is determined by plaque composition. Circulation 2002; 105: 1596–601.

10. Naghavi M, Madjid M, Gul K, et al. Thermography basket catheter: in vivo measurement of the temperature of atherosclerotic plaques for detection of vulnerable plaques. Catheter Cardiovasc Interv 2003; 59: 52–9.

11. Verheye S, De Meyer GR, Krams R, et al. Intravascular thermography: immediate functional and morphological vascular findings. Eur Heart J 2004; 25: 158–65.

12. Krams R, Verheye S, van Damme LC, et al. In vivo temperature heterogeneity is associated with plaque regions of increased MMP-9 activity. Eur Heart J 2005; 26: 2200–5.

13. Zarrabi A, Gul K, Willerson JT, Casscells W, Naghavi M. Intravascular thermography: a novel approach for detection of vulnerable plaque. Curr Opin Cardiol 2002; 17: 656–62.

14. Toutouzas K, Markou V, Drakopoulou M, et al. Increased heat generation from atherosclerotic plaques in patients with type 2 diabetes: an increased local inflammatory activation. Diabetes Care 2005; 28: 1656–61.

15. Toutouzas K, Drakopoulou M, Stefanadi E, Siasos G, Stefanadis C. Intracoronary thermography: does it help us in clinical decision making? J Interv Cardiol 2005; 18: 485–9.

16. Stefanadis C, Toutouzas K, Vavuranakis M, et al. Statin treatment is associated with reduced thermal heterogeneity in human atherosclerotic plaques. Eur Heart J 2002; 23: 1664–9.

17. Stefanadis C, Toutouzas K, Tsiamis E, et al. Increased local temperature in human coronary atherosclerotic plaques: an independent predictor of clinical outcome in patients undergoing a percutaneous coronary intervention. J Am Coll Cardiol 2001; 37: 1277–83.

18. Stefanadis C, Diamantopoulos L, Vlachopoulos C, et al. Thermal heterogeneity within human atherosclerotic coronary arteries detected in vivo: a new method of detection by application of a special thermography catheter. Circulation 1999; 99: 1965–71.

19. Toutouzas K, Vaina S, Tsiamis E, et al. Detection of increased temperature of the culprit lesion after recent myocardial infarction: the favorable effect of statins. Am Heart J 2004; 148: 783–8.

20. Toutouzas K, Tsiamis E, Drakopoulou M, et al. Impact of type 2 diabetes mellitus on diffuse inflammatory activation of de novo atheromatous lesions: implications for systemic inflammation. Diabetes Metab 2009; 35: 299–304.

21. Toutouzas K, Synetos A, Stefanadi E, et al. Correlation between morphologic characteristics and local temperature differences in culprit lesions of patients with symptomatic coronary artery disease. J Am Coll Cardiol 2007; 49: 2264–71.

22. Wainstein M, Costa M, Ribeiro J, Zago A, Rogers C. Vulnerable plaque detection by temperature heterogeneity measured with a guidewire system: clinical, intravascular ultrasound and histopathologic correlates. J Invasive Cardiol 2007; 19: 49–54.

23. Schmermund A, Rodermann J, Erbel R. Intracoronary thermography. Herz 2003; 28: 505–12.

24. Dudek D, Rzeszutko L, Legutko J, et al. High-risk coronary artery plaques diagnosed by intracoronary thermography. Kardiol Pol 2005; 62: 383–9.

25. Cuisset T, Beauloye C, Melikian N, et al. In vitro and in vivo studies on thermistor-based intracoronary temperature measurements: effect of pressure and flow. Catheter Cardiovasc Interv 2009; 73: 224–30.

26. Worthley S, Farouque MO, Worthley M, et al. The RADI PressureWire high-sensitivity thermistor and culprit lesion temperature in patients with acute coronary syndromes. J Invasive Cardiol 2006; 18: 528–31.

27. Takumi T, Lee S, Hamasaki S, et al. Limitation of angiography to identify the culprit plaque in acute myocardial infarction with coronary total occlusion utility of coronary plaque temperature measurement to identify the culprit plaque. J Am Coll Cardiol 2007; 50: 2197–203.

28. Stefanadis C, Toutouzas K, Vavuranakis M, et al. New balloon-thermography catheter for in vivo temperature measurements in human coronary atherosclerotic plaques: a novel approach for thermography? Catheter Cardiovasc Interv 2003; 58: 344–50.

29. Stefanadis C, Toutouzas K, Tsiamis E, et al. Thermal heterogeneity in stable human coronary atherosclerotic plaques is underestimated in vivo: the "cooling effect" of blood flow. J Am Coll Cardiol 2003; 41: 403–8.

30. Courtney BK, Nakamura M, Tsugita R, et al. Validation of a thermographic guidewire for endoluminal mapping of atherosclerotic disease: an in vitro study. Catheter Cardiovasc Interv 2004; 62: 221–9.

31. ten Have AG, Gijsen FJ, Wentzel JJ, et al. Temperature distribution in atherosclerotic coronary arteries: influence of plaque geometry and flow (a numerical study). Phys Med Biol 2004; 49: 4447–62.

32. Belardi JA, Albertal M, Cura FA, et al. Intravascular thermographic assessment in human coronary atherosclerotic plaques by a novel flow-occluding sensing catheter: a safety and feasibility study. J Invasive Cardiol 2005; 17: 663–6.

33. Yasuhiro H, Fitzgerald PJ. Frontiers in intravascular imaging technologies. Circulation 2008; 117: 2024–37.

34. Tearney GL, Yabushita H, Houser SL, et al. Quantification of macrophage content in atherosclerotic plaques by optical coherence tomography. Circulation 2006; 107: 113–9.

35. Toutouzas K, Riga M, Vaina S, et al. in acute coronary syndromes thin fibrous cap and ruptured plaques are associated with increased local inflammatory activation: a Combination of Intravascular Optical Coherence Tomography and Intracoronary Thermography Study. J Am Coll Cardiol 2008; 51: 1033.

36. Toutouzas K, Markou V, Drakopoulou M, et al. Patients with type two diabetes mellitus: increased local inflammatory activation in culprit atheromatous plaques. Hellenic J Cardiol 2005; 46: 283–8.

37. Webster M, Stewart J, Ruygrok P. Intracoronary thermography with a multiple thermocouple catheter: initial human experience. Am J Cardiol 2002: 90.

38. Toutouzas K, Drakopoulou M, Mitropoulos J, et al. Elevated plaque temperature in non-culprit de novo atheromatous lesions of patients with acute coronary syndromes. J Am Coll Cardiol 2006; 47: 301–6.

39. Stefanadis C, Diamantopoulos L, Dernellis J, et al. Heat production of atherosclerotic plaques and inflammation assessed by the acute phase proteins in acute coronary syndromes. J Mol Cell Cardiol 2000; 32: 43–52.

40. Toutouzas K, Drakopoulou M, Markou V, et al. Correlation of systemic inflammation with local inflammatory activity in non-culprit lesions: Beneficial effect of statins. Int J of Cardiol 2007; 119: 368–73.

41. Toutouzas K, Drakopoulou M, Markou V, et al. Increased coronary sinus blood temperature: correlation with systemic inflammation. Eur J Clin Invest 2006; 36: 218–23.

42. Toutouzas K, Grassos H, Synetos A, et al. A new non-invasive method for detection of local inflammation in atherosclerotic plaques: experimental application of microwave radiometry. Atherosclerosis 2011; 215: 82–9.

43. Toutouzas K, Grassos C, Drakopoulou M, et al. First in vivo application of microwave radiometry in human carotids: a new noninvasive method for detection of local inflammatory activation. J Am Coll Cardiol 2012; 59: 1645–53.

44. Stefanadis C, Tsiamis E, Vaina S, et al. Temperature of blood in the coronary sinus and right atrium in patients with and without coronary artery disease. Am J Cardiol 2004; 93: 207–10.

45. Rzeszutko L, Legutko J, Kaluza GL, et al. Assessment of culprit plaque temperature by intracoronary thermography appears inconclusive in patients with acute coronary syndromes. Arterioscler Thromb Vasc Biol 2006; 26: 1889–94.

17 Imaging of structure and composition of lipid core plaque with a combination NIRS-IVUS system: Current status and potential clinical applications

Emmanouil S. Brilakis, Zhihua He, Stephen T. Sum, Sean P. Madden, and James E. Muller

OUTLINE

Intracoronary near-infrared spectroscopy with intravascular ultrasonography (NIRS-IVUS) is a novel catheter-based combination technique that allows determination of both the structure and chemical composition of the coronary artery wall. This is accomplished by evaluating coronary anatomy by using intravascular ultrasonography and also measuring the proportion of near-infrared light diffusely reflected by the arterial wall after scattering and absorption have occurred. Histology and clinical studies have validated that NIRS can detect with high accuracy the presence of coronary lipid core plaques (LCPs) that form the substrate for a majority of acute coronary syndromes (ACSs) and complicate stenting procedures. Coronary NIRS-IVUS can be used to (*i*) risk stratify and optimize the outcomes of percutaneous coronary intervention (PCI), (*ii*) identify coronary lesions at risk for causing events and optimize their management, and (*iii*) evaluate novel anti-atherosclerotic treatments.

INTRODUCTION

The cause of most of the ACS is believed to be thrombosis in the coronary arteries resulting from rupture of a lipid-rich, necrotic core plaque with a thin fibrous cap (1,2). Unfortunately, the detection of such high-risk LCPs by vascular imaging techniques has been inadequate.

Over the last five decades, coronary angiography has been the primary diagnostic imaging method for assessing coronary artery disease (CAD) (3,4). This X-ray imaging modality provides an overall view of the coronary vasculature with respect to stenosis and luminal surface irregularity, presenting a map of potentially atherosclerotic regions. The angiogram, however, is significantly limited by the lack of information about the vessel wall regarding the structure and composition of the coronary plaque.

Numerous intravascular imaging methods have been developed to improve the assessment of CAD over angiography (5–19). Broadly speaking, the fundamental basis of each method can be categorized as either acquiring structural or compositional information. Methods for probing structure include intravascular ultrasound (IVUS), angioscopy, optical coherence tomography (OCT), and optical frequency domain imaging (OFDI) (10–13). Methods that can specifically assess composition include Raman spectroscopy (14,15) and near-infrared pectroscopy (NIRS). Hybrid methods attempting to extract compositional information from subtle characteristics of acoustic signals include IVUS virtual histology, integrated backscatter, elastography, and palpography

(5–9). The striking high-resolution structure achievable with OCT and OFDI can allow interpretation of structures consistent with certain composition. And colorimetry with angioscopy may offer some clues to plaque composition. While offering a number of advantages over angiography for plaque characterization, each modality possesses its own limitations (16–19). Table 17.1 summarizes the strengths and weaknesses of the different intra-coronary imaging methods (modified from Maehara et al. (20)).

NIRS in cardiovascular imaging analyzes the light reflected in a range of wavelengths to determine the chemical composition of tissue, including lipids such as cholesterol and cholesteryl esters. IVUS imaging maps the acoustic echo of the vessel wall, providing structural information such as lumen and vessel dimensions, plaque morphometry, vessel remodeling, side-branching, and stent strut expansion and apposition. This chapter describes a new dual-modality cardiovascular imaging system that combines NIRS and IVUS imaging in a single catheter. The chapter explains the basic principles of NIRS technology, delineates the rationale for the intravascular use of NIRS, summarizes the studies performed to validate NIRS detection of LCPs, and discusses the potential research and clinical utility of an NIRS-IVUS combination system.

PRINCIPLES OF DIFFUSE REFLECTANCE NEAR-INFRARED SPECTROSCOPY

In diffuse reflectance NIRS, light from the near-infrared region of the electromagnetic spectrum (approximately 800–2500 nm) is directed to a sample and the diffusely reflected light is collected. The proportion of light returned from the sample is dependent on wavelength and is a function of both scattering and absorption processes. Scattering occurs when light is randomly reflected by cellular and extracellular structures in the sample, while absorption results from the transformation of light into molecular energy primarily in the form of molecular vibrations of atoms about their chemical bonds. The infrared light used in this type of spectroscopy is termed 'near' due to the proximity of the near-infrared wavelength range to the visible region of the electromagnetic spectrum (mid- and far-infrared regions occur at wavelengths greater than 2500 nm) (Fig. 17.1).

With little to no sample preparation, NIRS provides direct and rapid measurements for qualitative and quantitative compositional analysis in an array of applications. Although NIRS spectral bands tend to be rather broad and featureless compared to those of the 'fingerprint' region of the mid-infrared, the near-infrared region is more appropriate for measurement due

Table 17.1 Strengths and Weaknesses of Intravascular Imaging Methods for Coronary Plaque Characterization and PCI

	Angiography	IVUS (40 MHz)	IVUS-VH (20 MHz)	Angioscopy	OCT/OFDI	Raman Spectroscopy	Near-Infrared Spectroscopy	NIRS-IVUS (40 MHz)
Axial resolution, μm	NA	100	200	10–50	10	NA	NA	100
Necrotic core	–	±	+	+	+	+	++	++
Calcium	–	++	++	–	++	–	–	++
Thin cap	–	±	+	+	++	–	*	*
Thrombus	±	±	–	++	+	–	*	*
Inflammation	–	–	–	–	±	–	–	–
Expansive remodeling	–	++	++	–	–	–	–	++
Measurement through blood	++	++	++	–	–	–	+	++
Stent tissue coverage	–	+	+	++	++	–	–	+
PCI (stent expansion and complications)	+	++	±	±	++	–	–	++

++, excellent; +, good; ±, possible; –, impossible; *, potential under investigation. *Abbreviations*: PCI, percutaneous coronary intervention; OCT, optical coherence tomography; OFDI, Optical Frequency Domain Imaging.
Source: Adapted from Ref. 20.

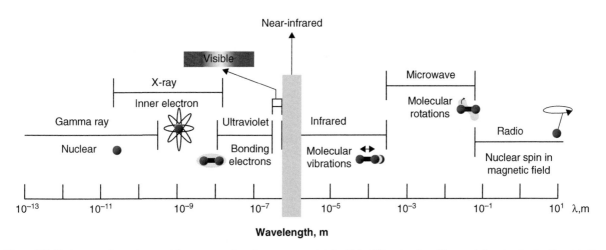

Figure 17.1 Electromagnetic spectrum and the energy-matter phenomena associated with its different regions. The near-infrared region is adjacent to the visible region at approximately 800–2500 nm.

to the relatively low water absorption, allowing NIRS to penetrate materials at depths suitable for analysis. NIRS has been widely adopted in many different areas including agriculture, food, petroleum, astronomy, pharmaceuticals, and medicine (21,22).

The broad-featured NIRS spectra of complex, multi-constituent samples are difficult to visually interpret, and thus require multivariate mathematical methods of analysis. The analysis is accomplished by mathematical modeling using calibration samples whose chemical and physical properties span the expected range of future samples. Reference values for the target components in these samples are obtained by an independent analytical method (e.g., histology). Models constructed from the calibration samples correlate the measured NIRS signals with the reference values, allowing qualitative or quantitative determination of unknown samples based on their NIRS spectra (23).

INTRAVASCULAR IMAGING USING NEAR-INFRARED SPECTROSCOPY

Rationale for Intravascular Near-Infrared Spectroscopy

NIRS is well-suited for the intravascular detection of LCPs in coronary vessels for a number of reasons. First, fiber optics can be used in a diagnostic cardiac catheter to deliver and collect near-infrared light in the coronary arteries. By coupling the catheter with a pullback and rotation device, the entire circumferential and longitudinal extent of the vessel can be scanned. Second, the low absorption of near-infrared light by water permits the light to penetrate blood and tissue at depths of several millimeters. The ability to transmit near-infrared light through flowing blood obviates the need to directly contact tissue or to clear the field of view with a saline flush or vessel occlusion. The ability to identify chemical components allows the detection of compositional features (e.g., lipid) characteristic of plaque. Finally, the use of an ultrafast laser as a near-infrared light source allows rapid generation and acquisition of spectra, thereby minimizing cardiac motion artifacts in the measurements. The NIRS catheter was demonstrated in the SPECTACL trial (NCT00330928) to have a similar safety profile as commercial IVUS catheters and since FDA approval, the catheter has been used safely in over 1500 patients.

Validation of LCP Detection by Near-Infrared Spectroscopy

The first studies in the application of NIRS to intravascular imaging of atherosclerosis employed off-the-shelf spectroscopic systems. A number of early investigators demonstrated that NIRS could detect cholesterol and collagen in rabbit and human aortic tissue (24–30). Other investigators also explored lipid detection by NIRS in human carotid and coronary tissue (31–33). In later studies, prototype NIRS intravascular diagnostic systems were developed and tested to assess the feasibility of lipid-rich plaque detection through variable blood depths in human aortic and coronary tissue (34–39).

The detection of LCPs by NIRS was validated in a large *ex vivo* study with human coronary autopsy specimens (40). For this study, arterial segments were scanned and then cut into 2-mm-thick cross-sectional blocks for histopathological analysis. The NIRS spectra and histological data were collected in a total of 84 autopsy hearts and 216 segments to build and validate an algorithm capable of automatically recognizing the NIRS spectral signals associated with LCPs.

The prospective validation was double-blinded with respect to both collection of the validation data and development of the algorithm. Prospective validation of the system for detection of LCPs in nearly 2000 individual blocks from 51 hearts yielded an area under the receiver operating characteristic (ROC) curve (AUC) of 0.80 for average lumen diameters of up to 3.0 mm. The detection of fibroatheroma of any size in an artery segment using the LCBI as a measure of lipid burden resulted in an AUC of 0.86 (40).

In order to develop and evaluate the LCP detection algorithm, a definition of LCP of interest was established. Specifically, LCP was defined as a fibroatheroma containing a necrotic core at least 200-μm thick with a circumferential span of at least 60 degrees on cross-section. The primary endpoint of the algorithm validation was the accuracy of detecting LCPs meeting this definition.

The LCP detection algorithm was also validated *in vivo* in several clinical studies. The first clinical studies demonstrated that spectra could be safely collected in patients and that these spectra carried information from the artery wall (2002 and 2006, Lahey Clinic, Burlington, MA). A subsequent pivotal study called SPECTroscopic Assessment of Coronary Lipid (SPECTACL) was performed to collect spectra in patients (in whom tissue is not available for validation) and show that these spectra were equivalent to the spectra recorded in autopsy specimens (in which histology was available for validation). This multicenter study showed prospectively that the spectral features of coronary arteries in patients were substantially equivalent to those of autopsy specimens. Demonstration of spectral similarity between NIRS measurements collected *in vivo* and *ex vivo* showed the applicability of the autopsy tissue-based LCP detection algorithm to patients (41).

More recently, in a prospective correlation study of NIRS with IVUS and coronary computed tomography angiography, good correlation was observed between the location of noncalcified plaques in computed tomography and VH-IVUS and cholesterol on NIRS. Plaque burden by computed tomography angiography correlated well with cholesterol deposition by NIRS (24). Noncalcified plaques, as well as low-and high-density noncalcified plaques, also correlated well with cholesterol on NIRS (24).

Near-Infrared–Intravascular Ultrasound Combination System

A clinical NIRS-IVUS system (TVC Imaging System, InfraReDx, Inc., Burlington, MA) consists of a console, a pullback and rotation device (Nexus™ controller), and an intravascular catheter (Fig. 17.2) (25). The console comprises a near-infrared scanning laser, computer, and power system, as well as two monitors (for operator and physician). The Nexus™ controller contains the electronic, optical, and mechanical components for delivering and detecting ultrasound and near-infrared light signals, as well as translating and rotating the imaging core of the catheter. The 3.2-Fr rapid exchange catheter consists of a tip with a 40-MHz ultrasound transducer and two mirrors, a core with two optical fibers, and a coax cable inside a drive cable. The delivery and collection fibers in the core are terminated by mirrors embedded in the tip for directing incident light through blood onto the artery wall and receiving the diffusely reflected light. The coax cable transmits and receives the electrical signal to and from the ultrasound transducer.

The catheter imaging core rotates at 960 rpm with automated pullback at a linear rate of 0.5 mm/s, interrogating tissue in a helical pattern. During rotation and pullback, the near-infrared laser scans across multiple wavelengths while the pulser simultaneously drives the ultrasound transducer. NIRS signals are generated at a rate of approximately 160 spectra per second, while ultrasound A-lines are created at 256 lines per frame.

In the NIRS modality, the resulting spectra are processed and interpreted by the LCP detection algorithm to generate a longitudinal image (chemogram) of the scanned artery segment (Fig. 17.3). Each spectral measurement is assigned a probability of LCP by the detection algorithm and displayed in a false color map known as a chemogram (Fig. 17.3A) with colors ranging from red (low probability of LCP) to yellow (high probability of LCP). From the chemogram, a summary metric of the probability that an LCP is present in a 2-mm interval of the pullback is computed and displayed in a supplementary false color map called a block chemogram (Fig. 17.3B). Blocks correspond to one of four discrete bins, each represented by a distinct color (red, orange, tan, and yellow, in increasing order of LCP probability).

An additional metric, the lipid core burden index (LCBI), quantifies the amount of LCPs in a scanned artery segment. The LCBI is defined as the proportion of yellow pixels in the chemogram on a scale of 0 to 1000. Figure 17.4 illustrates the computation of the LCBI.

In the IVUS component of the device, the transverse and longitudinal grayscale images are processed and displayed on the system monitor. The transverse IVUS image is overlaid with a chemogram ring taken from the corresponding longitudinal location in the chemogram. In addition, the longitudinal IVUS image is aligned with the chemogram and block chemogram (Fig. 17.2).

The principal strength of the NIRS-IVUS system is its ability to determine both the chemical composition and the structure of the artery wall through blood by simultaneously collecting co-registered NIRS and IVUS data in a single catheter pullback, rendering the system particularly well-suited for the detection of LCPs.

RESEARCH AND CLINICAL UTILITY OF THE NEAR-INFRARED SPECTROSCOPY AND INTRAVASCULAR ULTRASOUND CATHETER

Based on the results of the autopsy validation (40) and the demonstration of similarity between clinical and autopsy spectra (41), coronary NIRS was approved by the US Food and Drug Administration (FDA) for clinical use in the United States in April 2008 (26) for the detection of lipid core containing plaques of interest (LCP) and the assessment of lipid core burden in coronary arteries. The combination NIRS-IVUS system was approved by the FDA in June 2010. As of May 2011, the NIRS and NIRS-IVUS systems have been used in 2000 patients in 32 hospitals in the United States and the Netherlands.

The NIRS-IVUS catheter offers all the advantages of IVUS imaging and, in addition, provides easily interpretable information on vessel wall composition. It also has multiple clinical applications that are currently under investigation: (1) guiding PCI (2), identifying 'vulnerable' coronary lesions at risk for causing events and optimizing the medical management of such patients, and (3) evaluating novel anti-atherosclerotic treatments.

Optimization of PCI Outcomes

IVUS is currently routinely used in cardiac catheterization laboratories. IVUS imaging can assist with (1) evaluating whether pre-treatment of a coronary lesion is indicated, for example, in vessel with heavy calcification; (2) determining the optimum stent diameter and length for use in a specific target coronary lesion, by measuring the proximal and distal lumen reference diameter and the lesion length; (3) evaluating whether adequate stent expansion and stent strut apposition has been achieved; and (4) detecting the presence of edge

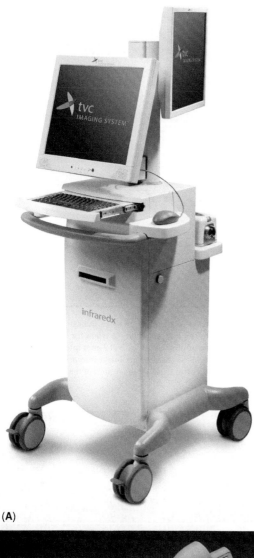

(A)

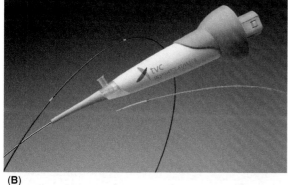

(B)

Figure 17.2 TVC combination NIRS and IVUS system. (**A**) The console includes two touch-screen monitors (for operator and physician) displaying the NIRS chemogram and IVUS images (*transverse* and *longitudinal*). (**B**) The catheter contains fiber optics and mirrors for near-infrared light, as well as a coax cable and a transducer for ultrasound.

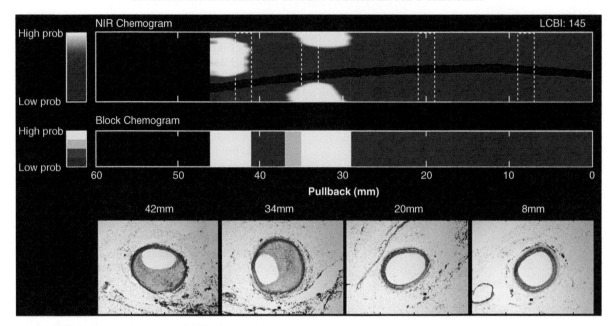

Figure 17.3 NIRS pullback and selected histologic findings from human coronary artery segment. (A) Chemogram image indicating LCP content by NIRS (*x*-axis = pullback distance in mm, *y*-axis = rotation angle in degrees). Pixel colors range from red for low probability to yellow for high probability of LCPs. Contiguous black region is guidewire. (B) Block chemogram image indicating summary metric of presence of LCPs at 2-mm intervals in four probability categories. (C) Movat cross-sections from locations along the artery indicated by dotted boxes in the chemogram. Image interpretation: The chemogram shows large LCP signals from 29 to 37 mm and from 41 to 46 mm. The block chemogram indicates that these are the regions of the strongest signals. Histology confirms the presence of fibroatheroma at these locations.

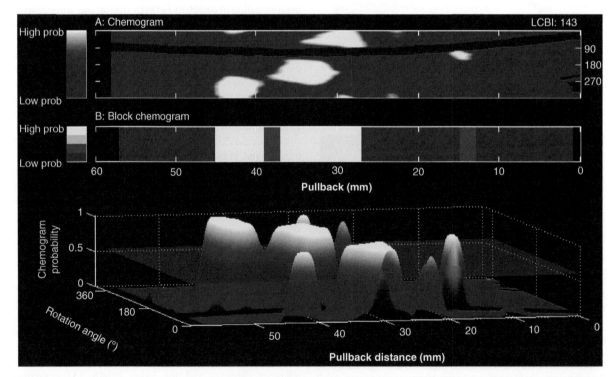

Figure 17.4 Illustration of the lipid core burden index (LCBI). The LCBI (*top right*) shows the proportion of lipid in a scanned artery on a 0–1,000 scale. The LCBI is calculated as the fraction of valid pixels in the chemogram that are yellow, multiplied by a factor of 1000. Yellow pixels are those whose values (probability of LCP) exceed a specified threshold, as indicated by the horizontal plane in the bottom panel.

dissection or possibly thrombus formation within a stent. Although not proven by a large randomized clinical trial, several retrospective studies have demonstrated that IVUS imaging may reduce the risk of in-stent restenosis or stent thrombosis (27,28).

The addition of NIRS can enhance the value of IVUS imaging for optimizing PCI results by (*i*) allowing easy and accurate prediction of the risk of peri-procedural complications, such as no-reflow and peri-procedural acute myocardial infarction (AMI) and (*ii*) helping to prevent such complications

Prediction of Post-PCI Complications

The safety and efficacy of PCI has markedly improved since 1977, yet complications such as peri-procedural myocardial infarction (MI) (29), distal embolization, in-stent restenosis, and stent thrombosis continued to occur (30).

Several reports have shown that PCI of a large LCP, as detected by NIRS, may be complicated by distal embolization and post-PCI MI (31–35).

Raghunathan et al. examined the association between the presence and extent of coronary LCPs detected by NIRS performed prior to PCI with post-procedural MI in 30 patients (35). Compared to patients who did not have post-PCI MI, those who did had similar clinical characteristics but received more stents and had more yellow blocks within the stented lesion. CK-MB level elevation >3× the upper limit of normal

was observed in 27% of patients with at least one yellow block vs. no patient without a yellow block within the stented lesion (*p* = 0.02). Similarly, Goldstein et al. examined 62 patients undergoing PCI from the COLOR registry (36). Peri-procedural MI was documented in 9/62 (14.5%) of cases. A maxLCBI4 mm of ≥500 identified seven patients in whom the risk of peri-procedural MI was 50%. Therefore, stenting of lipid-containing lesions is associated with an increased risk of post-procedural MI and that NIRS could help identify lesions that might benefit from aggressive preventive strategies.

Wood et al. demonstrated that ostial saphenous vein graft (SVG) lesions were less likely to have LCPs, as detected by NIRS, compared to body lesions (Fig. 17.5) (37). This finding could explain the lower likelihood of distal embolization and peri-procedural MI with treatment of ostial SVG lesions than body lesions (38,39).

Selvanaygam et al. used cardiac magnetic resonance imaging before and after PCI in 50 patients and described two patterns of myocardial injury: one adjacent to the area of stent, presumably due to epicardial side branch occlusion and one involving the

---

Focus Box 17.1

NIRS-IVUS is a powerful tool for prediction of the risk of myocardial infarction post PCI

Segment LCBI = 6 **Segment LCBI = 307**

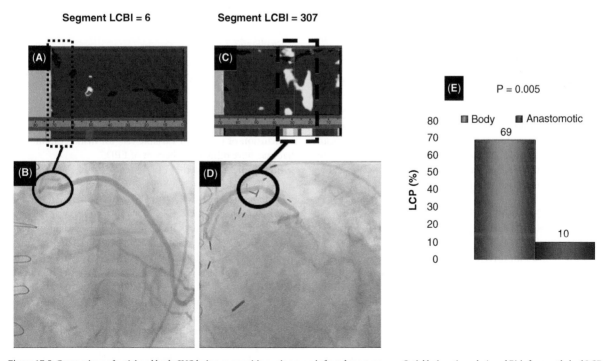

Figure 17.5 Comparison of ostial and body SVG lesion composition using near-infrared spectroscopy. Ostial lesions (panels A and B) infrequently had LCP, whereas the majority of body lesions (panels C and D) had LCP (panel E) (37). *Abbreviations*: LCBI, lipid core burden index; LCP, lipid core plaque.

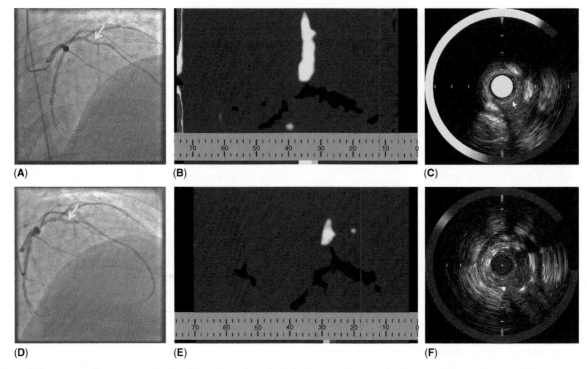

Figure 17.6 A 67-year-old man presented with stable angina and anterior ischemia on nuclear stress imaging. Diagnostic angiography demonstrated a mid left anterior descending artery lesion (*arrow*, panel A) between the first diagonal and first septal perforator artery, containing LCP (panels **B** and **C**). The lesion resolved after implantation of a 3.0 × 18 mm sirolimus-eluting stents (*arrow*, panel D) with significant reduction in the amount of the LCP (panels **E** and **F**).

distal myocardial segment supplied by the target coronary artery, likely due to distal embolization (42). NIRS may help in predicting both types of peri-procedural myocardial injury. First, PCI of large LCP lesions may cause plaque shift and side branch occlusion. This is currently being evaluated in the Lipid Core Shift Study (NCT00905671). Second, PCI of large LCPs may be more likely to result in release of debris and distal embolization. This is supported by studies showing a significant decrease in LCBI post stenting (Fig. 17.6) (43) and a high frequency of debris retrieval when a distal embolic protection device (EPD) is used during PCI (44).

Prevention of Post-PCI Complications

How can NIRS-IVUS help prevent or treat distal embolization? Although using a distal embolic protection device (EPD) appears to be an intuitive technique to prevent distal embolization, it was not beneficial in several trials of primary PCI for acute MI patients, such as the Enhanced Myocardial Efficacy and Removal by Aspiration of Liberalized Debris—EMERALD trial (45), the Drug Elution and Distal Protection in ST-Elevation Myocardial Infarction—DEDICATION trial (46), and the UpFlow MI trial. As a result, the use of EPD is currently only approved for use in the United States for SVG lesions (47). The lack of benefit, however, may have been due

Focus Box 17.2

Percutaneous coronary intervention of large LCP lesions carries high risk for distal embolization and in-stent thrombus formation

to inclusion of lesions of variable risk for distal embolization that may have diluted the benefit of EPD.

Pilot studies suggest that EPDs may be beneficial when used during PCI of LCP-rich lesions. Abdel-karim et al. reported the outcomes of EPD use in nine patients who underwent PCI of lesions with large LCPs (Fig. 17.7) (44). Debris was retrieved in eight of nine lesions. The debris mainly consisted of fibrin and platelet aggregates, but not lipids and macrophages, possibly due to the histologic preparation process. The mean target segment LCBI decreased from 395 ± 114 before stenting to 152 ± 106 after stenting ($p < 0.001$) and the lesion angular extent decreased from $312 \pm 70°$ to $240 \pm 90°$ ($p = 0.07$). The mean target vessel LCBI decreased from 173 ± 68 before stenting to 75 ± 25 after stenting (p = 0.04). Post-PCI MI occurred in two patients (22%), in one of whom two filters were required because of significant debris distal embolization causing 'clogging' of the filter.

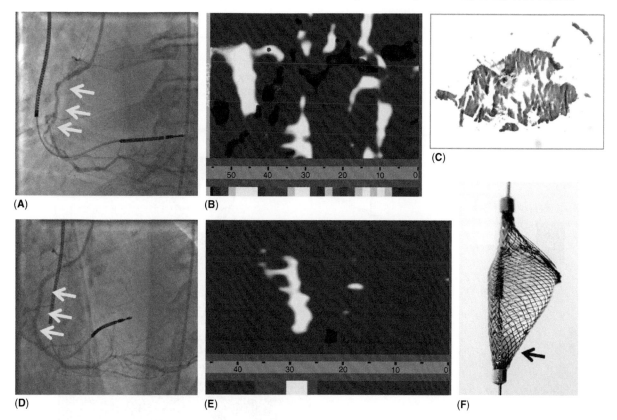

Figure 17.7 Example of distal embolization in a patient undergoing PCI. Coronary angiography demonstrated a severe right coronary artery lesion (panel A) with large LCP by near-infrared spectroscopy (panel B). Stenting of the right coronary artery was performed using a Spider (ev3, Plymouth Minnesota) filter. After stenting, the right coronary artery lesion resolved (panel D) with a marked reduction in the size of LCP (panel E). Debris was retrieved in the filter (that retrieved debris (*arrow*, panel F) that was shown to be composed of fibrin on histologic examination (panel C).

Papayannis et al. also reported that stenting of large lipid plaques (defined as at least three 2-mm yellow blocks on the NIRS block chemogram with >200 angular extent) was more likely to lead to in-stent thrombus formation (as detected by OCT) compared to stenting coronary lesions without large LCPs (48). Two of three patients with a large LCP (66%) developed intra-stent thrombus post stent implantation (Fig. 17.8) compared to none of six patients without large LCPs (0%, $p = 0.02$). This may be due to the high thrombogenicity of the lipid core with direct activation of platelets by the oxidized lipids, as well as the high content of active tissue factor in the lipid core, that can trigger the extrinsic clotting cascade (49). It is possible that the thrombus formed within the stent subsequently embolizes, and EPD use may prevent embolization not only of the LCP but also of the platelet or fibrin thrombus. Alternatively, more intensive antiplatelet and antithrombotic strategies could be utilized to prevent thrombus formation, such as administration of glycoprotein IIb/IIIa inhibitors when stenting lesions containing large LCPs.

The ability of NIRS to identify lesions at high risk of periprocedural rupture and distal embolization and the mitigation

Focus Box 17.3

Incomplete stent coverage of LCP lesions may be a predisposing factor for stent thrombosis

of this risk with an embolic protection device is currently being tested in the prospective, randomized Coronary Assessment by Near-infrared of Atherosclerotic Rupture-prone Yellow (CANARY NCT01268319) trial (Fig. 17.9). In the CANARY trial, patients found to be having large LCPs in a native coronary artery are randomized to either use of a Filterwire (Boston Scientific, Natick, Massachusetts) or placebo.

When drug-eluting stents (DES) are currently used for PCI, the operators usually attempt to cover from a proximal to a distal normal reference segment. However, occasionally these angiographically 'normal' sites may contain a large amount of LCPs that do not compromise the lumen due to positive remodeling. Disruption or incomplete coverage of such plaques could lead to stent thrombosis (50,51). Sakhuja et al. reported a case of acute stent thrombosis in a patient who underwent right

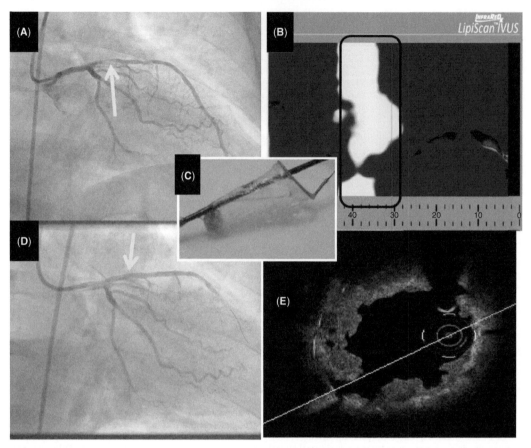

Figure 17.8 Example of in-stent thrombus formation post stenting of a large LCP. Coronary angiography showing a proximal left anterior descending artery lesion (*arrow*, panel **A**) due to a large circumferential LCP, as detected by near-infrared spectroscopy (panel **B**). Stenting was performed after insertion of a Filterwire (Boston Scientific, Natick, Massachusetts), resulting in yellow debris retrieval (panel **C**). In spite of an initially successful result (panel **D**), in-stent thrombus subsequently formed, confirmed by optical coherence tomography (panel **E**).

coronary stenting, in whom a large LCP was shown by NIRS imaging to extend proximal to the proximal stent edge (51). Use of coronary NIRS could aid selection of the appropriate stent length for complete lesion and adjacent LCP coverage that may help minimize the risk for stent thrombosis.

Identification of High-Risk Coronary Lesions and Optimization of Medical Management

The natural history of non-obstructive coronary artery lesions remains poorly studied. The Providing Regional Observations to Study Predictors of Events in the Coronary Tree (PROSPECT) study followed up 697 patients with ACS who underwent three-vessel coronary angiography and gray-scale and radiofrequency intravascular ultrasonographic imaging after PCI (52). During a median follow-up time of 3.4 years, the rate of major adverse cardiovascular events due to initially untreated lesions was 11.6%. Most of those lesions were angiographically mild and were either thin-cap fibroatheromas or

characterized by a large plaque burden, a small luminal area, or some combination of these characteristics, as determined by gray-scale and radiofrequency intravascular ultrasonography (52). However, only 17.2% of the highest-risk lesions progressed to causing symptoms, making pre-emptive lesion treatment impractical.

Identifying 'vulnerable plaques' that are at high risk for causing subsequent adverse clinical events and demonstrating that early treatment improves clinical outcomes remains challenging (53–55). The only group of plaques in which prophylactic stenting has been shown to be beneficial are intermediate SVG lesions. The Moderate VEin Graft LEsion Stenting With the Taxus Stent and Intravascular Ultrasound (VELETI) trial suggested that prophylactic stenting of intermediate SVG lesions with a paclitaxel-eluting stent may provide improved outcomes compared to medical therapy alone (56).

Coronary NIRS-IVUS could help identify high-risk non-obstructive coronary lesions and optimize the management of

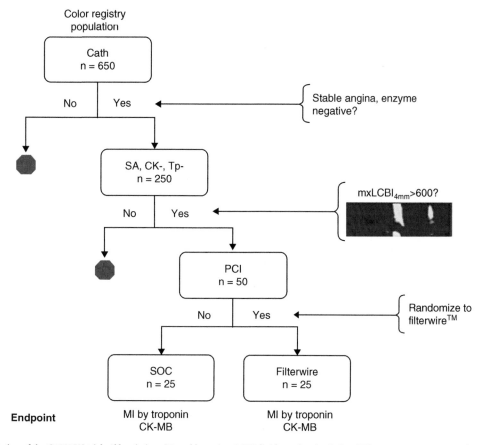

Figure 17.9 Design of the CANARY trial. *Abbreviations*: SA, stable angina; LCBI, lipid core burden index; PCI, percutaneous coronary intervention; SOC, standard of care.

Focus Box 17.4

NIRS-IVUS may help identify patients at high risk of coronary events and allow intensification of their medical therapy and appropriate lifestyle modifications

such patients (57). Preliminary observations from the COLOR registry have demonstrated that moderate lesions without LCPs are unlikely to progress (Fig. 17.10). Apart from mechanical treatments, patients with extensive LCP might benefit from aggressive pharmacologic therapies, such an intensive anti-thrombotic regimen, aggressive low-density lipoprotein cholesterol lowering, high-density lipoprotein infusion, low-density lipoprotein apheresis, or with medications such as niacin, fibrates, or, in the future, with novel compounds that are currently under clinical trial evaluation (58). NIRS-IVUS coronary imaging could also serve as a marker of

high coronary risk that could motivate patients to comply with the prescribed medical treatments and adopt beneficial lifestyle changes.

Evaluation of Novel Anti-Atherosclerotic Treatments

The combined NIRS-IVUS catheter is a powerful tool for the evaluation of novel anti-atherosclerotic treatments. Currently, the effect of such treatments on coronary plaques is based on IVUS imaging of a target coronary segment examining longitudinal changes in percent atheroma volume before and after treatment (59). Yet, fibrotic coronary plaques may be less likely to respond to lipid-lowering or anti-inflammatory treatments. Determination of the lipid core burden using NIRS, in a target coronary segment accurately outlined by IVUS, provides specific evaluation of the artery wall components that are at higher risk for causing subsequent events and are more likely to change in response to treatments.

The use of NIRS-IVUS for longitudinal coronary plaque composition changes is supported by the excellent reproducibility of

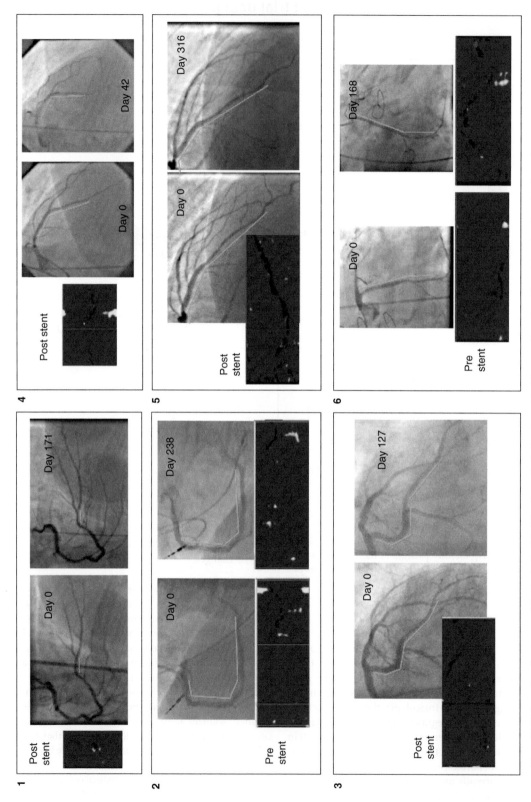

Figure 17.10 Examples of patients participating in the COLOR registry, who had angiographic follow-up of arteries without LCP at baseline, showing no lesion progression at follow-up.

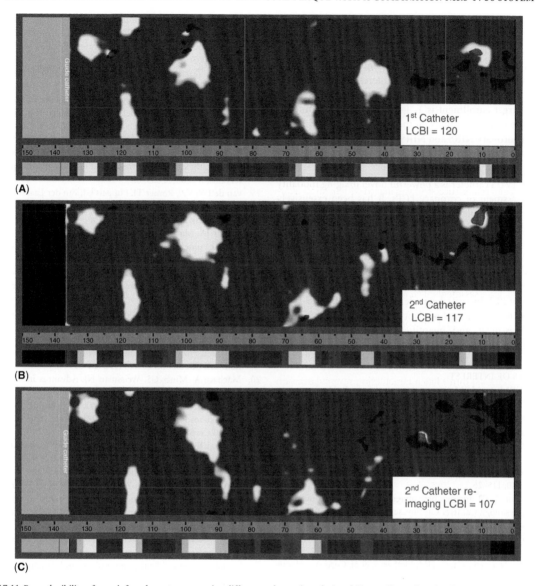

Figure 17.11 Reproducibility of near-infrared spectroscopy using different catheters (panels **A** and **B**) as well as re-imaging the same target vessel with the same catheter (panel **C**).

the NIRS findings during repeat pullbacks: Spearman's rho 0.927, intra-class correlation coefficient 0.925 in a 36-vessel analysis (43). Moreover, excellent inter-catheter NIRS measurement reproducibility (Spearman's rho 0.95) was found in an analysis of 10 coronary arteries by using two different NIRS catheters (Fig. 17.11) (60).

Several prospective coronary atherosclerosis studies are currently utilizing coronary NIRS as an endpoint, such as the AtheroREMO and the IBIS-3 trial. The Atherosclerosis Lesion Progression Intervention using Niacin Extended Release in Saphenous Vein Grafts (ALPINE-SVG) Pilot Trial is using multimodality imaging with IVUS, NIRS-IVUS, and OCT to assess

the impact of extended-release niacin in intermediate SVG lesions treated for 12 months (NCT01221402). The Cardiac CAtheterization for Bypass Graft Patency Rate Optimization (CABG-PRO, NCT01063491) study is randomizing patients undergoing coronary artery bypass graft surgery to early

Focus Box 17.5

NIRS-IVUS is a powerful tool for longitudinal assessment of coronary plaque morphology in response to various treatments.

(before dismissal) graft angiography versus no early graft angiography. NIRS is performed at early (before dismissal) angiography and at 12 months, to determine early changes in SVG composition. Finally, the ongoing Chemometric Observations of Lipid Core Containing Plaques of Interest in Native Coronary Arteries, NCT00831116 (COLOR) registry is enrolling patients (target enrollment is 1,500 patients) at 19 sites and will provide valuable insights on the clinical utility and implications of coronary NIRS and NIRS-IVUS imaging.

PERSONAL PERSPECTIVE

The NIRS-IVUS catheter is a powerful novel imaging modality for the assessment of coronary LCPs. It has been extensively validated and multiple studies are currently examining specific ways to implement the additional information obtained with the NIRS-IVUS catheter in clinical decision making. Using NIRS-IVUS to decide on the use of embolic protection devices, adjunctive pharmacologic therapy, and choice of the type and size of stents used could play a significant role in optimizing the outcomes of PCI. Increased experience with use of NIRS-IVUS can render it the preferred modality for longitudinal coronary plaque assessment and quantification of the response to advanced anti-atherosclerotic treatments.

CONFLICTS OF INTEREST

ZH, STS, SPM, and JEM are employees of InfraReDx, Inc.

REFERENCES

1. Clarke MC, Figg N, Maguire JJ, et al. Apoptosis of vascular smooth muscle cells induces features of plaque vulnerability in atherosclerosis. Nat Med 2006; 12: 1075–80.
2. Ross R. Atherosclerosis–an inflammatory disease. N Engl J Med 1999; 340: 115–26.
3. Goldstein JA. CT angiography: imaging anatomy to deduce coronary physiology. Catheter Cardiovasc Interv 2009; 73: 503–5.
4. Giroud D, Li JM, Urban P, Meier B, Rutishauer W. Relation of the site of acute myocardial infarction to the most severe coronary arterial stenosis at prior angiography. Am J Cardiol 1992; 69: 729–32.
5. Gonzalo N, Garcia-Garcia HM, Ligthart J, et al. Coronary plaque composition as assessed by greyscale intravascular ultrasound and radiofrequency spectral data analysis. Int J Cardiovasc Imaging 2008; 24: 811–8.
6. Nair A, Kuban BD, Tuzcu EM, et al. Coronary plaque classification with intravascular ultrasound radiofrequency data analysis. Circulation 2002; 106: 2200–6.
7. Okubo M, Kawasaki M, Ishihara Y, et al. Development of integrated backscatter intravascular ultrasound for tissue characterization of coronary plaques. Ultrasound Med Biol 2008; 34: 655–63.
8. de Korte CL, van der Steen AF, Cespedes EI, Pasterkamp G. Intravascular ultrasound elastography in human arteries: initial experience in vitro. Ultrasound Med Biol 1998; 24: 401–8.
9. Doyley MM, Mastik F, de Korte CL, et al. Advancing intravascular ultrasonic palpation toward clinical applications. Ultrasound Med Biol 2001; 27: 1471–80.
10. Ishibashi F, Aziz K, Abela GS, Waxman S. Update on coronary angioscopy: review of a 20-year experience and potential application for detection of vulnerable plaque. J Interv Cardiol 2006; 19: 17–25.
11. Patel NA, Stamper DL, Brezinski ME. Review of the ability of optical coherence tomography to characterize plaque, including a comparison with intravascular ultrasound. Cardiovasc Intervent Radiol 2005; 28: 1–9.
12. Yun SH, Tearney GJ, Vakoc BJ, et al. Comprehensive volumetric optical microscopy in vivo. Nat Med 2006; 12: 1429–33.
13. Bezerra HG, Costa MA, Guagliumi G, Rollins AM, Simon DI. Intracoronary optical coherence tomography: a comprehensive review clinical and research applications. JACC Cardiovasc Interv 2009; 2: 1035–46.
14. Brennan JF 3rd, Nazemi J, Motz J, Ramcharitar S. The vPredict optical catheter system: intravascular raman spectroscopy. EuroIntervention 2008; 3: 635–8.
15. van de Poll SW, Romer TJ, Puppels GJ, van der Laarse A. Imaging of atherosclerosis. Raman spectroscopy of atherosclerosis. J Cardiovasc Risk 2002; 9: 255–61.
16. Schaar JA, Mastik F, Regar E, et al. Current diagnostic modalities for vulnerable plaque detection. Curr Pharm Des 2007; 13: 995–1001.
17. Jan GK, Patrick S, Luc MVB. Identifying the vulnerable plaque: a review of invasive and non-invasive imaging modalities. 2008; 2: 21–34.
18. Escolar E, Weigold G, Fuisz A, Weissman NJ. New imaging techniques for diagnosing coronary artery disease. CMAJ 2006; 174: 487–95.
19. Honda Y, Fitzgerald PJ. Frontiers in intravascular imaging technologies. Circulation 2008; 117: 2024–37.
20. Maehara A, Mintz GS, Weissman NJ. Advances in intravascular imaging. Circ Cardiovasc Interv 2009; 2: 482–90.
21. Near-Infrared Technology in the Agriculture and Food Industries. In: Williams P, Norris KPaul ST. ed Minnesota: American Association of Cereal Chemists, Inc, 2001.
22. Ciurczak EW, Drennen JK. Pharmaceutical and Medical Applications of Near-Infrared Spectroscopy. New York: Marcel Dekker, 2002.
23. Lavine B, Workman J. Chemometrics. Anal Chem 2008; 80: 4519–31.
24. Voros S, Rinehart S, Qian Z, et al. Coronary atherosclerosis imaging by coronary CT angiography current status, correlation with intravascular interrogation and meta-analysis. JACC Cardiovasc Imaging 2011; 4: 537–48.
25. Garg S, Serruys PW, van der Ent M, et al. First use in patients of a combined near infra-red spectroscopy and intra-vascular ultrasound catheter to identify composition and structure of coronary plaque. EuroIntervention 2010; 5: 755–6.
26. U.S. Food and Drug Administration. [Available from: http://www.fda.gov/NewsEvents/Newsroom/PressAnnouncements/2008/ucm116888.html 2008]
27. Roy P, Steinberg DH, Sushinsky SJ, et al. The potential clinical utility of intravascular ultrasound guidance in patients undergoing percutaneous coronary intervention with drug-eluting stents. Eur Heart J 2008; 29: 1851–7.
28. Sera F, Awata M, Uematsu M, et al. Optimal stent-sizing with intravascular ultrasound contributes to complete neointimal coverage after sirolimus-eluting stent implantation assessed by angioscopy. JACC Cardiovasc Interv 2009; 2: 989–94.
29. Prasad A, Herrmann J. Myocardial infarction due to percutaneous coronary intervention. N Engl J Med 2011; 364: 453–64.
30. Prasad A, Rihal CS, Lennon RJ, et al. Trends in outcomes after percutaneous coronary intervention for chronic total occlusions: a 25-year experience from the Mayo Clinic. J Am Coll Cardiol 2007; 49: 1611–8.

31. Goldstein JA, Grines C, Fischell T, et al. Coronary embolization following balloon dilation of lipid-core plaques. JACC Cardiovasc Imaging 2009; 2: 1420–4.

32. Maini B, Brilakis E, Kim M, et al. Association of large lipid core plaque detected by near infrared spectroscopy with post percutaneous coronary intervention myocardial infarction. J Am Coll Cardiol 2010; 55: A179, E1672.

33. Schultz C, Serruys P, van der Ent M, et al. Prospective identification of a large lipid core coronary plaque with a novel near-infrared spectroscopy and intravascular ultrasound (NIR-IVUS) catheter: Infarction following stenting possibly due to distal embolization of plaque contents. J Am Coll Cardiol 2010; 56: 314.

34. Saeed B, Banerjee S, Brilakis ES. Slow flow after stenting of a coronary lesion with a large lipid core plaque detected by near-infrared spectroscopy. EuroIntervention 2010; 6: 545.

35. Raghunathan D, Abdel Karim AR, DaSilva M, et al. Association between the presence and extent of coronary lipid core plaques detected by near-infrared spectroscopy with post percutaneous coronary intervention myocardial infarction. Am J Cardiol 2011; 107: 1613–18.

36. Goldstein JA, Maini B, Dixon SR, et al. Detection of lipid-core plaques by intracoronary near-infrared spectroscopy identifies high risk of periprocedural myocardial infarction. Circ Cardiovasc Interv 2011; 4: 429–37.

37. Wood FO, Badhey N, Garcia B, et al. Analysis of saphenous vein graft lesion composition using near-infrared spectroscopy and intravascular ultrasonography with virtual histology. Atherosclerosis 2010; 212: 528–33.

38. Hong MK, Mehran R, Dangas G, et al. Creatine kinase-MB enzyme elevation following successful saphenous vein graft intervention is associated with late mortality. Circulation 1999; 100: 2400–5.

39. Sdringola S, Assali AR, Ghani M, et al. Risk assessment of slow or no-reflow phenomenon in aortocoronary vein graft percutaneous intervention. Catheter Cardiovasc Interv 2001; 54: 318–24.

40. Gardner CM, Tan H, Hull EL, et al. Detection of lipid core coronary plaques in autopsy specimens with a novel catheter-based near-infrared spectroscopy system. JACC Cardiovasc Imaging 2008; 1: 638–48.

41. Waxman S, Dixon SR, L'Allier P, et al. In vivo validation of a catheter-based near-infrared spectroscopy system for detection of lipid core coronary plaques: initial results of the SPECTACL study. JACC Cardiovasc Imaging 2009; 2: 858–68.

42. Selvanayagam JB, Porto I, Channon K, et al. Troponin elevation after percutaneous coronary intervention directly represents the extent of irreversible myocardial injury: insights from cardiovascular magnetic resonance imaging. Circulation 2005; 111: 1027–32.

43. Garcia BA, Wood F, Cipher D, Banerjee S, Brilakis ES. Reproducibility of near-infrared spectroscopy for the detection of lipid core coronary plaques and observed changes after coronary stent implantation. Catheter Cardiovasc Interv 2010; 76: 359–65.

44. Abdel-Karim AR, Papayannis AC, Rangan BV, Banerjee S, Brilakis ES. Stenting of native coronary artery lesions with large lipid core plaques as detected by near-infrared spectroscopy is associated with high frequency of debris retrieval using embolic protection devices. Cathet Cardiovasc Interv 2011; in press.

45. Stone GW, Webb J, Cox DA, et al. Distal microcirculatory protection during percutaneous coronary intervention in acute ST-Segment elevation myocardial infarction: a randomized controlled trial. JAMA 2005; 293: 1063–72.

46. Kelbaek H, Terkelsen CJ, Helqvist S, et al. Randomized comparison of distal protection versus conventional treatment in primary percutaneous coronary intervention: the drug elution and distal protection in ST-elevation myocardial infarction (DEDICATION) trial. J Am Coll Cardiol 2008; 51: 899–905.

47. Banerjee S, Brilakis ES. Embolic protection during saphenous vein graft interventions. J Invasive Cardiol 2009; 21: 415–7.

48. Papayannis AC, Abdel-Karim AR, Mahmood A, et al. Association of coronary lipid core plaque with intra-stent thrombus formation: a Near-Infrared Spectroscopy and Optical Coherence Tomography study. Cathet Cardiovasc Interv 2012; e-pub ahead of print.

49. Reininger AJ, Bernlochner I, Penz SM, et al. A 2-step mechanism of arterial thrombus formation induced by human atherosclerotic plaques. J Am Coll Cardiol 2010; 55: 1147–58.

50. Farb A, Burke AP, Kolodgie FD, Virmani R. Pathological mechanisms of fatal late coronary stent thrombosis in humans. Circulation 2003; 108: 1701–6.

51. Sakhuja R, Suh WM, Jaffer FA, Jang IK. Residual thrombogenic substrate after rupture of a lipid-rich plaque: possible mechanism of acute stent thrombosis? Circulation 2010; 122: 2349–50.

52. Stone GW, Maehara A, Lansky AJ, et al. A prospective natural-history study of coronary atherosclerosis. N Engl J Med 2011; 364: 226–35.

53. Muller JE, Abela GS, Nesto RW, Tofler GH. Triggers, acute risk factors and vulnerable plaques: the lexicon of a new frontier. J Am Coll Cardiol 1994; 23: 809–13.

54. Naghavi M, Libby P, Falk E, et al. From vulnerable plaque to vulnerable patient: a call for new definitions and risk assessment strategies: part II. Circulation 2003; 108: 1772–8.

55. Naghavi M, Libby P, Falk E, et al. From vulnerable plaque to vulnerable patient: a call for new definitions and risk assessment strategies: part I. Circulation 2003; 108: 1664–72.

56. Rodes-Cabau J, Bertrand OF, Larose E, et al. Comparison of plaque sealing with paclitaxel-eluting stents versus medical therapy for the treatment of moderate nonsignificant saphenous vein graft lesions. The moderate VEin Graft LEsion stenting with the taxus stent and intravascular ultrasound (VELETI) Pilot Trial. Circulation 2009; 120: 1978–86.

57. Muller JE, Tawakol A, Kathiresan S, Narula J. New opportunities for identification and reduction of coronary risk: treatment of vulnerable patients, arteries, and plaques. J Am Coll Cardiol 2006; 47: C2–6.

58. Sacks FM, Rudel LL, Conner A, et al. Selective delipidation of plasma HDL enhances reverse cholesterol transport in vivo. J Lipid Res 2009; 50: 894–907.

59. Bose D, von Birgelen C, Erbel R. Intravascular ultrasound for the evaluation of therapies targeting coronary atherosclerosis. J Am Coll Cardiol 2007; 49: 925–32.

60. Abdel-Karim AR, Rangan BV, Banerjee S, Brilakis ES. Intercatheter reproducibility of near-infrared spectroscopy for the in vivo detection of coronary lipid core plaques. Catheter Cardiovasc Interv 2011; 77: 657–61.

18 Role of endothelial shear stress in the destabilization of coronary plaque: Acute coronary syndromes and rapid plaque progression

Antonios P. Antoniadis, Michail I. Papafaklis, Saeko Takahashi, Charles L. Feldman, and Peter H. Stone

OUTLINE

Local endothelial shear stress (ESS) triggers vascular phenomena which synergistically exacerbate atherosclerosis toward an unstable phenotype. Specifically, low ESS augments lipid uptake and catabolism, induces plaque inflammation and oxidation, downregulates the production and upregulates the degradation of extracellular matrix, and increases cellular apoptosis ultimately leading to thin-cap fibroatheromas and/or endothelial erosions. Increases in blood thrombogenicity that result from either high or low ESS, also contribute to plaque destabilization. A destabilized plaque manifests clinically as either abrupt luminal occlusion and acute coronary syndrome, or accelerated atherosclerosis progression via repeated cycles of subclinical partial luminal occlusion and healing which causes worsening ischemia.

INTRODUCTION

Atherosclerosis research has advanced significantly over recent decades, leading to major clinical benefits. However, coronary artery disease (CAD) remains a major cause of morbidity and mortality. In 2007, coronary disease caused about 1 of 6 deaths in the United States and accounted for 1,572,000 inpatient hospital discharges (1). These data underscore the shortcomings of current preventive, diagnostic, and therapeutic strategies, and emphasize the need for better insight into the underlying etiologic factors.

Atherosclerosis exhibits significant heterogeneity. First, the topographic localization of plaques in the coronary tree is typically asymmetrical, showing a predilection for the lateral walls of bifurcations or branching points and the inner aspect of curved segments, while other areas are less frequently affected (2–4). Second, the progression rate of each lesion is variable and independent, as plaques of different size and composition routinely co-exist within the same subject, indeed even inside a single artery. Third, the natural history of individual lesions is diverse. Some plaques are non-obstructive, remain clinically

Focus Box 18.1

Atherosclerosis exhibits significant morphological and clinical heterogeneity
Disturbed local hemodynamics, in particular, low ESS, lead to plaque initiation, progression, and destabilization
Destabilized plaques, with either plaque rupture or erosion, account for the majority of adverse cardiovascular events, in the form of either acute coronary syndromes or worsening ischemia

quiescent and may only become evident by chance during coronary imaging. Others encroach into the lumen and limit blood flow in a fixed manner presenting with stable angina. A small proportion of plaques may spontaneously activate the blood coagulation cascade and manifest as worsening ischemia or acute coronary syndrome (ACS) (5).

Locally disturbed blood flow is a major modulator of the atherogenic process and contributes significantly to the regional, constitutional, and clinical variability of atherosclerosis (6,7). Specifically, low endothelial shear stress (ESS) provokes molecular, cellular, and vascular responses in atherosclerosis-prone sites, leading to plaque initiation and progression (5). The local ESS microenvironment further contributes to plaque evolution toward a stable or unstable phenotype via a multitude of mechanisms and interactions (8). This chapter will focus on the role of ESS in the pathobiologic processes responsible for plaque destabilization, leading either to accelerated plaque growth or acute coronary events. We will also discuss the clinical perspective of *in vivo* ESS calculation in the early identification of high-risk lesions.

PLAQUE DESTABILIZATION: DEFINITIONS AND MORPHOLOGICAL DESCRIPTORS

The terms vulnerable, unstable, or high-risk plaque are used interchangeably to denote an atheromatous region with propensity to trigger adverse cardiovascular events (9). Plaque rupture or fissuring is the most common pathophysiological substrate for atherothrombosis and luminal occlusion, yet in a smaller fraction of cases, endothelial erosion may be the provoking factor and even less frequently calcified nodules overlying plaques are the culprit lesions (10–12). Moreover, some incidents of plaque disruption are clinically silent, because of only partial blood flow obstruction. These events of asymptomatic rupture and healing can incite rapid plaque progression and result in adverse clinical outcomes (13,14).

While no consensus exists on all attributes of high-risk plaque, the histological hallmarks most commonly distinctive of this entity are a large lipid core (>40% of cross-sectional area), a thin fibrous cap (<65 μm), and intense inflammatory cell infiltration (15–17). These plaques are commonly called thin-cap fibroatheromas (TCFAs) and account for the majority of unfavorable coronary outcomes. The recent PROSPECT study reinforced this concept, demonstrating that TCFA, as assessed by radiofrequency intravascular ultrasound (IVUS) was an independent predictor of subsequent lesion-related

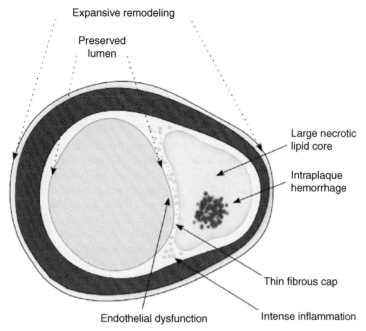

Figure 18.1 The vulnerable plaque. Prominent features are a large lipid core, a thin fibrous cap, intense inflammatory cell infiltration, lumen preservation with expansive remodeling, endothelial dysfunction, and intraplaque hemorrhage.

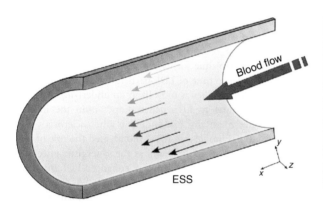

Figure 18.2 Definition of endothelial shear stress (ESS). ESS is the tangential component of the mechanical stress exerted on the endothelium by the flowing blood.

major adverse cardiovascular events (18). However, a significant proportion of TCFAs may heal spontaneously during the natural course of atherosclerosis, which underscores the complexity of relating high-risk plaque to clinical events (19). Other features suggestive of a high-risk plaque profile are endothelial denudation with superimposed platelet aggregation, disruption of the cap integrity, intraplaque hemorrhage, endothelial dysfunction, and expansive remodeling (Fig. 18.1) (20–22).

BASIC CONCEPTS RELATED TO ESS
Endothelial shear stress is the tangential component of the mechanical stress exerted on the endothelium by the flowing

---

Focus Box 18.2

ESS is the tangential component of the mechanical stress exerted on the endothelium by the flowing blood
Normal or physiologic ESS is present in regions with undisturbed laminar flow
Low and/or oscillatory ESS is found at atherosclerosis-prone regions, at the inner side of curvatures, downstream of stenoses, the lateral walls of bifurcations, and areas contiguous to side-branch take-off
High ESS is common in the areas of luminal narrowing, with associated increased local blood velocity

---

blood (Fig. 18.2). ESS is calculated as the product of blood viscosity (μ) and the spatial gradient of blood velocity (dv/dy), and is expressed in force per area units (1 Pascal = 1 N/m² = 10 dyne/cm²).

$$ESS = \mu \frac{dv}{dy}$$

The composite effects of geometrical complexities, cardiac motion, and pulsatile blood flow cause considerable variations in the direction and magnitude of ESS within the coronaries, both spatially and temporally. The physiologic ESS range lies between 1 and 2.5 Pascal. However, ESS values vary significantly across different species and are subject to systemic regulation (23).

213

Normal or physiologic ESS is present in regions with undisturbed laminar flow. Oscillatory ESS denotes changes in the direction of force along the endothelium because of blood flow fluctuation. Low and/or oscillatory ESS typically predominates on sites where atherosclerosis preferentially develops, that is, the inner side of arterial curvatures, downstream of stenoses, the lateral walls of bifurcations, and areas contiguous to side-branch take-off (5,24,25). High ESS is typically observed in areas of luminal narrowing, with associated increased local blood velocity (26).

In vivo ESS calculation in the coronary arteries is accomplished with the use of computational fluid dynamics in geometrically correct, three-dimensional representations similar to the true anatomic structures. Fusion of biplane angiography and IVUS is the principal technique for the reconstruction of these coronary models, and this method has proven feasible, accurate, and reproducible (27–32). Novel reconstruction approaches using non-invasive modalities, such as multi-detector computed tomography, will likely become more widely applicable, and thus shed further light into the role of ESS in atherosclerosis (33–35).

THE ROLE OF ESS IN THE DEVELOPMENT OF HIGH-RISK PLAQUES

ESS, Vascular Endothelium, and Atherosclerosis Initiation

Rather than a simple lining structure, the endothelial layer is an active tissue elaborating numerous molecules that determine vascular homeostasis (36). Normal endothelium synthesizes nitric oxide (NO) from L-arginine via endothelial nitric oxide synthase (eNOS). NO has a prominent atheroprotective role as it not only maintains vascular tone, but decisively counteracts endothelial permeability, cellular proliferation, inflammation, apoptosis, and thrombosis (37). Endothelial dysfunction is recognized as the initial critical step in the atherosclerotic process (38). Specific receptors in the glycocalyx, a surface proteoglycan layer in endothelial cells, sense ESS (mechanosensing) and translate biomechanical forces into biochemical signals (mechanotransduction) (39–41). The mechanosensing process involves expression of sensors in endothelial caveolae, opening of transmembrane ion channels, activation of heterotrimeric G-proteins, and phosphorylation of the transmembrane platelet endothelial cell adhesion molecule (PECAM)-1 (42,43). The sensitivity of endothelial response to ESS is to the order of 0.025 Pascal over a length of approximately 10 cells (44). ESS subsequently activates several intra- and inter-cellular signaling pathways and, via complex molecular interactions, affects protein expression and, ultimately, cellular behavior within the arterial wall (45). On the basis of different ESS values, low-ESS-induced activation of nuclear factor-kappa B (NF-κB) promotes atherogenesis while physiologic-ESS-induced transcription factor Kruppel-like factor-2 (KLF-2) mediates atheroprotection (46).

Low and/or oscillatory ESS generates structural and functional conformational changes in endothelial cells. Instead of being spindle-shaped and aligned parallel to blood flow, endothelial cells become polygonal with an irregular and disorganized orientation (47). Provision of L-arginine is suppressed and eNOS is downregulated (48–50). The resulting reduced NO levels render the endothelial layer susceptible to systemic risk factors and set the stage for the initiation of atherosclerosis. Conversely, higher ESS values mediate atheroprotection via eNOS upregulation (51,52). Low ESS further accentuates atherosclerosis by augmenting endothelin-1 and suppressing prostacyclin production in endothelial cells (53).

ESS, Lipid Accumulation, and Plaque Growth

Lipid plaque growth with necrotic core expansion is an important element of vulnerability. Low ESS is associated with increased plaque size and lipid content. Low ESS augments cholesterol influx across the endothelial layer by increasing membrane permeability, and by disrupting intercellular tight junctions via induction of endothelial apoptosis (54–57). Moreover, disturbed flow upregulates oxidized low-density lipoprotein (oxLDL) receptors and oxLDL catabolizing enzymes produced by macrophages, as lipoprotein-associated phospholipase-A$_2$ (58). Additionally, low ESS triggers vascular smooth muscle cell apoptosis, which in turn exacerbates macrophage and monocyte death through multiple feedback mechanisms (59). Death of lipid-laden foam cells in combination with ineffective clearance of the necrotic material, leads to accumulation of cellular debris and plaque expansion (60).

In computational models of coronary circulation, low ESS increases focal subendothelial low-density lipoprotein (LDL) accumulation (61–63). High LDL concentration correlates well with subsequent plaque formation in these regions (64). The increased residence time of LDL particles in this low-velocity, low-ESS coronary milieu is most likely an underlying etiologic factor predisposing to LDL penetration within the intima, which initiates, maintains, and augments atherosclerosis.

In vivo animal models readily demonstrated the role of low ESS in plaque progression as well as the synergistic effects of low ESS and hypercholesterolemia in enhanced LDL build-up within plaques, leading to the formation of TCFAs (51,65–67). Hence, low-ESS-induced lipid enrichment of coronary plaques contributes to an increasingly unstable phenotypic profile.

ESS and Inflammation

The intensity of inflammation in atherosclerotic plaques determines the transition of early fibroatheromas into advanced plaques with large lipid cores and thin fibrous caps, and in this manner directly leads to vulnerability (68,69). Low and/or oscillatory ESS contributes to recruitment of leukocytes in plaque regions by inducing synthesis of adhesion molecules [intracellular adhesion molecule (ICAM)-1, vascular cell adhesion molecule (VCAM)-1, E-selectin], chemoattractant chemokines [monocyte chemoattractant protein (MCP)-1, interleukin (IL)-8], and pro-inflammatory cytokines [tumor necrosis factor (TNF)-α, IL-1, interferon (IFN)-γ] (44,47,70–74). These mediators facilitate circulating leukocyte (predominantly monocyte) tethering in the endothelial membrane and diapedesis into the intima. After reaching the subendothelial layer, monocytes differentiate to macrophages, engulf oxLDL, and transform into foam cells. Foam cells produce cytokines, growth factors, reactive oxygen species, and matrix-degrading enzymes, sustaining atherosclerosis progression (75). On the other hand, physiologic ESS protects against endothelial leukocyte infiltration by reducing pseudopod projection via mechanosensing pathways (76). Normal laminar flow antagonizes leukocyte recruitment, vascular endothelial growth factor (VEGF)-1 induction, and E-selectin expression mediated by TNF-α, thus conferring atheroprotection (77,78).

Animal studies assessed the *in vivo* effects of low ESS in plaque progression and risk profile. Mouse carotid regions exposed to low ESS showed increased expression of inflammatory mediators and accommodated vulnerable plaques (51,79). Furthermore, in swine models of atherosclerosis, the magnitude of low ESS related in a time- and dose-dependent manner to plaque inflammatory cell infiltration and ultimately led to the formation of TCFAs (66,67).

ESS and Oxidative Stress

Oxidation is critical to many aspects of the atherosclerotic process as it augments the production of oxLDL in the subendothelium, promotes inflammation, stimulates smooth muscle cell proliferation and migration to the intima, and upregulates matrix degradation, leading to advanced and destabilized plaques (80). ESS locally modulates redox balance via numerous molecular interactions. Low and/or oscillating ESS exacerbates oxidation within the intima by upregulating oxidative enzymes [nicotinamide adenine dinucleotide phosphate (NADPH) oxidase, xanthine oxidase] while suppressing antioxidant ones (superoxide dismutase, glutathione peroxidase) (81–87). Low-ESS-generated reactive oxygen species in the intima react with NO to form peroxynitrite, which is an additional oxidant (88). In addition, reactive oxygen species lead to oxidation of the eNOS co-factor tetrahydrobiopterin to dihydrobiopterin. In the absence of tetrahydrobiopterin, eNOS uncoupling occurs and superoxide formation rather than NO is induced, thus accentuating oxidation (89). Thus, low ESS enhances oxidation, which not only diminishes the vasculoprotective effects of NO but also further aggravates oxidative stress. Conversely, normal ESS activates the transcription factor nuclear factor (erythroid-derived 2)-like 2 (Nrf2), leading to increased intracellular antioxidant levels (90). Physiologic ESS downregulates angiotensin type 1 receptors in endothelial cells, offsetting the angiotensin II-mediated oxidative stress (91). Another potential mechanism of the antioxidant effects of physiologic ESS is an increase in the mitochondrial membrane potential, low values of which are linked to oxidative stress (92,93).

ESS and Matrix Degradation

Extracellular matrix (ECM) is ubiquitous in biological tissues and consists of collagen and elastin fibers interspersed with proteoglycans and glycosaminoglycans (94). ECM is the predominant constituent of both the vessel wall and the fibrous cap of the plaque. A dynamic equilibrium between ECM synthesis and breakdown controls the amount of ECM in the arterial wall. In areas containing plaque, vascular smooth muscle cells and fibroblasts produce ECM, while endothelial cells, macrophages, smooth muscle cells, T-lymphocytes, and mast cells secrete ECM-degrading enzymes, namely, metalloproteinases, cathepsins, serine proteases, chymase, and tryptase (95). In the progression of atherosclerosis, ECM degradation augments lesion formation by introducing internal elastic lamina fragmentation. This facilitates migration of vascular smooth muscle cells and macrophages to plaques and signals a shift from moderate to severe lesions (66). In developed plaques, collagen provides biomechanical strength to the fibrous cap and safeguards its integrity. Thus, ECM degradation predisposes to instability. A porcine model of native atherosclerosis confirmed this concept by showing increased metalloproteinase and cathepsin expression levels in TCFAs (66).

Low ESS *in vivo* is associated with an enhanced expression and activity of metalloproteinases and cathepsins (51,66). Low ESS induces pro-inflammatory cytokines, which in turn stimulate the release of ECM-degrading enzymes (96). Low-ESS-induced reactive oxygen species further augment the activity of proteolytic enzymes via numerous inflammatory mediators (97,98). Combined coronary flow and histopathological studies in a swine model of native atherosclerosis showed that in coronary regions of low ESS, the internal elastic lamina undergoes local fragmentation by metalloproteinases and cathepsins. Moreover, exposure to low ESS induces the activity of ECM-catabolizing enzymes and leads to formation of TCFAs (66). Indeed, cap thickness was inversely associated with ESS, as regions exposed to lower ESS had plaques with thinner caps (67). ECM degradation is particularly evident at the plaque shoulders and renders these regions more prone to disruption (67).

In addition to contributing to ECM breakdown, ESS variably influences ECM generation. Low ESS attenuates ECM production by smooth muscle cells by promoting vascular smooth muscle cell apoptosis (99,100). In an animal model of carotid atherosclerosis, plaques with low ESS showed a reduced density of vascular smooth muscle cells and less collagen (51). In contrast, the role of high ESS in ECM homeostasis is less well understood. It has been reported that high ESS upregulates collagen synthesis and downregulates metalloproteinase activity contributing to plaque stabilization (101). Other studies, however, indicate that high ESS suppresses collagen synthesis and stimulates metalloproteinase activity via an inappropriately high induction of NO (102–104). The translation of these studies and the integrated role of high ESS in the pathogenesis of plaque destabilization will be discussed in a subsequent section.

With regard to proteoglycans of the ECM, heparan sulfate has anti-atherogenic properties due to reduced affinity to LDL and monocytes, as opposed to chondroitin and dermatan sulfate, which are pro-atherogenic. Low ESS upregulates heparanase, an enzyme that destroys heparan sulfate chains in ECM, and which co-localizes with intense inflammatory infiltration and formation of TCFAs (105).

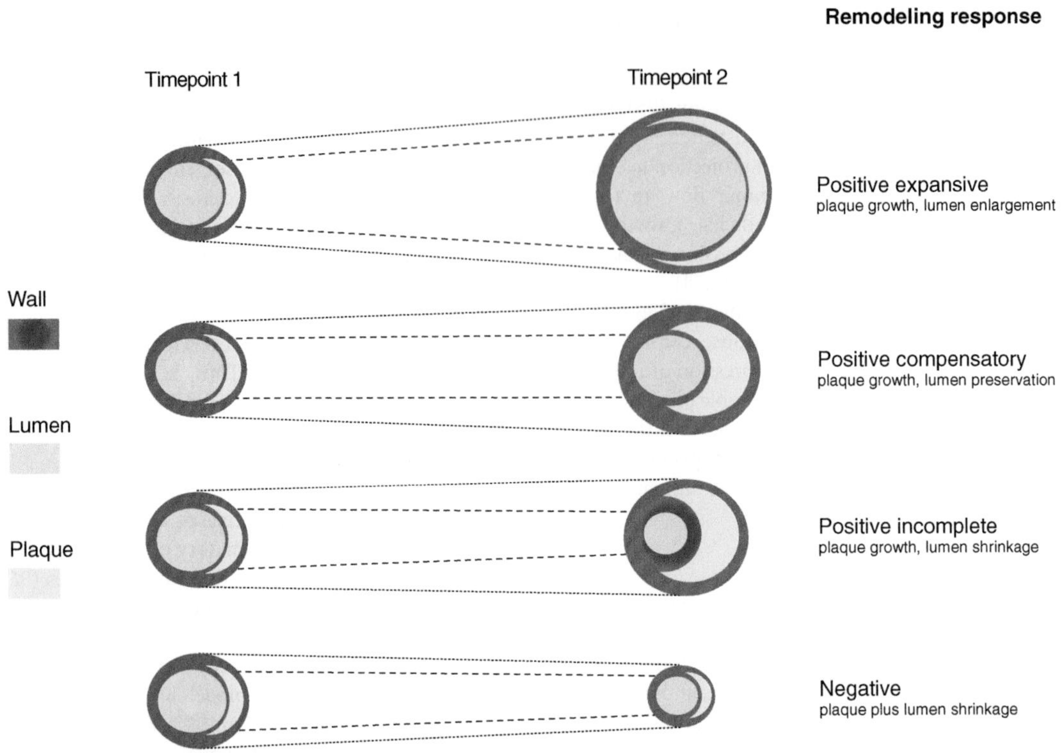

Figure 18.3 Arterial remodeling patterns. Cross-sectional arterial views illustrating different remodeling responses. In positive remodeling, the external elastic membrane (EEM) area increases, while in negative remodeling, the EEM area decreases. Positive remodeling further divides into three categories: in expansive positive remodeling, the EEM increase exceeds the plaque increase, leading to lumen enlargement; in compensatory positive remodeling, the EEM increase equals the plaque increase, leading to lumen preservation; in incomplete positive remodeling, the EEM increase falls behind the plaque increase, leading to lumen shrinkage.

ESS and Coronary Remodeling

Remodeling is an inherent arterial feature referring to the ability of vessels to adjust their shape in response to plaque growth or flow alterations. Generally, positive remodeling means that the arterial dimensions increase, while negative remodeling signifies that the arterial size decreases. Under physiologic conditions, lumen size and blood flow rate act synergistically to retain ESS within normal range. In non-diseased arteries, high ESS stimulates positive remodeling, while low ESS induces negative remodeling, in order to restore normal flow (106). In diseased segments, however, the interactions are more complex and decisively affected by the molecular processes of atherosclerosis. Figure 18.3 presents a contemporary classification scheme for remodeling in diseased arteries, incorporating the nomenclature of a recent expert consensus report on IVUS (107). Remodeling is positive when the external elastic membrane (EEM) area increases, while it is negative when the EEM area decreases in the temporal course of atherosclerosis. Positive remodeling is further categorized on the basis of the relationship between EEM and plaque area change. Where EEM area increases equally to plaque area, the lumen is preserved (compensatory positive remodeling). Expansive positive remodeling occurs when EEM area increases more than the plaque area, leading to lumen

enlargement (over-compensation). Incomplete positive remodeling occurs when plaque area increases more than EEM area, leading to lumen shrinkage.

The relationship between plaque growth and vascular remodeling is not stereotypical and easily predictable, but represents a dynamic continuum of adaptive mechanisms (108,109). Expansive remodeling is associated with indices of plaque vulnerability, unstable clinical presentation, and long-term adverse outcome (110–113). Remodeling tightly relies upon the local dynamic ECM turnover. Low ESS, via induction of inflammation and intense ECM degradation as previously discussed, leads to TCFAs with corresponding expansive remodeling (51,66,67,114,115). This finding highlights the distinction between compensatory and expansive remodeling in low-ESS regions. While compensatory remodeling is a corrective process destined to maintain physiologic vasculoprotective ESS, expansive remodeling is an exaggerated response, likely related to intense local inflammation, plaque growth, and excessive wall destruction as a result of profoundly low ESS. As the plaque and arterial wall expand because of intense local inflammation, ESS actually further decreases in these excessively enlarged regions. Under these circumstances, a vicious cycle seems to follow: low ESS causes intense inflammation, plaque growth, and expansive remodeling, which increases lumen size leading to perpetuation or even aggravation of low ESS and further plaque growth (5,67).

The natural history trajectory of each lesion may involve switching to a different remodeling pattern over time not only once, but numerous times. A recent multiple time-point IVUS natural history study in swine demonstrated that regions exposed to low ESS culminated in high-risk expansive remodeling. In contrast, coronary segments with compensatory remodeling showed higher baseline ESS values than those with expansive remodeling (65). Other studies reported that low ESS in expansively remodeled arteries is associated with increased elasticity, yet another marker of plaque instability (116,117). A further consideration to be taken into account is that most coronary plaques are eccentric, and thus in the same cross-section diseased areas with low ESS are contiguous with healthy segments with higher ESS. One could speculate that the expansive remodeling response to plaque growth in such regions is the synergistic effect of intense ECM degradation resulting from low ESS in diseased parts and luminal dilatation in response to high ESS in the plaque-free wall (118). A study showing that coronary segments with expansive remodeling have larger plaque-free wall areas than regions with constriction supports such a mechanism (119).

Overall, by affecting ECM turnover, ESS likely determines the point beyond which the favorable effects of compensatory remodeling in response to plaque growth convert to a more hazardous profile related to expansive remodeling.

ESS, Neovascularization, and Intraplaque Hemorrhage

Intimal extension and proliferation of the vasa vasorum network is an important feature of advanced and ruptured plaques (120). Neovessels contribute to plaque growth by supplying inflammatory cells and mediators from the perivascular tissue. Spontaneous rupture of structurally immature and brittle vasa vasorum causes intraplaque hemorrhage (21,121,122). Increased metalloproteinase activity weakens the structural scaffolding of neovessels and causes extravasation of erythrocytes and bleeding within plaques (123). Other potential sources of intraplaque hemorrhage include subclinical plaque rupture as well as local injury of the endothelium and fibrous cap overlying the plaque (14). Bleeding within plaques contributes in turn to plaque growth, possibly, by providing cholesterol from erythrocyte membranes (124).

Low ESS induces neovascularization by causing intimal thickening, and thus subintimal ischemia, and by upregulating VEGF and other angiogenic stimuli (125,126). Low ESS areas were the exclusive sites of intraplaque hemorrhage in experimental atherosclerosis. In addition, high blood pressure-induced intraplaque hemorrhage occurs in low-ESS segments only (51).

ESS AND ENDOTHELIAL EROSION

Either mechanical or functional destruction of the endothelial layer directly exposes the underlying procoagulant material, most notably von Willebrand factor and tissue factor, to circulating blood cells and plasma components. Subsequently, platelet aggregation and fibrin formation ensue. As noted previously, low and/or oscillatory ESS induces endothelial cell apoptosis, increased endothelial cell turnover, and thus likely accounts for a preponderance of the respective arterial regions to erode (43,56,57,127–129). High endothelial cell turnover is postulated to relate to endothelial stem and progenitor cell senescence and exhaustion, thus reducing the vascular regenerative potential (130). Apoptotic endothelial cells are highly proadhesive and procoagulant further favoring thrombosis (131,132). Conversely, physiologic laminar flow contributes toward endothelial repair by enhancing stem cell proliferation and differentiation into endothelial cells (133,134). In rabbit femoral arteries, oscillatory ESS led to erosive injury and endothelial detachment, leading to local thrombus formation (135). In a porcine model of atherosclerosis, low ESS was associated with reduced endothelial coverage of the respective coronary regions (67). Low ESS, via heparanase induction may also damage the endothelial glycocalyx, which covers the luminal surface of the endothelium, and may provide the molecular substrate for endothelial erosion (40,105).

The role of high ESS on endothelial erosion is controversial. A preliminary study showed that acute exposure to high ESS leads to endothelial cell disintegration and luminal erosion (136). This finding was corroborated in some subsequent reports, (137,138) although other studies did not confirm the above concept and showed that disturbed flow in the form of oscillatory ESS is the critical factor inducing intimal erosion in diseased arteries (135,139). Similar inconsistency is noted with regard to the effects of high ESS on endothelial apoptosis, as some studies report that high ESS induces endothelial apoptosis (140,141), while other studies suggest that it suppresses apoptosis (142,143).

ESS-PLAQUE INTERACTIONS, PLAQUE MECHANICS, AND THE LOCAL ROLE OF HIGH ESS

The dynamic interplay between ESS and plaque at flow obstruction sites largely determines plaque stability. Low ESS induces plaque growth, but such plaque affects ESS by modifying arterial geometry and altering blood flow. ESS increases at the throat of substantial stenoses, low ESS is more prevalent in the upstream region, while low/oscillatory ESS predominates in the downstream shoulder (Fig. 18.4) (26). The plaque region downstream of minimal luminal area contains considerably more smooth muscle cells, whereas the upstream portion is more inflamed, encompassing more macrophages and more frequently shows ECM degradation and intraplaque hemorrhage (144,145). In animal models, the downstream regions exhibited stable plaques, while the upstream segments developed vulnerable lesions (51). Overall, it is postulated that low and/or oscillatory ESS in the downstream plaque portion induces a feedback mechanism, leading to downstream plaque extension, while a high-risk plaque profile predominates in the upstream portion (Fig. 18.4). Plaque rupture may ensue from ordinary hemodynamic stress in this fragile upstream area.

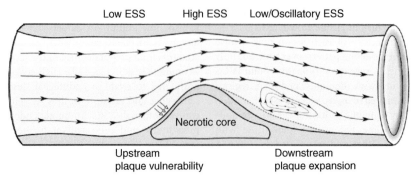

Figure 18.4 Flow pattern along a lumen-protruding plaque. The upstream shoulder of the plaque encounters low endothelial shear stress (ESS). ESS is high at the throat and low/oscillatory at the downstream shoulder where disturbed flow occurs. These local ESS conditions promote the formation of a vulnerable, rupture-prone plaque in the upstream region (*white arrows*), and additional growth (*dashed line*) downstream of the plaque.

Increased ESS values have been associated with plaque rupture or ulceration in some reports (146–148). Vascular areas exposed to high flow rates may be associated with smooth muscle cell atrophy, increased macrophage infiltration, and ECM degradation (149–151). High ESS pathophysiologically is linked to increased strain, which is a potential marker of instability (152,153). There is recent evidence that exposure to high ESS sensitizes platelets, so that when they subsequently reach the low ESS area they are activated at least 20-fold faster (154). Newly published studies further show that platelets respond to high ESS by cellular polarization, cytoskeletal reorganization, and flow-directed migration, and that even brief passage through very high ESS stenotic regions triggers platelet aggregation (155,156). Also, high ESS causes platelets to secrete connective tissue growth factor, which mediates platelet adherence, and to attach to von Willebrand factor leading to the formation of platelet-rich thrombus (157–159). A recent serial human study found that high ESS is responsible for the transition of plaques toward an unstable phenotype characterized by necrotic core expansion, dense calcium accumulation, and regression of fibrous and fibrofatty tissue as assessed by radio-frequency IVUS (160). However, it is uncertain if such a high-risk plaque profile would actually lead to clinical events.

Furthermore, it is not yet clear if high ESS is the cause of plaque disruption, or it is simply an epiphenomenon. Increased flow rate through a site of abrupt partial luminal compromise due to plaque rupture may account for high ESS, which in this case would be the result and not the cause of rupture. From a biomechanical standpoint, the order of magnitude of ESS values is considerably smaller than that of the blood-pressure-induced circumferential tensile stress in the coronary wall. Conceivably, the circumferential tensile stress is more likely to exceed the highest force that the plaque can withstand and cause rupture. In eccentric lesions, fibrous cap disruption most commonly occurs at areas exposed to the highest tensile stress as the lateral plaque shoulders (161,162). Long-standing circumferential strain in these regions as well as substantial axial strain resulting from flow impediment is thought to introduce

cap fatigue reducing tissue mechanical strength and, ultimately, causing cap fracture (163).

ESS AND BLOOD THROMBOGENICITY

The presence of a vulnerable plaque is not the sole factor responsible for adverse outcomes in the natural history of atherosclerosis. An increased responsiveness of the clotting mechanism to loss of vascular integrity is also required (164). Low ESS promotes local blood thrombogenicity by suppressing anti-thrombotic and anti-coagulant factors such as NO, prostacyclin, thrombomodulin, and tissue plasminogen activator (48,165–169). Also, low ESS induces tissue factor, a strong procoagulant molecule (170,171). Regional low ESS leads to increased thrombin generation (170) and increased platelet activation (172,173). As already mentioned, low-ESS-induced endothelial apoptosis may further contribute to an increased local thrombogenic potential (131,132). These effects in turn stimulate a plethora of proatherogenic and plaque-destabilizing actions (174). Interestingly, high ESS also activates platelets as discussed in the previous section. In the setting of an acute fibrous cap disruption or endothelial denudation, this ESS-mediated enhanced clotting tendency likely leads to significant fibrin formation, which gives rise either to rapid plaque progression or abrupt luminal occlusion.

EFFECTS OF MEDICATIONS ON ESS

The modification of the local ESS microenvironment and plaque stabilization may partly account for the favorable effects of established medications for coronary disease. Chronic administration of valsartan or a valsartan/simvastatin combination attenuated the pro-atherogenic influence of low ESS in an animal model. This effect was mediated via reduced inflammation, ECM degradation, and expansive remodeling independent of their antihypertensive and hypolipidemic action (175). Statins upregulate atheroprotective transcriptional factors, and hence are likely to counterbalance the detrimental effects of low ESS (176,177). Both aspirin and ticlopidine significantly inhibit platelet aggregation under high shear stress conditions (178). In an animal model of vulnerable plaque, metoprolol treatment

Focus Box 18.3

Low and/or oscillatory ESS causes endothelial dysfunction and exacerbates local inflammation and oxidative stress

Low-ESS-induced molecular mediators trigger the pathobiologic vascular manifestations of lipid uptake and catabolism, extracellular matrix degradation, cellular apoptosis, and angiogenesis

These pathobiologic manifestations cause the development of TCFAs and/or endothelial erosions

Both high- and low-ESS-mediated increases in blood thrombogenicity in regions with TCFAs and/or endothelial erosions lead to plaque destabilization, which causes either acute complete luminal occlusion or partial occlusion and healing

increased ESS to physiological values, and this was associated with a reduction in inflammatory cytokines, attenuation of expansive remodeling, reduced histopathological indices of vulnerability, and a trend toward reduced plaque size and rate of rupture (179).

IN VIVO ASSESSMENT OF ESS IN THE DETECTION OF

HIGH-RISK PLAQUE: RESEARCH AND CLINICAL IMPLICATIONS

As discussed above, ESS is a critical determinant of vascular behavior and orchestrates several responses that lead to plaque destabilization. Destabilized plaques are likely to experience rapid progression of fixed, flow-impeding lesions manifesting as worsening ischemia or abrupt luminal occlusion presenting as ACS (Fig. 18.5). Prevention of plaque destabilization is a major challenge in current cardiovascular medicine. Early identification of high-risk lesions is still problematic with the current diagnostic modalities. ACS in a previously asymptomatic individual is a common clinical scenario, often with catastrophic consequences. In addition, residual cardiovascular morbidity exists post ACS despite intensive risk-factor modification, pharmacological, and interventional therapy. For stable ischemia, coronary interventions currently apply only to significantly flow-limiting or occlusive lesions, overlooking potentially hazardous but non-stenotic plaques (180).

Identification of coronary regions with disturbed flow could prompt measures to prevent adverse future sequelae. *In vivo* assessment of ESS and remodeling using catheter-based or noninvasive vascular profiling may allow identification of coronary regions with an unfavorable rheological profile. Low ESS and expansive remodeling may not only assist to distinguish vulnerable plaques, but also, most importantly, foretell the development of lesions likely to exhibit accelerated atherosclerosis or trigger an ACS. Vigorous systemic or local treatment focused on high-risk early plaques may be prophylactic against future adverse cardiovascular events. Novel pharmacologic agents as well as innovative interventional devices (i.e., drug-eluting and bioabsorbable stents) portend satisfactory outcomes with a low risk of adverse events (181,182). To justify the rationale for pre-emptive intervention in high-risk regions without overt disease, the *in vivo* role

of ESS in human coronary atherosclerosis needs to be firmly established. A large-scale multicenter clinical natural history study of atherosclerosis (the PREDICTION study) is the first-in-man study investigating the predictive value of low ESS and expansive remodeling in atherosclerosis progression and plaque vulnerability. The study results are awaited with great interest.

CONCLUSIONS

Low ESS leads to mechanisms that synergistically promote the conversion of early atherosclerotic plaques toward an unstable phenotype. Low ESS stimulates local inflammation, oxidation, reduced production, and increased breakdown of ECM, and fosters plaque growth and expansive remodeling, a high-risk structural wall response that further exacerbates the adverse low-ESS stimulus. Early lesions persistently exposed to this deleterious milieu may, thereby, progress to high-risk TCFAs. Endothelial erosion and increased blood thrombogenicity also contribute to plaque destabilization.

The *in vivo* measurement of ESS may enable early recognition of lesions destined to acquire a vulnerable phenotype. Early identification of such high-risk plaques before they cause adverse outcomes could be a breakthrough in the management of patients with coronary artery disease, as it may set the stage for highly selective prophylactic treatment strategies to avert future coronary events, a possibility that may be both clinically invaluable and cost-effective.

PERSONAL PERSPECTIVE

Coronary atherosclerosis progresses both as a slow, gradual enlargement of focal plaque and a more dynamic process with periodic abrupt changes of plaque geometry, size, and morphology. These pathobiologic processes develop in a subclinical manner within the arterial wall until the magnitude of disturbance of coronary blood flow becomes so substantial that clinical manifestations are evident. Abrupt plaque changes may result from local rupture or erosion and lead to either acute luminal occlusion manifesting as ACS or rapid plaque growth presenting as exacerbation of stable angina. These events clearly do not occur in a random manner, but as a result of numerous pathobiologic and biomechanical processes, acting alone and in concert. An understanding of the actively evolving vascular phenomena, as well as development of *in vivo* imaging methodologies to identify the presence and severity of the different processes, may enable early identification of a coronary plaque destined to acquire a high-risk state and allow for pre-emptive intervention to avert the adverse natural history of that particular plaque.

In vivo technologies are evolving to accurately assess high-risk plaque. Since most imaging can realistically be performed only at a single timepoint, these methods will need to accomplish two tasks: (*i*) identify the current state of an individual plaque, and (*ii*) determine whether ongoing pathobiologic processes are present, which are likely to lead to further deterioration of plaque stability in the near future. Current *in vivo* modalities can define the plaque constituents and characteristics at a snapshot in time: coronary angiography, IVUS,

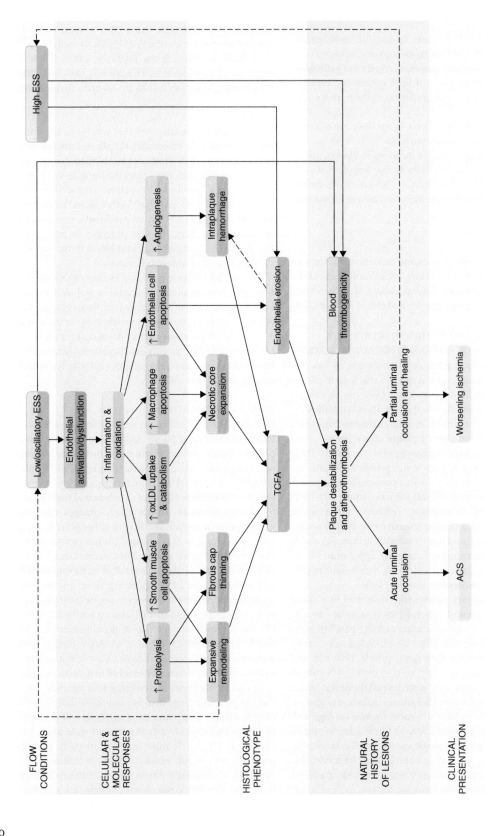

Figure 18.5 Mechanisms of endothelial shear stress (ESS)-mediated plaque destabilization. Low and/or oscillatory ESS orchestrates molecular, cellular, and vascular responses in atherosclerosis-prone regions favoring plaque initiation and leads toward thin–cap fibroatheroma (TCFA) formation, endothelial erosion, and increased blood thrombogenicity, factors likely to cause plaque destabilization and atherothrombosis. Atherothrombosis causes either abrupt luminal occlusion and acute coronary syndrome (ACS) or accelerated plaque progression via repeated cycles of subclinical partial luminal occlusion and healing, which presents as worsening ischemia. Increased luminal stenosis relates to high ESS, which aggravates blood-clotting tendency and may induce endothelial erosion, further contributing to plaque destabilization. *Abbreviations*: ECM, Extracellular matrix; oxLDL, oxidized low-density lipoprotein.

radiofrequency IVUS, optical coherence tomography, near-infrared spectroscopy, angioscopy, etc. Complementary and potentially synergistic methodologies now exist to evaluate the underlying pathophysiologic driving mechanism responsible for ongoing progression of each plaque, such as the assessment of local ESS, and may add incremental insight concerning the natural history of that individual plaque. Future methodologies may also be able to characterize the inflammatory state more directly, such as with targeted nanotechnology and advanced imaging techniques, and may also be able to distinguish the mechanical properties of plaque.

There is, undoubtedly, a large denominator of theoretically high-risk coronary plaques, but the number of these plaques that actually go on to trigger a new vascular and clinical event is very low. The challenges for investigators at this time are to identify the specific constellation of high-risk features that characterize the truly highest-risk plaques, and screen out the vast majority of plaques and patients that are not in the highest-risk category. These objectives must be accomplished in a manner where the clinical and cost-effectiveness benefits substantially outweigh the risks and costs of the procedures. An enormous payback for society is anticipated if these tasks are achieved, and thus these goals are worth our continued pursuit.

REFERENCES

1. Roger VL, Go AS, Lloyd-Jones DM, et al. Heart disease and stroke statistics–2011 update: a report from the American Heart Association. Circulation 2011; 123: e18–e209.
2. Asakura T, Karino T. Flow patterns and spatial distribution of atherosclerotic lesions in human coronary arteries. Circ Res 1990; 66: 1045–66.
3. Giannoglou GD, Soulis JV, Farmakis TM, Farmakis DM, Louridas GE. Haemodynamic factors and the important role of local low static pressure in coronary wall thickening. Int J Cardiol 2002; 86: 27–40.
4. Malek AM, Alper SL, Izumo S. Hemodynamic shear stress and its role in atherosclerosis. JAMA 1999; 282: 2035–42.
5. Chatzizisis YS, Coskun AU, Jonas M, et al. Role of endothelial shear stress in the natural history of coronary atherosclerosis and vascular remodeling: molecular, cellular, and vascular behavior. J Am Coll Cardiol 2007; 49: 2379–93.
6. Richter Y, Edelman ER. Cardiology is flow. Circulation 2006; 113: 2679–82.
7. Gimbrone MA Jr, Topper JN, Nagel T, Anderson KR, Garcia-Cardena G. Endothelial dysfunction, hemodynamic forces, and atherogenesis. Ann NY Acad Sci 2000; 902: 230–9.
8. Koskinas KC, Chatzizisis YS, Baker AB, et al. The role of low endothelial shear stress in the conversion of atherosclerotic lesions from stable to unstable plaque. Curr Opin Cardiol 2009; 24: 580–90.
9. Ambrose JA, Srikanth S. Vulnerable plaques and patients: improving prediction of future coronary events. Am J Med 2010; 123: 10–6.
10. Davies MJ. Anatomic features in victims of sudden coronary death. Coronary artery pathology. Circulation 1992; 85: I19–24.
11. Farb A, Burke AP, Tang AL, et al. Coronary plaque erosion without rupture into a lipid core. A frequent cause of coronary thrombosis in sudden coronary death. Circulation 1996; 93: 1354–63.
12. Virmani R, Kolodgie FD, Burke AP, Farb A, Schwartz SM. Lessons from sudden coronary death: a comprehensive morphological classification scheme for atherosclerotic lesions. Arterioscler Thromb Vasc Biol 2000; 20: 1262–75.
13. Mann J, Davies MJ. Mechanisms of progression in native coronary artery disease: role of healed plaque disruption. Heart 1999; 82: 265–8.
14. Burke AP, Kolodgie FD, Farb A, et al. Healed plaque ruptures and sudden coronary death: evidence that subclinical rupture has a role in plaque progression. Circulation 2001; 103: 934–40.
15. Burke AP, Farb A, Malcom GT, et al. Coronary risk factors and plaque morphology in men with coronary disease who died suddenly. N Engl J Med 1997; 336: 1276–82.
16. Davies MJ. The composition of coronary-artery plaques. N Engl J Med 1997; 336: 1312–4.
17. Virmani R, Burke AP, Farb A, Kolodgie FD. Pathology of the vulnerable plaque. J Am Coll Cardiol 2006; 47: C13–8.
18. Stone GW, Maehara A, Lansky AJ, et al. A prospective natural-history study of coronary atherosclerosis. N Engl J Med 2011; 364: 226–35.
19. Kubo T, Maehara A, Mintz GS, et al. The dynamic nature of coronary artery lesion morphology assessed by serial virtual histology intravascular ultrasound tissue characterization. J Am Coll Cardiol 2010; 55: 1590–7.
20. Fichtlscherer S, Breuer S, Zeiher AM. Prognostic value of systemic endothelial dysfunction in patients with acute coronary syndromes: further evidence for the existence of the "vulnerable" patient. Circulation 2004; 110: 1926–32.
21. Kolodgie FD, Gold HK, Burke AP, et al. Intraplaque hemorrhage and progression of coronary atheroma. N Engl J Med 2003; 349: 2316–25.
22. Schoenhagen P, Ziada KM, Kapadia SR, et al. Extent and direction of arterial remodeling in stable versus unstable coronary syndromes: an intravascular ultrasound study. Circulation 2000; 101: 598–603.
23. Cheng C, Helderman F, Tempel D, et al. Large variations in absolute wall shear stress levels within one species and between species. Atherosclerosis 2007; 195: 225–35.
24. Soulis JV, Giannoglou GD, Chatzizisis YS, et al. Spatial and phasic oscillation of non-Newtonian wall shear stress in human left coronary artery bifurcation: an insight to atherogenesis. Coron Artery Dis 2006; 17: 351–8.
25. Lee SW, Antiga L, Spence JD, Steinman DA. Geometry of the carotid bifurcation predicts its exposure to disturbed flow. Stroke 2008; 39: 2341–7.
26. Davies PF. Hemodynamic shear stress and the endothelium in cardiovascular pathophysiology. Nat Clin Pract Cardiovasc Med 2009; 6: 16–26.
27. Slager CJ, Wentzel JJ, Schuurbiers JC, et al. True 3-dimensional reconstruction of coronary arteries in patients by fusion of angiography and IVUS (ANGUS) and its quantitative validation. Circulation 2000; 102: 511–6.
28. Krams R, Wentzel JJ, Oomen JA, et al. Evaluation of endothelial shear stress and 3D geometry as factors determining the development of atherosclerosis and remodeling in human coronary arteries in vivo. Combining 3D reconstruction from angiography and IVUS (ANGUS) with computational fluid dynamics. Arterioscler Thromb Vasc Biol 1997; 17: 2061–5.

29. Feldman CL, Ilegbusi OJ, Hu Z, et al. Determination of in vivo velocity and endothelial shear stress patterns with phasic flow in human coronary arteries: a methodology to predict progression of coronary atherosclerosis. Am Heart J 2002; 143: 931–9.

30. Coskun AU, Yeghiazarians Y, Kinlay S, et al. Reproducibility of coronary lumen, plaque, and vessel wall reconstruction and of endothelial shear stress measurements in vivo in humans. Catheter Cardiovasc Interv 2003; 60: 67–78.

31. Feldman CL, Stone PH. Intravascular hemodynamic factors responsible for progression of coronary atherosclerosis and development of vulnerable plaque. Curr Opin Cardiol 2000; 15: 430–40.

32. Ilegbusi OJ, Hu Z, Nesto R, et al. Determination of blood flow and endothelial shear stress in human coronary artery in vivo. J Invasive Cardiol 1999; 11: 667–74.

33. Ramkumar PG, Mitsouras D, Feldman CL, Stone PH, Rybicki FJ. New advances in cardiac computed tomography. Curr Opin Cardiol 2009; 24: 596–603.

34. van der Giessen AG, Schaap M, Gijsen FJ, et al. 3D fusion of intravascular ultrasound and coronary computed tomography for in-vivo wall shear stress analysis: a feasibility study. Int J Cardiovasc Imaging 2010; 26: 781–96.

35. van der Giessen AG, Wentzel JJ, Meijboom WB, et al. Plaque and shear stress distribution in human coronary bifurcations: a multislice computed tomography study. EuroIntervention 2009; 4: 654–61.

36. Libby P, Aikawa M, Jain MK. Vascular endothelium and atherosclerosis. In: Moncada S, Higgs A, eds. The Vascular Endothelium II, Handbook of Experimental Pharmacology, Springer Berlin Heidelberg 2006; 176: 285–306.

37. Li H, Forstermann U. Prevention of atherosclerosis by interference with the vascular nitric oxide system. Curr Pharm Des 2009; 15: 3133–45.

38. Giannotti G, Landmesser U. Endothelial dysfunction as an early sign of atherosclerosis. Herz 2007; 32: 568–72.

39. Pahakis MY, Kosky JR, Dull RO, Tarbell JM. The role of endothelial glycocalyx components in mechanotransduction of fluid shear stress. Biochem Biophys Res Commun 2007; 355: 228–33.

40. Reitsma S, Slaaf DW, Vink H, van Zandvoort MA, oude Egbrink MG. The endothelial glycocalyx: composition, functions, and visualization. Pflugers Arch 2007; 454: 345–59.

41. Tarbell JM, Weinbaum S, Kamm RD. Cellular fluid mechanics and mechanotransduction. Ann Biomed Eng 2005; 33: 1719–23.

42. Milovanova T, Chatterjee S, Hawkins BJ, et al. Caveolae are an essential component of the pathway for endothelial cell signaling associated with abrupt reduction of shear stress. Biochim Biophys Acta 2008; 1783: 1866–75.

43. Collins C, Tzima E. Hemodynamic forces in endothelial dysfunction and vascular aging. Exp Gerontol 2011; 46: 185–8.

44. Tsou JK, Gower RM, Ting HJ, et al. Spatial regulation of inflammation by human aortic endothelial cells in a linear gradient of shear stress. Microcirculation 2008; 15: 311–23.

45. Dhawan SS, Avati Nanjundappa RP, Branch JR, et al. Shear stress and plaque development. Expert Rev Cardiovasc Ther 2010; 8: 545–56.

46. Nigro P, Abe J, Berk BC. Flow shear stress and atherosclerosis: a matter of site specificity. Antioxid Redox Signal 2011; 15: 1405–14.

47. Cicha I, Goppelt-Struebe M, Yilmaz A, Daniel WG, Garlichs CD. Endothelial dysfunction and monocyte recruitment in cells exposed to non-uniform shear stress. Clin Hemorheol Microcirc 2008; 39: 113–9.

48. Mun GI, Kim IS, Lee BH, Boo YC. Endothelial argininosuccinate synthetase 1 regulates nitric oxide production and monocyte adhesion under static and laminar shear stress conditions. J Biol Chem 2011; 286: 2536–42.

49. Andrews AM, Jaron D, Buerk DG, Kirby PL, Barbee KA. Direct, real-time measurement of shear stress-induced nitric oxide produced from endothelial cells in vitro. Nitric Oxide 2010; 23: 335–42.

50. Thacher TN, Silacci P, Stergiopulos N, da Silva RF. Autonomous effects of shear stress and cyclic circumferential stretch regarding endothelial dysfunction and oxidative stress: an ex vivo arterial model. J Vasc Res 2010; 47: 336–45.

51. Cheng C, Tempel D, van Haperen R, et al. Atherosclerotic lesion size and vulnerability are determined by patterns of fluid shear stress. Circulation 2006; 113: 2744–53.

52. Cheng C, van Haperen R, de Waard M, et al. Shear stress affects the intracellular distribution of eNOS: direct demonstration by a novel in vivo technique. Blood 2005; 106: 3691–8.

53. White SJ, Hayes EM, Lehoux S, et al. Characterization of the differential response of endothelial cells exposed to normal and elevated laminar shear stress. J Cell Physiol 2011; 226: 2841–8.

54. Chien S. Molecular and mechanical bases of focal lipid accumulation in arterial wall. Prog Biophys Mol Biol 2003; 83: 131–51.

55. Himburg HA, Grzybowski DM, Hazel AL, et al. Spatial comparison between wall shear stress measures and porcine arterial endothelial permeability. Am J Physiol Heart Circ Physiol 2004; 286: H1916–22.

56. Tricot O, Mallat Z, Heymes C, et al. Relation between endothelial cell apoptosis and blood flow direction in human atherosclerotic plaques. Circulation 2000; 101: 2450–3.

57. Cancel LM, Tarbell JM. The role of apoptosis in LDL transport through cultured endothelial cell monolayers. Atherosclerosis 2010; 208: 335–41.

58. Papafaklis MI, Koskinas KC, Baker AB, et al. Low endothelial shear stress upregulates atherogenic and inflammatory genes extremely early in the natural history of coronary artery disease in diabetic hyperlipidemic juvenile swine. Eur Heart J 2011; 32(Abstract Supplement): 156.

59. Cai Q, Lanting L, Natarajan R. Interaction of monocytes with vascular smooth muscle cells regulates monocyte survival and differentiation through distinct pathways. Arterioscler Thromb Vasc Biol 2004; 24: 2263–70.

60. Seimon T, Tabas I. Mechanisms and consequences of macrophage apoptosis in atherosclerosis. J Lipid Res 2009; 50(Suppl): S382–7.

61. Olgac U, Kurtcuoglu V, Poulikakos D. Computational modeling of coupled blood-wall mass transport of LDL: effects of local wall shear stress. Am J Physiol Heart Circ Physiol 2008; 294: H909–19.

62. Soulis JV, Fytanidis DK, Papaioannou VC, Giannoglou GD. Wall shear stress on LDL accumulation in human RCAs. Med Eng Phys 2010; 32: 867–77.

63. Sun N, Wood NB, Hughes AD, Thom SA, Yun Xu X. Effects of transmural pressure and wall shear stress on LDL accumulation in the arterial wall: a numerical study using a multilayered model. Am J Physiol Heart Circ Physiol 2007; 292: H3148–57.

64. Olgac U, Knight J, Poulikakos D, et al. Computed high concentrations of low-density lipoprotein correlate with plaque locations in human coronary arteries. J Biomech 2011; 44: 2466–71.

65. Koskinas KC, Feldman CL, Chatzizisis YS, et al. Natural history of experimental coronary atherosclerosis and vascular remodeling

in relation to endothelial shear stress: a serial, in vivo intravascular ultrasound study. Circulation 2010; 121: 2092–101.

66. Chatzizisis YS, Baker AB, Sukhova GK, et al. Augmented expression and activity of extracellular matrix-degrading enzymes in regions of low endothelial shear stress colocalize with coronary atheromata with thin fibrous caps in pigs. Circulation 2011; 123: 621–30.

67. Chatzizisis YS, Jonas M, Coskun AU, et al. Prediction of the localization of high-risk coronary atherosclerotic plaques on the basis of low endothelial shear stress: an intravascular ultrasound and histopathology natural history study. Circulation 2008; 117: 993–1002.

68. Hosokawa T, Kumon Y, Kobayashi T, et al. Neutrophil infiltration and oxidant-production in human atherosclerotic carotid plaques. Histol Histopathol 2011; 26: 1–11.

69. Erbel C, Dengler TJ, Wangler S, et al. Expression of IL-17A in human atherosclerotic lesions is associated with increased inflammation and plaque vulnerability. Basic Res Cardiol 2011; 106: 125–34.

70. Urschel K, Worner A, Daniel WG, Garlichs CD, Cicha I. Role of shear stress patterns in the TNF-alpha-induced atherogenic protein expression and monocytic cell adhesion to endothelium. Clin Hemorheol Microcirc 2010; 46: 203–10.

71. Rouleau L, Copland IB, Tardif JC, Mongrain R, Leask RL. Neutrophil adhesion on endothelial cells in a novel asymmetric stenosis model: effect of wall shear stress gradients. Ann Biomed Eng 2010; 38: 2791–804.

72. Shaik SS, Soltau TD, Chaturvedi G, et al. Low intensity shear stress increases endothelial ELR+ CXC chemokine production via a focal adhesion kinase-p38{beta} MAPK-NF-{kappa}B pathway. J Biol Chem 2009; 284: 5945–55.

73. Fu Y, Hou Y, Fu C, et al. A novel mechanism of gamma/delta T-lymphocyte and endothelial activation by shear stress: the role of ecto-ATP synthase beta chain. Circ Res 2011; 108: 410–7.

74. Boisvert WA, Curtiss LK, Terkeltaub RA. Interleukin-8 and its receptor CXCR2 in atherosclerosis. Immunol Res 2000; 21: 129–37.

75. Zhu CH, Ying DJ, Mi JH, et al. Low shear stress regulates monocyte adhesion to oxidized lipid-induced endothelial cells via an IkappaBalpha dependent pathway. Biorheology 2004; 41: 127–37.

76. Makino A, Prossnitz ER, Bunemann M, et al. G protein-coupled receptors serve as mechanosensors for fluid shear stress in neutrophils. Am J Physiol Cell Physiol 2006; 290: C1633–9.

77. Chiu JJ, Lee PL, Chen CN, et al. Shear stress increases ICAM-1 and decreases VCAM-1 and E-selectin expressions induced by tumor necrosis factor-[alpha] in endothelial cells. Arterioscler Thromb Vasc Biol 2004; 24: 73–9.

78. Sheikh S, Rainger GE, Gale Z, Rahman M, Nash GB. Exposure to fluid shear stress modulates the ability of endothelial cells to recruit neutrophils in response to tumor necrosis factor-alpha: a basis for local variations in vascular sensitivity to inflammation. Blood 2003; 102: 2828–34.

79. Cheng C, Tempel D, van Haperen R, et al. Shear stress-induced changes in atherosclerotic plaque composition are modulated by chemokines. J Clin Invest 2007; 117: 616–26.

80. Hulsmans M, Holvoet P. The vicious circle between oxidative stress and inflammation in atherosclerosis. J Cell Mol Med 2010; 14: 70–8.

81. Dimmeler S, Hermann C, Galle J, Zeiher AM. Upregulation of superoxide dismutase and nitric oxide synthase mediates the apoptosis-suppressive effects of shear stress on endothelial cells. Arterioscler Thromb Vasc Biol 1999; 19: 656–64.

82. Hwang J, Ing MH, Salazar A, et al. Pulsatile versus oscillatory shear stress regulates NADPH oxidase subunit expression: implication for native LDL oxidation. Circ Res 2003; 93: 1225–32.

83. McNally JS, Davis ME, Giddens DP, et al. Role of xanthine oxidoreductase and NAD(P)H oxidase in endothelial superoxide production in response to oscillatory shear stress. Am J Physiol Heart Circ Physiol 2003; 285: H2290–7.

84. Resnick N, Yahav H, Shay-Salit A, et al. Fluid shear stress and the vascular endothelium: for better and for worse. Prog Biophys Mol Biol 2003; 81: 177–99.

85. Dai G, Kaazempur-Mofrad MR, Natarajan S, et al. Distinct endothelial phenotypes evoked by arterial waveforms derived from atherosclerosis-susceptible and -resistant regions of human vasculature. Proc Natl Acad Sci USA 2004; 101: 14871–6.

86. Davies PF, Civelek M. Endoplasmic reticulum stress, redox, and a proinflammatory environment in athero-susceptible endothelium in vivo at sites of complex hemodynamic shear stress. Antioxid Redox Signal 2011; 15: 1427–32.

87. Takeshita S, Inoue N, Ueyama T, Kawashima S, Yokoyama M. Shear stress enhances glutathione peroxidase expression in endothelial cells. Biochem Biophys Res Commun 2000; 273: 66–71.

88. Hsiai TK, Hwang J, Barr ML, et al. Hemodynamics influences vascular peroxynitrite formation: implication for low-density lipoprotein apo-B-100 nitration. Free Radic Biol Med 2007; 42: 519–29.

89. Crabtree MJ, Channon KM. Synthesis and recycling of tetrahydrobiopterin in endothelial function and vascular disease. Nitric Oxide 2011; 25: 81–8.

90. Takabe W, Warabi E, Noguchi N. Anti-atherogenic effect of laminar shear stress via Nrf2 activation. Antioxid Redox Signal 2011; 15: 1415–26.

91. Ramkhelawon B, Vilar J, Rivas D, et al. Shear stress regulates angiotensin type 1 receptor expression in endothelial cells. Circ Res 2009; 105: 869–75.

92. Fariss MW, Chan CB, Patel M, Van Houten B, Orrenius S. Role of mitochondria in toxic oxidative stress. Mol Interv 2005; 5: 94–111.

93. Li R, Beebe T, Cui J, et al. Pulsatile shear stress increased mitochondrial membrane potential: implication of Mn-SOD. Biochem Biophys Res Commun 2009; 388: 406–12.

94. Karangelis DE, Kanakis I, Asimakopoulou AP, et al. Glycosaminoglycans as key molecules in atherosclerosis: the role of versican and hyaluronan. Curr Med Chem 2010; 17: 4018–26.

95. Rouis M. Matrix metalloproteinases: a potential therapeutic target in atherosclerosis. Curr Drug Targets Cardiovasc Haematol Disord 2005; 5: 541–8.

96. Dollery CM, Libby P. Atherosclerosis and proteinase activation. Cardiovasc Res 2006; 69: 625–35.

97. Galis ZS, Khatri JJ. Matrix metalloproteinases in vascular remodeling and atherogenesis: the good, the bad, and the ugly. Circ Res 2002; 90: 251–62.

98. Ketelhuth DF, Back M. The role of matrix metalloproteinases in atherothrombosis. Curr Atheroscler Rep 2011; 13: 162–9.

99. Shukla S, Fujita K-i, Xiao Q, et al. A shear stress responsive gene product PP1201 protects against Fas-mediated apoptosis by reducing Fas expression on the cell surface. Apoptosis 2010; 16: 162–73.

100. Qi YX, Qu MJ, Long DK, et al. Rho-GDP dissociation inhibitor alpha downregulated by low shear stress promotes vascular smooth muscle cell migration and apoptosis: a proteomic analysis. Cardiovasc Res 2008; 80: 114–22.

101. Yamane T, Mitsumata M, Yamaguchi N, et al. Laminar high shear stress up-regulates type IV collagen synthesis and down-regulates MMP-2 secretion in endothelium. A quantitative analysis. Cell Tissue Res 2010; 340: 471–9.

102. Dumont O, Loufrani L, Henrion D. Key role of the NO-pathway and matrix metalloprotease-9 in high blood flow-induced remodeling of rat resistance arteries. Arterioscler Thromb Vasc Biol 2007; 27: 317–24.

103. Kolpakov V, Gordon D, Kulik TJ. Nitric oxide-generating compounds inhibit total protein and collagen synthesis in cultured vascular smooth muscle cells. Circ Res 1995; 76: 305–9.

104. Death AK, Nakhla S, McGrath KC, et al. Nitroglycerin upregulates matrix metalloproteinase expression by human macrophages. J Am Coll Cardiol 2002; 39: 1943–50.

105. Baker AB, Chatzizisis YS, Beigel R, et al. Regulation of heparanase expression in coronary artery disease in diabetic, hyperlipidemic swine. Atherosclerosis 2010; 213: 436–42.

106. Korshunov VA, Schwartz SM, Berk BC. Vascular remodeling: hemodynamic and biochemical mechanisms underlying Glagov's phenomenon. Arterioscler Thromb Vasc Biol 2007; 27: 1722–8.

107. Mintz GS, Garcia-Garcia HM, Nicholls SJ, et al. Clinical expert consensus document on standards for acquisition, measurement and reporting of intravascular ultrasound regression/progression studies. EuroIntervention 2011; 6: 1123–30; 1129.

108. Feldman CL, Coskun AU, Yeghiazarians Y, et al. Remodeling characteristics of minimally diseased coronary arteries are consistent along the length of the artery. Am J Cardiol 2006; 97: 13–16.

109. Papafaklis MI, Koskinas KC, Chatzizisis YS, Stone PH, Feldman CL. In-vivo assessment of the natural history of coronary atherosclerosis: vascular remodeling and endothelial shear stress determine the complexity of atherosclerotic disease progression. Curr Opin Cardiol 2010; 25: 627–38.

110. Kroner ES, van Velzen JE, Boogers MJ, et al. Positive remodeling on coronary computed tomography as a marker for plaque vulnerability on virtual histology intravascular ultrasound. Am J Cardiol 2011; 107: 1725–9.

111. Alviar CL, Tellez A, Wallace-Bradley D, et al. Impact of adventitial neovascularisation on atherosclerotic plaque composition and vascular remodelling in a porcine model of coronary atherosclerosis. EuroIntervention 2010; 5: 981–8.

112. Kashiwagi M, Tanaka A, Kitabata H, et al. Relationship between coronary arterial remodeling, fibrous cap thickness and high-sensitivity C-reactive protein levels in patients with acute coronary syndrome. Circ J 2009; 73: 1291–5.

113. Okura H, Kobayashi Y, Sumitsuji S, et al. Effect of culprit-lesion remodeling versus plaque rupture on three-year outcome in patients with acute coronary syndrome. Am J Cardiol 2009; 103: 791–5.

114. Stone PH, Coskun AU, Kinlay S, et al. Effect of endothelial shear stress on the progression of coronary artery disease, vascular remodeling, and in-stent restenosis in humans: in vivo 6-month follow-up study. Circulation 2003; 108: 438–44.

115. Stone PH, Coskun AU, Kinlay S, et al. Regions of low endothelial shear stress are the sites where coronary plaque progresses and vascular remodelling occurs in humans: an in vivo serial study. Eur Heart J 2007; 28: 705–10.

116. Duivenvoorden R, Vanbavel E, de Groot E, et al. Endothelial shear stress: a critical determinant of arterial remodeling and arterial stiffness in humans–a carotid 3.0-T MRI study. Circ Cardiovasc Imaging 2010; 3: 578–85.

117. Baldewsing RA, Schaar JA, Mastik F, van der Steen AF. Local elasticity imaging of vulnerable atherosclerotic coronary plaques. Adv Cardiol 2007; 44: 35–61.

118. Slager CJ, Wentzel JJ, Gijsen FJ, et al. The role of shear stress in the generation of rupture-prone vulnerable plaques. Nat Clin Pract Cardiovasc Med 2005; 2: 401–7.

119. Wentzel JJ, Janssen E, Vos J, et al. Extension of increased atherosclerotic wall thickness into high shear stress regions is associated with loss of compensatory remodeling. Circulation 2003; 108: 17–23.

120. Moreno PR, Purushothaman KR, Fuster V, et al. Plaque neovascularization is increased in ruptured atherosclerotic lesions of human aorta: implications for plaque vulnerability. Circulation 2004; 110: 2032–8.

121. Sluimer JC, Kolodgie FD, Bijnens AP, et al. Thin-walled microvessels in human coronary atherosclerotic plaques show incomplete endothelial junctions: relevance of compromised structural integrity for intraplaque microvascular leakage. J Am Coll Cardiol 2009; 53: 1517–27.

122. Virmani R, Kolodgie FD, Burke AP, et al. Atherosclerotic plaque progression and vulnerability to rupture: angiogenesis as a source of intraplaque hemorrhage. Arterioscler Thromb Vasc Biol 2005; 25: 2054–61.

123. de Nooijer R, Verkleij CJN, von der Thüsen JH, et al. Lesional overexpression of matrix metalloproteinase-9 promotes intraplaque hemorrhage in advanced lesions but not at earlier stages of atherogenesis. Arterioscler Thromb Vasc Biol 2006; 26: 340–6.

124. Giannoglou GD, Koskinas KC, Tziakas DN, et al. Total cholesterol content of erythrocyte membranes and coronary atherosclerosis: an intravascular ultrasound pilot study. Angiology 2009; 60: 676–82.

125. Hohberg M, Knochel J, Hoffmann CJ, et al. Expression of ADAMTS1 in endothelial cells is induced by shear stress and suppressed in sprouting capillaries. J Cell Physiol 2011; 226: 350–61.

126. Chu TJ, Peters DG. Serial analysis of the vascular endothelial transcriptome under static and shear stress conditions. Physiol Genomics 2008; 34: 185–92.

127. Davies PF, Remuzzi A, Gordon EJ, Dewey CF Jr, Gimbrone MA Jr. Turbulent fluid shear stress induces vascular endothelial cell turnover in vitro. Proc Natl Acad Sci USA 1986; 83: 2114–7.

128. Xu Q. Disturbed flow-enhanced endothelial turnover in atherosclerosis. Trends Cardiovasc Med 2009; 19: 191–5.

129. Vasa M, Breitschopf K, Zeiher AM, Dimmeler S. Nitric oxide activates telomerase and delays endothelial cell senescence. Circ Res 2000; 87: 540–2.

130. Kovacic JC, Moreno P, Hachinski V, Nabel EG, Fuster V. Cellular senescence, vascular disease, and aging: part 1 of a 2-part review. Circulation 2011; 123: 1650–60.

131. Bombeli T, Schwartz BR, Harlan JM. Endothelial cells undergoing apoptosis become proadhesive for nonactivated platelets. Blood 1999; 93: 3831–8.

132. Potapova IA, Cohen IS, Doronin SV. Apoptotic endothelial cells demonstrate increased adhesiveness for human mesenchymal stem cells. J Cell Physiol 2009; 219: 23–30.

133. Zeng L, Xiao Q, Margariti A, et al. HDAC3 is crucial in shear- and VEGF-induced stem cell differentiation toward endothelial cells. J Cell Biol 2006; 174: 1059–69.

134. Zhou B, Margariti A, Zeng L, Xu Q. Role of histone deacetylases in vascular cell homeostasis and arteriosclerosis. Cardiovasc Res 2011; 90: 413–20.

135. Sumi T, Yamashita A, Matsuda S, et al. Disturbed blood flow induces erosive injury to smooth muscle cell-rich neointima and promotes thrombus formation in rabbit femoral arteries. J Thromb Haemost 2010; 8: 1394–402.

136. Fry DL. Acute vascular endothelial changes associated with increased blood velocity gradients. Circ Res 1968; 22: 165–97.

137. Bernardo A, Ball C, Nolasco L, et al. Platelets adhered to endothelial cell-bound ultra-large von Willebrand factor strings support leukocyte tethering and rolling under high shear stress. J Thromb Haemost 2005; 3: 562–70.

138. Wechezak AR, Coan DE, Viggers RF, Sauvage LR. Dextran increases survival of subconfluent endothelial cells exposed to shear stress. Am J Physiol 1993; 264: H520–5.

139. Langille LB. Integrity of arterial endothelium following acute exposure to high shear stress. Biorheology 1984; 21: 333–46.

140. Dolan JM, Meng H, Singh S, Paluch R, Kolega J. High fluid shear stress and spatial shear stress gradients affect endothelial proliferation, survival, and alignment. Ann Biomed Eng 2011; 39: 1620–31.

141. Macario DK, Entersz I, Abboud JP, Nackman GB. Inhibition of apoptosis prevents shear-induced detachment of endothelial cells. J Surg Res 2008; 147: 282–9.

142. Metaxa E, Meng H, Kaluvala SR, et al. Nitric oxide-dependent stimulation of endothelial cell proliferation by sustained high flow. Am J Physiol Heart Circ Physiol 2008; 295: H736–42.

143. Zeng Y, Qiao Y, Zhang Y, et al. Effects of fluid shear stress on apoptosis of cultured human umbilical vein endothelial cells induced by LPS. Cell Biol Int 2005; 29: 932–5.

144. Segers D, Helderman F, Cheng C, et al. Gelatinolytic activity in atherosclerotic plaques is highly localized and is associated with both macrophages and smooth muscle cells in vivo. Circulation 2007; 115: 609–16.

145. Fagerberg B, Ryndel M, Kjelldahl J, et al. Differences in lesion severity and cellular composition between in vivo assessed upstream and downstream sides of human symptomatic carotid atherosclerotic plaques. J Vasc Res 2010; 47: 221–30.

146. Fukumoto Y, Hiro T, Fujii T, et al. Localized elevation of shear stress is related to coronary plaque rupture: a 3-dimensional intravascular ultrasound study with in-vivo color mapping of shear stress distribution. J Am Coll Cardiol 2008; 51: 645–50.

147. Groen HC, Gijsen FJ, van der Lugt A, et al. Plaque rupture in the carotid artery is localized at the high shear stress region: a case report. Stroke 2007; 38: 2379–81.

148. Tang D, Teng Z, Canton G, et al. Sites of rupture in human atherosclerotic carotid plaques are associated with high structural stresses: an in vivo MRI-based 3D fluid-structure interaction study. Stroke 2009; 40: 3258–63.

149. Kenagy RD, Min SK, Mulvihill E, Clowes AW. A link between smooth muscle cell death and extracellular matrix degradation during vascular atrophy. J Vasc Surg 2011; 54: 182–91 e124.

150. Kenagy RD, Fischer JW, Davies MG, et al. Increased plasmin and serine proteinase activity during flow-induced intimal atrophy in baboon PTFE grafts. Arterioscler Thromb Vasc Biol 2002; 22: 400–4.

151. Min SK, Kenagy RD, Jeanette JP, Clowes AW. Effects of external wrapping and increased blood flow on atrophy of the baboon iliac artery. J Vasc Surg 2008; 47: 1039–47.

152. Gijsen FJ, Mastik F, Schaar JA, et al. High shear stress induces a strain increase in human coronary plaques over a 6-month period. EuroIntervention 2011; 7: 121–7.

153. Gijsen FJ, Wentzel JJ, Thury A, et al. Strain distribution over plaques in human coronary arteries relates to shear stress. Am J Physiol Heart Circ Physiol 2008; 295: H1608–14.

154. Sheriff J, Bluestein D, Girdhar G, Jesty J. High-shear stress sensitizes platelets to subsequent low-shear conditions. Ann Biomed Eng 2010; 38: 1442–50.

155. Kraemer BF, Schmidt C, Urban B, et al. High shear flow induces migration of adherent human platelets. Platelets 2011; 22: 415–21.

156. Para A, Bark D, Lin A, Ku D. Rapid platelet accumulation leading to thrombotic occlusion. Ann Biomed Eng 2011; 39: 1961–71.

157. Cicha I, Yilmaz A, Suzuki Y, et al. Connective tissue growth factor is released from platelets under high shear stress and is differentially expressed in endothelium along atherosclerotic plaques. Clin Hemorheol Microcirc 2006; 35: 203–6.

158. Cicha I, Garlichs CD, Daniel WG, Goppelt-Struebe M. Activated human platelets release connective tissue growth factor. Thromb Haemost 2004; 91: 755–60.

159. Reininger AJ, Heijnen HF, Schumann H, et al. Mechanism of platelet adhesion to von Willebrand factor and microparticle formation under high shear stress. Blood 2006; 107: 3537–45.

160. Samady H, Eshtehardi P, McDaniel MC, et al. Coronary artery wall shear stress is associated with progression and transformation of atherosclerotic plaque and arterial remodeling in patients with coronary artery disease. Circulation 2011; 124: 779–88.

161. Richardson PD, Davies MJ, Born GV. Influence of plaque configuration and stress distribution on fissuring of coronary atherosclerotic plaques. Lancet 1989; 2: 941–4.

162. Kumar RK, Balakrishnan KR. Influence of lumen shape and vessel geometry on plaque stresses: possible role in the increased vulnerability of a remodelled vessel and the "shoulder" of a plaque. Heart 2005; 91: 1459–65.

163. Doriot PA. Estimation of the supplementary axial wall stress generated at peak flow by an arterial stenosis. Phys Med Biol 2003; 48: 127–38.

164. Naghavi M, Libby P, Falk E, et al. From vulnerable plaque to vulnerable patient: a call for new definitions and risk assessment strategies: part I. Circulation 2003; 108: 1664–72.

165. Kolluru GK, Sinha S, Majumder S, et al. Shear stress promotes nitric oxide production in endothelial cells by sub-cellular delocalization of eNOS: a basis for shear stress mediated angiogenesis. Nitric Oxide 2010; 22: 304–15.

166. Di Francesco L, Totani L, Dovizio M, et al. Induction of prostacyclin by steady laminar shear stress suppresses tumor necrosis factor-alpha biosynthesis via heme oxygenase-1 in human endothelial cells. Circ Res 2009; 104: 506–13.

167. Sjogren LS, Gan L, Doroudi R, et al. Fluid shear stress increases the intra-cellular storage pool of tissue-type plasminogen activator in intact human conduit vessels. Thromb Haemost 2000; 84: 291–8.

168. Rossi J, Rouleau L, Tardif JC, Leask RL. Effect of simvastatin on Kruppel-like factor2, endothelial nitric oxide synthase and thrombomodulin expression in endothelial cells under shear stress. Life Sci 2010; 87: 92–9.

169. Lin Z, Kumar A, SenBanerjee S, et al. Kruppel-like factor 2 (KLF2) regulates endothelial thrombotic function. Circ Res 2005; 96: e48–57.

170. Yin W, Shanmugavelayudam SK, Rubenstein DA. The effect of physiologically relevant dynamic shear stress on platelet and endothelial cell activation. Thromb Res 2011; 127: 235–41.

171. Tedgui A, Mallat Z. Apoptosis as a determinant of atherothrombosis. Thromb Haemost 2001; 86: 420–6.

172. Lu Q, Malinauskas RA. Comparison of two platelet activation markers using flow cytometry after in vitro shear stress exposure of whole human blood. Artif Organs 2011; 35: 137–44.

173. Rubenstein DA, Yin W. Quantifying the effects of shear stress and shear exposure duration regulation on flow induced platelet activation and aggregation. J Thromb Thrombolysis 2010; 30: 36–45.

174. Borissoff JI, Spronk HM, ten Cate H. The hemostatic system as a modulator of atherosclerosis. N Engl J Med 2011; 364: 1746–60.

175. Chatzizisis YS, Jonas M, Beigel R, et al. Attenuation of inflammation and expansive remodeling by Valsartan alone or in combination with Simvastatin in high-risk coronary atherosclerotic plaques. Atherosclerosis 2009; 203: 387–94.

176. Sen-Banerjee S, Mir S, Lin Z, et al. Kruppel-like factor 2 as a novel mediator of statin effects in endothelial cells. Circulation 2005; 112: 720–6.

177. Ali F, Hamdulay SS, Kinderlerer AR, et al. Statin-mediated cytoprotection of human vascular endothelial cells: a role for Kruppel-like factor 2-dependent induction of heme oxygenase-1. J Thromb Haemost 2007; 5: 2537–46.

178. Matsumoto M, Kawaguchi S, Ishizashi H, et al. Platelets treated with ticlopidine are less reactive to unusually large von Willebrand factor multimers than are those treated with aspirin under high shear stress. Pathophysiol Haemost Thromb 2005; 34: 35–40.

179. Liang C, Xiaonan L, Xiaojun C, et al. Effect of metoprolol on vulnerable plaque in rabbits by changing shear stress around plaque and reducing inflammation. Eur J Pharmacol 2009; 613: 79–85.

180. Kushner FG, Hand M, Smith SC Jr, et al. 2009 focused updates: ACC/AHA guidelines for the management of patients with ST-elevation myocardial infarction (updating the 2004 guideline and 2007 focused update) and ACC/AHA/SCAI guidelines on percutaneous coronary intervention (updating the 2005 guideline and 2007 focused update) a report of the American College of Cardiology Foundation/American Heart Association Task Force on Practice Guidelines. J Am Coll Cardiol 2009; 54: 2205–41.

181. Silber S, Gutierrez-Chico JL, Behrens S, et al. Effect of paclitaxel elution from reservoirs with bioabsorbable polymer compared to a bare metal stent for the elective percutaneous treatment of de novo coronary stenosis: the EUROSTAR-II randomised clinical trial. EuroIntervention 2011; 7: 64–73.

182. Reifart N, Hauptmann KE, Rabe A, Enayat D, Giokoglu K. Short and long term comparison (24 months) of an alternative sirolimus-coated stent with bioabsorbable polymer and a bare metal stent of similar design in chronic coronary occlusions: the CORACTO trial. EuroIntervention 2010; 6: 356–60.

19 Tissue characterization using virtual histology and iMAP: Current status and potential clinical applications

Salvatore Brugaletta and Hector M. Garcia-Garcia

OUTLINE

Coronary angiography, depicting coronary contrast-filled lumen, does not provide any information about the atherosclerosis of the coronary vessel wall. Conversely, grayscale IVUS is the modality that has been established as the gold standard for in vivo imaging of the coronary vessel wall. Nevertheless, it is still limited to qualitatively identify the plaque morphology similar as histopathology. To overcome this limitation, new innovative IVUS-based methods, such as virtual histology IVUS and iMAP-IVUS, based on interpretation of the raw radiofrequency analysis, have been developed. This chapter reviews the role of these intra-coronary imaging techniques either in the assessment of coronary plaques or in the evaluation of the drugs and stents efficacy in atherosclerosis treatment.

INTRODUCTION

Coronary angiography depicts arteries as a planar silhouette of the contrast-filled lumen. Importantly, angiography does not provide visualization of the vessel wall and is not suitable for complete assessment of atherosclerosis. Angiographic disease assessment is based on comparison of the stenotic segment with the adjacent, 'normal-appearing' coronary, which is often an incorrect assumption due to the diffuse nature of atherosclerosis, as shown by pathological and intravascular ultrasound (IVUS) studies (1).

Grayscale IVUS is the modality established as the gold standard for in vivo imaging of the vessel wall of the coronary arteries (2). However, the grayscale representation of the coronary vessel wall and plaque morphology in combination with the limited resolution of current IVUS catheters makes difficult, if not impossible, to identify qualitatively (e.g., visually) the

---

Focus Box 19.1

1. Angiography is limited in the evaluation of coronary plaque. It only provides information on the lumen
2. IVUS and IVUS-based modalities can help us not only to fully assess the coronary vessel wall, but also to characterize plaque tissue components

---

Focus Box 19.2

IVUS-VH, based on backscattering signal interpretation, enables characterization of fibrous and fibrofatty tissues, necrotic core, and dense calcium in coronary plaques

---

plaque morphology in a manner similar to that afforded by histopathology, the gold standard to characterize and quantify coronary plaque tissue components (3).

Recently, this limitation has been partially overcome by new innovative IVUS-based methods such as: virtual histology IVUS (4–6) (IVUS-VH, Volcano Therapeutics, Rancho Cordova, CA, USA) and iMAP-IVUS (7,8) (Boston Scientific, Santa Clara, CA, USA), based on interpretation of the raw radiofrequency analysis.

Tissue Characterization Using Virtual Histology IVUS (IVUS-VH)

The first commercial available radiofrequency (RF) signal-based tissue composition analysis tool was the so-called virtual histology (IVUS-VH, Volcano Therapeutics) software. It uses in-depth analysis of the backscattered RF-signal in order to provide a more detailed description of atheromatous plaque composition and is performed with either a 20-MHz, 2.9-Fr phased array transducer catheter (Eagle Eye™ Gold, Volcano Therapeutics) or 45-MHz 3.2-Fr rotational catheter (Revolution, Volcano Therapeutics) that acquires electrocardiogram gated IVUS data.(6). The main principle of this technique is that it uses not only the envelope amplitude of the reflected RF signals (as grayscale IVUS does), but also the underlying frequency content to analyze the tissue components present in coronary plaques (Fig. 19.1). This combined information is processed using autoregressive models and thereafter in a classification tree that determines four basic plaque tissue components (4): (*i*) fibrous tissue (dark green), (*ii*) fibrofatty tissue (light green), (*iii*) necrotic core (red), and (*iv*) dense calcium (white). The current software version assumes the presence of a media layer, which is artificially added and positioned just inside the outer vessel contour. This technique has been compared in several studies with histology in humans and other species (Table 19.1).

Natural History of Atherosclerosis

Acute coronary syndromes (ACS) are often the first manifestation of coronary atherosclerosis, making the identification of plaques at a high risk of provoking future clinical events an important component of strategies to reduce mortality and morbidity associated with atherosclerosis. Our current understanding of plaque biology suggests that ~60% of clinically evident plaque ruptures originate within an inflamed thin-capped fibroatheroma (9,10). Pathological studies have demonstrated that ruptured plaques are mainly located in the proximal portions of the left anterior descending and circumflex arteries, and are more widely dispersed in the right coronary artery (11). This

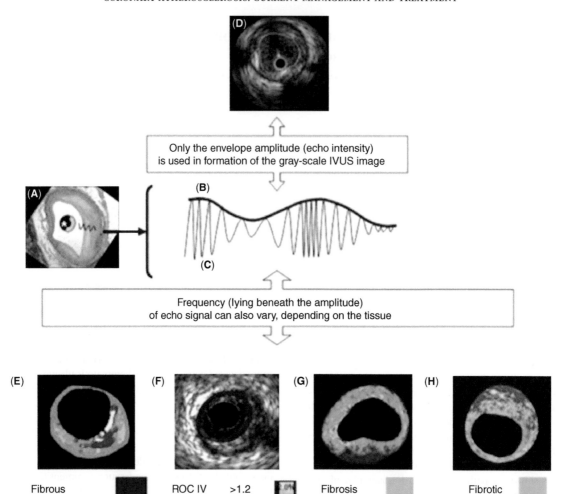

Figure 19.1 Intravascular ultrasound signal is obtained from the vessel wall (**A**). Grayscale intravascular ultrasound imaging is formed by the envelope (amplitude) (**B**) of the radiofrequency signal (**C**). By grayscale, atherosclerotic plaque can be classified into four categories: soft, fibrotic, calcified, and mixed plaques. Part (**D**) shows a cross-sectional view of a grayscale image. The blue lines limit the actual atheroma. The frequency and power of the signal commonly differ between tissues, regardless of similarities in the amplitude. From the backscatter radiofrequency data, different types of information can be retrieved: virtual histology (**E**), palpography (**F**), integrated backscattered intravascular ultrasound (**G**), and iMAP (**H**). Virtual histology is able to detect four tissue types: necrotic core, fibrous, fibrofatty, and dense calcium. Plaque deformability at palpography is reported in strain values, which are subsequently categorized into four grades according to the Rotterdam Classification (ROC). The tissues characterized by integrated backscattered intravascular ultrasound are lipidic, fibrous, and calcified; iMAP detects fibrotic, lipidic, necrotic, and calcified. *Source:* From Ref. 1.

tendency for advanced plaques to develop preferentially in these locations has been explained by the low shear stress conditions generated in areas with tortuosity or those that are the site of multiple branches. Low shear stress may induce the migration of lipid and monocytes into the vessel wall leading to lesion progression toward a plaque with a high risk of rupture (12).

Although a description of the development of atherosclerosis and the details of plaque composition is beyond the scope of this chapter, some important concepts are briefly addressed to support the use of tissue characterization imaging modalities for plaque characterization. In brief, an atheromatous plaque is formed by an intricate sequence of events, not necessarily in

Table 19.1 IVUS-VH Validation Studies

Reference	Type of study	Year	Aim	Results
(4)	*Ex vivo*	2002	Coronary plaque classification with intravascular ultrasound radiofrequency data analysis	Autoregressive classification schemes performed better than those from classic Fourier spectra with accuracies of 90.4% for fibrous, 92.8% for fibrolipidic, 90.9% for calcified, and 89.5% for calcified-necrotic regions in the training dataset and 79.7%, 81.2%, 92.8%, and 85.5% in the test data, respectively.
(46)	*In vivo*	2006	Accuracy of in vivo coronary plaque morphology assessment: a validation study of in vivo virtual histology compared with in vitro histopathology	Predictive accuracy from the overall patient cohort: 87.1% for FT, 87.1% for FF, 88.3% for NC, and 96.5% for DC regions. Sensitivities: NC 67.3%, FT 86%, FF 79.3%, DC 50%. Specificities: NC 92.9%, FT 90.5%, FF 100%, DC 99%
(5)	*Ex vivo*	2007	Automated coronary plaque characterization with intravascular ultrasound backscatter: ex vivo validation	The overall predictive accuracies were 93.5% for FT, 94.1% for FF, 95.8% for NC, and 96.7% for DC. Sensitivities: NC 91.7%, FT 95.7%, FF 72.3%, DC 86.5%. Specificities: NC 96.6%, FT 90.9%, FF 97.9%, DC 98.9%.
(47)	*Ex vivo*	2007	In vivo plaque characterization using intravascular ultrasound-virtual histology in a porcine model of complex coronary lesions	Compared with histology, IVUS-VH correctly identified the presence of FT, FF, and necrotic tissue in 58.33%, 38.33%, and 38.33% of lesions, respectively. Sensitivities: FT 76.1%, FF 46%, and NC 41.1%
(48)	*Ex vivo*	2009	Validation of in vivo plaque characterization by virtual histology in a rabbit model of atherosclerosis	IVUS-VH had a high sensitivity, specificity, and positive predictive value for the detection of non-calcified thin cap fibroatheroma (88%, 96%, and 87%, respectively) and calcified thin-cap fibroatheroma (95%, 99%, and 93%, respectively). These values were, respectively, 82%, 94%, and 85% for non-calcified fibroatheroma and 78%, 98%, and 84% for calcified fibroatheroma. The lowest values were obtained for pathological intimal thickening (74%, 92%, and 70%, respectively). For all plaque types, IVUS-VH had a kappa-value of 0.79.
(49)	*Ex vivo*	2010	Unreliable Assessment of necrotic core by VH™ IVUS in porcine coronary artery disease	No correlation was found between the size of the NC determined by IVUS-VH and that seen on histology. VH IVUS suggested the presence of NC in lesions lacking cores by histology.

Abbreviations: NC, necrotic core; DC, dense calcium; FF, fibrofatty; FT, fibrous.

a linear chronologic order, that involves extracellular lipid accumulation, endothelial dysfunction, leucocyte recruitment, intracellular lipid accumulation (foam cells), smooth muscle cell migration and proliferation, expansion of extracellular matrix, neo-angiogenesis, tissue necrosis, and mineralization at later stages (13,14). The characteristics of an atherosclerotic plaque at any given time depend on the relative contribution of each of these determinants (13). Thus, in histological cross-sections, pathologic intimal thickening is rich in proteoglycans and lipid pools, but no trace of necrotic core is seen. Conversely, the necrotic core appears in the fibroatheroma (FA), that is, the precursor lesion of symptomatic heart disease. Thin-capped fibroatheroma (TCFA) is a lesion characterized by a large necrotic core containing numerous cholesterol clefts, cellular debris, and microcalcifications. The overlying fibrous cap is thin and rich in inflammatory cells, macrophages, and T-lymphocytes, along with a few smooth muscle cells.

Plaque Type Characterization by IVUS-VH

Using IVUS-VH, it is possible to define the various stages of atherosclerosis (Fig. 19.2). The definition of an IVUS-derived TCFA, for example, is a lesion fulfilling the following criteria in at least three consecutive frames: (*i*) plaque burden ≥40%; (*ii*)

confluent necrotic core ≥10% in direct contact with the lumen (i.e., no visible overlying tissue) (15). Using this definition of IVUS-derived TCFA, in patients with acute coronary syndrome (ACS) who underwent IVUS of all three epicardial coronaries, on average, two IVUS-derived TCFAs per patient were found, with half of them showing outward remodelling (15).

Hong et al. reported the frequency and distribution of TCFA identified by IVUS-VH in ACS (105 pts) and SAP (107 pts) in a three-vessel IVUS-VH study (16). There were 2.5 ± 1.5 in ACS and 1.7 ± 1.1 in SAP TCFAs per patient ($p < 0.001$). Presentation with an ACS was the only independent predictor of the presence of multiple VH-derived TCFAs (VH-TCFA) ($p = 0.011$). Eighty-three percent of VH-TCFAs were located within 40 mm of the ostium.

The potential value of IVUS-VH-derived plaque characterization in the prediction of adverse coronary events was evaluated in an international multicenter prospective study, the Providing Regional Observations to Study Predictors of Events in the Coronary Tree (PROSPECT) study (17). The PROSPECT trial was a multicenter, natural history study of ACS patients. All patients underwent percutaneous coronary intervention in their culprit lesion at baseline, followed by an angiogram and IVUS virtual histology of the three major coronary arteries. A TCFA with a

Lesion type

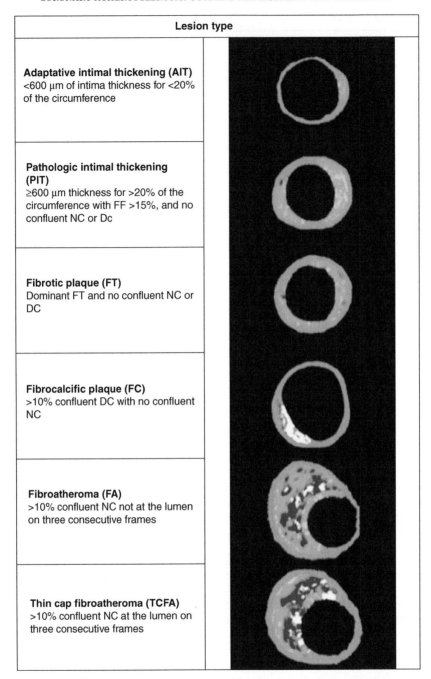

Adaptative intimal thickening (AIT)
<600 μm of intima thickness for <20% of the circumference

Pathologic intimal thickening (PIT)
≥600 μm thickness for >20% of the circumference with FF >15%, and no confluent NC or Dc

Fibrotic plaque (FT)
Dominant FT and no confluent NC or DC

Fibrocalcific plaque (FC)
>10% confluent DC with no confluent NC

Fibroatheroma (FA)
>10% confluent NC not at the lumen on three consecutive frames

Thin cap fibroatheroma (TCFA)
>10% confluent NC at the lumen on three consecutive frames

Figure 19.2 Virtual histology plaque types. *Source:* From Ref. 1.

minimum lumen area of ≤4 mm² and a large plaque burden (≥70%) had a 17.2% likelihood of causing an event within three years. Interestingly, the anticipated high frequency of acute thrombotic cardiovascular events did not occur, with only a 1% rate of myocardial infarction and no deaths directly attributable to non-culprit vessels over three years of follow-up. These results suggest that non-culprit, yet obstructive, coronary plaques are most likely to be associated with increasing symptoms rather than thrombotic acute events, with 8.5% of patients presenting with worsening angina and 3.3% with unstable angina. The conclusions of the PROSPECT study were recently reinforced by the publication of the VIVA study (18).

Serial changes in plaque components have been also investigated with IVUS-VH. In particular, Kubo et al. showed that

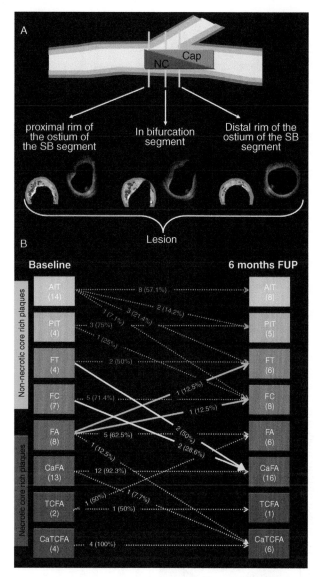

Figure 19.3 Panel (**A**): At bifurcations, plaque were analyzed only in the main coronary arteries at the proximal rim of the ostium of the side branch (the first frame proximal to the takeoff of the side branch), at the in-bifurcation site (the frame with the largest ostial diameter of the side branch) and at the distal rim of the ostium of the side branch (the first frame distal to the takeoff of the side branch). VH and OCT frames were selected. Panel (**B**): Changes in bifurcation plaque type at 6-month follow-up. For each plaque type, the number and percent of changes are reported. *Abbreviations*: AIT, adaptive intimal thickening; CaFA, calcified fibroathroma; CaTCFA, calcified thin-cap fibroatheroma; FA, fibroatheroma; FC, fibrocalcific plaque; FT, fibrotic plaque; PIT, pathological intimal thickening; TCFA, thin-cap fibroatheroma.

most VH-TCFAs healed during 12-month follow-up. However, during this time, new VH-TCFAs developed and in general pathologic intimal thickening and necrotic core plaques progressed significantly compared with fibrotic and fibrocalcific plaques in terms of increase in plaque and decrease in lumen area (19). At the site of coronary bifurcations, using a combined approach with VH/optical coherence tomography (OCT), we previously showed that most of the necrotic core-rich plaques remained unchanged (Fig. 19.3) (20).

Focus Box 19.3

IVUS-VH TCFA has been correlated with long-term clinical outcome in the PROSPECT trial

Although plaque characteristics (i.e., tissue characterization) do not yet influence current therapeutic guidelines, the available clinical imaging modalities, IVUS and IVUS-based tissue characterization techniques such as virtual histology

Table 19.2 Similarities and Differences of IVUS and IVUS-based Imaging Modalities

	IVUS	VH	i-MAP	Integrated Backscatter	Echogenicity
Type of device	Mechanical and electrical	Mechanical and electrical	Mechanical	Mechanical	Mechanical and electrical
Transducer Frequency	20–40 MHz	20–45 MHz	40MHz	40 MHz	20–40 MHz
Color code	Grayscale	Fibrous: green Necrotic core: Red Calcium: White Fibrofatty: Light green	Fibrous: light green Necrotic core: Pink Calcium: Blue Fibrofatty: Yellow	Fibrous: Green Necrotic core: Blue Calcium: Red Fibrofatty: Yellow	Red for hyperechogenic areas and green for hypoechogenic areas
Backscatter Radiofrequency signal analysis	Amplitude (dB)	Autoregressive model	Fast Fourier Transformation	Fast Fourier Transformation	It does not use backscatter radiofrequency but the amplitude of the signal

and iMAP, have the ability to identify some of the pathological fingerprints of atheroma, described above; moreover, these will help us to further advance our understanding of the complex interaction between atherosclerosis and the occurrence of clinical events.

Tissue Characterization Using iMAP-IVUS

Recently, another RF-based processing method, iMAP-IVUS (Boston Scientific), has become commercially available for coronary plaque tissue characterization (7). In principle, this software is comparable, from a methodological point of view, to IVUS-VH or other IVUS-based technique for tissue characterization (Table 19.2). However, by design, these two IVUS catheters have different capabilities for tissue characterization. Unlike VH, the iMAP uses a 40-MHz single rotational transducer on a drive shaft and can acquire radiofrequency data continuously; VH uses a similar catheter but is also available in an electronic-based catheter (20 MHz). Virtual histology acquires only Electrocardiogram-gated data. In addition, VH feeds the spectra that are obtained from the radiofrequency data by using autoregressive models into a classification tree that has reported diagnostic accuracies of over 90% for each plaque component as compared to histology (5). The iMAP uses a pattern recognition algorithm on spectra obtained from a fast Fourier transformation and a histology-derived database (7). Taken together, these distinctive features may lead to differences in the tissue characteristics of the images of coronary plaque obtained. iMAP and VH (40 MHz vs. 45/20 MHz) have relative advantages and disadvantages in displaying grayscale images. iMAP has higher resolution, but has specific artifacts such as non-uniform rotational distortion, because it is a rotational catheter. In addition, far-field imaging can be more problematic with high-frequency catheters due to amplified attenuation and enhanced blood backscatter.

The color code for tissue types is different. iMAP depicts fibrotic (light green), lipidic (yellow), necrotic (pink), and calcified tissue (blue), while VH depicts fibrous (green), fibrofatty (yellow green), necrotic core (red), and dense calcium (white).

Shin et al. compared in vivo the findings of these two IVUS-based tissue characterization systems, and showed significant and systematic variability in the assessment of plaque composition (8). iMAP classified plaque as necrotic tissue in signal-poor areas, such as those with guidewire artifact or acoustic shadowing, while VH displays fibrofatty (Fig. 19.4). VH showed external elastic membrane as a gray medial stripe, while iMAP always provided plaque composition results even for very thin plaques. VH tended to overestimate metallic stent struts, and iMAP showed thinner stent thickness than VH. Also peri-stent and calcium necrotic core halo on VH was not seen on iMAP.

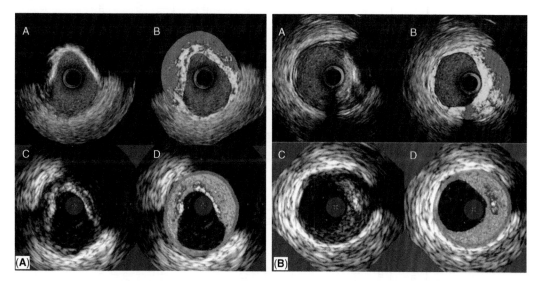

Figure 19.4 Corresponding cross-section of iMap (*top*) and VH images (*bottom*). iMap shows large amounts of necrotic tissue behind calcium, while with VH the same area is reported as fibrous or fibrofatty tissue. In panel (B), iMAP shows necrotic tissue also because of the wire artifact. *Source*: From Ref. 8.

Table 19.3 IVUS-based tissue characterization studies

References	Type of study	Year	Treatment	Number of patients	Time of follow-up	Primary endpoint	Results
Yokoyama (39)	RCT	2005	Atorvastatin Control	25 25	6 months	Overall plaque size and tissue characterization by IB IVUS	Atorvastatin reduced plaque size and changed plaque composition
Kawasaki (40)	RCT	2005	Pravastatin, Atorvastatin Diet	17 18 17	6 months	Overall tissue characterization by IB IVUS	Statins reduced lipid without changes in plaque size
IBIS 2 (13)	RCT	2008	Darapladib Placebo	175 155	12 months	Necrotic core volume by IVUS-VH	Darapladib significantly reduced necrotic core
Nasu (4)	Observational	2009	Fluvastatin Control	40 40	12 months	Overall tissue characterization by IVUS-VH	Fluvastatin reduced plaque and fibro-fatty volume
Hong (5)	RCT	2009	Simvastatin Rosuvastatin	50 50	12 months	Overall tissue characterization by IVUS-VH	Both reduced necrotic core and increased fibro-fatty volume
Toi (41)	RCT	2009	Atorvastatin Pivastatin	80 80	2–3 weeks	Overall tissue characterization by IVUS-VH	Pitavastatin reduced plaque volume and fibro-fatty
Miyagi (42)	Observational	2009	Statin (pravastatin, pitavastatin, atorvastatin, fluvastatin, simvastatin) Non statin	44 56	6 months	Overall tissue characterization by IB IVUS	Statins reduced lipid and increased fibrous

Total plaque volume = [External elastic membrane (EEM) $_{cross\ sectional\ area\ (CSA)}$] − [Lumen$_{CSA}$].

PAV = (EEM$_{CSA}$ − Lumen$_{CSA}$)/(EEM$_{CSA}$) *100.

Abbreviations: RCT, randomized controlled trial; PAV, percent atheroma volume; IVUS, intravascular ultrasound; IB, integrated backscatter; VH, virtual histology.

* $p < 0.05$ between groups.

‡ $p < 0.05$ vs. baseline.

†*%Change in plaque volume* = [Total plaque volume $_{FOLLOW-UP}$ − Total plaque volume $_{BASELINE}$]/[Total plaque volume $_{BASELINE}$] *100.

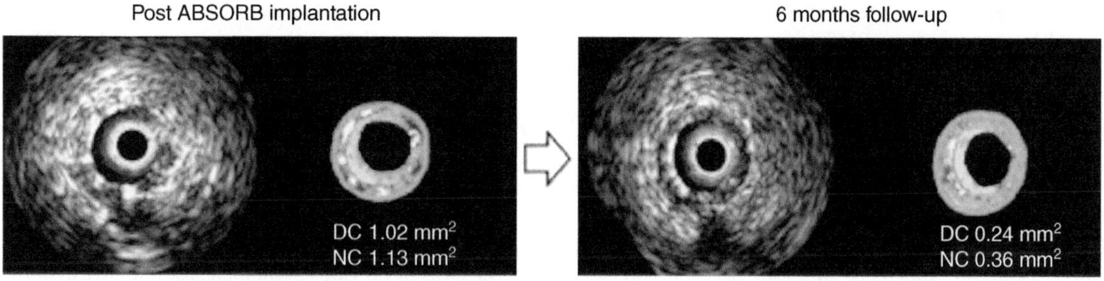

Post ABSORB implantation   6 months follow-up

DC 1.02 mm² \
NC 1.13 mm²

DC 0.24 mm² \
NC 0.36 mm²

Figure 19.5 IVUS-VH recognizes the polymeric struts of the ABSORB scaffold as dense calcium (DC), surrounded by a red halo of necrotic core (NC). At follow-up, a reduction in DC and NC can be appreciated. In order to pick up all the struts, the lumen contour has been drawn surrounding the catheter, according to Shin's method.

Taken together, these findings warrant further exploration of these imaging techniques in a large population to find particular areas of clinical usefulness.

Assessment of Drug Effect on Atherosclerosis by IVUS-VH

IVUS-VH has been used in several studies in order to show serial changes of plaque composition in patients treated with various statin treatments (Table 19.3).

In one of them, patients with stable angina pectoris ($n = 80$) treated with fluvastatin for one year had significant regression in plaque volume and changes in the atherosclerotic plaque composition with a significant reduction in fibrofatty volume ($p < 0.0001$). These changes in fibrofatty volume were significantly correlated with changes in LDL-cholesterol ($r = 0.703$, $p < 0.0001$) and hs-C-reactive protein levels ($r = 0.357$, $p = 0.006$) (21). Of note, necrotic core volume did not change significantly.

In a second study, Hong et al. randomized 100 patients with stable angina and ACS to either rosuvastatin 10 mg or simvastatin 20 mg for 1 year. The overall necrotic core volume significantly decreased ($p = 0.010$) and the fibrofatty plaque volume increased ($p = 0.006$) after statin treatments. There was a particularly significant decrease in the necrotic core volume ($p = 0.015$) in the rosuvastatin-treated subgroup. By multiple stepwise logistic regression analysis, they showed that the only independent clinical predictor of decrease in the necrotic core volume was the baseline HDL-cholesterol level ($p = 0.040$, OR: 1.044, 95% CI 1.002–1089) (22).

The IBIS 2 study compared the effects of 12-month treatment with darapladib (oral Lp-PLA2 inhibitor, 160 mg daily) or placebo in 330 patients (23). Endpoints included changes in necrotic core size (IVUS-VH) and atheroma size (IVUS-grayscale). Background therapy was comparable between groups, with no difference in LDL-cholesterol at 12 months (placebo: 88 ± 34 and darapladib: 84 ± 31 mg/dL, $p = 0.37$). In the placebo-treated group, however, necrotic core volume increased significantly, whereas darapladib halted this increase, resulting in a significant treatment difference of $-5.2\,\text{mm}^3$ ($p = 0.012$). These intra-plaque compositional changes occurred without a significant treatment difference in total atheroma volume.

Despite all these studies, there is no single report describing a clear direct association between reduction in plaque size and/or plaque composition with a reduction in clinical events. The best attempt was a pooled analysis of 4137 patients from six clinical trials that used serial IVUS: the relationship between baseline and change in percent atheroma volume with the incidence of major adverse cardiovascular events (MACE) was investigated. Each standard deviation increase in percent atheroma volume was associated with a 1.32-fold (95% CI: 1.22 to 1.42; $p < 0.001$) greater likelihood of experiencing a MACE (24).

Assessment of Stent by IVUS-VH

Polymeric Scaffolds

Kim et al. have previously shown that metallic stents eluting sirolimus and paclitaxel introduce artifacts in IVUS-VH images, interfering with the classification of plaque behind the struts (25). Normally, drug-eluting stent struts appear as dense calcium, surrounded by a red halo. Although the ABSORB scaffold is made of non-metallic materials, it is also recognized by IVUS-VH software as dense calcium and necrotic core. Moreover, the presence of 'pseudo' dense calcium and necrotic core could be used as a quantitative surrogate for the presence of the polymeric material of the scaffold and may help evaluate the bioresorption process during follow-up (26–29). We have already shown, in a sub-study of ABSORB cohort A trial, that polymeric struts are identified with radiofrequency backscattering signal as calcific structures, and that the ability of IVUS-VH to recognize polymeric struts is important not only to study imaging of the scaffold post-implantation, but also to potentially follow the changes in mechanical support and the bioresorption process (Fig. 19.5) (27). The absence of validation to recognize polymeric material by VH should be, however, acknowledged.

Analysis of Changes in Scaffolded Plaque Composition

IVUS-VH can also be used to analyze the changes in composition of the plaque scaffolded by a metallic or a bioresorbable scaffold.

Kubo et al. analyzed the long-term effects of drug-eluting stent (DES) and bare-metal stent (BMS) on coronary arterial wall morphology by IVUS-VH, and showed that DES-treated lesions had a greater frequency of unstable lesion morphology at follow-up compared to BMS (30). In particular, assessing the total amount of the four-color-VH components, including contribution of the stent, they found that DES-treated lesions showed a significantly higher incidence of necrotic core abutting the lumen at follow-up compared to BMS-treated lesions, although there was not a significant difference in mean necrotic core area between groups. This was due to suppression of the protective neointimal hyperplasia layer in DES compared with BMS.

Aoki et al. have demonstrated in vivo that plaque volume behind the metallic stent eluting sirolimus increases slightly at four-month follow-up and then significantly decreases at four-yearfollow-up compared to post-implantation, and that change in echogenicity suggests a change in plaque composition (31). They also documented a significant increase in plaque area outside a metallic stent eluting paclitaxel at six months, with regression at two years (32). In these situations, it would be interesting to know what type of tissue contributed to this process and, from a quantitative standpoint, to develop a third (stent) contour in the VH software in order to characterize selectively intimal hyperplasia and peri-stent tissue. The potential lack of validation of VH in the assessment of in-stent restenosis should be, however, acknowledged.

Sarno et al. analyzed IVUS-VH plaque characterization behind the first-generation ABSORB scaffold and found a reduction in necrotic core component between six-month and two-year follow-up, probably related to a synergistic effect of the bioresorption process and the anti-inflammatory action of everolimus (33).

Nevertheless, considering that the stent struts are recognized by IVUS-VH as dense calcium and necrotic core, careful evaluation of the plaque behind the stent should be done to avoid any misclassification of the actual tissue (25,28). Recently, customized software has been developed and used to introduce, in a semi-automatic fashion, a third contour behind the stent, allowing the analysis to focus only on the plaque behind the struts (34).

Stent Thrombosis

Another possible application of IVUS-VH for stent evaluation is its potential to elucidate the mechanisms of stent thrombosis. It is known that one of the proposed pathological mechanisms of coronary stent thrombosis is stenting of necrotic core-rich plaques with extensive tissue prolapse and plaque disruption in the proximity of the stented arterial segment (35,36). Thus, pre-stenting imaging using IVUS-VH can give us an insight not only into the extent of plaque, but also on the extent of necrotic core within and beyond the intended stented segment. In this context, 24 patients, in whom 26 segments were stented, were assessed using IVUS-VH. No stent thrombosis was observed, where necrotic core-rich areas were

left unstented (36). Ramcharitar et al. presented the first clinical case of a patient with a non-culprit IVUS-VH-derived thin-cap fibroatheroma, successfully treated with percutaneous coronary intervention, with a good six-month angiographic follow-up (37). A large trial in which patients are randomized to IVUS-VH or angiography guided optimal coronary stenting is required to draw firm conclusions.

Edge Effects Assessed by IVUS-VH

On the basis of previous pathological studies, we hypothesized that the tissue associated with an increase in plaque at the edges of the paclitaxel stent is mainly fibrofatty tissue as assessed by IVUS-VH. Fibrofatty, on IVUS-VH, has been described as loosely packed bundles of collagen fibers with regions of lipid deposition and extracellular matrix without necrotic areas (5).

In the BETAX study (38), 24 patients (26 paclitaxel-eluting stents) were studied. Serial expansive vascular remodeling was observed at the proximal and distal edges of the stent to accommodate fibrofatty and fibrous tissue growth. More specifically, proximal and distal segments were divided into five sub-segments of 1-mm. In the first two sub-segments adjacent to the proximal edge of the stent, the vessel wall grew to compensate the plaque growth without affecting the lumen size. In the following three sub-segments, overcompensation (vessel wall increased more than plaque size) was observed. Consequently, the lumen size increased. At the distal edge, overcompensation was observed in all five sub-segments, followed by an increase in lumen size. In summary, proximal and distal growth patterns were characterized by an increase in fibrofatty tissue ($p < 0.001$ and $p < 0.001$, respectively), decrease in necrotic core ($p = 0.014$ and $p < 0.001$, respectively), and decrease in dense calcium content ($p < 0.001$ and $p < 0.001$, respectively).

Combined Assessment of Coronary Atherosclerosis by Using VH and Other Imaging Modalities

In the future, integration of multiple image technologies in a single catheter is likely to provide a more comprehensive assessment of the coronary vasculature. The combined use of IVUS-VH analysis and OCT seems to improve the accuracy for TCFA detection (39,40). IVUS-VH has a limited axial resolution (100–200 μm), not allowing a precise measurement of the fibrous thin cap; on the contrary, OCT is a high-resolution imaging technique (10–20 μm) that can be used in the assessment of microstructure, but using only OCT in plaque-type characterization can result in misclassification. In fact, OCT signals have low penetration, limited to 1–2 mm, and cannot detect lipid pools or calcium behind thick fibrous caps, thus producing inaccurate detection of signal poor areas (41). The combined use of IVUS-VH analysis and OCT seems to improve the accuracy for TCFA detection (39,40). Recently, the combined use of IVUS-VH and a direct measurement of the physiological significance of a coronary lesion, fractional flow reserve (FFR) has been also explored: no differences

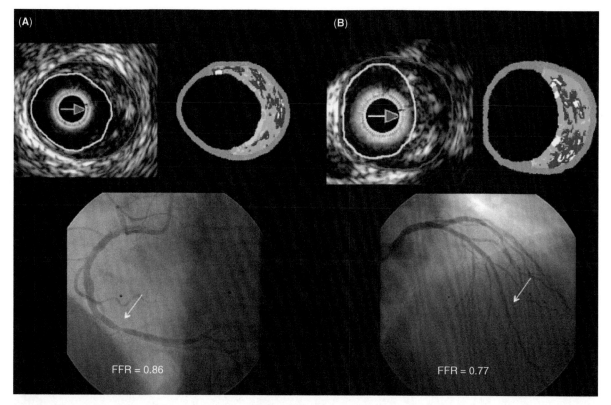

Figure 19.6 Example of two fibroatheromas at the level of two different lesions (white arrows) with an FFR >0.80 (Panel A) and ≤0.80 (Panel B). Red and yellow contours in the IVUS images indicate vessel and lumen contours, respectively. *Source*: Adapted from Ref. 42.

were found in terms of plaque composition and virtual histology plaque types in coronary lesions with FFR more or less than 0.80 (Fig. 19.6) (42).

IVUS-VH has been compared with near infra-red spectroscopy (NIRS) for the detection of lipid/necrotic core rich-plaques: although large plaques were more often associated with either elevated VH-NC and NIRS-lipid core, the correlation between the detection of lipid core by NIRS and necrotic core by VH was weak (Fig. 19.7) (43).

Furthermore, several lines of investigation have validated plaque imaging by coronary computed tomography angiography against other imaging modalities, such as IVUS-VH or OCT (44). In particular, low-density non-calcified plaques correlated with the sum of necrotic core and fibrofatty tissue by IVUS-VH (45).

PERSONAL PERSPECTIVE

In recent years, IVUS-VH has been widely used as a tool to study the natural history of coronary plaques in vivo and to assess the efficacy of new drugs or devices. To date, much has been achieved: (*i*) VH-derived TCFAs have been strongly correlated with future coronary events; (*ii*) VH has prompted the suggestion that pharmacological or mechanical treatments for coronary atherosclerosis may modify plaque composition in a positive fashion; (*iii*) in addition, IVUS-VH can be used to explore causes of DES limitations and has tremendous potential in the promising field of new bio-absorbable vascular scaffolds.

Despite the clear potential of the technology in these areas, its role in daily clinical practice remains unclear. It is currently being studied whether screening for the presence of VH-TCFA, with the aim of treatment to prevent future adverse events, is warranted. For treatment, efficacious pharmacological or mechanical strategies would be needed. Randomized trials to address these issues would be difficult and costly.

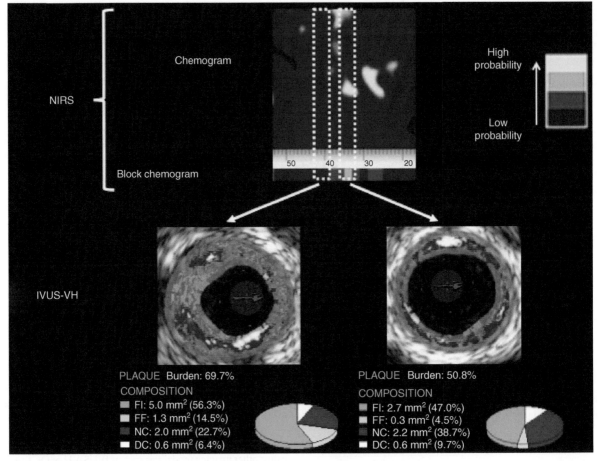

Figure 19.7 Near-infrared spectroscopy displays the probability of lipid core plaque in a false color scale from red (low probability) to yellow (high probability). In this example, two VH-necrotic core-rich plaques are displayed with two different colors on the NIRS output.

Focus Box 19.7

A combined approach using IVUS-VH and other imaging modalities should be considered for a comprehensive evaluation of a coronary plaque

REFERENCES

1. Garcia-Garcia HM, Costa MA, Serruys PW. Imaging of coronary atherosclerosis: intravascular ultrasound. Eur Heart J 2010; 31: 2456–69.
2. Mintz GS, Nissen SE, Anderson WD, et al. American college of cardiology clinical expert consensus document on standards for acquisition, measurement and reporting of intravascular ultrasound studies (ivus). A report of the american college of cardiology task force on clinical expert consensus documents. J Am Coll Cardiol 2001; 37: 1478–92.
3. Garcia-Garcia HM, Gogas BD, Serruys PW, Bruining N. Ivus-based imaging modalities for tissue characterization: Similarities and differences. Int J Cardiovasc Imaging 2011; 27: 215–24.
4. Nair A, Kuban BD, Tuzcu EM, et al. Coronary plaque classification with intravascular ultrasound radiofrequency data analysis. Circulation 2002; 106: 2200–6.
5. Nair A, Margolis MP, Kuban BD, Vince DG. Automated coronary plaque characterisation with intravascular ultrasound backscatter: ex vivo validation. EuroIntervention 2007; 3: 113–20.
6. Garcia-Garcia HM, Mintz GS, Lerman A, et al. Tissue characterisation using intravascular radiofrequency data analysis: Recommendations for acquisition, analysis, interpretation and reporting. EuroIntervention 2009; 5: 177–89.
7. Sathyanarayana S, Carlier S, Li W, Thomas L. Characterisation of atherosclerotic plaque by spectral similarity of radiofrequency intravascular ultrasound signals. EuroIntervention 2009; 5: 133–9.
8. Shin ES, Garcia-Garcia HM, Ligthart JM, et al. In vivo findings of tissue characteristics using imap ivus and virtual histology ivus. EuroIntervention 2011; 6: 1017–9.
9. Virmani R, Burke AP, Farb A, Kolodgie FD. Pathology of the vulnerable plaque. J Am Coll Cardiol 2006; 47: C13–18.
10. Schaar JA, Muller JE, Falk E, et al. Terminology for high-risk and vulnerable coronary artery plaques. Report of a meeting on the

vulnerable plaque, 17 and 18 June 2003, Santorini, Greece, Eur Heart J 2004; 25: 1077–82.

11. Cheruvu PK, Finn AV, Gardner C, et al. Frequency and distribution of thin-cap fibroatheroma and ruptured plaques in human coronary arteries: a pathologic study. J Am Coll Cardiol 2007; 50: 940–9.

12. Cunningham KS, Gotlieb AI. The role of shear stress in the pathogenesis of atherosclerosis. Lab Invest 2005; 85: 9–23.

13. Virmani R, Kolodgie FD, Burke AP, Farb A, Schwartz SM. Lessons from sudden coronary death: a comprehensive morphological classification scheme for atherosclerotic lesions. Arterioscler Thromb Vasc Biol 2000; 20: 1262–75.

14. Ross R. Atherosclerosis–an inflammatory disease. N Engl J Med 1999; 340: 115–26.

15. Garcia-Garcia HM, Goedhart D, Schuurbiers JC, et al. Virtual histology and remodeling index allow in vivo identification of allegedly high risk coronary plaques in patients with acute coronary syndromes: a three vessel intravascular ultrasound radiofrequency data analysis. EuroIntervention 2006; 2: 338–44.

16. Hong MK, Mintz GS, Lee CW, et al. A three-vessel virtual histology intravascular ultrasound analysis of frequency and distribution of thin-cap fibroatheromas in patients with acute coronary syndrome or stable angina pectoris. Am J Cardiol 2008; 101: 568–72.

17. Stone GW, Maehara A, Lansky AJ, et al. A prospective natural-history study of coronary atherosclerosis. N Engl J Med 2011; 364: 226–35.

18. Calvert PA, Obaid DR, O'Sullivan M, et al. Association between ivus findings and adverse outcomes in patients with coronary artery disease the viva (IVUS-VH in vulnerable atherosclerosis) study. JACC. Cardiovascular imaging 2011; 4: 894–901.

19. Kubo T, Maehara A, Mintz GS, et al. The dynamic nature of coronary artery lesion morphology assessed by serial virtual histology intravascular ultrasound tissue characterization. J Am Coll Cardiol 2010; 55: 1590–7.

20. Diletti R, Garcia-Garcia HM, Gomez-Lara J, et al. Assessment of coronary atherosclerosis progression and regression at bifurcations using combined ivus and oct. JACC. Cardiovascular Imaging 2011; 4: 774–80.

21. Nasu K, Tsuchikane E, Katoh O, et al. Effect of fluvastatin on progression of coronary atherosclerotic plaque evaluated by virtual histology intravascular ultrasound. JACC Cardiovasc Interv 2009; 2: 689–96.

22. Hong MK, Park DW, Lee CW, et al. Effects of statin treatments on coronary plaques assessed by volumetric virtual histology intravascular ultrasound analysis. JACC Cardiovasc Interv 2009; 2: 679–88.

23. Serruys PW, Garcia-Garcia HM, Buszman P, et al. Effects of the direct lipoprotein-associated phospholipase a(2) inhibitor darapladib on human coronary atherosclerotic plaque. Circulation 2008; 118: 1172–82.

24. Nicholls SJ, Hsu A, Wolski K, et al. Intravascular ultrasound-derived measures of coronary atherosclerotic plaque burden and clinical outcome. J Am Coll Cardiol 2010; 55: 2399–407.

25. Kim SW, Mintz GS, Hong YJ, et al. The virtual histology intravascular ultrasound appearance of newly placed drug-eluting stents. Am J Cardiol 2008; 102: 1182–6.

26. Serruys PW, Ormiston JA, Onuma Y, et al. A bioabsorbable everolimus-eluting coronary stent system (absorb): 2-year outcomes and results from multiple imaging methods. Lancet 2009; 373: 897–910.

27. Garcia-Garcia HM, Gonzalo N, Pawar R, et al. Assessment of the absorption process following bioabsorbable everolimus-eluting stent implantation: temporal changes in strain values and tissue composition using intravascular ultrasound radiofrequency data analysis. A substudy of the absorb clinical trial. EuroIntervention 2009; 4: 443–8.

28. Sarno G, Onuma Y, Garcia Garcia HM, et al. Ivus radiofrequency analysis in the evaluation of the polymeric struts of the bioabsorbable everolimus-eluting device during the bioabsorption process. Catheter Cardiovasc Interv 2010; 75: 914–8.

29. Ormiston JA, Serruys PW, Regar E, et al. A bioabsorbable everolimus-eluting coronary stent system for patients with single de-novo coronary artery lesions (absorb): a prospective open-label trial. Lancet 2008; 371: 899–907.

30. Kubo T, Maehara A, Mintz GS, et al. Analysis of the long-term effects of drug-eluting stents on coronary arterial wall morphology as assessed by virtual histology intravascular ultrasound. Am Heart J 2010; 159: 271–7.

31. Aoki J, Abizaid AC, Serruys PW, et al. Evaluation of four-year coronary artery response after sirolimus-eluting stent implantation using serial quantitative intravascular ultrasound and computer-assisted grayscale value analysis for plaque composition in event-free patients. J Am Coll Cardiol 2005; 46: 1670–6.

32. Aoki J, Colombo A, Dudek D, et al. Peristent remodeling and neo-intimal suppression 2 years after polymer-based, paclitaxel-eluting stent implantation: Insights from serial intravascular ultrasound analysis in the taxus ii study. Circulation 2005; 112: 3876–83.

33. Sarno G, Onuma Y, Garcia Garcia HM, et al. Ivus radiofrequency analysis in the evaluation of the polymeric struts of the bioabsorbable everolimus-eluting device during the bioabsorption process. Catheter Cardiovasc Interv 2010; 75: 914–8.

34. Brugaletta S, Garcia-Garcia HM, Garg S, et al. Temporal changes of coronary artery plaque located behind the struts of the everolimus eluting bioresorbable vascular scaffold. Int J Cardiovasc Imaging 2011; 27: 859–66.

35. Farb A, Burke AP, Kolodgie FD, Virmani R. Pathological mechanisms of fatal late coronary stent thrombosis in humans. Circulation 2003; 108: 1701–6.

36. Garcia-Garcia HM, Goedhart D, Serruys PW. Relation of plaque size to necrotic core in the three major coronary arteries in patients with acute coronary syndrome as determined by intravascular ultrasonic imaging radiofrequency. Am J Cardiol 2007; 99: 790–2.

37. Ramcharitar S, Gonzalo N, van Geuns RJ, et al. First case of stenting of a vulnerable plaque in the secritt i trial-the dawn of a new era? Nat Rev Cardiol 2009; 6: 374–8.

38. Garcia-Garcia HM, Gonzalo N, Tanimoto S, et al. Characterization of edge effects with paclitaxel-eluting stents using serial intravascular ultrasound radiofrequency data analysis: The betax (beside taxus) study. Rev Esp Cardiol 2008; 61: 1013–9.

39. Sawada T, Shite J, Garcia-Garcia HM, et al. Feasibility of combined use of intravascular ultrasound radiofrequency data analysis and optical coherence tomography for detecting thin-cap fibroatheroma. Eur Heart J 2008; 29: 1136–46.

40. Gonzalo N, Garcia-Garcia HM, Regar E, et al. In vivo assessment of high-risk coronary plaques at bifurcations with combined intravascular ultrasound and optical coherence tomography. JACC Cardiovasc Imaging 2009; 2: 473–82.

41. Manfrini O, Mont E, Leone O, et al. Sources of error and interpretation of plaque morphology by optical coherence tomography. Am J Cardiol 2006; 98: 156–9.

42. Brugaletta S, Garcia-Garcia HM, Shen ZJ, et al. Morphology of coronary artery lesions assessed by virtual histology intravascular

ultrasound tissue characterization and fractional flow reserve. Int J Cardiovasc Imaging 2012; 28: 221–8.

43. Brugaletta S, Garcia-Garcia HM, Serruys PW, et al. Nirs and ivus for characterization of atherosclerosis in patients undergoing coronary angiography. J Am Coll Cardiol Imaging 2011; 4: 647–55.

44. Voros S, Rinehart S, Qian Z, et al. Coronary atherosclerosis imaging by coronary ct angiography: Current status, correlation with intravascular interrogation and meta-analysis. JACC Cardiovascular Imaging 2011; 4: 537–48.

45. Voros S, Rinehart S, Qian Z, et al. 3rd. Prospective validation of standardized, 3-dimensional, quantitative coronary computed tomographic plaque measurements using radiofrequency backscatter intravascular ultrasound as reference standard in intermediate coronary arterial lesions: results from the atlanta (assessment of tissue characteristics, lesion morphology, and hemodynamics by angiography with fractional flow reserve, intravascular ultrasound and virtual histology, and noninvasive computed tomography in athero-

sclerotic plaques) i study. JACC Cardiovascular Interventions 2011; 4: 198–208.

46. Nasu K, Tsuchikane E, Katoh O. Accuracy of in vivo coronary plaque morphology assessment: a validation study of in vivo virtual histology compared with in vitro histopathology. JACC 2006; 47: 2405–12.

47. Granada JF, Wallace-Bradley D, Win HK, et al. In vivo plaque characterization using intravascular ultrasound-virtual histology in a porcine model of complex coronary lesions. Arterioscler Thromb Vasc Biol 2007; 27: 387–93.

48. Van Herck J, De Meyer G, Ennekens G, et al. Validation of in vivo plaque characterisation by virtual histology in a rabbit model of atherosclerosis. EuroIntervention 2009; 5: 149–56.

49. Thim T, Hagensen MK, Wallace-Bradley D, et al. Unreliable assessment of necrotic core by VH™ IVUS in porcine coronary artery disease. Circ Cardiovasc Imaging 2010; 3: 384–91.

20 The role of angioscopy in the assessment of the atherosclerotic plaque: Current status and potential clinical applications

Yasunori Ueda and Kazuhisa Kodama

OUTLINE

Angioscopy allows direct visualization of intracoronary structures. Multiple angioscopic studies have shown that yellow plaques, often with associated thrombus, are present in patients whose initial presentation is an acute coronary syndrome (ACS). On the other hand, many such plaques remain clinically silent. Thus, their presence appears to be a necessary but not sufficient prerequisite for the occurrence of a clinical event. Additional systemic and local factors must also play a role and future studies will be needed to refine the role of angioscopy in risk stratification and treatment planning in this subset of patients with de novo lesions.

Angioscopy has provided unique insights into the mechanisms of ACS at stented sites in patients with previously implanted bare metal stents (BMS) or drug-eluting stents (DES). Thrombus at stented sites has mainly been observed at uncovered stent struts, unhealed disrupted yellow plaques under the stent struts or adjacent to the stent, new disruption of yellow plaques already present at stent implantation, or new disruption of yellow plaques that have formed after stent implantation. Therefore, we may be able to evaluate the risk of stent thrombosis from the angioscopic evaluation of the extent of neointimal coverage, yellow plaques, and thrombus. We believe dual antiplatelet therapy is not required for DES completely covered by white neointima without thrombus that also covers yellow plaques under the stent, although this hypothesis requires validation in clinical trials.

INTRODUCTION

Angioscopy is the only technique that can directly visualize intracoronary structures. It allows direct visual assessment of the luminal surface of the vessel and the lumen itself. The wall of the coronary artery is white and smooth in a normal vessel. Atherosclerotic plaques are yellow in color; they may be raised or ulcerated, may protrude into the lumen, and often have superimposed thrombus. Angioscopy has a very high sensitivity to detect thrombus. Thrombus can appear as white or red material, in the lumen or adhering to the wall, with a cotton-like or ragged appearance. Although accurate and reproducible quantitative evaluation of angioscopic images has not yet been achieved, the images have abundant information that has not yet been fully exploited. Angioscopic examination could be described as the macroscopic equivalent of histopathology that can be performed in living patients. Important findings derived from angioscopy and potential hypotheses based on the findings are summarized in Table 20.1.

APPLICATIONS, LIMITATIONS, TECHNICAL ASPECTS, PROPER EVALUATION (TIPS AND TRICKS), AND POTENTIAL COMPLICATIONS

Detection of Thrombus and Disrupted Plaques

The most important role of angioscopy is in the detection and classification of disrupted plaques. Disrupted plaques can be subclassified into ruptured plaques with a distinct crater and plaques with surface erosions. Because thrombosis at a disrupted plaque is the most frequent mechanism of acute coronary syndrome (ACS) (1–3), the detection of disrupted plaques is very important both for the identification of the culprit lesion(s) in ACS and for investigating the mechanisms that lead a minority of such disrupted plaques to provoke a clinical event (Fig. 20.1; Video clip 20.1). We know from angioscopic studies that there are many disrupted plaques with active thrombus formation but without any clinical consequences; therefore, the disruption of vulnerable plaques must not be the only key step in the pathogenesis of an ACS. Other important factors involved in the process may be blood thrombogenicity (4) and the degree of luminal stenosis. However, we are still far from a comprehensive understanding of the pathophysiological mechanisms leading to ACS. To date, it is apparent that the majority of ACS events are caused by thrombosis at disrupted plaques, excluding a small percentage of events caused by vasospasm. Therefore, angioscopy has the potential to ascertain which lesion is the true culprit when patients with suspected symptoms of ACS have multiple stenotic lesions. In addition, the disrupted plaque is not always located at the site of the minimal lumen area (MLA) on angiography but is often found at a site somewhat proximal to the MLA site. The site of the disrupted plaque is called the "culprit site" of the "culprit lesion." It has been suggested that it is important to implant a stent placing its both edges at angiographically normal segments in order to ensure complete lesion coverage rather than placing the stent edge in the midst of the disrupted plaque in order to minimize the risk of stent thrombosis or of stenosis progression at the stent edges.

Should Disrupted Plaques be an Indication for PCI?

The main indication for percutaneous coronary intervention (PCI) in stable patients is to treat a stenosis that is flow-limiting and responsible for symptoms or ischemia. The situation may be somewhat different for unstable coronary syndromes. An early aggressive strategy for the treatment of unstable angina is associated with better outcomes than a conservative strategy; and systematic stenting at the culprit lesion in the setting of acute myocardial infarction (STEMI) is associated with a better outcome than either plain old balloon angioplasty or thrombolysis alone. These results suggest that disrupted plaques have

a risk of thrombotic coronary occlusion that is associated with adverse outcomes and that systematic stenting may improve outcomes. We can determine whether a stenotic lesion is severe enough to cause myocardial ischemia using a pressure wire to measure fractional flow reserve (FFR). However, the validity of this technique in the setting of an ACS is limited by the fact that microvascular obstruction will lead to an overestimation of the FFR. The risk of future events in this setting may relate more to the inherent potential of a lesion to occlude (or re-occlude) rather than to its intrinsic anatomic severity. This suggests that a more liberal approach to stenting at stenotic lesions in ACS may be warranted given that scaffolding the lesion with a stent should mechanically passivate the lesion. We believe that stenotic lesions with disrupted plaques, which are culprit lesions in unstable angina or acute MI patients, should be stented even if the stenosis is not severe enough to cause ischemia. Furthermore, this policy can be extended to intermediate stenotic lesions in a variety of clinical presentations that have disrupted plaques. Controlled clinical trials would help determine whether the presence of disrupted plaques on angioscopy is an appropriate tool for risk stratification and to guide individual therapy in the circumstances described above.

Table 20.1 Findings on Angioscopy and Potential Implications

Target	Findings and suggestions
ACS	Disrupted yellow plaque and thrombus is common at ACS culprit lesions
	White thrombus adheres directly to the vessel wall
	Thrombus becomes more reddish in the center of the occluded site
	Disrupted yellow plaques exist in non-culprit segments (silent disruptions)
Risk evaluation	PCI at disrupted yellow plaque has a higher risk of a no reflow phenomenon
	The number of yellow plaques may reflect future risk of ACS events
DES	Neointima coverage is less extensive with DES than BMS
	Stent and yellow plaque are not fully covered by neointima
	Thrombus is observed on angioscopic follow-up in around 20% of first-generation DES
	Dual antiplatelet therapy may not be required for DES completely covered by white neointima

Focus Box 20.2

The presence of disrupted plaques with thrombosis might be a potential indication for PCI in selected patients with ACS despite the fact that the degree of stenosis is not severe enough to cause ischemia.

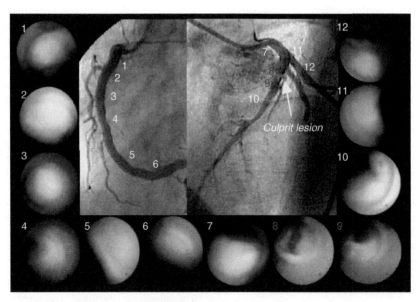

Figure 20.1 Angioscopic findings in the coronary arteries of a patient with an acute myocardial infarction. Yellow plaques are present in all three major epicardial coronary vessels. The culprit lesion has disrupted yellow plaques (#8 and #9). *Source:* From Ref. 2.

Detection of Vulnerable Plaques and Vulnerable Patients

Based on observations in multiple studies, >90% of culprit lesions in patients presenting with ACS have disrupted yellow plaques. Thus, yellow plaque color could be regarded as an angioscopic marker of plaque vulnerability. This is supported by the observation that plaques with a higher yellow color grade (5) have a higher incidence of thrombus, that is, disruption (Fig. 20.2). OCT studies have recently demonstrated that the fibrous cap is thinner at yellow plaques of higher yellow color intensity (6). Furthermore, both ruptured and eroded yellow plaques have similar atherosclerotic lesion features including VH-TCFA (7). Both rupture-prone and erosion-prone vulnerable plaques are detected on angioscopy as yellow plaques. However, as there is no way to identify the occurrence of asymptomatic plaque disruption in the general population, it is impossible to determine the elusive link between plaque vulnerability and clinical events. Based on a prospective angioscopic study (8), patients with more yellow plaques in their coronary arteries have a higher risk of future ACS events (Fig. 20.3), that is, are vulnerable patients, although the incidence of ACS events occurring from each yellow plaque is very low.

Evaluation of Plaque Stabilization

Statin therapy is an established treatment to decrease the risk of future ACS events and reduce coronary plaque volume as evaluated by intravascular ultrasound (IVUS) imaging. We have demonstrated in a prospective trial (the TWINS study (9))

using both angioscopy and IVUS that statin therapy reduces both the yellow color intensity and the volume of coronary plaques (Fig. 20.4). Because yellow plaques are the primary substrate for the occurrence of ACS and the intensity of their yellow color appears to be proportional to their vulnerability, as discussed above, a reduction in yellow color intensity would be a potentially valuable surrogate endpoint to evaluate the stabilization of vulnerable plaques and assess risk reduction in vulnerable patients. Plaque volume reduction and yellow color intensity reduction of the plaque may reflect different pathophysiological processes, and it has not been established which of these two processes is more directly associated with a reduction in ACS risk. Although statins have been shown to reduce plaque volume and decrease the intensity of yellow plaque color, some other treatments may affect only one of these two variables.

Evaluation of the Risk of Stent Thrombosis

Another thrombotic event in the coronary artery that has increasing clinical importance is stent thrombosis, particularly very late stent thrombosis (VLST) after drug-eluting stent (DES) implantation. Angioscopic studies have shown evidence of thrombus formation at stented sites in about 20% of cases at follow-up after DES implantation, while the rate is very low after bare metal stent (BMS) implantation (10). Thrombus formation at the stented lesion is usually associated with the presence

---

Focus Box 20.3

Yellow plaques are vulnerable plaques and patients with many yellow plaques are vulnerable patients.

Focus Box 20.4

The extent of the reduction in color intensity may be a marker for the degree of stabilization of yellow plaques.

Prevalence (%) of thrombus in non-stenotic yellow plaques

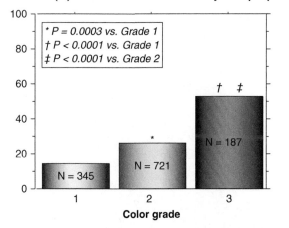

Figure 20.2 Incidence of thrombus formation on yellow plaques as a function of color grade. Yellow plaques detected in non-stenotic segments were evaluated. Yellow plaques with a higher yellow color grade had a higher prevalence of thrombus (disruption) and thus might be potentially more vulnerable. *Source*: From Ref. 5.

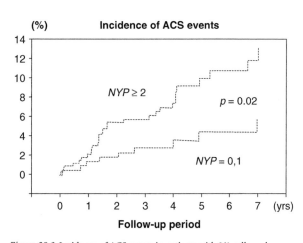

Figure 20.3 Incidence of ACS events in patients with 0/1 yellow plaque vs. those with ≥2 yellow plaques per coronary vessel. Patients with coronary heart disease were divided into two groups depending on the number of yellow plaques per vessel (NYP): NYP = 0/1 vs. NYP ≥ 2. The incidence of ACS events was significantly higher in patients with NYP ≥ 2 than in those with NYP = 0/1. *Source*: From Ref. 8.

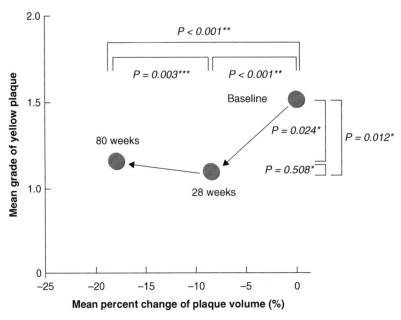

Figure 20.4 Changes in plaque volume and color by statin therapy in the TWINS study. During treatment with atorvastatin, the yellow color grade of plaques decreased significantly from baseline to 28 weeks, with no further significant change from 28 to 80 weeks. Plaque volume decreased by about 10% from baseline to 28 weeks, with an additional 10% decrease from 28 to 80 weeks. The early beneficial effect of statins demonstrated in clinical trials may be reflected in the early reduction of yellow color grade demonstrated in this trial. *Source*: From Ref. 9.

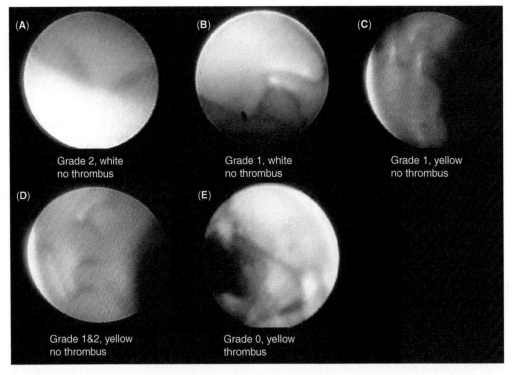

Figure 20.5 Illustrative angioscopic images, at follow-up, of lesions treated with DES. The extent of neointimal coverage (grade 0–2), lesion color (*yellow* or *white*), and the presence of thrombus are evaluated at the stented lesions. Thrombus is usually detected at yellow lesions as illustrated in panel E. Thrombus is rarely detected on white grade-2 neointima (**A**); white neointima is commonly seen after BMS implantation. *Source*: From Ref. 11.

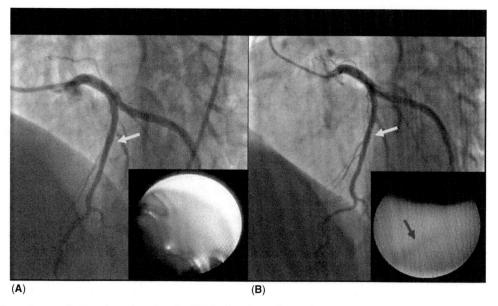

(A)   **(B)**

Figure 20.6 Illustrative case of yellow plaque formation after DES implantation. Yellow neointima is apparent overlying the struts of a DES at follow-up (**B**) although no yellow plaque was apparent beneath the stent immediately after DES implantation (**A**). DES implantation may promote the formation of atherosclerotic yellow plaques; this hypothesis is consistent with pathological observations that new atherosclerotic lesions may occur early after DES implantation. The yellow arrow indicates the site of stent implantation. The red arrow indicates a stent strut buried under yellow neointima. *Source:* From Ref. 11.

of yellow plaques at the lesion and poor neointimal coverage of the stent (Fig. 20.5; Video clips 20.2 and 20.3). In other words, yellow plaques or uncovered stent struts appear to be powerful stimuli for thrombus formation. Furthermore, DES implantation, when compared with BMS, has been shown to promote (11) the formation of yellow plaques at the stented lesion (Fig. 20.6) and disrupted yellow plaques are often detected at the site of VLST. Therefore, possible mechanisms of VLST are thrombosis caused by (*i*) uncovered stent struts, (*ii*) unhealed disrupted yellow plaques under the struts or adjacent to the stent, (*iii*) new disruption of yellow plaques already present at stent implantation, and (*iv*) new disruption of yellow plaques that have formed after stent implantation. Pathological studies (12,13) have also demonstrated that atherosclerotic lesions appear at an earlier stage within the neointima at sites of DES implantation as opposed to sites of BMS implantation. OCT studies have also demonstrated the presence of ruptured plaques at the site of VLST. When all of these findings are taken into consideration, a major difference between DES and BMS seems to be the speed of atherosclerosis progression at the stented site, which appears to play an important role in the higher rate of VLST observed with DES. After BMS implantation (14,15), thick, white, non-atherosclerotic neointima formed over the stent has a sealing effect and becomes a thick fibrous cap for the yellow plaque that is usually present before stenting. Therefore, it takes a long time for vulnerable yellow plaques to form on the surface of the new vessel wall. However, after DES implantation, the very thin neointima does not protect the pre-existing vulnerable yellow plaques and therefore yellow plaque formation is

---

Focus Box 20.5

The presence of uncovered stent struts, yellow plaques, and/ or thrombus may be a marker of the risk of subsequent stent thrombosis. We believe that dual antiplatelet therapy is no longer required for a DES that is completely covered by white neointima without thrombus or yellow plaques.

---

promoted. As a result, new disruption of yellow plaques and subsequent thrombosis occur earlier after DES implantation than after BMS implantation. In the BMS era, acute MI that occurred at the stented site about 10 years after stent implantation was the subject of many case reports. In those cases, the culprit lesion had an angioscopic appearance identical to that observed at the culprit lesion of acute MI occurring in native unstented coronary arteries. It was generally accepted, in those days, that this long time frame (of 10 years) after BMS implantation was required for atherosclerosis to progress to such an extent that it could once again become a substrate for ACS. Angioscopic evaluation of neointima after DES implantation may be useful to evaluate the risk of VLST. White smooth neointima without thrombus that completely covers both the stent struts and any pre-existing yellow plaques under the stent might be regarded as an indicator of lesion stability, for the subsequent decade, until new atherosclerotic lesions form within the neointima. Angioscopic evaluation of neointima may be a useful tool for comparisons among DES or to customize antiplatelet therapy in individual patients.

Limitations of Angioscopy

Angioscopic catheters have not undergone any major techno-logical improvements over time and are not easy to handle. Blood needs to be replaced with transparent liquids such as 3% dextran-40 to acquire clear images of the vessel wall. This is achieved by intracoronary injection with or without balloon occlusion of the vessel. Without balloon occlusion, clear images may not be acquired due to the inadequate clearance of blood in some cases. With balloon occlusion, myocardial ischemia is induced and the time for observation is relatively limited. A complete 360-degree view may not be acquired in all cases. However, these limitations pertain to the current devices and are not of angioscopy itself. Therefore, advances in technology are eagerly awaited.

Technical Issues and Possible Complications of Angioscopy

There are two basic types of angioscopy catheters. One is based on balloon occlusion while the other is non-occlusive. With the occlusion-based angioscope, the major potential for complica-tion relates to ischemia (e.g., angina and arrhythmia), so the observation time should be short enough to prevent this compli-cation. On the other hand, with the non-occlusion-type angio-scope, we can continuously observe the entire target vessel from the distal bed to the ostium by pulling back the catheter while injecting 3% dextran-40. Myocardial ischemia is not induced unless the catheter (4 Fr) occludes the stenotic lesion. For safer exploration of severely stenotic lesions, an aspiration catheter can be used. With this system, we can observe the lesion while advancing the catheter from the proximal end and can prevent occlusion at the lesion site by the catheter before observation.

Classification, Semi-Quantitative Evaluation, and Quantitative Evaluation of Angioscopic Images

Thrombus is defined as white or red material with a cotton-like or ragged appearance or with fragmentation with or without protrusion into the lumen or adherent to the luminal surface (Fig. 20.7). Thrombus is classified as red thrombus, white thrombus, or mixed thrombus. The majority of thrombus is classified as mixed thrombus. White thrombus is commonly detected directly adhering to the vessel wall, and it becomes more and more reddish as a function of the disturbance of the blood flow and probably also as a function of the amount of red blood cells incorporated into the fibrin network of white thrombus (16). In ruptured plaques, white thrombus some-times contains lipid material protruding from the necrotic core and looks yellow (i.e., yellow thrombus).

Plaques are classified as non-disrupted or disrupted based on the absence or presence of thrombus. Disrupted plaques are classified as ruptured (7,17) or erosive plaques based on the presence or absence of yellow material protruding into the lumen, which comes from the ruptured necrotic core. This is an angioscopic classification and is not always consistent with pathological classification; pathologically, small ruptures may be classified as erosive by angioscopy.

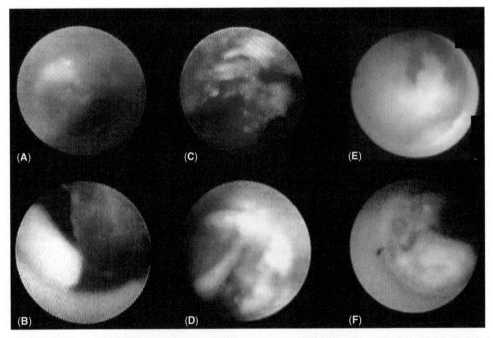

Figure 20.7 Angioscopic classification of thrombus. Thrombus is classified as red (A and B), white (E and F), or mixed thrombus (C and D). Thrombus that contains lipid material appears yellow (D) and is frequently present in ruptured plaques. Red thrombus is a common feature in occlusive lesions in acute MI patients (A). Red thrombus with a smooth surface in an otherwise normal vessel (B) may be an embolized thrombus from an extracoronary source.

Plaque color (5) is classified into four grades by comparison with standard colors (Fig. 20.8): grade 0 (white), grade 1 (slightly yellow), grade 2 (yellow), and grade 3 (intense yellow). Plaque color can be evaluated quantitatively using the LCH color space (18) system that uses three parameters [lightness (L), chrome (C), and hue (H)]. According to the increase in the yellow color grade, C becomes larger and H becomes smaller. Although quantitative evaluation provides greater objectivity and grading provides greater subjectivity, a single picture is required to perform quantitative color analysis while grading is usually performed by viewing the whole movie. Choosing a single picture from the movie is a key but ultimately subjective step that determines the result of the color analysis. If the image of the blood flow is superimposed on the image of a yellow plaque, the plaque color would become more reddish. On the other hand, grading is usually done comprehensively by viewing the whole movie of the plaque, thus lessening the effect of blood flow that is sometimes seen over the plaque to affect classification. As a result, grading is often more consistent and reliable than quantitative color analysis.

Neointimal coverage (10,19) of stents is classified into three or four grades: grade 0 (stent is not covered), grade 1 (stent is on the vessel wall but covered by a thin layer), and grade 2 (stent is completely buried under the neointima and is below the level of the vessel surface). Grade 2 can be divided into two grades according to whether or not the stent is visible through the neointima: grade 2 (visible) and grade 3 (invisible).

PITFALLS: CLINICAL EFFECTIVENESS

It is difficult to translate angioscopic findings into clinical practice because there are no clinical trials that have demonstrated the clinical implications of specific angioscopic observations. For example, we believe that dual antiplatelet therapy is no longer mandatory for a DES that is completely covered by white neointima without thrombus formation. This suggestion is based on the hypothesis that vessel walls without thrombogenic potential never cause ACS. Many cardiologists may agree with this hypothesis. On the other hand, we believe that a DES with

evidence of persistent ruptured yellow plaques under or adjacent to the stent, or with thrombus formation on the struts, has an ongoing high risk of stent thrombosis. This suggestion is based on the hypothesis that the presence of a thrombogenic lesion is a marker of the risk of a future thrombotic event. Obviously this hypothesis, based on intuition, needs to be tested in clinical trials. In native vessels, potentially thrombogenic lesions such as ruptured plaques often remain silent and do not cause ACS. Thus, the mere presence of thrombogenic lesions does not necessarily result in an ACS and the factors that link ruptured plaques to the occurrence of a clinical event remain elusive. Furthermore, vessel walls without thrombogenic lesions but with intact vulnerable yellow plaques may potentially have a similar risk of causing ACS as vessel walls with already ruptured plaques. Therefore, we should be very careful in interpreting angioscopic findings; however, the observations themselves contain a wealth of information that have the potential to refine our understanding of the mechanisms of ACS and may ultimately help in risk stratification and in guiding individual patient management.

PERSONAL PERSPECTIVE

Angioscopic findings have provided remarkable insights into the pathophysiology of coronary disease based on observations in native and stented coronary lesions. These findings have generated many hypotheses that have potentially important clinical relevance both for risk stratification and treatment in individual patients. However, the paucity of prospective controlled randomized trials has meant that the evidence base required to integrate angioscopy into daily practice is lacking. Based on our experience with angioscopy, there are several potentially important hypotheses that merit further exploration in randomized trials.

First, complete coverage of stent struts with white neointima at follow-up after DES implantation may be an indication that dual antiplatelet therapy can be discontinued. Conversely, the presence of thrombus or of yellow plaque formation may indicate a continuing risk of stent thrombosis that warrants continued dual antiplatelet therapy. Second, the angioscopic

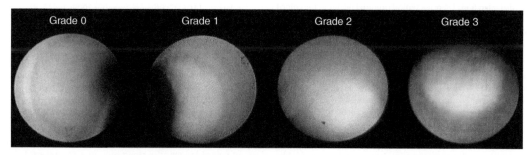

Figure 20.8 Standard classification of plaque color. Plaque color is classified into four grades: grade 0 (white), grade 1 (slightly yellow), grade 2 (yellow), and grade 3 (intense yellow). As the plaques with higher grade yellow color have a higher incidence of thrombus detected on the plaques, they might be regarded as potentially more vulnerable. *Source:* From Ref. 1.

documentation of disrupted yellow plaques in angiographically intermediate stenotic lesions may be an indication for stent implantation rather than medical therapy alone in an attempt to reduce future clinical events. Third, target lesions for PCI that have yellow plaques, especially ruptured yellow plaques, may have a high risk of a no reflow phenomenon after stent implantation that might be reduced by the systematic use of specifically designed stents or distal protection devices.

Angioscopy is useful to identify the true culprit lesion (i.e., the lesion responsible for the thrombotic event) in ACS patients but evidence for its use as an adjunctive imaging modality, to guide intervention, is lacking. Many patients with ACS have multiple stenotic lesions and are treated by dilating and stenting the severely stenotic lesions on the angiogram. However, angioscopy often reveals that ruptured yellow plaques with thrombus is not completely covered by the stent despite an acceptable angiographic result. Such ruptured plaques are often detected near the edge of the stent but are sometimes detected in a remote segment with or without stenosis. Whether complete coverage of disrupted plaques adjacent to the stent or at other sites would reduce future clinical events ought to be investigated in a controlled trial.

As an investigational tool, angioscopy might prove useful to evaluate the stabilization of vulnerable plaques using changes in the yellow color intensity of the plaques as a surrogate endpoint. In many clinical trials to evaluate the drug effect of statins, reduction of plaque volume evaluated by IVUS is already used as a surrogate endpoint of the trials. However, a causal association between reduction of plaque volume and reduction of cardiovascular events has not been established in general, although there is some convincing evidence from statin trials. We believe that changes in the yellow color intensity of plaques may have a more direct association with plaque stabilization and reduction of ACS events than reduction of plaque volume.

To conclude, angioscopic images provide abundant information and are a source of inspiration for future research. However, refinements in device technology and controlled trials are required before the device can be incorporated into daily clinical practice.

VIDEO CLIPS

Video clip 20.1 Angioscopic images of the culprit lesion in a patient with an acute myocardial infarction. There is a typical ruptured plaque at the culprit lesion before intervention. The protruding necrotic core with mixed white and red thrombus is clearly visible. This is a typical case of a ruptured plaque with superimposed thrombus leading to an acute coronary event. The coronary lumen is filled with cotton-like mixed (white and red) thrombus.

Video clip 20.2 Angioscopic appearance of a first-generation sirolimus-eluting stent (Cypher™) 1 year after implantation. The struts are not completely covered by neointima and are apposed to the vessel wall. White and red thrombus is observed adhering both to the ruptured yellow plaques below the stent and to the stent struts.

Video clip 20.3 Angioscopic images 1 year after implantation of a zotarolimus-eluting DES (Endeavor). The stent struts are almost completely covered by smooth white neointima. There is no evidence of thrombus. Such complete

neointimal coverage resembles that described with BMS and is in marked contrast to the angioscopic appearance reported with the first-generation sirolimus- and paclitaxel-eluting DES.

REFERENCES

1. Ueda Y, Asakura M, Yamaguchi O, et al. The healing process of infarct-related plaques. Insights from 18 months of serial angioscopic follow-up. J Am Coll Cardiol 2001; 38: 1916–22.
2. Asakura M, Ueda Y, Yamaguchi O, et al. Extensive development of vulnerable plaques as a pan-coronary process in patients with myocardial infarction: an angioscopic study. J Am Coll Cardiol 2001; 37: 1284–8.
3. Masumura Y, Ueda Y, Matsuo K, et al. Frequency and location of yellow and disrupted coronary plaques in patients as detected by angioscopy. Circ J 2011; 75: 603–12.
4. Matsuo K, Ueda Y, Nishio M, et al. Thrombogenic potential of whole blood is higher in patients with acute coronary syndrome than in patients with stable coronary diseases. Thromb Res 2011; 128: 268–73.
5. Ueda Y, Ohtani T, Shimizu M, Hirayama A, Kodama K. Assessment of plaque vulnerability by angioscopic classification of plaque color. Am Heart J 2004; 148: 333–5.
6. Kubo T, Imanishi T, Takarada S, et al. Implication of plaque color classification for assessing plaque vulnerability: a coronary angioscopy and optical coherence tomography investigation. JACC Cardiovasc Interv 2008; 1: 74–80.
7. Sanidas EA, Maehara A, Mintz GS, et al. Angioscopic and virtual histology intravascular ultrasound characteristics of culprit lesion morphology underlying coronary artery thrombosis. Am J Cardiol 2011; 107: 1285–90.
8. Ohtani T, Ueda Y, Mizote I, et al. Number of yellow plaques detected in a coronary artery is associated with future risk of acute coronary syndrome: detection of vulnerable patients by angioscopy. J Am Coll Cardiol 2006; 47: 2194–200.
9. Hirayama A, Saito S, Ueda Y, et al. Qualitative and quantitative changes in coronary plaque associated with atorvastatin therapy. Circ J 2009; 73: 718–25.
10. Oyabu J, Ueda Y, Ogasawara N, et al. Angioscopic evaluation of neointima coverage: sirolimus drug-eluting stent versus bare metal stent. Am Heart J 2006; 152: 1168–74.
11. Higo T, Ueda Y, Oyabu J, et al. Atherosclerotic and thrombogenic neointima formed over sirolimus drug-eluting stent: an angioscopic study. JACC Cardiovasc Imaging 2009; 2: 616–24.
12. Nakazawa G, Vorpahl M, Finn AV, Narula J, Virmani R. One step forward and two steps back with drug-eluting-stents: from preventing restenosis to causing late thrombosis and nouveau atherosclerosis. JACC Cardiovasc Imaging 2009; 2: 625–8.
13. Nakazawa G, Otsuka F, Nakano M, et al. The pathology of neoatherosclerosis in human coronary implants bare-metal and drug-eluting stents. J Am Coll Cardiol 2011; 57: 1314–22.
14. Ueda Y, Nanto S, Komamura K, Kodama K. Neointimal coverage of stents in human coronary arteries observed by angioscopy. J Am Coll Cardiol 1994; 23: 341–6.
15. Asakura M, Ueda Y, Nanto S, et al. Remodeling of in-stent neointima, which became thinner and transparent over 3 years: serial angiographic and angioscopic follow-up. Circulation 1998; 97: 2003–206.
16. Ueda Y, Asakura M, Hirayama A, et al. Intracoronary morphology of culprit lesions after reperfusion in acute myocardial infarction: serial angioscopic observations. J Am Coll Cardiol 1996; 27: 606–10.

17. Mizote I, Ueda Y, Ohtani T, et al. Distal protection improved reperfusion and reduced left ventricular dysfunction in patients with acute myocardial infarction who had angioscopically defined ruptured plaque. Circulation 2005; 112: 1001–7.

18. Okada K, Ueda Y, Oyabu J, et al. Plaque color analysis by the conventional yellow-color grading system and quantitative measurement using LCH color space. J Interv Cardiol 2007; 20: 324–34.

19. Kotani J, Awata M, Nanto S, et al. Incomplete neointimal coverage of sirolimus-eluting stents: angioscopic findings. J Am Coll Cardiol 2006; 47: 2108–11.

21   What is the optimal imaging tool for coronary atherosclerosis?
Takashi Kubo and Takashi Akasaka

OUTLINE

Recently developed intravascular imaging techniques can reveal information about coronary atherosclerosis beyond that provided by traditional angiography. Grayscale intravascular ultrasound (IVUS) is a widely accepted catheter-based diagnostic tool that allows assessment of plaque area, plaque distribution, lesion length, and coronary remodeling. When combined with spectral analysis of radiofrequency data, IVUS enables a more detailed analysis of plaque composition. Coronary angioscopy permits direct visualization of both the coronary artery lumen and wall. Therefore, angioscopy is the most reliable tool for detecting intraluminal thrombus, while diagnosis of thrombus by other imaging techniques is considered presumptive. Optical coherence tomography is a high-resolution imaging technique that allows excellent characterization of atherosclerotic plaques. Although this technique is limited by a shallow depth of penetration, its higher resolution with respect to IVUS has the ability to detect thin-cap fibroatheroma. Given the complementary information acquired from diverse imaging modalities, a combination of techniques may represent the optimal approach to a comprehensive evaluation of coronary atherosclerosis.

INTRODUCTION

Imaging of coronary atherosclerosis has contributed to the understanding of the natural history of coronary artery disease (CAD), the processes leading to luminal narrowing, and the phenomenon of plaque rupture. The conventional method for imaging atherosclerosis is X-ray angiography. Selective coronary angiography reliably identifies the luminal dimension of the epicardial artery and remains the gold standard for detecting stenotic lesions. The development of intravascular ultrasound (IVUS) offered cross-sectional images of both the arterial wall and the lumen, thus providing additional information about atherosclerotic plaques and precise measurements of vessel dimensions that enhanced the understanding of the natural history of the disease. Spectral analysis of radiofrequency ultrasound signals allows more detailed assessment of plaque composition. Coronary angioscopy is a unique imaging method that permits direct visualization of thrombus, plaque rupture, and the color of the coronary arterial wall. Optical coherence tomography (OCT) is an optical analogue of IVUS and provides cross-sectional images with ultrahigh resolution. However, in spite of the development of imaging technologies, there is no widely accepted diagnostic method to prospectively identify vulnerable plaques. The challenge for the future is to identify vulnerable plaques before clinical events, generally mediated by plaque rupture, and subsequent thrombus formation occur.

Many of the invasive imaging techniques are able to detect different features of the vulnerable plaques. The purpose of this chapter is to briefly outline the advantages and disadvantages of each imaging technique to assess coronary atherosclerosis.

ADVANTAGES AND DISADVANTAGES OF EACH TECHNIQUE
Angiography

Coronary angiography is the standard method for assessing the exact location and severity of obstructive luminal narrowing, and serves as a clinical decision-making tool to evaluate the need for an intracoronary interventional procedure. Computerized quantitative coronary angiography has been widely used in many trials of atherosclerotic progression and regression. Angiographic classifications, such as the American College of Cardiology/American Heart Association Task Force (ACC/AHA) classification (1) and the Ambrose classification (2), are useful to assess the complexity of CAD and are helpful in anticipating the risks of percutaneous or surgical revascularization, taking into account the impact of the presence of bifurcations, total occlusions, thrombus, calcification, and small vessels. The number of diseased vessels provides a simple index of the risk of future events. Angiographic features, such as intraluminal filling defects compatible with thrombus and the presence of contrast with hazy contour beyond the vessel lumen compatible with plaque ulceration, are associated with vulnerable lesion morphologies.

Although invaluable for assessing CAD, coronary angiography has several limitations. First, the severity of stenosis is generally estimated visually in the clinical setting and estimation is limited by the fact that interobserver variability may range from 30% to 60% (3). Second, the presence of diffuse disease, common in diabetic patients, may lead to underestimation of stenosis because the narrowed segments are expressed as a percentage of the luminal diameter compared with adjacent normal coronary segments, and, in diffuse disease, no such segments exist. Third, early-stage CAD will not be detected unless there is a visible narrowing of the vessel lumen on the angiogram. Fourth, in the presence of complex branching and vessel overlapping, or tortuosity, the lumen narrowing may be underestimated or not detected at all given the limitations of the views that can be obtained with a rotating X-ray tube. Finally, angiography does not provide information about plaque burden or plaque components (4,5). Acute coronary syndrome (ACS) is known to develop at (<50%) plaques in most patients. Angiography, therefore, has a low discriminatory power to identify vulnerable plaques prone to cause an acute event.

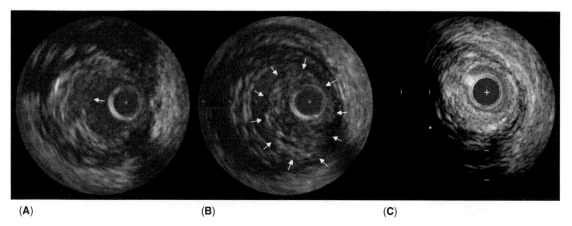

Figure 21.1 Grayscale IVUS images of coronary atherosclerotic plaques showing a ruptured plaque (arrow) (A), intracoronary thrombus (arrows) (B), and hypoechoic plaque with high attenuation (*) (C).

Focus Box 21.1

Angiography does not provide information about plaque burden or plaque components.

Grayscale IVUS

Grayscale IVUS is an intravascular imaging technique that renders two-dimensional cross-sectional views of the coronary arteries. Depending on the distance of the vessel wall from the catheter, the current IVUS provides 100–200 μm axial resolution with >5 mm penetration. IVUS allows qualitative assessments of the coronary vessel wall and quantitative measurements of the external elastic membrane, lumen, plaque, and media cross-sectional area (6). IVUS can demonstrate plaque rupture (Fig. 21.1A) and intracoronary thrombus (Fig. 21.1B) much more clearly than angiography. A hypoechoic plaque with high attenuation is considered to be related to the lipid-rich necrotic core (Fig. 21.1C). Ostial lesions and diffuse diseased segments can be well characterized using IVUS. Assessment of vascular remodeling by IVUS might help to identify plaques at high risk of spontaneous rupture and subsequent thrombosis. Furthermore, serial IVUS analysis is useful to evaluate the change in plaque volume, and therefore IVUS has the potential to assess progression and regression of coronary atherosclerosis in a relatively small number of patients and over a relatively short time period compared with angiography (7).

However, grayscale IVUS has limited power to provide information on plaque composition. Indeed, both calcified and dense fibrotic tissues have strong echo reflections with shadowing and are, therefore, not easy to differentiate. In addition, areas with low echo reflections may represent different tissue components such as foam cells or necrotic core, fibrotic tissue, intraplaque hemorrhage, and fresh or "still-organizing" intraluminal thrombus. IVUS studies use the external elastic membrane and lumen cross-sectional areas to create a surrogate for

Focus Box 21.2

Grayscale IVUS allows qualitative assessment of the coronary vessel wall and quantitative measurements of the external elastic membrane, lumen, plaque, and media cross-sectional area.

Focus Box 21.3

The prognostic implication of the change in plaque volume, which has been used to assess progression and regression of coronary atherosclerosis in a number of IVUS studies, is yet to be determined.

the actual plaque load. However, quantitative assessment of the plaque lacks accuracy because IVUS cannot quantify precisely the media and thereby the true histologic features of the plaque. Finally, the prognostic implication of a change in plaque volume, which has been used to assess progression and regression of coronary atherosclerosis in a number of IVUS studies, is yet to be determined.

Virtual Histology IVUS

Virtual histology (VH) IVUS (Volcano Corporation, Rancho Cordova, CA, USA) uses advanced radiofrequency analysis of ultrasound signals and is able to overcome the main limitation of grayscale IVUS by providing a more detailed analysis of plaque composition (8). The VH-IVUS technology allows in vivo quantitative evaluation of four coronary plaque components, namely fibrous, fibro-fatty, dense calcium, and necrotic core, in real time (Fig. 21.2). The reported sensitivity and specificity of VH-IVUS are 91.7% and 96.6%, respectively, for identification of the lipid-rich necrotic core. The high accuracy of detecting the necrotic core supports the argument that VH-IVUS is a potentially valuable tool for the identification of vulnerable plaques. While thin-cap fibroatheroma (TCFA) with a

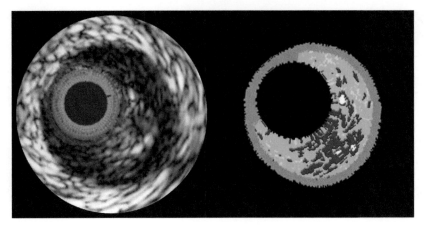

Figure 21.2 Grayscale IVUS and VH-IVUS images of a thin-cap fibroatheroma (TCFA). VH-IVUS analysis codes tissue as green (fibrotic), yellow-green (fibrofatty), white (dense calcium), and red (necrotic core). VH-IVUS-derived TCFA is defined as a lesion that has a confluent necrotic core (>10%) without any evidence of a fibrous cap and a minor amount of calcium (<10%).

Focus Box 21.4

The VH-IVUS technology allows in vivo quantitative evaluation of four coronary plaque components, namely fibrous, fibro-fatty, dense calcium, and necrotic core, in real time.

Focus Box 21.5

The axial resolution of VH-IVUS is insufficient (100–200 μm) to detect critical fibrous cap thickness of TCFA.

---

large necrotic core and an overlying thin fibrous cap of <65 μm thickness is considered to be prone to plaque rupture, VH-IVUS-derived TCFA is defined as a lesion that has a confluent necrotic core (>10%) without any evidence of a fibrous cap and a minor amount of calcium (<10%) (9). Using this definition, a number of studies have investigated the frequency, distribution, and outcome of VH-IVUS-derived TCFA (10). Recently, a prospective VH-IVUS study with 3 years of clinical follow-up reported that the presence of VH-IVUS-derived TCFA was an independent predictor of subsequent lesion-related major adverse cardiovascular events (hazard ratio, 3.35; 95% CI, 1.77 to 6.36; $p < 0.001$) (11). VH-IVUS has the potential to detect high-risk lesions and can provide new insights into the pathophysiology of CAD. The in vivo specific histological analysis of coronary atherosclerosis might allow better stratification of treatment of patients with CAD.

Although VH-IVUS is a promising plaque-imaging platform, some technical limitations must be acknowledged. Current VH-IVUS techniques have poor ability for automated vessel and lumen border detection. Accurate border detection is critically important for qualitative and quantitative VH analysis. Manual correction of the automated border detection needs experience in grayscale IVUS imaging and it is time consuming for the assessment of long coronary segments. Moreover, VH-IVUS suffers from a poor longitudinal resolution due to electrocardiogram-gated image acquisition. The end-diastolic point (peak R-wave) is chosen to acquire the frame for the VH analysis. Capturing only one frame per cardiac cycle with a constant pullback speed significantly decreases the longitudinal

resolution of IVUS imaging. In addition, the axial resolution of VH-IVUS is insufficient (100–200 μm) to detect critical fibrous cap thickness of TCFA (12). VH-IVUS-derived TCFA includes fibroatheroma with a fibrous-cap of >65 μm thickness. Finally, intracoronary thrombus cannot be detected and, therefore, has to be excluded from current VH-IVUS analyses. Thrombus seems to be misclassified as fibrous and fibro-fatty plaque in the VH-IVUS analysis.

iMAP-IVUS

iMAP-IVUS (Boston Scientific Corporation, Maple Grove, Minnesota, USA) is another radiofrequency-based processing method for plaque characterization that is compatible with the latest 40-MHz mechanical IVUS imaging system (as opposed to VH-IVUS with a 20-MHz solid-state IVUS system). Unlike VH-IVUS which uses a classification tree, iMAP discriminates tissue types (fibrotic, necrotic, lipidic, and calcified tissues) based on the degree of spectral similarity between the received signals versus the reference library data obtained from known tissue types (Fig. 21.3). Ex vivo validation demonstrated accuracies at the highest level of confidence as: 97%, 98%, 95%, and 98% for necrotic, lipidic, fibrotic, and calcified regions, respectively (13). Although VH-IVUS cannot provide tissue composition results for very thin plaques, less than the thickness of the artificial gray medial stripe, iMAP allows plaque characterization without imposing any media area.

A major limitation of iMAP is misclassification induced by guide-wire artifacts, not seen in VH-IVUS. iMAP classifies signal poor areas such as guide-wire artifacts as necrotic tissues.

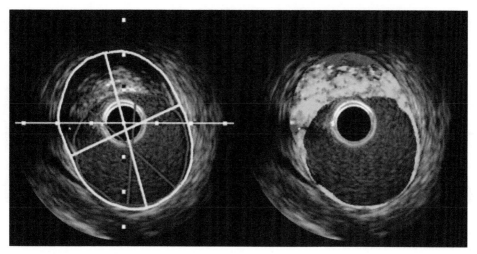

Figure 21.3 Grayscale IVUS and iMAP-IVUS images that are classified as fibroatheroma. iMAP-IVUS codes tissue as green (fibrotic), yellow (lipidic), red (necrotic), and blue (calcified). * = guide wire.

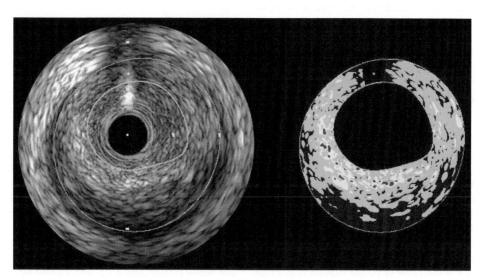

Figure 21.4 Grayscale IVUS and IB-IVUS images that are classified as fibroatheroma. IB-IVUS analysis codes tissue as green (fibrous), yellow (dense fibrosis), blue (lipid), and red (calcification). * = guide wire.

This imaging artifact due to the guide wire decreases the diagnostic accuracy of iMAP. To eliminate this problem, removal of the guide wire may be necessary in clinical studies.

Integrated Backscatter IVUS

Integrated backscatter (IB) IVUS (Terumo Corporation, Tokyo, Japan) is an alternative approach using radiofrequency signal analysis to characterize coronary plaque tissue components. Different tissue components reflect the radiofrequency signals at different power levels, which are used to differentiate various tissue components in IB-IVUS. Similar to VH-IVUS and iMAP, the IB-IVUS system constructs color-coded tissue maps, providing a quantitative visual readout for four types of plaque composition: calcification, fibrosis, dense fibrosis, and lipid pool (Fig. 21.4). Using histological images as a gold standard, the sensitivity and specificity of IB-IVUS for characterizing the lipid pool is reported to be 95% and 98%, respectively (14–16).

There are some limitations to the IB-IVUS technique. First, the angle dependence of the ultrasound signal makes tissue characterization unstable when lesions are not perpendicular to the axis. An in vitro study reported that angular scattering behavior is large in calcified and fibrous tissues, whereas it is slight to null in normal and fatty plaque. Second, calcification is a perfect reflector of ultrasound, resulting in the acoustic shadows that are typical of IVUS images. The ultrasound signals cannot penetrate the calcified layer and are

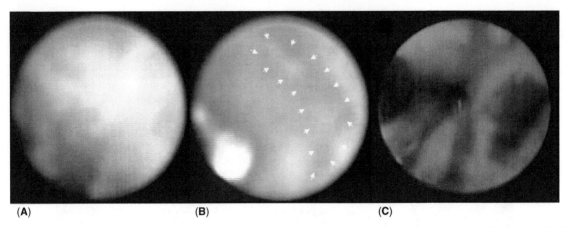

Figure 21.5 Angioscopic images of coronary atherosclerotic plaques. Coronary angioscopy demonstrates rupture of glistening yellow plaque (**A**), plaque erosion (arrows) (**B**), and intracoronary thrombus (**C**).

reflected back toward the transducer. Therefore, accurate tissue characterization of the areas behind calcification is not possible as with conventional IVUS and this may also decrease the diagnostic accuracy. Finally, IB-IVUS cannot discriminate TCFA consisting of a thin fibrous cap of <65 μm thickness because of the limited resolution of current ultrasound imaging technologies.

Angioscopy

Coronary angioscopy is an intravascular technique that allows direct visualization of the internal surface of the coronary arteries. The angioscopy system consists of a 4.5-Fr imaging catheter, 300 W xenon light source, a color monitor, and a recorder. The illumination source provides high intensity cold light to avoid thermal damage within the vessel wall. Angioscopy is especially suitable for detecting plaque rupture, erosion, and thrombus. When the surface of the lesion has a rough, ulcerated, or irregular appearance with visible cracks, fissures, or intimal flaps, it is indicative of plaque rupture (Fig. 21.5A) (17). Plaque erosion is characterized as a reddening on the surface of the plaque with no evidence of dissection, cleft, or depressed ulceration (Fig. 21.5B) (18). Thrombus is defined as a red, white, or mixed intraluminal, superficial, or protruding mass (Fig. 21.5C) (17). The white thrombus is platelet-rich, whereas the red thrombus contains an abundance of fibrin mixed with erythrocytes and platelets. Using histology as the gold standard, the sensitivity of angioscopy to detect plaque rupture was 73%, while the specificity and positive predictive value were >90% (19). On the other hand, the specificity, accuracy, and predictive value were >93% and the sensitivity was 100% for detecting thrombus (19).

Angioscopy identifies coronary atherosclerotic plaque as a protrusion into the lumen that is in continuity with the normal vessel wall. The normal vessel wall appears white, whereas atherosclerotic plaque is categorized on the basis of its yellow color intensity. A pale yellow color of the plaque indicates that the

plaque consists of fibrous tissue alone or that the fibrous cap covering the necrotic core is thick. A deep yellow color of the plaque reflects yellow atheroma seen through the thin fibrous cap. The fibrous cap in a glistening yellow plaque is extremely thin (20). The yellow color intensity of the plaque is related to plaque burden, compensatory positive remodeling, and serum C-reactive protein level (21,22). Indeed, the deep yellow or glistening yellow plaque is frequently observed in the culprit lesion of acute coronary syndrome. Moreover, the number of yellow plaques in a coronary artery is an independent risk factor for the future occurrence of an acute coronary syndrome. Patients with more than two yellow plaques and those with more than five yellow plaques have a 2.2- and 3.8-fold higher incidence of acute coronary syndrome, respectively, than those with no or only one yellow plaque (23). The evaluation of yellow color intensity might be useful to estimate plaque instability and find vulnerable patients with a high risk of future presentation with an acute coronary syndrome.

However, coronary angioscopy has certain drawbacks. First, angioscopy requires coronary artery occlusion and lactate Ringer's irrigation to remove the blood from the viewing field for image acquisition, which occasionally induces significant myocardial ischemia. Moreover, occlusion balloon inflation may cause coronary artery dissection and intimal damage. Second, only a limited part of the vessel tree can be investigated, due to the almost twofold difference in catheter size for angioscopy compared with IVUS. Third, since angioscopic observation is limited to the luminal surface, information about the degree of plaque extension into the vessel wall is not provided. Finally, angioscopic interpretation is entirely subjective, and

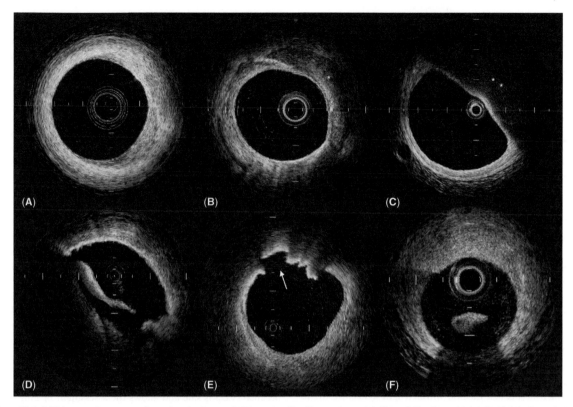

Figure 21.6 OCT images of coronary atherosclerotic plaques. OCT can visualize fibrous plaque (**A**), fibrocalcific plaque (*) (**B**), lipid-rich plaque (**) (**C**), plaque rupture (**D**), plaque erosion (arrow) (**E**), and intracoronary thrombus (**F**).

> **Focus Box 21.7**
>
> Since angioscopic observation is limited to the luminal surface, information about the degree of plaque extension into the vessel wall is not provided.

plaque color is not assessed quantitatively. In addition to plaque components, several factors such as the intensity of light, angle, and distance can affect color perception.

Optical Coherence Tomography

OCT is a recently developed intravascular imaging modality that uses near infrared light to create images. The wavelength used is 1310 nm, which minimizes absorption of the light waves by water, proteins, lipids, and hemoglobin without tissue damage. The current time-domain OCT system employs a 0.016-inch fiber-optic imaging wire. Compared with various other coronary imaging modalities, the main advantage of OCT is its high resolution of up to 10 μm (axial) and 20 μm (lateral), which is approximately 10 times higher than that of IVUS. OCT can clearly differentiate the three layers of the coronary artery wall comprising the intima as the signal-rich layer nearest the lumen, the media as the signal-poor middle layer, and the adventitia as the signal-rich layer surrounding the media. For plaque characterization, OCT demonstrates fibrous plaques as signal-rich homogenous lesions (Fig 21.6A), fibrocalcific plaques as signal-poor sharp-border lesions (Fig. 21.6B), and lipid-rich plaques as signal-poor diffuse border lesions (Fig. 21.6C), with good intra- and interobserver reliability ($\kappa = 0.83$–0.84) as well as excellent sensitivity and specificity (71–98%) (24). Furthermore, OCT can visualize vulnerable lesion morphologies including plaque rupture (Fig. 21.6D), erosion (Fig. 21.6E), and intracoronary thrombus (Fig. 21.6F) (25,26). Using a measurement of the OCT signal attenuation, thrombi can be classified as white or red. White thrombi were identified as signal-rich, low-backscattering protrusions, while red thrombi were identified as high backscattering protrusions inside the lumen of the artery with signal-free shadow. Since OCT has near-histological grade resolution, OCT might be the best tool available to detect TCFA (25). A good correlation is seen for the measurements of the fibrous cap thickness between OCT and histological examination ($r = 0.90$; $p < 0.001$) (27). Another unique feature of OCT is its ability to visualize macrophages. A high degree of positive correlation is found between OCT and histological measurements of fibrous cap macrophage density ($r = 0.84$, $p < 0.0001$) (28).

Focus Box 21.8

Since OCT has near-histological grade resolution, OCT might be the best tool available to detect TCFA.

Focus Box 21.9

OCT is not appropriate for the visualization of the entire cross-sectional vessel architecture or the evaluation of plaque remodeling.

Recently, a second-generation OCT technology, termed Fourier-domain OCT (FD-OCT), has been developed. The imaging catheter for FD-OCT, which is designed for rapid exchange delivery, has a 2.5–2.8 Fr crossing-profile and can be delivered over a 0.014-inch guide wire through a 6 Fr or larger guide catheter. Injecting angiographic contrast media through the guide catheter can achieve effective clearing of blood for FD-OCT imaging. The high frame rate (100 frames/s) and fast pullback speeds (20 mm/s) of FD-OCT allow imaging of long coronary segments with minimal ischemia, eliminating the need for proximal vessel balloon occlusion during image acquisition (29). FD-OCT enables imaging of the three-dimensional microstructure of coronary arteries and facilitates the acquisition of spectroscopic and polarization, Doppler, and other imaging modes for plaque characterization (30). When FD-OCT is fully exploited, it has the potential to dramatically change the way physicians and researchers understand CAD, which in turn will result in better diagnosis and treatment.

The current OCT system has some limitations for clinical use. First, an inherent limitation of OCT is the need for a blood-free imaging zone, because the near-infrared light signals are attenuated by red blood cells. Second, the rate of flush may carry a risk of underestimating the size of the vessel lumen. Third, OCT has a relatively low axial penetration depth of 2 mm. The penetration depth of OCT depends on tissue characteristics. The OCT signal is attenuated rapidly in the lipidic plaque and thrombi. OCT is not appropriate for the visualization of the whole cross-sectional area of the vessel or for the evaluation of vessel remodeling. Fourth, OCT cannot yield a quantitative assessment of the lipid-core size, which was semiquantified as the number of quadrants involved on the cross-sectional image in the previous study. Finally, OCT-derived TCFA is not yet a validated surrogate for plaque prone to thrombosis. The natural history of OCT-derived TCFA remains unknown.

CONCLUSION

Several invasive imaging techniques to investigate coronary atherosclerosis are emerging. The ideal technique would allow us to assess coronary artery obstruction, plaque composition, and lesion vulnerability, guiding the appropriate therapeutic approach. Identification of vulnerable plaques before rupture might help reduce the incidence of acute coronary events. Recent advances in imaging techniques have provided a greater understanding of the pathophysiology of acute coronary syndromes and have shown the potential to identify TCFA. Most techniques currently assess only one feature of the vulnerable plaque, so multimodality imaging might be useful for the detection of high risk plaques. Furthermore, research to explore the predictive value of vulnerable features on future adverse coronary events is important to validate the new imaging techniques as clinical tools in the management of CAD. Although further development of imaging technologies and clinical studies with greater numbers of subjects are required, catheter-based coronary imaging will play an important role in the future of cardiology.

PERSONAL PERSPECTIVE

Table 21.1 summarizes some of the advantages and disadvantages of the techniques discussed. During the last decade several imaging techniques have been developed to overcome the limitations of angiography. The ideal coronary imaging technology would be capable of identifying not only vessel narrowing but also plaque characteristics. Assessment of the plaque characteristics might in particular be important for identifying vulnerable plaques and stratifying the risk of future coronary events. Plaque burden and vessel remodeling is well evaluated by IVUS, which is widely accepted and routinely used for coronary imaging in daily clinical practice. The longitudinal extent of atherosclerotic plaque is also assessed using this technique because IVUS is safe and allows the assessment of long coronary segments of coronary vessels. Plaque rupture is obviously much more reliably visualized by angioscopy and OCT compared with IVUS. Although angioscopic evaluation is subjective due to a limited viewing field, OCT allows quantitative measurements of disrupted fibrous cap thickness and ruptured core-cavity size. Plaque erosion without lipid core rupture may be detected by angioscopy and OCT. Although the angioscopic and OCT characteristics of erosion have never been validated against histology, the appearances of the lesions with those techniques appear to support the assumption. The presence of thrombus is clearly documented by angioscopy and OCT. Angioscopy permits direct visualization of intracoronary thrombi; therefore, it is recognized to be the best tool for detecting both red cell and platelet-rich thrombus. OCT is also useful in thrombus detection; however, mural red thrombi covering the plaque surface may be misdiagnosed as lipid-rich fibroatheromas because they have similar appearances on OCT. Grayscale IVUS and coronary angiography may underestimate the presence of intracoronary thrombus. VH-IVUS is more limited than grayscale IVUS in thrombus identification. The lipid-rich necrotic core can be quantitatively determined by VH-IVUS. In grayscale IVUS and OCT, signal-poor regions with high attenuation seem to be related to the presence of the necrotic core and their presence is a strong predictor of slow flow during percutaneous coronary intervention. TCFA is thought to be the precursor of plaque rupture, which is histopathologically characterized by a fibrous cap thickness of <65 μm with prominent macrophage infiltration. OCT is well

Table 21.1 Advantages and Disadvantages of Each Imaging Technique

	Angiography	Grayscale IVUS	VH-IVUS	Angioscopy	OCT	IVPA/US
Image	Images of blood flow	Tomogram	Tomogram	Surface imaging only	Subsurface tomogram	Tomogram
Axial resolution (μm)	100–200	100	200	1–50	10	100
Type of radiation	X-ray	Ultrasound	Ultrasound	Visible light	Near-IR light	(Near-IR) light + ultrasound
Lumen area	−	++	++	−	++	++
Plaque burden	−	++	++	−	−	++
Positive remodeling	−	++	++	−	−	++
Necrotic core	−	±	++	±	−	++
Fibrous-cap thickness	−	−	±	±	++	±
TCFA	−	−	±	±	++	±
Plaque rupture	±	+	+	++	++	+
Erosion	−	−	−	+	+	−
Thrombus	±	±	±	++	+	±

Intravascular imaging techniques such as grayscale and VH-IVUS, coronary angioscopy, andOCT can be used to assess the characteristics of coronary atherosclerotic plaques.

Abbreviations: IVUS, intravascular ultrasound; VH, virtual histology; OCT, optical coherence tomography; IVPA/US, combined intravascular photoacoustics and ultrasound; IR, infrared; TCFA, thin-cap fibroatheroma; ++, excellent; +, good; ±, possible; −, impossible.

suited for the assessment of the thin fibrous cap and has the capability to identify macrophages within the cap. On angioscopy, the yellow color intensity increased inversely with the thickness of the cap located above the necrotic core, and the glistening yellow plaque is recognized as TCFA. Although the thickness of the thin fibrous cap is below the resolution of IVUS, VH-derived TCFA is a useful surrogate for histologic TCFA. Nevertheless, no single diagnostic modality is available that unequivocally identifies the vulnerable plaque. As each individual imaging modality is suited to identify different characteristics of a plaque, a combination of techniques may be necessary for comprehensive evaluation of the coronary vessel. Although the use of multiple techniques may not be practical during daily practice, these various techniques truly complement each other.

REFERENCES

1. Ellis SG, Vandormael MG, Cowley MJ, et al. Coronary morphologic and clinical determinants of procedural outcome with angioplasty for multivessel coronary artery disease: implications for patient selection. Circulation 1990; 82: 1193–202.
2. Ambrose JA, Israel DH. Angiography in unstable angina. Am J Cardiol 1991; 68: 78B–84B.
3. Zir LM, Miller SW, Dinsmore RE, et al. Interobserver variability in coronary angiography. Circulation 1976; 53: 627–32.
4. Little WC, Constantinescu M, Applegate RJ, et al. Can coronary angiography predict the site of a subsequent myocardial infarction in patients with mild-to-moderate coronary artery disease? Circulation 1988; 78: 1157–66.
5. Ambrose JA, Tannenbaum MA, Alexopoulos D, et al. Angiographic progression of coronary artery disease and the development of myocardial infarction. J Am Coll Cardiol 1988; 12: 56–62.
6. Mintz GS, Nissen SE, Anderson WD, et al. American College of Cardiology Clinical Expert Consensus Document on Standards for Acquisition, Measurement and Reporting of Intravascular Ultrasound Studies (IVUS). A report of the American College of Cardiology Task Force on Clinical Expert Consensus Documents. J Am Coll Cardiol 2001; 37: 1478–92.
7. Nissen SE, Tuzcu EM, Brown BG, et al. Effect of intensive compared with Moderate Lipid-Lowering Therapy on progression of coronary atherosclerosis – a randomized controlled trial. JAMA 2004; 291: 1071–80
8. König A, Margolis MP, Virmani R, et al. Technology insight: in vivo coronary plaque classification by intravascular ultrasonography radiofrequency analysis. Nat Clin Pract Cardiovasc Med 2008; 5: 219–29.
9. Rodriguez-Granillo GA, García-García HM, McFadden EP, et al. In vivo intravascular ultrasound-derived thin-cap fibroatheroma detection using ultrasound radiofrequency data analysis. J Am Coll Cardiol 2005; 46: 2038–42.
10. Kubo T, Maehara A, Mintz GS, et al. The dynamic nature of coronary artery lesion morphology assessed by serial virtual histology intravascular ultrasound tissue characterization. J Am Coll Cardiol 2010; 55: 1590–7.
11. Stone GW, Maehara A, Lansky AJ, et al. A prospective natural-history study of coronary atherosclerosis. N Engl J Med 2011; 364: 226–35.
12. Kubo T, Nakamura N, Matsuo Y, et al. Virtual histology intravascular ultrasound compared with optical coherence tomography for identification of thin-cap fibroatheroma. Int Heart J 2011; 52: 175–9.
13. Sathyanarayana S, Carlier S, Li W, et al. Characterisation of atherosclerotic plaque by spectral similarity of radiofrequency intravascular ultrasound signals. EuroIntervention 2009; 5: 133–9.
14. Kawasaki M, Takatsu H, Noda T, et al. In vivo quantitative tissue characterization of human coronary arterial plaques by use of

integrated backscatter intravascular ultrasound and comparison with angioscopic findings. Circulation 2002; 105: 2487–92.

15. Okubo M, Kawasaki M, Ishihara Y, et al. Development of integrated backscatter intravascular ultrasound for tissue characterization of coronary plaques. Ultrasound Med Biol 2008; 34: 655–63.

16. Kawasaki M, Bouma BE, Bressner J, et al. Diagnostic accuracy of optical coherence tomography and integrated backscatter intravascular ultrasound images for tissue characterization of human coronary plaques. J Am Coll Cardiol 2006; 48: 81–8.

17. Nesto RW, Waxman S, Mittleman M, et al. Angioscopy of culprit lesions in unstable angina: correlation of clinical presentation with plaque morphology. Am J Cardiol 1998; 81: 225–8.

18. Hayashi T, Kiyoshima T, Matsuura M, et al. Plaque erosion in the culprit lesion is prone to develop a smaller myocardial infarction size compared with plaque rupture. Am Heart J 2005; 149: 284–90.

19. Siegel RJ, Ariani M, Fishbein M, et al. Histopathologic validation of angioscopy and intravascular ultrasound. Circulation 1991; 84: 109–17.

20. Kubo T, Imanishi T, Takarada S, et al. Implication of plaque color classification for assessing plaque vulnerability: A coronary angioscopy and optical coherence tomography investigation. JACC Cardiovasc Interv 2008; 1: 74–80.

21. Takano M, Mizuno K, Okamatsu K, et al. Mechanical and structural characteristics of vulnerable plaques: Analysis by coronary angioscopy and intravascular ultrasound. J Am Coll Cardiol 2001; 38: 99–104.

22. Nishikawa K, Satomura K, Miyake T, et al. Relation between plasma fibrinogen level and coronary plaque morphology in patients with stable angina pectoris. Am J Cardiol 2001; 87: 1401–4.

23. Ohtani T, Ueda Y, Mizote I, et al. Number of yellow plaques detected in a coronary artery is associated with future risk of acute coronary syndrome: detection of vulnerable patients by angioscopy. J Am Coll Cardiol 2006; 47: 2194–200.

24. Yabushita H, Bouma BE, Houser SL, et al. Characterization of human atherosclerosis by optical coherence tomography. Circulation 2002; 106: 1640–5.

25. Kubo T, Imanishi T, Takarada S, et al. Assessment of culprit lesion morphology in acute myocardial infarction. Ability of optical coherence tomography compared with intravascular ultrasound and coronary angioscopy. J Am Coll Cardiol 2007; 50: 933–9.

26. Ino Y, Kubo T, Tanaka A, et al. Difference of culprit lesion morphologies between ST-segment elevation myocardial infarction and non-ST-segment elevation acute coronary syndrome: an optical coherence tomography study. JACC Cardiovasc Interv 2011; 4: 76–82.

27. Kume T, Akasaka T, Kawamoto T, et al. Measurement of the thickness of the fibrous cap by optical coherence tomography. Am Heart J 2006; 152: 755; e1– e4.

28. Tearney GJ, Yabushita H, Houser SL, et al. Quantification of macrophage content in atherosclerotic plaques by optical coherence tomography. Circulation 2003; 107: 113–19.

29. Takarada S, Imanishi T, Liu Y, et al. Advantage of next-generation frequency-domain optical coherence tomography compared with conventional time-domain system in the assessment of coronary lesion. Catheter Cardiovasc Interv 2010; 75: 202–6.

30. Tearney GJ, Waxman S, Shishkov M, et al. Three-dimensional coronary artery microscopy by intracoronary optical frequency domain imaging. JACC Cardiovasc Imaging 2008; 1: 752–61.

22   Optimization of primary and secondary prevention

Katerina K. Naka, Aris Bechlioulis, and Lampros K. Michalis

OUTLINE

Coronary artery disease (CAD) is the leading cause of morbidity and mortality worldwide. Preventive interventions have been proven efficient in reducing morbidity, mortality, and health costs globally both for patients with established CAD (secondary prevention) and asymptomatic subjects without CAD (primary prevention). In secondary prevention, the role of aspirin and other specific medications is essential. In both primary and secondary prevention, several risk factors for CAD have been identified and have been shown to account for a large number of acute CAD events. Four major modifiable risk factors (dyslipidemia, hypertension, diabetes mellitus, and smoking) have been well established and their management should follow detailed guidelines issued from scientific societies. Other modifiable risk factors (e.g. obesity, physical inactivity, poor diet) may be targeted mainly via lifestyle and public health measures. Less well-established risk factors (e.g. inflammation, psychosocial stress, genetic factors) are currently investigated. Future targeted research and implementation of established knowledge by both physicians and the community are needed to further optimize primary and secondary prevention.

INTRODUCTION—DEFINITIONS

Coronary artery disease (CAD) is the leading cause of morbidity and mortality in developed and developing countries. Effective prevention of CAD is therefore of paramount importance in reducing morbidity, mortality, and health costs globally.

Epidemiology of Coronary Atherosclerosis

Based on United States' (US) data published in 2011 (1), CAD causes ≈1 of every 6 deaths in the US. About every 25 seconds, an American will experience a CAD event, and approximately every minute, someone will die of one. Based on data from Europe and the US (1,2), CAD mortality and morbidity rates have fallen in most western high-income countries in the last 40–50 years, while they continue to increase in low- and middle-income countries. This decrease in CAD mortality and morbidity has been attributed partly (approximately 45–50%) to life-saving, evidence-based medical therapies applied to patients with acute CAD events, especially acute myocardial infarction (MI), as well as secondary preventive therapies after MI or revascularization. The other 50% of the decrease has been attributed to recognition of cardiovascular (CV) risk factors and efficient interventions to manage most of them. Nevertheless, these favorable improvements in risk factors were offset partly by increases in the prevalence of obesity and diabetes mellitus (DM) (1). A decrease in age-adjusted CAD mortality rate has also been reported in the United Kingdom (UK) (3)

from 1984 to 2004. However, it has to be noted that this decrease was apparent mainly in older subjects >55 years, while in younger subjects (45–54 years) the decline was slower or there was even in increase in men 35–44 years. These unfavorable trends in younger subjects have been also attributed to an increase in obesity and DM.

Primary and Secondary Prevention

Currently, most scientific and health resources go toward treatment of CAD. However, it is increasingly widely accepted that interventions aiming to prevent CAD may reduce deaths, nonfatal events, and hospitalizations that may be related to coronary but also non-coronary atherosclerosis, and undoubtedly a large proportion of the tremendous health-related costs. This explains why primary and secondary prevention of CAD (and inevitably also cardiovascular diseases—CVD) have attracted increasing attention by physicians, the general public as well as governments and policy makers.

Secondary Prevention

Secondary prevention consists of therapeutic interventions that aim to reduce CV risk in patients with known or documented CVD (CAD, peripheral arterial disease, cerebrovascular disease, abdominal aortic aneurysm). The great majority of these patients, about 80%, will die of CVD as opposed to subjects without known CVD, of whom only 40% are expected to die of CVD.

Primary Prevention

Primary prevention consists of interventions that aim to reduce risk in subjects without a history of any CVD. As CVD has a long asymptomatic latent period, it provides an opportunity for early preventive interventions. Primary prevention is a complex process that involves: (*i*) identification of CV risk factors, (*ii*) assessment of global CV risk, (*iii*) decision for interventions that are expected to reduce CV risk (at an individual and a population level) at a known and acceptable risk and cost.

Cardiovascular Risk Factors

A CV risk factor, a term widely used currently in cardiology, is a factor that has a causal association with CVD, while some risk factors may also be used also to predict CV risk. For each risk factor, it is important to know whether it can be modified, the intervention by which this can be achieved, whether modification is associated with a reduction of risk and at which level this may be proven, the cost and potential risks of the intervention. CVD is most often the consequence of complex interaction of multiple risk factors. Thus, multiple interventions are usually needed to reduce CV risk.

Risk factors for CAD may be classified into: (*i*) established and non-established or emerging depending on our knowledge on how these are related to CV risk and (*ii*) modifiable, potentially modifiable and non-modifiable depending on whether they can be modified with various interventions (Focus Box 22.1). Furthermore, the term 'risk factor' has been increasingly used lately to include parameters that may predict CV risk and future CV events, but are not causally associated with CAD. These risk markers are shown in Focus Box 22.2.

Non-Modifiable Risk Factors
These include age, family history, and male gender.

Ageing undoubtedly increases the risk for CAD. Although the average age at first MI is about 65 years for men and 70 for women, there is no clear age cut-off point for the occurrence of increased CV risk. Furthermore, it is well known that atherosclerosis begins in childhood and progresses into adulthood. To maximize the benefits of preventive interventions, especially those involving lifestyle changes, it is recommended that guidelines should be applied in asymptomatic persons beginning at age 20, although CV risk is usually estimated for ages >35–40 (4).

A family history of premature CAD, defined most often as occurring in a first-degree male relative <55 years or in a female relative <65 years, has long been considered an important risk factor for CAD; a family history is associated with a 1.5–2.0-fold increased risk for a first CVD event even after adjusting for coexistent risk factors (4). Family history is currently recommended to be obtained for CV risk assessment in all asymptomatic adults (4). Although intensive interventions have been shown to improve modifiable risk factors in subjects with a family history of CAD, the influence on CAD events has not been proven.

Although CAD remains the leading cause of death in both genders, the epidemiology of CAD events differs between men and women (1). Men have a higher risk for CAD and tend to have CAD events at a younger age; the incidence in women lags behind men by 10 years for total CAD and by 20 years for more serious events such as MI and sudden death (1). CAD mortality

Focus Box 22.1 Risk Factors for Coronary Artery Disease

Established risk factors	Non-established or emerging risk factors
Non-modifiable	
1. Age	1. Specific genetic polymorphisms
2. Male gender	2. Low socioeconomic status
3. Family history of premature CAD	
4. Previous history of CVD (Coronary, cerebrovascular or peripheral arterial disease, abdominal aortic aneurysm)	
5. Chronic kidney disease	
Modifiable	*Modifiable or potentially modifiable*
1. Dyslipidemia (increased total and LDL cholesterol)	1. Obesity/Metabolic syndrome/ Insulin resistance/Pre-diabetes
2. Hypertension	2. Low/no alcohol intake
3. DM	3. Low or no physical activity
4. Smoking	4. Other types of dyslipidemia: increased Lp(a), reduced HDL, increased TRG
	5. Menopause
	6. Increased homocysteine
	7. Inflammation/oxidative stress
	8. Mental stress, personality type

Focus Box 22.2 Markers of CV Risk—AHA/ACC Recommendations on CV Risk Assessment in Asymptomatic Adults (4)

Modality	Marker	Recommendations
Electrocardiogram	Left ventricular hypertrophy	Hypertensives or diabetics or even all asymptomatic adults
Echocardiogram	• Left ventricular hypertrophy	→ Hypertensives
	• Diastolic dysfunction	
	• Wall motion abnormalities at rest/systolic dysfunction	
Biochemistry	• High sensitivity C-reactive protein	→ Adults at intermediate risk
	• Microalbuminuria (urinalysis)	→ Hypertensives or diabetics
Imaging of atherosclerosis	• Carotid intima-media thickness	→ Adults at intermediate risk
	• Coronary artery calcium score	→ Adults at intermediate risk or even low-to-intermediate risk
	• Extracoronary atherosclerosis (carotid plaques, peripheral limb arteries, aorta)	
Assessment of peripheral vessels	• Ankle-brachial index	→ Adults at intermediate risk
	• Endothelial function	
	• Aortic pulse wave velocity	
	• Compliance or distensibility	
Functional tests of ischemia	• Exercise electrocardiography	→ Adults at intermediate risk
	• Stress echocardiography	
	• Myocardial perfusion imaging	→ Diabetics or strong family history

is higher in women (1-year mortality after a first MI 38% and 25% in women and men, respectively); this is probably because of the older age in women at first event and the fact that CV risk factors as well as CAD still remain under diagnosed and under treated in women (5). To underline this, American Heart Association (AHA) has issued specific evidence-based guidelines for CV prevention in women (5) that follow those for the general population.

Modifiable Risk Factors

Robust epidemiological data have identified four easily measured and modifiable risk factors that are associated with the development of clinical CAD in asymptomatic individuals ≥40 years old: smoking, cholesterol, blood pressure (BP), and diabetes (4). Lack of control of these four risk factors was recently estimated to account for 29% of CVD risk (6). According to the World Health Organization (7), seven risk factors (the four classical ones and also overweight and obesity, physical inactivity, low fruit, and vegetable intake), are the leading risks of mortality accounting for 61% of CV deaths and >75% of CAD. Reducing exposure to these seven risk factors would be expected to increase global life expectancy by almost 5 years. Similar results were reported by the INTERHEART study (8) that revealed nine common modifiable risk factors that accounted for ≈90% of the MIs observed worldwide. Apart from the factors mentioned above, two other factors were also identified: phychosocial factors and very low or no alcohol consumption.

Assessment of Global Cardiovascular Risk—Risk Scores

As suggested by most scientific societies today, the absolute CV risk of an individual should always be assessed for the appropriate intervention that aims to target a specific risk factor to be decided. The importance of any intervention (especially in terms of cost-efficacy) varies depending on the level of the absolute risk; the higher the risk, the more cost-efficient the intervention.

There are certain conditions on the basis of which subjects are categorized as being at *very high risk* according to ESC (9) or at *high risk* according to the AHA/American College of Cardiology (ACC) classification (4): (*i*) Patients with any clinically overt or documented CVD by invasive or non-invasive testing, (*ii*) Patients with DM (type 2 or type 1 with target organ damage such as microalbuminuria), and (*iii*) Patients with chronic kidney disease (CKD) (glomerular filtration rate <60 mL/min/1.73 m²). According to the European Society of Cardiology (ESC) (9), patients with markedly elevated single risk factors such as familial dyslipidemias and severe hypertension are considered to be at high risk.

In the absence of known CVD or any of the above factors, CV risk is assessed using various scores or tools for CV risk prediction. To optimize primary prevention, risk scores should be obtained for all asymptomatic adults without a clinical history of CAD (4). Several risk scores exist and many are also available in the Internet and can be downloaded in order to help the physician. The most popular risk tools are the Framingham Risk Score (FRS—derived from US population) (Fig. 22.1) (10) and the

European Systematic Coronary Risk Evaluation (SCORE—derived from European populations, tailored for individual countries, with two versions available, for high- and low-risk countries) (Fig. 22.2) (2). Other popular tools (4) not discussed in detail here are the Reynolds, PROCAM (derived from a German male population), and the QRISK score (from the UK). In addition, longer-term prediction tools of CV risk are being prepared (FRS) to offer additional risk burden information, which is particularly important for younger people and female populations.

Factors mainly included in risk scores are: age, gender, total or low density lipoprotein cholesterol (LDL-c), high density lipoprotein cholesterol (HDL-c) (or HDL-to-LDL ratio), systolic blood pressure (SBP), diastolic blood pressure (DBP), and smoking. DM may be incorporated in the score (e.g. FRS) or patients with DM may a priori be considered as high-risk individuals. Some risk scores have also included family history, and high sensitivity C-reactive protein (CRP).

Apart from estimating absolute risk of either fatal and non-fatal CAD events (FRS) or CVD death (SCORE) in the next 10 years, CV risk may be categorized in four categories, that is, low, intermediate or moderate, high, and very high risk (4,9) as shown in Table 22.1. According to the latest guidelines issued by the AHA/ACC (4) or the ESC (2), if a patient is at very high risk or high risk intensive preventive interventions are warranted and there is no incremental benefit of added testing. If an asymptomatic adult is at low risk, no further testing is necessary. If an asymptomatic adult is at intermediate or moderate risk, additional testing may further be used to define risk status. Additional testing consists of detection of CV risk markers as outlined in Focus Box 22.2. The selection of the method to be used for further screening depends on the patient profile (4).

Interventions to Reduce CV Risk

Before a preventive intervention may be used and established in everyday clinical practice to target a specific modifiable risk factor that is causally associated with CV risk, a clear benefit of the intervention in reducing long-term or intermediate CV risk that is expected to exceed any potential risks and cost related to the intervention must be proven. This evidence is being gathered via appropriately designed and performed research projects such as clinical investigations and various types of epidemiological studies (mainly randomized controlled trials and meta-analyses). Based on the amount and quality of evidence to prove the above, interventions targeting specific modifiable risk factors for primary or secondary CV prevention have been classified (11) into three categories (Fig. 22.3).

Two distinct approaches in CV prevention may be described. The first approach is based on reduction of the individual CV risk by targeting a small population that is at high absolute risk. This approach consists of (*i*) secondary prevention measures in patients with known CVD and (*ii*) screening for high-risk individuals who are most likely to benefit from primary prevention measures. The second approach is based on reduction of population-based risk by targeting much greater population that is at small

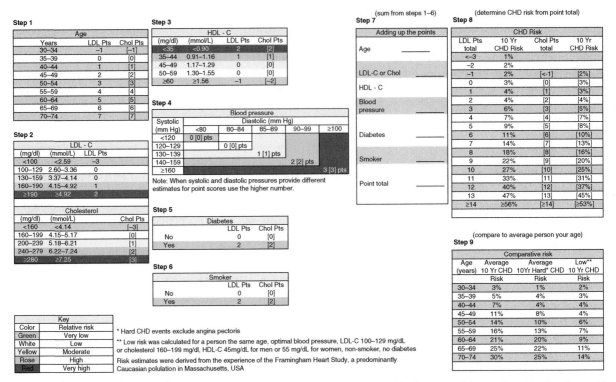

Figure 22.1 Framingham CAD score sheet for men using age, total cholesterol (or LDL-c), HDL-c, blood pressure, diabetes and smoking. It estimates risk for CAD over a period of 10 years based on Framingham experience in men 30–74 years old at baseline. Pts indicates points.

Table 22.1 Categories of CV Risk

	10-year absolute risk of	
	CAD events (fatal and non-fatal) (Framingham risk score)	CVD death (SCORE)
Low risk	< 10%	< 1%
Inter mediate or moderate	10–20%	≥ 1–< 5%
High risk	> 20%	5–< 10%
Very high risk	–	≥ 10%

absolute risk. This approach involves primary prevention interventions targeting the whole population regardless of each individual's risk and potential benefit, that is, public health programs such as smoking ban, advertising for smoking harms, campaign for physical exercise, or healthy diet. It is widely recognized that prevention at a public health level should start very early in life. Population-based strategies need legislation initiatives, financial incentives, health-promotion campaigns and although the potential gains are substantial, the challenges in implementing such changes are great.

The two primary prevention strategies are considered to be complementary and have been estimated to have contributed equally to the 50% reduction in US mortality due to MI between 1980 and 2000. However, control of classical risk factors remains poor in a large proportion of patients. It is estimated that by consistently implementing proven, effective, inexpensive preventive interventions in both the clinic and the community, a large number (probably >50%) of fatal and non-fatal CAD and CV events could have been prevented in small periods of time. Overall, the most important and cost-efficient interventions in CV prevention

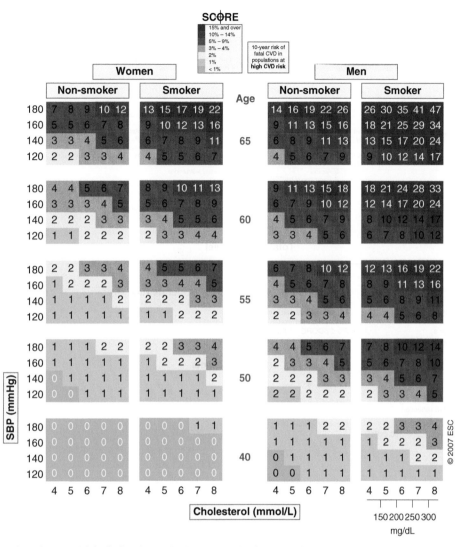

Figure 22.2 SCORE chart of 10-year risk for fatal cardiovascular diseases in high risk regions of Europe by age, gender, SBP, total cholesterol, and smoking status.

appear to be: (*i*) Aspirin for appropriately selected high-risk patients, (*ii*) blood-pressure control, (*iii*) cholesterol management, and (*iv*) smoking cessation. Apart from aspirin, all other three targets need the involvement of physicians but more importantly community-based programs to reduce smoking, improve nutrition, and increase physical activity. Such simple interventions are part of a huge public prevention policy very recently launched in the US (12) aiming to prevent 1 million MIs and strokes over the next 5 years that is estimated to save more than 100,000 lives a year.

GUIDELINES—CURRENT STATUS—EVOLVING TARGETS

Guidelines and expert consensus documents on CAD prevention issued in the last 10 years by several medical societies and organizations worldwide have evaluated and summarized all available evidence with the aim of assisting the optimization of primary and secondary CAD prevention in clinical practice taking into account the impact on outcome, as well as the risk–benefit ratio of specific diagnostic means and therapeutic measures.

Established Major Risk Factors—Interventions
Dyslipidemia

The most recently issued guidelines by ESC/European Atherosclerotic Society (EAS) joint committee on dyslipidemia management for CVD prevention consider lipid profile screening in all adult men ≥40 and in women ≥50 years of age or those who are postmenopausal. In addition, irrespective of age, lipid profiling is indicated in all subjects with evidence of subclinical atherosclerosis in any vascular bed, type 2 diabetes, a family history of premature CVD, arterial hypertension, central obesity, autoimmune

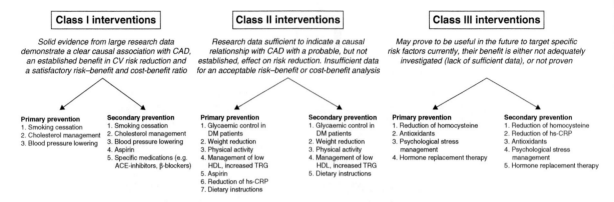

Figure 22.3 Interventions in cardiovascular prevention.

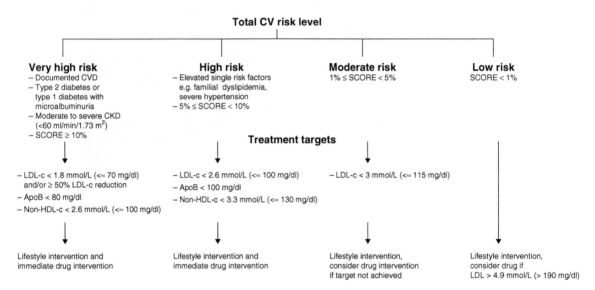

Figure 22.4 Treatment targets for dyslipidemia management based on total cardiovascular risk of patients according to ESC/EAS 2011 guidelines.

chronic inflammatory conditions, CKD, and family history of familial dyslipidemia. LDL-c is the primary lipid target for screening and risk estimation, but HDL-c and triglycerides levels are also considered important for risk stratification. Apolipoprotein B (apoB) and non-HDL-c cholesterol are alternative lipid risk markers especially in combined dyslipidemias, diabetes, metabolic syndrome or CKD. Lipoprotein (a) (Lp(a)) is recommended for screening in selected high-risk subjects with a family history of premature CAD (9).

Based on results from clinical trials, LDL-c remains the primary therapeutic target in dyslipidaemia management. The most recent Cholesterol Treatment Trialists' Collaboration meta-analysis involving >170,000 patients confirmed the dose-dependent reduction in CVD with LDL-c lowering. Every 1.0 mmol/L (≈ 40 mg/dL) reduction in LDL-c is associated with a corresponding 20% reduction in CAD events (13). Secondary treatment targets are apoB and non-HDL-c, while HDL-c is not

considered as a treatment target. The intensity of the preventive intervention is recommended to be modulated according to the level of the total CV risk (Fig. 22.4). Of note, in diabetics without established CVD, the American Diabetes Association (ADA) 2011 position statement for diabetes management (14) suggests that the target LDL-c should be <100 mg/dl, in contrast to the ESC/EAS 2011 guidelines for dyslipidemia management that suggest the more stringent level of <70 mg/dl.

In the management of dyslipidemias, lifestyle modifications should always come first. The most important lifestyle changes currently recommended are: (i) reduced intake of saturated and trans fat, cholesterol and carbohydrates, (ii) increased dietary intake of fibers, foods enriched with phytosterols and soy products, (iii) reduce excessive body weight with concomitant increased habitual physical exercise, and (iv) reduced alcohol intake. However, most patients will ultimately require drug therapy to reach treatment targets. Statins are the first choice for LDL-c reduction while other pharmacological treatment modalities, such as bile acid sequestrants, nicotinic acid, and cholesterol absorption inhibitors should be considered in case of statin intolerance or when target level is not reached. The use of drugs to lower triglycerides should be considered only in subjects with triglycerides >2.3 mmol/L (>200 mg/dL) who cannot lower them by lifestyle measures, and if the subject is at high total CV risk. Fibrates, nicotinic acid, and n-3 fatty acid supplements and their combinations with statins are currently recommended for lowering triglycerides in these patients. It has to be noted that LDL-c control should remain the primary goal in these patients. According to ESC/EAS 2011 guidelines nicotinic acid is considered the most efficient drug to raise HDL-c, while statins and fibrates also raise HDL-c but to a lesser magnitude. To date, no specific targets for HDL-c or triglycerides levels have been determined in clinical trials (9).

Evolving Targets
Recently, a number of promising new drugs have been reported to lower LDL-c effectively in severe or familial forms of hypercholesterolemias and may further help in achieving therapeutic targets. Future studies are needed to clarify the role of HDL-c and triglycerides lowering in reduction of CV risk. Major developments in the search for efficacious agents to raise HDL-c and apolipoprotein A1 will help in defining the benefit of HDL-c lowering on prevention of atherosclerosis and CV events.

Hypertension
Hypertension is clearly associated with an increased risk for all types of CVD, especially for cerebrovascular disease, but also for CAD, heart failure, and CKD. Death from both CAD and stroke increases progressively and linearly from levels as low as 115 mmHg SBP and 75 mmHg DBP upward for all ages between 40 and 89 years (15). Each 2 mmHg rise in SBP is associated with a 7% increase in risk of mortality from CAD (16). Data from the US during 2005–2008 showed that of those with hypertension who were >20 years of age, 79.6% were aware of their condition, 70.9% were under current treatment, but only 47.8% had their hypertension controlled (1).

The most recent guidelines (16–18) on management of hypertension recommend that diagnosis (Focus Box 22.3) and management of hypertension should be related to estimation of global CV risk based on the fact that only a small fraction of the hypertensive population has an elevation of blood pressure alone, with the great majority exhibiting additional CV risk factors. Emphasis has also been given to identification of target organ damage (Focus Box 22.4), since hypertension-related subclinical alterations in several organs indicate progression in the CVD continuum which markedly increases the risk beyond that caused by the simple presence of risk factors. Presence of target organ damage mandates a more aggressive management of hypertension.

On the whole, it is recommended that SBP should be lowered <140 mmHg and DBP <90 mmHg in all hypertensive patients who are at low, moderate or high risk (18). The benefit of lowering SBP <140 mmHg in the elderly hypertensive

---

Focus Box 22.3 Classification of Hypertension Based on Blood Pressure Levels

Optimal	SBP <120 and/or DBP <80 mmHg
Normal	SBP 120–129 and/or DBP 80–84 mmHg
High normal	SBP 130–139 and/or DBP 85–89 mmHg
Grade 1 hypertension	SBP 140–159 and/or DBP 90–99 mmHg
Grade 2 hypertension	SBP 160–179 and/or DBP 100–109 mmHg
Grade 3 hypertension	SBP ≥180 and/or DBP ≥110 mmHg
Isolated systolic hypertension	SBP >140 and DBP <90 mmHg

Grade 1 Hypertension corresponds to stage 1 hypertension of AHA classification.
Grades 2 and 3 hypertension correspond to stage 2 hypertension of AHA classification.

Focus Box 22.4 Target Organ Damage in Hypertension

Electrocardiographic—left ventricular hypertrophy;
echocardiographic—left ventricular hypertrophy (particularly concentric);
vascular ultrasound—carotid wall thickening (IMT >0.9 mm) or plaque;
increased arterial stiffness—carotid femoral pulse wave velocity >12 m/sec;
ankle-brachial index <0.9;
slight increase in serum creatinine: ♂1.3–1.5 mg/dl (115–133 mmol/l);
♀1.2–1.4 mg/dl (107–124 mmol/l);
low estimated glomerular filtration rate <60 ml/min/1.73 m^2 or creatinine clearance <60 ml/min;
microalbuminuria 30–300 mg/24 h
or albumin/creatinine ratio ♂ ≥22 mg/g creatinine, ♀ ≥31 mg/g creatinine

---

patients (i.e. >80 years old) has not been tested extensively in randomized trials and National Institute for Health and Clinical Excellence (NICE) guidelines recommend a target of BP <150/90 mmHg (16). The BP goal traditionally recommended in diabetes and patients with previous CV events (<130/80 mmHg) is not supported by outcome evidence from trials, while it has been very difficult to achieve in the majority of patients. Indeed, there has been some withdrawal from an aggressive BP lowering, based on data of trials that have raised the doubt of an increase (rather than a further reduction) in the incidence of CAD events in patients at high cardiovascular risk treated with regimens that reduced SBP to values close or below 120–125 mmHg and DBP <70–75 mmHg. Besides, it is well known that the additional benefit arising from reducing BP at very low values is rather small (18).

In all grade 1–3 hypertensives, lifestyle instructions should be given as soon as hypertension is diagnosed or suspected, while promptness in the initiation of pharmacological therapy depends

Table 22.2 Management of Blood Pressure According to Total CV Risk

CV risk	Normal BP	High normal BP	Grade 1 Hypertension	Grade 2 Hypertension	Grade 3 Hypertension
Low SCORE <1%	No BP intervention	No BP intervention	Lifestyle changes for several months then drug treatment	Lifestyle changes + immediate drug treatment	Lifestyle changes + immediate drug treatment
Moderate SCORE 1–4%	Lifestyle changes	Lifestyle changes	Lifestyle changes for several weeks then drug treatment	Lifestyle changes + immediate drug treatment	Lifestyle changes + immediate drug treatment
High SCORE 5–10% or target organ damage	Lifestyle changes	Lifestyle changes	Lifestyle changes + immediate drug treatment	Lifestyle changes + immediate drug treatment	Lifestyle changes + immediate drug treatment
Very high SCORE >10% or CVD, diabetes, renal disease	Lifestyle changes	Lifestyle changes + Consider drug treatment	Lifestyle changes + immediate drug treatment	Lifestyle changes + immediate drug treatment	Lifestyle changes + immediate drug treatment

on the level of total cardiovascular risk (Table 22.2). In brief, drug treatment should be initiated immediately in grade 2 and 3 hypertension, as well as in grade 1 when total cardiovascular risk is high or very high (16,18). In grade 1 hypertensives, drug treatment may be delayed for several weeks in those with moderate total cardiovascular risk, and for several months in those with low risk. In patients with high normal BP and high cardiovascular risk, no trial evidence is available for treatment benefits, except for a delayed onset of hypertension (18). In patients with high normal BP and associated very high CV risk, administration of BP lowering drugs should be considered together with intense lifestyle changes (17). However, in diabetic patients at the high normal BP range, initiation of treatment is at present not sufficiently supported by outcome evidence from trials. Drug treatment could be recommended in these patients, particularly when microalbuminuria is present, based on the evidence of its favorable effect on regression and progression of this sign of organ damage (18).

Lifestyle measures widely agreed to lower BP or CV risk, and that should be considered in all patients are: (*i*) smoking cessation, (*ii*) weight reduction in the overweight, (*iii*) moderation of alcohol consumption, (*iv*) physical activity, (*v*) reduction of salt intake, (*vi*) increase in fruit and vegetable intake, and (*vii*) decrease in saturated and total fat intake. Five major classes of antihypertensive agents—thiazide diuretics, calcium antagonists, angiotensin converting enzyme inhibitors (ACE-I), angiotensin receptor antagonists (ARBs) and β-blockers—are suitable for the initiation and maintenance of antihypertensive treatment, alone or in combination. Treatment algorithms based on ESC/European Society of Hypertension (ESH) 2007 and NICE 2011 guidelines are summarized in Figure 22.5. Monotherapy could be the initial treatment in grade 1 hypertensives with a low or moderate total CV risk, but achieves BP target in only a limited number of patients. Use of more than one agent is necessary to achieve target BP in the majority of patients and should be preferred as first step treatment when initial BP is in the grade 2 or 3 range or total CV risk is high or very high. Fixed combinations of two drugs can simplify treatment schedule and favor the compliance of patients (18).

Focus Box 22.5 Preferred Antihypertensive Medications According to Patient's CV Risk Profile and Other Concomitant Conditions

Previous stroke	Any blood pressure lowering agent
Previous myocardial infarction	β-blocker, ACE-I, ARB
Angina pectoris	β-blocker, calcium antagonist
Peripheral artery disease	Calcium antagonist
Asymptomatic atherosclerosis	ACE-I, calcium antagonist
Heart failure	Diuretics, β-blocker, ACE-I, ARB, antialdosterone agents
Left ventricular hypertrophy	ACE-1, calcium antagonists, ARB
Permanent atrial fibrillation	β-blocker, non-dihydropyridine calcium antagonist
Renal failure/proteinuria	ACE-1, ARB, loop diuretics
Renal dysfunction	ACE-1, ARB
Microalbuminuria	ACE-1, ARB
Isolated systoilic hypertension (elderly)	Diuretics, calcium antagonists
Diabetes mellitus	ACE-1, ARB
Metabolic syndrome	ACE-1, ARB, calcium antagonist
Pregnancy	Calcium antagonist, methyldopa, β-blocker
Blacks	Diuretics, calcium antagonists

The main benefits of antihypertensive therapy are due to lowering of BP per se, irrespective of the agent used to achieve this. However, each of the recommended classes may have specific properties and advantages that favor its use in specific conditions shown in Focus Box 22.5.

Evolving Targets

Many important decisions on hypertension management must currently be taken without the support of evidence from large randomized controlled trials. Future studies are needed to clarify whether antihypertensive drugs should be prescribed to (*i*) all patients with grade 1 hypertension, even when total cardiovascular risk is relatively low or moderate because of the very low rate of CV events expected in these patients, (*ii*) the elderly with grade 1 hypertension to achieve a goal of below

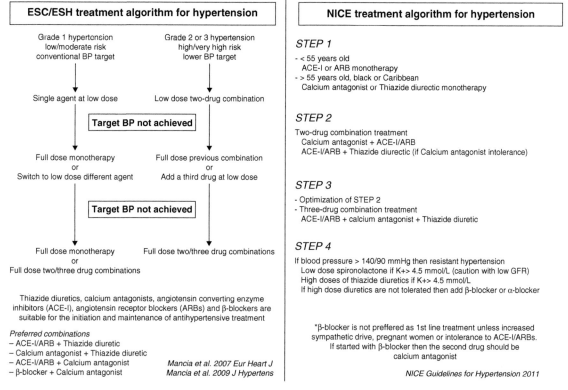

ESC/ESH treatment algorithm for hypertension

Grade 1 hypertension
low/moderate risk
conventional BP target

Grade 2 or 3 hypertension
high/very high risk
lower BP target

Single agent at low dose

Low dose two-drug combination

Target BP not achieved

Full dose monotherapy
or
Switch to low dose different agent

Full dose previous combination
or
Add a third drug at low dose

Target BP not achieved

Full dose monotherapy
or
Full dose two/three drug combinations

Full dose two/three drug combinations

Thiazide diuretics, calcium antagonists, angiotensin converting enzyme inhibitors (ACE-I), angiotensin receptor blockers (ARBs) and β-blockers are suitable for the initiation and maintenance of antihypertensive treatment

Preferred combinations
– ACE-I/ARB + Thiazide diuretic
– Calcium antagonist + Thiazide diuretic
– ACE-I/ARB + Calcium antagonist
– β-blocker + Calcium antagonist

Mancia et al. 2007 Eur Heart J
Mancia et al. 2009 J Hypertens

NICE treatment algorithm for hypertension

STEP 1

- < 55 years old
   ACE-I or ARB monotherapy
- > 55 years old, black or Caribbean
   Calcium antagonist or Thiazide diurectic monotherapy

STEP 2

Two-drug combination treatment
   Calcium antagonist + ACE-I/ARB
   ACE-I/ARB + Thiazide diurectic (if Calcium antagonist intolerance)

STEP 3

- Optimization of STEP 2
- Three-drug combination treatment
   ACE-I/ARB + calcium antagonist + Thiazide diuretic

STEP 4

If blood pressure > 140/90 mmHg then resistant hypertension
   Low dose spironolactone if K+> 4.5 mmol/L (caution with low GFR)
   High doses of thiazide diuretics if K+> 4.5 mmol/L
   If high dose diuretics are not tolerated then add β-blocker or α-blocker

*β-blocker is not preffered as 1st line treatment unless increased sympathetic drive, pregnant women or intolerance to ACE-I/ARBs. If started with β-blocker then the second drug should be calcium antagonist

NICE Guidelines for Hypertension 2011

Figure 22.5 Treatment algorithms of hypertension according to ESC/ESH 2007 (updated 2009) and NICE 2011 guidelines.

140/90 mmHg, and (*iii*) diabetic patients or patients with previous CVD when BP is still in the high normal level. Furthermore, the lowest safe BP target values should be defined in different clinical conditions, that is, should BP goal be below 130/80 mmHg in very high risk patients? Finally, there are no randomized trials to prove the effectiveness of various lifestyle measures known to reduce BP in reducing also morbidity and mortality.

Management of DM

CVD is the major cause of morbidity and mortality for patients with DM, and the largest contributor to the direct and indirect costs of DM. DM itself confers an important independent risk for CVD even after adjustment for the coexisting common CV risk factors (14). CVD risk for patients with overt DM is considered to be increased by 2–3 times for men and 3–5 times for women compared to subjects without DM, although more recent data suggest that this risk is probably lower than believed 10 years earlier (1). The relationship between hyperglycemia and CVD should be seen as a continuum, that is, for each 1% increase of glycated hemoglobin (HbA1c), there is a defined increased risk for CVD. DM is currently diagnosed based on specific criteria (Focus Box 22.6) defined by the relation to its microvascular complications.

Focus Box 22.6 Criteria Used for Glucometabolic Classification According to the ADA (2011) (14)

Increased risk for diabetes – Prediabetes
impaired fasting glucose:
fasting plasma glucose 100–125 mg/dl (5.6–6.9 mmol/l)

or

Impaired glucose tolerance: 2-h plasma glucose in the 75-g oral glucose tolerance test 140–199 mg/dl (7.8–11.0 mmol/l)

or

glycated hemoglobin - HbA1c 5.7–6.4%

Diabetes
glycated hemoglobin - HbA1c ≥ 6.5 %

or

fasting plasma glucose ≥ 126 mg/dl (7.0 mmol/l)

or

2-h plasma glucose in the 75-g oral glucose tolerance test ≥ 200 mg/dl (11.1 mmol/l)

or

In a patient with classic symptoms of hyperglycemia or hyperglycemic crisis, a random plasma glucose ≥ 200 mg/dl (11.1 mmol/l)

However, macrovascular diseases such as CAD and stroke are the major causes of death in type 2 DM patients and subjects with impaired glucose tolerance (14).

Recent guidelines for CVD management in DM are based on the premise that most DM patients are at high risk for future CVD events even in the absence of established CVD. Numerous studies have shown large benefits in preventing or slowing CVD when multiple risk factors are addressed globally in DM patients (14). For primary and secondary CV risk reduction in DM, providers should follow the evidence-based recommendations for blood pressure and dyslipidemia treatment as discussed above.

The major focus of lifestyle interventions should be on improving glycemic control and controlling other major CV risk factors. Weight control remains an important component of lifestyle management. Reeducation of the patient about food selection (regulation of calories and fat intake), smoking cessation, and regular physical activity may be the most successful approach to improve long-term outcomes (19).

The recommended goals for glycemic control in DM patients are shown in Focus Box 22.7. The risk of microvascular complications (retinopathy, nephropathy and neuropathy) can be reduced by intensive glycemic control in patients with types 1 and 2 DM and the relationship between glucose control and risk of complications was extended down to the normal HbA1c range (<6%) with no threshold noted. Despite reports on the link between microvascular and macrovascular complications in DM, intensive versus standard glycaemic control has not shown a significant reduction in macrovascular CVD outcomes in either type 1 or 2 DM (19). In type 1 DM, the gold standard of glycemic control is intensified insulin therapy. In type 2 DM, a common pharmacologic treatment approach is less well-accepted; detailed instructions and treatment algorithms may be found elsewhere (14) but are beyond the scope of this text. In brief, early, stepwise increase of therapy towards pre-defined treatment targets has been shown to improve a composite of morbidity and mortality in type 2 DM. Metformin is recommended as first line drug in overweight type 2 diabetics. Early initiation of insulin should be considered in type 2 DM patients with failing glucose target, and in patients with excessive post-prandial glucose excursions.

Evolving Targets

Despite successful implementation of evidence-based strategies, many DM patients are not properly identified before their first event or continue to experience CV events despite optimal management. Although the proportion of DM patients achieving recommended levels of HbA1c, blood pressure, and LDL cholesterol has steadily improved in the last 10 years, disappointingly only a minority of patients ($\approx$12%) achieve the desirable targets to reduce global CV risk during long-term follow-up. Optimal management of DM requires an organized, systematic approach and involvement of a coordinated multi-disciplinary team of dedicated health care professionals. Future studies are needed to clarify the

---

Focus Box 22.7 Treatment Goals in Glycemic Control in Diabetic Patients

- Lowering glycated hemoglobin <7% can reduce microvascular and neuropathic complications of types 1 and 2 DM and is currently considered the reasonable general goal
- Even lower HbA1c goals (<6.0–6.5%), provided that this can be achieved without significant hypoglycemia or other adverse effects of treatment, might be reasonably suggested for selected patients with
  - short duration of diabetes
  - long life expectancy
  - no significant CV disease
- Less stringent glycated hemoglobin goals than the general goal of <7% may be appropriate for selected patients in whom the general goal is difficult to attain, such as those with
  - history of severe hypoglycemia
  - limited life expectancy
  - advanced microvascular or macrovascular complications
  - extensive comorbid conditions or
  - long-standing diabetes

---

safety and efficacy of antidiabetic medications on CV prognosis in the shadow of the concerns about the CV effects of thiazolidinediones.

Smoking

Despite a substantial reduction in smoking rates in the last 60 years, smoking appears to be an important risk factor for both males and females. Smoking is second only to dyslipidemia as a risk factor for MI (8) and the 10-year fatal CV risk is approximately doubled for smokers for any given age, systolic blood pressure, and cholesterol level. Smoking-associated CV risk is greater for females than males and appears to be greatest among younger smokers. A strong dose-response relationship between duration/extent of smoking and CAD death rate has been observed. Exposure to environmental tobacco smoke is also a significant CV risk factor (2,20).

Smoking cessation should be a priority in primary and secondary CV prevention. In CAD patients, smoking cessation reduces mortality by 36% and re-infarction by 32% compared with continuing smoking. In secondary prevention, mortality from CAD is reduced more via smoking cessation than by other preventive therapies such as aspirin, β-blockers, ACE-I, or cholesterol lowering drugs. In primary prevention, smoking cessation therapy has been proposed to be the most cost-effective intervention, followed by aspirin and hypertensives, while statin is still the least cost-effective treatment option. Stopping smoking leads to a quicker reduction in the risk of subsequent CAD events in patients with established CAD than in asymptomatic individuals; in CAD patients the risk falls within 2–3 years to the level of those CAD patients who never smoked, whereas in asymptomatic individuals up to 10 years are needed to reach the risk level of never-smokers (2).

Smoking and the subsequent nicotine addiction should be viewed as a chronic, relapsing medical condition which, like other major CV risk factors, requires treatment, close follow-up, and repeated assessment and intervention. Systematic approaches to the identification and treatment of smokers, can dramatically enhance the likelihood of cessation. It is strongly recommended that identification of smoking status and provision of cessation assistance should be provided in every professional setting. There are currently three first-line classes of pharmacotherapy for smoking cessation: nicotine-replacement therapy, bupropion, and varenicline, while nor-triptyline and clonidine are second-line choices. The safety and efficacy of these pharmacotherapies in CV patients has been demonstrated in several studies. Their effectiveness is further accentuated when accompanied by strategic and practical counselling concerning the settings, circumstances and difficulties commonly associated with smoking cessation as well as the advantages of ensuring support from family and friends. For smokers hospitalized with an acute CAD event, smoking cessation interventions should commence during hospitalization since they appear to be more effective than those initiated thereafter (2,20).

Evolving Targets

Despite the known health risks of smoking and the desire of smokers to stop, quit rates are very low. Smoking is not recognized as a medical condition, but rather as a "lifestyle choice" by patients; surveys have shown that physicians offer advice on smoking cessation in <50% of all consultations. Preventing smoking and increasing cessation rates need to remain priorities of all public health professionals. Innovative approaches for the follow-up and management of patients engaged in smoking-cessation attempts include structured primary care programs, community cessation resources (e.g. quitlines), and ongoing follow-up using sophisticated telephone techniques. Comprehensive public health tobacco-control programs that include smoking ban in public places, reduction of smoking advertisements, increasing the real price of tobacco products, and increasing health insurance coverage for effective cessation interventions could be implemented at a wider scale. In secondary prevention, encouraging physicians to invest time and effort in patient's counseling and wider implementation of nurse-led programs for in-hospital counseling as part of cardiac rehabilitation soon after the event, could be useful.

Other (Potentially) Modifiable Risk Factors—Interventions
Aspirin—Acetyl Salicylic Acid (ASA)
Low-dose aspirin (75–162 mg/day), as anti-platelet therapy is still the drug of choice in both primary and secondary prevention of CV events and despite its very long-term use, ASA is considered to be a highly cost-efficient intervention. For all patients with an acute coronary syndrome who survive to hospital discharge or patients with chronic stable CAD, indefinite treatment with low-dose ASA is recommended unless contraindications exist (2,21). After percutaneous coronary intervention with stent placement or the first year following an acute coronary syndrome, specific recommendations on double anti-platelet therapy apply (presented in the following chapters). In case of allergies or intolerance to ASA, other anti-platelet agents such as clopidogrel may be used at greater cost.

The benefits of ASA therapy in primary prevention depend substantially on an individual's risk of CVD and of adverse treatment effects (most often are gastrointestinal bleed and hemorrhagic stroke). ASA has been shown to reduce the risk for a MI by 30% in healthy men but not in women. In contrast, in healthy women, a beneficial 17% decrease in risk for stroke has been reported with ASA use. The underlying biological reasons for differences in the aspirin effect between the two genders are not well understood. ESC and AHA guidelines recommend the use of low-dose ASA in asymptomatic high-risk individuals with low bleeding risk provided that blood pressure is well controlled (Table 22.3) (2,22). The US Preventive Services Task Force (23) in 2009 has issued more detailed guidelines on the use of ASA in primary prevention. Decision on ASA use lies on 3 important factors: gender, age and estimated CV risk (Table 22.3). Most recently issued guidelines from ADA/ACC/AHA recommend also low-dose ASA for primary CV prevention in adults with DM who are at high or intermediate CV risk after assessment of their Framingham risk score (Table 22.3) (19).

Evolving Targets

Further investigation is needed to clarify the effectiveness of aspirin use in primary prevention of CAD especially in certain subgroups of patients such as diabetics at intermediate risk and older people (i.e. >80 years old).

Specific Medications in Secondary Prevention
β-Blockers
A number of trials have demonstrated the long-term efficacy of β-blockers following MI in reducing by 20–25% all-cause and CV mortality as well as non-fatal reinfarction. It is currently recommended that β-blockers should be started and continued indefinitely in all patients who have had MI, acute coronary syndrome or left ventricular dysfunction with or without heart failure unless contraindicated. β-blockers should be also considered for chronic therapy in patients with stable CAD (24,25).

ACE-I–ARBs
Several trials have established that ACE-I improve CV outcome in patients with CAD, especially in those with impaired left ventricular function. It is strongly recommended that ACE-I should be started and continued indefinitely in all patients after MI or acute coronary syndrome with left ventricular ejection fraction ≤40% and in patients with heart failure, DM, hypertension, or CKD, unless contraindicated. ACE-I may also be considered for all other post-MI patients to prevent recurrence of ischemic events, with preference given to agents and doses of

Table 22.3 Recommendations on the Use of Low-dose Aspirin in Primary Cardiovascular Prevention

ESC 2007 and AHA 2002 guidelines	USPTF 2009 guidelines	ADA/ACC/AHA 2011 guidelines in DM patients
ASA is recommended for prevention of coronary events in those patients whose risk is sufficiently high for the benefits to outweigh the risks associated with treatment *i.e. Framingham risk score for CHD > 10% or SCORE >10%* and provided that blood pressure is well controlled	ASA is recommended <ul><li>for men aged 45–79 years when the potential benefit due to a reduction in myocardial infarction outweighs the potential harm due to an increase in gastrointestinal hemorrhage</li><li>for women aged 55–79 years when the potential benefit due to a reduction in stroke outweighs the potential harm due to an increase in gastrointestinal hemorrhage</li></ul> ASA use is NOT recommended for stroke prevention in women <55 years and for myocardial infarction prevention in men <45 years Current evidence is insufficient to assess the balance of benefits and harms of ASA for cardiovascular disease prevention in men and women ≥80 years	ASA is recommended in diabetic patients who are not at increased risk for bleeding and are: <ul><li>at increased CV risk</li></ul> *Most men >50 years and women >60 years who have additionally ≥1 of the following risk factors: smoking, hypertension, dyslipidemia, family history of premature CVD, and albuminuria.or* <ul><li>at intermediate CV risk until further research is available</li></ul> *Younger patients with ≥1 risk factors, or older patients with no risk factors, or patients with 10-year Framingham CV risk 5–10%.* Aspirin should NOT be recommended for adults with diabetes at low CV risk (*men <50 years and women <60 years with no major additional CV risk factors; 10-year Framingham CV risk <5%*) as the potential adverse effects from bleeding offset the potential benefits

proven efficacy. In patients with ACE-I intolerance, an ARB is an established alternative with preference given to agents and doses of proven efficacy (24,25).

Aldosterone Blockers
Aldosterone antagonists, namely eplerenone, have been shown to reduce CV mortality after MI in patients with reduced left ventricular function even in only mildly symptomatic patients. Therefore, aldosterone antagonists are recommended to be used in patients after MI who are already being treated with ACE-I and β-blockers and who have a left ventricular ejection fraction ≤35–40% and either DM or heart failure but without significant renal dysfunction (i.e. serum creatinine >221 µmol/L (>2.5 mg/ dL) and >177 µmol/L (>2.0 mg/dL) for men and women respectively) or hyperkalemia (serum potassium >5.0 mEq/L). Routine monitoring of serum potassium is warranted and should be particularly careful when other potential potassium-sparing agents are used (24,25).

Seasonal influenza represents a major preventable threat to the health of CVD patients. Vaccination against influenza is associated with significantly reduced risk of CV death and nonfatal events and is thus recommended as a component of secondary prevention for patients with CAD and other atherosclerotic vascular conditions unless they have a contraindication to the vaccine. Vaccination is also currently recommended for persons with DM (21).

Evolving Targets
Many patients remain undertreated for CAD despite the known benefits of medical secondary prevention strategies; this refers particularly to females. Barriers to optimizing management are usually multifactorial and related to several patient, physician, and health system determinants. The implementation of multidisciplinary management programs may improve medication compliance, reduce hospitalizations, and improve quality of life in patients with CAD. Further research, ideally in a randomized trial setting, should be conducted to study the effects of such an approach on CAD management and clinical outcomes.

Diet and Nutrition
Improving diet is a critical component of primary and secondary CV prevention strategies. Although the vast majority of research studies have focused on individual nutrients and foods, it is well recognized that multiple dietary factors (dietary patterns or diets) influence major CV risk factors and the risk of developing CVD. The two main goals of a dietary intervention should be a change toward healthier nutritional components and a balance between energy intake and expenditure to achieve bodyweight goals (Focus Box 22.8). In general, it is recommended that fat should be reduced to <30–35% of the total energy intake, while proteins and carbohydrates to 10–35% and 45–65%, respectively. Daily sodium intake should be reduced to <2.3 g (≈ 1 teaspoon of salt); further reductions to 1.5 g are considered for persons ≥51 years, or irrespective of age if they are African-American or have hypertension, DM, or CKD. Several diets such as the Dietary Approaches to Stop Hypertension (DASH) or the Mediterranean diet, have been proven beneficial in reducing specific risk factors (e.g. DASH for hypertension) or even CAD risk (Table 22.4) (2,26–28).

Alcohol Intake
Moderate alcohol intake (wine but also other alcoholic beverages) has been associated with reduced CV events although its overall (although protective) contribution to CV risk is rather small (8). On the other hand, alcohol can be addictive, and high intake can be associated with serious adverse health and social consequences, including hypertriglyceridemia,

Table 22.4 Recommended Dietary Patterns According to Underlying Risk Factors

Diabetes (AHA/ACC 2007)	Dyslipidemia (ESC/EAS 2011)	Hypertension – DASH eating plan (NIH/NHLBI)	Mediterranean diet (Basic components)
• Total fat: 25–35% of total calories (mainly of MUFAs and PUFAs)	• Total fat 25–35% of total calories (mainly of MUFAs and PUFAs)	• Total fat 27% and saturated fat 6% of calories	• Plant-based foods (e.g., fruits, vegetables, breads, cereals, potatoes, legumes, nuts)
• Saturated fats <7% of energy intake, cholesterol <200 mg/d, *trans*-unsaturated fatty acids <1% of energy intake[a]	• Saturated fat <7% of energy intake, cholesterol ideally <300 mg/day, trans fats <1% of energy intake	• Cholesterol 150 mg • Dietary fiber 30 g/d • Carbohydrate 55% of calories • Protein 18% of calories	• Locally grown, minimally processed food • Fish and poultry (at least twice a week)
• Ample fiber >14 g/1000 calories consumed	• Dietary fibers 25–40 g including >7–13 g soluble fibers	• Daily sodium 2.3 g (or 1.5 g)	• Infrequent red meat intake (once a week)
• If individuals choose to drink alcohol, this should be limited to 1 drink/daily for women and 2 drinks/daily for men.	• Carbohydrate 45–55% of total energy	• Increase potassium[c] to 4.7 g/day	• Up to four whole eggs per week • Moderate amount of dairy products
• Reduce sodium intake to 2.3 g/d (or even 1.5 g/d)	• Added sugars[b] <10% of total energy	• Calcium 1.25 g, Magnesium 0.5 g	• Olive oil as the principal source of fat • Moderate amount of red wine with meals • Desserts primarily of fresh fruits

[a]Limited consumption of foods made with processed sources of trans fats, such as partially hydrogenated oils, and by limiting other solid fats, provides the most effective means of reducing.
[b]Not those found in sugars present in natural foods such as fruit and dairy products; more restrictive advice concerning sugars may be useful for those who need to lose weight or have with high triglycerides.
[c]Patients with stage 3 or 4 chronic kidney disease should restrict their intake of potassium.

Focus Box 22.8 Diet Recommendations for CVD Risk Reduction

- Balance calorie intake and physical activity to achieve/maintain a healthy body weight
- Consume a diet rich in vegetables and fruits
- Choose whole-grain, high-fiber foods
- Choose a variety of protein foods (seafood, lean meat and poultry, eggs, beans and peas, soy products, and unsalted nuts and seeds)
- Consume fish, especially oily fish, at least twice a week
- Limit your intake of saturated fat to <7% of energy, trans fat to <1% of energy, and cholesterol to <300 mg per day by
  - choosing lean meats and vegetable alternatives
  - selecting fat-free, 1%-fat, and low-fat dairy products
  - minimizing intake of partially hydrogenated fats
- Minimize your intake of beverages and foods with added sugars
- Prepare foods with little or no salt
- If you consume alcohol, do so in moderation

hypertension, obesity, liver damage, physical abuse, vehicular and work accidents, and increased risk of cancer. For these reasons, it is not recommended that nondrinkers should start consuming alcohol solely for CVD prevention but if alcoholic beverages are consumed, these should be limited to ≤2 drinks/day for men and ≤1 drink/day for women, and ideally during meals. Individuals who choose to consume alcoholic beverages should also be aware that alcohol has a high caloric density (21,28).

Antioxidant Supplements

Antioxidant vitamin supplements to prevent CVD are not recommended. Although observational studies have suggested that high intakes of antioxidant vitamins from food and supplements are associated with a lower CVD risk, clinical trials of antioxidant vitamin supplementation have not confirmed this (27).

Plant Stanols/Sterols

Plant stanols/sterols lower LDL-c levels by up to 15% and therefore are seen as a therapeutic option, in addition to diet and lifestyle modification, for individuals with elevated LDL-c levels. To sustain LDL-c reductions from these products, individuals need to consume them daily, just as they would use lipid-lowering medications (27).

Fish Oil Supplements

Fish intake has been associated with decreased risk of CVD. Patients without documented CAD are encouraged to eat a variety of fish, preferably oily fish, at least twice a week. Patients with CAD are advised to consume >1 g of omega-3 polyunsaturated fatty acids (PUFAs) daily, preferably from oily fish, although supplements could be considered. For hypertriglyceridemia, 2–4 g of omega-3 PUFAs daily are recommended (9,27).

Soy Protein

Although earlier research has suggested that soy protein has clinically important favorable effects on LDL-c levels and other CV risk factors, more recent studies have not confirmed those results. Nevertheless, consumption of soy protein-rich foods may indirectly reduce CV risk if these replace animal and dairy products containing saturated fat and cholesterol (27).

Focus Box 22.9 Physical activity Recommendations for Adults Aged 18–65 yr

- Moderate-intensity aerobic activity ≥30 min (preferably 45–60 min) at least 5 days/week or vigorous-intensity aerobic activity ≥20 min for 3 days/week (in addition to any light intensity activities performed during daily life)
- Activities that maintain/increase muscular strength and endurance ≥2 days/week - 8–10 exercises (8–12 repetitions) using major muscle groups
- Participation in physical activities above minimum recommendations provides additional health benefits and results in higher levels of physical fitness
- Adults >65 years, or those with disabilities: follow recommendations if possible or be as physically active as possible
- High-risk CAD patients (e.g. recent acute coronary syndrome or revascularization, heart failure): medically supervised programs
- Previously obese people: 60–90 min activity daily to maintain weight loss
- Hypertensive patients: avoid intensive isometric exercise, for example, heavy weight lifting (marked pressor effect). If hypertension is poorly controlled, heavy physical exercise should be discouraged or postponed until appropriate drug treatment has been instituted and blood pressure lowered

Focus Box 22.10 Classification of Disease Risk by Body Mass Index (BMI) and Waist Circumference (WC)

Classification	BMI (kg/m^2)	♂ WC 94–102 cm ♀ WC 80–88 cm	♂ WC > 102 cm ♀ WC > 88 cm
Overweight	25.0–29.9	Increased	High
Obese			
Mild – Class I	30.0–34.9	High	Very High
Moderate – Class II	35.0–39.9	Very High	Very High
Extreme – Class III	≥ 40.0	Extremely high	Extremely high

Disease risk for type 2 diabetes, hypertension, and cardiovascular disease relative to normal weight and waist circumference.

Increased WC can also be a marker for increased risk even in subjects with normal weight.

Evolving Targets

Recent studies suggest that focusing on formulating nutrient-dense diets provides a greater CV benefit than attempting to consume nutrient-based foods. The current challenge to healthcare providers but also government officials is to develop and implement effective clinical and public health strategies that may lead to sustained lifestyle and diet changes among individuals and among populations. Meeting this goal will require comprehensive and coordinated approaches that engage every level of the society and reshape the environment so that the healthy choices are the easy, accessible and desirable choices for all. Legislative initiatives are needed, for example, to reduce sodium content in processed foods especially in public places and importantly schools, to replace artificial trans fat with heart-healthy oils, to establish listing of trans fat content on food labels and menu-labeling in restaurants so that people make more informed choices.

Physical Activity

Physical inactivity is a significant public health problem in western countries and a strong predictor of CV mortality independent of other risk factors. A sedentary lifestyle is associated with a doubling of risk of premature death and an increased CV risk. Longitudinal studies report a graded, inverse association of physical activity level and duration with incident CAD. Avoiding a sedentary lifestyle during adulthood may extend life expectancy and CVD-free life expectancy by about 1.3–3.5

years (1,2). Regular exercise has been shown to improve blood glucose control and insulin resistance, reduce triglycerides and increase HDL-c (probably without an effect on LDL-c), reduce blood pressure, body weight, body fat and waist circumference, and improve well-being (2,9,14,17,29). The recommendations for engagement in various physical activities are essentially the same in primary and secondary CV prevention (Focus Box 22.9) (2,9,14,17,30,31). Physical activity counseling and exercise training are central components of cardiac rehabilitation as a part of secondary prevention strategies; many of the risk factor improvements required in the rehabilitation process are mediated through exercise training (31).

Evolving Targets

For all health professionals, the challenge is to enroll increasing numbers of participants in physical activity programs that are designed to sustain long-term adherence. Using effective behavioral management and environmental change strategies, many more individuals will realize the benefits provided by a physically active lifestyle.

Obesity and Weight Reduction

Obesity is a growing epidemic worldwide; nearly 70% of adults in western countries are classified as overweight or obese. In adults, overweight is defined by an increased body mass index (BMI) 25–29.9 kg/m^2 and obesity by BMI ≥30 kg/m^2. Obesity is recognized as a major risk factor for CVD while it has been also related to increased incidence of established CV risk factors such as type 2 DM, hypertension, dyslipidemia and the metabolic syndrome. Whether the increased CV risk attributed to obesity may be related to the clustering of these risk factors or is an independent effect of obesity per se is not clear. Waist circumference, a measure of central obesity, in addition to BMI gives additional information for CV risk estimation (Focus Box 22.10). Waist-to-hip ratio may also be a useful predictor of DM and CV risk, but is more difficult to measure than waist circumference (32,33).

Interventions should be implemented in patients with BMI >25 kg/m^2 but weight loss targets and intervention strategies should be realistic and individualized to the patient's associated co-morbidities. In patients with BMI 25–35 kg/m^2, obesity-related co-morbidities are less likely to be present and a 5–10% weight loss (about 5–10 kg) is required for CV and metabolic risk reduction. In patients with BMI>35 kg/m^2, obesity-related co-morbidities are more likely and thus weight loss interventions should be targeted to >15–20% weight loss (always >10 kg) (33).

It is generally recommended to implement a combined diet, physical activity/exercise, and behavioral program designed to reduce total caloric intake, maintain appropriate intake of nutrients and fiber, and increase energy expenditure. Daily energy deficit should be tailored to approximately 500–1000 kcal/day to achieve weight goals. Low and very low calorie diets (1000–1600 and < 1000 kcal/day, respectively) may also be considered for people who are obese and have reached a plateau in weight loss but are less likely to be nutritionally complete. Adults should be encouraged to increase their physical activity, as described previously in detail, because of the other health benefits (reduced risk of DM and CVD) (32). Drug treatment for weight reduction (orlistat, rimonabant) has shown modest results and some products may have serious side effects. Drug therapy should be considered as an adjunct to lifestyle interventions for weight loss in patients with BMI ≥28 kg/m^2 (and comorbidities) or BMI ≥30 kg/m^2 and always on an individual case basis following assessment of risk and benefit (2,33).

Despite the established positive association of obesity with increased CV risk in primary prevention, a paradoxical improved prognosis in obese patients with known CAD, post coronary angioplasty, heart failure or multiple risk factors, compared to lean patients has been repeatedly described (as obesity paradox), leading to doubt upon deciding for weight loss strategies in secondary prevention (34). However, these observations have not been validated in prospective randomized trials and are not included in any guideline or position statement document issued so far.

Metabolic Syndrome

The metabolic syndrome describes the clustering of CV risk factors (Focus Box 22.11) in individuals with obesity or insulin resistance with a prevalence of 35–40% in US adults. These individuals are at increased CV risk in accordance with the clustering of risk factors but it is not clear whether metabolic syndrome may be related to an increased CV risk over and above the effects of associated risk factors (35). The diagnosis of metabolic syndrome is of greatest importance in non-diabetic subjects as an indicator of increased risk of type 2 DM and CVD. The main emphasis in the management of metabolic syndrome patients should be given in efforts to reduce weight and increase physical activity while the recommendations for management of risk factors and aspirin administration should follow corresponding guidelines according to the individual's level of risk (2,36).

Evolving Targets

There are currently no prospective studies demonstrating that intentional weight loss may increase survival and decrease CV hard outcomes (i.e. CVD non-fatal and fatal events). Further research is needed to evaluate the efficacy and safety of obesity treatments (lifestyle interventions, drugs or even bariatric surgery) and their impact on CV prognosis in various populations and especially in secondary CV prevention. Identification of optimal biomarkers and genetic determinants that would predict which of the obese individuals are at highest risk is also important.

Inflammation—Reduction of High-Sensitivity C-Reactive Protein

CRP is the most intensively studied inflammatory biomarker associated with CV risk. A meta-analysis of 22 studies performed recently by the US Preventive Services Task Force showed that CRP concentrations >3.0 mg/dl were associated with roughly 60% excess risk of incident CAD (37). However, despite the robust statistical association between CRP and CV events, evidence from multiple studies indicates that CRP measurements provide only modest improvements in predictive accuracy on top of traditional risk factors (37). It is currently recommended that CRP measurement may be reasonable for CV risk assessment in asymptomatic intermediate-risk men ≤50 years or women ≤60 years of age, but not in low- or high-risk subjects (4). Furthermore, a recent clinical trial in primary prevention (JUPITER) (38) showed that statin use was associated with a significant reduction in CV events in low or moderate risk non-diabetic subjects with LDL-c <130 mg/dl and CRP >2 mg/dl. Despite the criticism that the trial was not designed to assess the use of CRP to identify candidates for statin therapy, the most recent guidelines for primary CV prevention in asymptomatic adults recommend the measurement of CRP to decide upon statin use in selected populations (4).

Evolving Targets

The JUPITER trial left a number of questions unanswered about the use of CRP levels in CV risk assessment. Future studies are needed to clarify the effects of statins in subjects with low CRP as well as to assess whether a CRP-based strategy may be efficient and cost-effective for primary CV prevention.

Homocysteine Lowering

Homocysteine is an amino acid derived from normal methionine metabolism in the liver. It is widely accepted that increased plasma homocysteine is associated with increased CV risk, independently of other risk factors. Although single studies have previously reported an increased risk for CAD up to a 25–30% for each 5 μmol/l increase in homocysteine levels (39), a recent meta-analysis from the US Preventive Services Task Force has demonstrated a much smaller effect (approximately 9% increase) (37). Therefore, measurement of plasma homocysteine are not currently recommended in the evaluation of CV risk at least in low- or intermediate-risk populations (37). Treatment with folate alone or in combination with other

Focus Box 22.11 The New Definition of Metabolic Syndrome (IDF/AHA/NHLBI 2009) (36)

≥3 of the following 5 criteria	
Increased waist circumference	♂ ≥ 94 cm and ♀ ≥ 80 cm
Increased triglycerides (or drug treatment for increased triglycerides)	≥ 150 mg/dL (1.7 mmol/L)
Decreased HDL-c (or drug treatment for decreased HDL-c)	♂ ≥ 40 mg/dL (1.0 mmol/L) and ♀ ≥ 50 mg/dL (1.3 mmol/L)
Increased blood pressure (or drug treatment in patient with a history of hypertension)	Systolic ≥ 130 and/or diastolic ≥ 85 mm Hg
Increased fasting glucose (or drug for increased glucose)	≥ 100 mg/dL

Focus Box 22.12 Psychosocial Risk Factors with or Without Established Prognostic Role in CVD

Established risk factors
  Social isolation
  Lack of quality social support
  Depression
  Low socioeconomic status
  Catastrophic life events of a highly stressful nature (e.g. earthquake, terrorist attacks)

Non- established risk factors
  Work stress
  Family stress
  Anxiety or panic attacks
  Type A personality
  Hostility

B-vitamins has been shown to reduce homocysteine levels but without any established beneficial effect in primary or secondary CV prevention (37,40).

Evolving Targets
As most of the clinical trials on the CV effects of homocysteine-lowering therapies have included patients regardless of homocysteine levels, future studies are needed to clarify whether such treatment would be beneficial for patients with elevated homocysteine, at what level it would be appropriate to start treatment, the appropriate treatment target and the most effective means to reduce homocysteine (diet vs supplements).

Management of Psychosocial Factors/Stress
Psychosocial factors are increasingly recognized as independent determinants of CV health. The INTERHEART study reported that psychosocial stress accounted for approximately 30% of the attributable risk of acute MI. In addition to increasing risk of CV events and worsening prognosis in CAD, these factors may act as barriers to treatment adherence and efforts to improve lifestyle (2,8,41). Psychosocial risk factors that have been shown to influence CV risk and prognosis are shown in Focus Box 22.12. It has become clear that psychosocial risk factors do not occur in isolation from one another, but tend to cluster in individuals and patient groups. In patients at high risk or with established CVD, multimodal, behavioral intervention involving counseling for psychosocial risk factors and coping with stress and illness should be considered, while patients with clinically significant emotional distress should be referred to a specialist. Cognitive behavioral strategies to reduce or manage stress and clinical approaches to help people change behavior and lifestyle have not consistently shown benefits in terms of reducing CV risk and improving prognosis in primary or secondary CV prevention (2,42,43).

Evolving Targets
Future research is needed to clarify the effects of behavioral interventions as well as drug therapy for psychosocial factors in CV prognosis especially in secondary prevention strategies. It is important to develop and implement simple and user-friendly clinical models that may help apply psychosocial screening and treatment to appropriate patients in clinical cardiology practice.

Menopause - Hormone Replacement Therapy
The majority of CVD in women occurs during the menopause, or after age 55, suggesting that menopause and the subsequent loss of endogenous estrogen may be causally related to an increased risk for CAD. The role of female sex hormones on CVD has been debated for decades. Early and more recent observational studies showed that hormone replacement therapy (HRT) reduced the risk for CV events by 30–50%. However, randomized trials of HRT published in the last 10–15 years showed overall no benefit for HRT in the primary or secondary prevention of CAD (44). Consequently, the latest guidelines for CV prevention in women do not recommend initiation of HRT for CV prevention in menopause (5,45). HRT is currently approved for the management of menopausal symptoms and osteoporosis but is recommended to be taken at the lowest effective dose and for the shortest period of time (44).

Evolving Targets
Most of the randomized trials of HRT involved women at high CV risk (primary prevention) or established CVD, conditions that favor the prothrombotic and proinflammatory effects of HRT. There is evidence mainly from observational studies and subgroup analyzes of large randomized studies that younger perimenopausal/menopausal (50–59 years old) early after menopause (<10 years in menopause) may have CV benefits from HRT use. Future studies are needed to clarify the effects of HRT on primary CV prevention in early menopausal women at low or moderate risk.

Genetic Factors

It has been suggested that the implementation of genetic information (multiple common genetic variants) may have a predictive value beyond measures of risk factors in CV risk assessment of an individual. The first widely replicated genetic variant for CAD was recently discovered by a genome-wide association study on chromosome 9p21.3; risk increases by 1.3–2.0 times for individual single nucleotide polymorphisms (SNPs) (46). However, given the small incremental risk information of the individual polymorphisms, genotype testing for CAD risk assessment in asymptomatic adults is not currently recommended since it offers no proven benefit in risk assessment when added to a global risk score (4). More recently, genetic scores based on multiple SNPs from genome-wide association studies for CAD have been reported to improve risk reclassification especially in subjects at intermediate risk (47) but this finding was not consistent in all studies (48). Furthermore, there are no available data as to whether the results of genotype testing could improve management and outcomes for CAD prevention.

Evolving Targets

There is currently an increasing set of candidate genes/variants with established modest associations with increased risk of CAD but there is no information on which of the gene/variant associations identified might benefit from further validation and/or analysis to improve their credibility. Furthermore, it is likely that a large number of validated SNPs (>40) will be required to improve the clinical utility of risk prediction. More importantly, an understanding at the molecular level of the mechanisms of the additive and interactive effects between genetic polymorphisms as well as between genetic and environmental factors may be the foundation for developing novel therapeutic strategies for CV prevention.

PERSONAL PERSPECTIVE

CAD is the leading cause of death worldwide. Most of the fatal and non fatal CAD events are due to recognizable CV risk factors. To reduce the global burden of CAD, physicians and the community need to focus on improving both primary and secondary prevention. In primary prevention, integration of population-based and clinician-orientated interventions to prevent the occurence of CV events in asymptomatic individuals with a satisfactory cost-effectiveness and benefit–harm ratio, is very important. Public health strategies aiming to improve diet (reduced salt and transfat consumption), discourage or ban smoking, encourage regular physical activity and maintain healthy weight need to be implemented at a larger scale and target the whole community, including subpopulations such as women and children. Prevention of the largely increasing incidence of obesity and DM at an early age is of paramount importance. Population-based interventions are strongly advocated by the large scientific cardiological societies both in the US and Europe. Furthermore, the feasibility of interventions at a population level, the extent of their implementation, and the assessment of their performance and cost-effectiveness in reducing CV events, is a matter of research. At an individual level, identification of all CV risk factors (established and novel, modifiable and non-modifiable) that may increase individual's CV risk and reliable assessment of an individual's global CV risk, that is, risk for CV events in the future, should be regularly performed. Existing guidelines from scientific societies have set the goals to be achieved by physicians and patients focusing mainly on management of CV risk factors, but on the basis of global CV risk rather than isolated RFs. However, apart from the medical treatment that has been well adopted by physicians, careful attention should be given to instructions regarding non-medical treatment, i.e lifestyle change, a goal much more difficult to achieve. New medications for residual risk reduction, especially to increase HDL, reduce triglycerides, improve glycaemic control, are needed and currently investigated. Further research is also needed to explore the significance of "novel" risk factors, mainly inflammation and genetic factors, and their role in CV risk and also to identify better tools and more efficient methods (imaging, biomarkers, etc.) that could be incorporated in risk prediction tools in order to predict CV risk more reliably especially in subjects considered to be at moderate CV risk.

In secondary prevention, existing guidelines for patients who are known to have CAD and have suffered a CV event already offer very clear messages to both physicians and patients regarding management of risk factors, use of medications, lifestyle measures, medical counselling and follow-up. Specific drug treatments have been well documented to increase patient survival and reduce CV events. Ways to improve patient education and compliance (especially for non-medical measures), and to assess performance of guidelines' implementation are evolving targets. Finally, larger implementation of well organised, physician- or nurse-led, cardiac rehabilitation programs is expected to improve quality of life in patients with CAD.

REFERENCES

1. Roger VL, Go AS, Lloyd-Jones DM, et al. Heart disease and stroke statistics–2011 update: a report from the American Heart Association. Circulation 2011; 123: e18–e209.
2. Graham I, Atar D, Borch-Johnsen K, et al. European guidelines on cardiovascular disease prevention in clinical practice: full text. Fourth Joint Task Force of the European Society of Cardiology and other societies on cardiovascular disease prevention in clinical practice (constituted by representatives of nine societies and by invited experts). Eur J Cardiovasc Prev Rehabil 2007; 14(Suppl 2): S1–113.
3. O'Flaherty M, Ford E, Allender S, Scarborough P, Capewell S. Coronary heart disease trends in England and Wales from 1984 to 2004: concealed levelling of mortality rates among young adults. Heart 2008; 94: 178–81.
4. Greenland P, Alpert JS, Beller GA, et al. 2010 ACCF/AHA guideline for assessment of cardiovascular risk in asymptomatic adults: a report of the American College of Cardiology Foundation/American Heart Association Task Force on Practice Guidelines. J Am Coll Cardiol 2010; 56: e50–103.
5. Mosca L, Benjamin EJ, Berra K, et al. Effectiveness-based guidelines for the prevention of cardiovascular disease in women–2011

update: a guideline from the american heart association. Circulation 2011; 123: 1243–62.

6. Guallar E, Banegas JR, Blasco-Colmenares E, et al. Excess risk attributable to traditional cardiovascular risk factors in clinical practice settings across Europe – The EURIKA Study. BMC Public Health 2011; 11: 704.

7. World Health Organization Global Health Risks – Mortality and burden of diseae attributable to selected major risks. 2009. [Available from: www.who.int/healthinfo/global_burden_disease/global_health_risks/en/index.html]

8. Yusuf S, Hawken S, Ounpuu S, et al. Effect of potentially modifiable risk factors associated with myocardial infarction in 52 countries (the INTERHEART study): case-control study. Lancet 2004; 364: 937–52.

9. Reiner Z, Catapano AL, De Backer G, et al. ESC/EAS Guidelines for the management of dyslipidaemias: the Task Force for the management of dyslipidaemias of the European Society of Cardiology (ESC) and the European Atherosclerosis Society (EAS). Eur Heart J 2011; 32: 1769–818.

10. Wilson PW, D'Agostino RB, Levy D, et al. Prediction of coronary heart disease using risk factor categories. Circulation 1998; 97: 1837–47.

11. Gaziano JM, Manson JE, Ridker PM. Primary and Secondary Prevention of Coronary Heart Disease, in Braunwald's Heart Disease. In: Zipes DP, et al. eds. A textbook of Cardiovascular Medicine. 7th edn. Philadelphia, Pennsylvania: Elsevier Saunders, 2005: 1057–84.

12. Frieden TR, Berwick DM. The "Million Hearts" initiative – preventing heart attacks and strokes. N Engl J Med 2011; 365: e27.

13. Baigent C, Blackwell L, Emberson J, et al. Efficacy and safety of more intensive lowering of LDL cholesterol: a meta-analysis of data from 170,000 participants in 26 randomised trials. Lancet 2010; 376: 1670–81.

14. American Diabetes Association. Standards of medical care in diabetes - 2011. Diabetes Care 2011; 34(Suppl 1): S11–61.

15. Chobanian AV, Bakris GL, Black HR, et al. The Seventh Report of the Joint National Committee on Prevention, Detection, Evaluation, and Treatment of High Blood Pressure: the JNC 7 report. JAMA 2003; 289: 2560–72.

16. National Institute for Health and Clinical Excellence – Hypertension – Clinical management of primary hypertension in adults. 2011. [Available from: www.nice.org.uk/guidance/CG127]

17. Mancia G, De Backer G, Dominiczak A, et al. 2007 Guidelines for the management of arterial hypertension: the Task Force for the Management of Arterial Hypertension of the European Society of Hypertension (ESH) and of the European Society of Cardiology (ESC). Eur Heart J 2007; 28: 1462–536.

18. Mancia G, Laurent S, Agabiti-Rosei E, et al. Reappraisal of European guidelines on hypertension management: a European Society of Hypertension Task Force document. J Hypertens 2009; 27: 2121–58.

19. Skyler JS, Bergenstal R, Bonow RO, et al. Intensive glycemic control and the prevention of cardiovascular events: implications of the ACCORD, ADVANCE, and VA Diabetes Trials: a position statement of the American Diabetes Association and a Scientific Statement of the American College of Cardiology Foundation and the American Heart Association. J Am Coll Cardiol 2009; 53: 298–304.

20. Erhardt L. Cigarette smoking: an undertreated risk factor for cardiovascular disease. Atherosclerosis 2009; 205: 23–32.

21. Smith SC Jr, Allen J, Blair SN, et al. AHA/ACC guidelines for secondary prevention for patients with coronary and other atherosclerotic vascular disease: 2006 update: endorsed by the National Heart, Lung, and Blood Institute. Circulation 2006; 113: 2363–72.

22. Pearson TA, Blair SN, Daniels SR, et al. AHA guidelines for primary prevention of Cardiovascular disease and stroke: 2002 Update: Consensus Panel Guide to Comprehensive Risk Reduction for adult patients without coronary or Other Atherosclerotic Vascular diseases. American Heart Association Science Advisory and Coordinating Committee. Circulation 2002; 106: 388–91.

23. Aspirin for the prevention of cardiovascular disease: U.S. Preventive Services Task Force recommendation statement. Ann Intern Med 2009; 150: 396–404.

24. Van de Werf F, Bax J, Betriu A, et al. Management of acute myocardial infarction in patients presenting with persistent ST-segment elevation: the task force on the management of ST-Segment Elevation Acute Myocardial Infarction of the European Society of Cardiology. Eur Heart J 2008; 29: 2909–45.

25. Hamm CW, Bassand JP, Agewall S, et al. ESC Guidelines for the management of acute coronary syndromes in patients presenting without persistent ST-segment elevation: The Task Force for the management of acute coronary syndromes (ACS) in patients presenting without persistent ST-segment elevation of the European Society of Cardiology (ESC). Eur Heart J 2011; 32: 2999–3054.

26. Trichopoulou A, Costacou T, Bamia C, Trichopoulos D. Adherence to a Mediterranean diet and survival in a Greek population. N Engl J Med 2003; 348: 2599–608.

27. Lichtenstein AH, Appel LJ, Brands M, et al. Diet and lifestyle recommendations revision 2006: a scientific statement from the American Heart Association Nutrition Committee. Circulation 2006; 114: 82–96.

28. Flock MR, Kris-Etherton PM. Dietary Guidelines for Americans 2010: implications for Cardiovascular disease. Curr Atheroscler Rep 2011; 13: 499–507.

29. Marwick TH, Hordern MD, Miller T, et al. Exercise training for type 2 diabetes mellitus: impact on cardiovascular risk: a scientific statement from the American Heart Association. Circulation 2009; 119: 3244–62.

30. Haskell WL, Lee IM, Pate RR, et al. Physical activity and public health: updated recommendation for adults from the American College of Sports Medicine and the American Heart Association. Circulation 2007; 116: 1081–93.

31. Corrà U, Piepoli MF, Carré F, et al. Secondary prevention through cardiac rehabilitation: physical activity counselling and exercise training: key components of the position paper from the Cardiac Rehabilitation Section of the European Association of Cardiovascular Prevention and Rehabilitation. Eur Heart J 2010; 31: 1967–74.

32. Poirier P, Giles TD, Bray GA, et al. Obesity and cardiovascular disease: pathophysiology, evaluation, and effect of weight loss: an update of the 1997 American Heart Association Scientific Statement on Obesity and Heart Disease from the Obesity Committee of the Council on Nutrition, Physical Activity, and Metabolism. Circulation 2006; 113: 898–918.

33. Scottish Intercollegiate Guidelines Network – Management of Obesity – A national clinical guideline. 2010. [Available from: www.sign.ac.uk/guidelines/fulltext/115/index.html]

34. Morse SA, Gulati R, Reisin E. The obesity paradox and cardiovascular disease. Curr Hypertens Rep 2010; 12: 120–6.

35. Mottillo S, Filion KB, Genest J, et al. The metabolic syndrome and cardiovascular risk a systematic review and meta-analysis. J Am Coll Cardiol 2010; 56: 1113–32.

36. Alberti KG, Eckel RH, Grundy SM, et al. Harmonizing the metabolic syndrome: a joint interim statement of the International Diabetes Federation Task Force on Epidemiology and Prevention; National Heart, Lung, and Blood Institute; American Heart Association; World Heart Federation; International Atherosclerosis Society; and International Association for the Study of Obesity. Circulation 2009; 120: 1640–5.

37. Helfand M, Buckley DI, Freeman M, et al. Emerging risk factors for coronary heart disease: a summary of systematic reviews conducted for the U.S. Preventive Services Task Force. Ann Intern Med 2009; 151: 496–507.

38. Ridker PM, Danielson E, Fonseca FA, et al. Rosuvastatin to prevent vascular events in men and women with elevated C-reactive protein. N Engl J Med 2008; 359: 2195–207.

39. Wald DS, Law M, Morris JK. Homocysteine and cardiovascular disease: evidence on causality from a meta-analysis. BMJ 2002; 325: 1202.

40. Clarke R, Halsey J, Lewington S, et al. Effects of lowering homocysteine levels with B vitamins on cardiovascular disease, cancer, and cause-specific mortality: Meta-analysis of 8 randomized trials involving 37 485 individuals. Arch Intern Med 2010; 170: 1622–31.

41. Das S, O'Keefe JH. Behavioral cardiology: recognizing and addressing the profound impact of psychosocial stress on cardiovascular health. Curr Hypertens Rep 2008; 10: 374–81.

42. Berkman LF, Blumenthal J, Burg M, et al. Effects of treating depression and low perceived social support on clinical events after myocardial infarction: the Enhancing Recovery in Coronary Heart Disease Patients (ENRICHD) Randomized Trial. JAMA 2003; 289: 3106–16.

43. Gulliksson M, Burell G, Vessby B, et al. Randomized controlled trial of cognitive behavioral therapy vs standard treatment to prevent recurrent cardiovascular events in patients with coronary heart disease: Secondary Prevention in Uppsala Primary Health Care project (SUPRIM). Arch Intern Med 2011; 171: 134–40.

44. Bechlioulis A, Naka KK, Calis KA, et al. Cardiovascular effects of endogenous estrogen and hormone therapy. Curr Vasc Pharmacol 2010; 8: 249–58.

45. Schenck-Gustafsson K, Brincat M, Erel CT, et al. EMAS position statement: Managing the menopause in the context of coronary heart disease. Maturitas 2011; 68: 94–7.

46. McPherson R, Pertsemlidis A, Kavaslar N, et al. A common allele on chromosome 9 associated with coronary heart disease. Science 2007; 316: 1488–91.

47. Ripatti S, Tikkanen E, Orho-Melander M, et al. A multilocus genetic risk score for coronary heart disease: case-control and prospective cohort analyses. Lancet 2010; 376: 1393–400.

48. Paynter NP, Chasman DI, Paré G, et al. Association between a literature-based genetic risk score and cardiovascular events in women. JAMA 2010; 303: 631–7.

23 Anti-ischemic pharmacotherapy in patients with established coronary artery disease

Dimitrios Alexopoulos and Ioanna Xanthopoulou

OUTLINE

Medical management continues to play an essential role in the treatment of patients with established coronary artery disease (CAD), particularly in patients with stable CAD and in a subgroup of patients who, for various reasons, are not suitable candidates for a revascularization procedure. β-blockers are considered as first-line therapy as they combine anti-anginal properties with survival benefit. Nitrates and calcium-channel blockers are useful as adjuncts to β-blockade or when β-blockade fails or is poorly tolerated. Novel agents have become available that may prove useful where conventional anti-anginal agents have failed or are poorly tolerated. In this chapter we review the main categories of anti-ischemic drugs and the current guidelines for their use in the various clinical presentations of CAD.

INTRODUCTION/DEFINITIONS

CAD is a major determinant of mortality in Europe and in the United States. In 2006, nearly 33% of cardiovascular deaths occurred before the age of 75 years, while the average life expectancy was 77.7 years. In 2010, an estimated 785,000 Americans had an inaugural myocardial infarction and approximately 470,000 had a further infarct. Mortality data show that cardiovascular death accounted for 34.3% (831272) of all 2,426,264 deaths in 2006, or 1 of every 2.9 deaths in the United States (1).

Myocardial ischemia may result from increased myocardial oxygen demand, decreased oxygen supply, or a combination of both factors.

Decreased myocardial oxygen supply may result from progression of coronary atherosclerosis, coronary artery spasm, intracoronary thrombus formation at the site of a ruptured or eroded atherosclerotic plaque, or microvascular disease (syndrome X, vasculitis, etc.). Rare causes include myocardial bridges, coronary embolism, and a coronary slow flow phenomenon. Increased myocardial oxygen demand may be the result of increased heart rate, elevated arterial pressure, or left ventricular hypertrophy.

Although the most common cause of myocardial ischemia is coronary atherosclerosis, it may also be the result of other conditions such as hypertrophic or dilated cardiomyopathy or aortic stenosis, in the absence of obstructive CAD.

Myocardial ischemia encompasses a wide spectrum of clinical presentations including effort angina, unstable angina (UA), and acute myocardial infarction (MI). Acute MI is defined as the detection of a typical rise and fall in cardiac biomarkers with at least one value above the 99th percentile of the upper reference limit, together with evidence of ischemia, according to a consensus document published in 2007 (2). Unstable angina/Non ST-elevation myocardial infarction (NSTEMI) is defined by electrocardiographic ST segment depression or prominent T-wave inversion and/or positive biomarkers of necrosis (e.g., troponin) in the absence of ST-segment elevation and in an appropriate clinical setting (chest discomfort or anginal equivalent) (3). Stable angina is a clinical syndrome characterized by discomfort in the chest or adjacent areas, typically brought on by exertion or emotional stress and relieved by rest or nitroglycerin.

Over the past years, remarkable progress has been achieved in the management of CAD by new interventional and medical therapies and strategies of care, resulting in a significant improvement in survival. The aim of medical treatment is to reduce the risk of death, relieve symptoms, improve quality of life, and prevent future ischemic complications. Optimal medical treatment has become of particular importance for patients with stable CAD because of the results of the BARI 2D (4) and COURAGE (5) trials, which showed that a strategy of initial pharmacological therapy, in low or intermediate risk patients, is as effective as an initial strategy of coronary artery bypass grafting or percutaneous coronary revascularization in terms of long-term mortality. In particular, anti-ischemic pharmacotherapy plays a pivotal role in the management of patients with CAD. These agents reduce myocardial ischemia by several mechanisms; the major classes of drugs employed are nitrates, β-blockers, and calcium channel blockers.

NITRATES

Mechanism of Action

Nitrates are prodrugs which are converted to nitric oxide (NO), a free radical that activates guanylate cyclase leading to intracellular elevation of cyclic guanosine monophosphate (cGMP) levels. In turn, this causes relaxation of smooth muscle cells and vasodilation.

The main effect of nitrates in ischemia is a decrease in myocardial oxygen consumption through their venodilatory action in the extremities, which causes a reduction in preload and in cardiac filling. This leads to decreased left-ventricular (LV) end-diastolic pressure, LV wall-stress, and myocardial oxygen consumption. Nitrates also reduce afterload through arterial dilation and a reduction in wave reflexion from the peripheral vascular bed back to the ascending aorta (6). Additionally, nitrates dilate large coronary arteries and arterioles >100 μm in diameter (7) resulting in a decrease in coronary vasomotor tone and an increased blood supply to ischemic territories.

Pharmacokinetics

Nitrates are absorbed from the gastrointestinal tract, skin, and mucus membranes. Nitroglycerin has a very short half-life of a few minutes with extrahepatic sites of metabolism including red blood cells and vascular walls. Isosorbide dinitrate is subjected to liver metabolism after oral administration and conversion to active mononitrates with a half-life of 4–6 hours. Isosorbide mononitrate does not undergo hepatic conversion, therefore, is almost 100% bioavailable. Table 23.1 summarizes doses, onset, and duration of action of commonly used nitrate preparations.

Use of Nitrates in STEMI

Nitrates do not seem to improve short-term survival after MI. The GISSI-3 trial tested a strategy of intravenous nitrate administration for the first 24 hours followed by transdermal glyceryl trinitrate (GTN) 10 mg daily versus selected administration because of ongoing ischemia in more than 19,000 patients. No significant reduction in 6-week mortality was observed with the systematic use of nitrate. (8). Likewise, in the ISIS-4 trial, 58,000 patients with suspected acute MI (both STEMI and NSTEMI) were randomly assigned to receive either 1 month of oral controlled-release mononitrate (30 mg initial dose

titrated up to 60 mg once daily) for 1 month versus matching placebo. With nitrate use, there was no significant reduction in 5-week mortality either overall or in any pre-specified subgroup (9). However, pre- and in-hospital nitrate use in the control groups is a potential confounding factor in the interpretation of these trials. According to the ACC/AHA STEMI guidelines (10) patients with ongoing ischemic discomfort should receive sublingual nitroglycerin (0.4 mg) every 5 minutes for a total of 3 doses, after which an assessment should be performed regarding the need for intravenous nitroglycerin. (Class I, level of evidence: C). Intravenous nitroglycerin is indicated in the first 48 hours after STEMI for treatment of persistent ischemia, congestive heart failure (CHF), or hypertension. In any case, their use should not preclude therapy with other proven mortality-reducing interventions such as beta-blockers or ACE inhibitors. Beyond the first 48 hours after STEMI, nitrates should be administered for treatment of recurrent angina or persistent CHF (Class I, level of evidence B). Nitrates should not be administered to patients with systolic blood pressure less than 90 mm Hg or greater than or equal to 30 mm Hg below baseline, severe bradycardia (less than 50 bpm), tachycardia (more than 100 bpm), or RV infarction. (Class III, level of evidence C). Nitrates are also contraindicated in patients who have received a phosphodiesterase inhibitor for erectile dysfunction within the last 24 hours (48 hours for tadalafil). (Class III, level of evidence: B).

Table 23.1 Doses, Onset, and Duration of Action of Commonly Used Nitrate Preparations

Drug	Route	Dose	Onset of action	Duration of action	Comments
Amyl nitrite	Inhalation	2–5 mg	Within 30 seconds	1–10 min	For the diagnosis of LVOT obstruction in hypertrophic cardiomyopathy
Nitroglycerin	Sublingual tablet	0.3–0.6 mg	2–5 min	10–30 min	Should be stored in a tightly capped dark bottle in the refrigerator, lasts 3–6 months
Nitroglycerin	Sublingual spray	0.4 mg	2–5 min	10–30 min	Lasts 2–3 years
Nitroglycerin	Intravenous	5–200 μg/min	seconds	mins	Rapid tolerance, as may precipitate a significant drop in blood pressure
Nitroglycerin	Buccal (trans-mucosal)	1–3 mg × 3	within 2–3 min	3–5 h	
Nitroglycerin	Transdermal patch	0.2–0.8 mg/h	Within minutes	3–5 h	Remove for 12 hours per day in order to avoid tolerance
Nitroglycerin	Oral extended-release	2.5–13 mg	60 min	Up to 12 h	
Isosorbide dinitrate	Sublingual	2.5–10 mg	5–10 min	30–60 min	
Isosorbide dinitrate	Oral (immediate release)	5–40 mg 2–3 times daily	Within 15 to 30 minutes	3–6 hours	
Isosorbide dinitrate	Oral (slow release)	40 mg 1–2 times daily		Up to 6–8 hours	
Isosorbide-5-mononitrate	Oral	20–60 mg every 12 hours	Within 30 minutes	6–8 hours	Extended release preparations are preferable. Starting dose is 30 mg once daily can be titrated to 120 mg once daily as needed.

Use of Nitrates in UA/NSTEMI

The two large randomized trials on nitrate therapy, conducted in patients with suspected acute MI (both STEMI and NSTEMI) failed to show any survival benefit of these drugs on short-term mortality in the overall population or in the subgroup of patients with NSTEMI (8,9). Therefore, the use of nitrates seems justified purely on the basis of symptom relief. In patients with UA, there are no randomized controlled trials on nitrate us and the ACC/AHA N-STEMI/UA recommendations (3) regarding the use of nitrates in patients with UA/NSTEMI are similar to those discussed above for STEMI patients.

Use of Nitrates in Stable Angina

In patients with stable exertional angina, nitrates improve exercise-induced myocardial ischemia and may increase exercise tolerance (11,12). A survival benefit of long-term therapy with nitrates in patients with chronic stable angina remains unproven. Short-acting nitrate preparations provide rapid symptom relief from acute effort angina, whereas use of long-acting nitrates improves compliance and provides prophylaxis from angina attacks.

The ACC/AHA guidelines for the management of patients with chronic stable angina (13) recommend sublingual nitroglycerin or nitroglycerin spray for the immediate relief of angina (Class I, level of evidence: B). Long-acting nitrates can be given as initial therapy for reduction of symptoms when beta-blockers are contraindicated. (Class I, level of evidence: B), in combination with beta-blockers when initial treatment with beta-blockers is not successful (Class I, level of evidence: B), or as a substitute for beta-blockers if initial treatment with beta-blockers leads to unacceptable side effects. (Class I, level of evidence: C).

Side Effects and Interactions with Other Drugs

Headache is the most common side effect associated with nitrate use, usually occurs at the onset of treatment, and tends to decrease in severity with continued use or with a reduction in dose. Severe hypotension can occur, due to reduction in both preload and afterload. Other side effects include flushing, dizziness, weakness, and rarely methemoglobinemia (only with high doses).

The concomitant use of other vasodilators (ACE inhibitors, hydralazine, calcium channel blockers, sildenafil) can exacerbate nitrate-induced hypotension. High doses of intravenous nitroglycerin (>200 µg/min) can induce resistance to heparin treatment by displacement of heparin from antithrombin III.

Nitrate Tolerance

Prolonged therapy with nitrates (with constant maintenance of their levels above a certain threshold level) leads to an attenuation of their efficacy with time. Impaired conversion to active metabolite and increased oxidative stress, are both likely implicated to this phenomenon. Patients treated with long-acting nitrates should have a "nitrate-free" interval each day to preserve the therapeutic effects. A rebound of angina can occur during intermittent therapy with nitrates, which has been more strongly associated with the use of transdermal nitroglycerin (11). The principles of nitrates use in patients with CAD are summarized in Focus Box 23.1.

β-BLOCKERS

Beta-adrenoceptor blocking agents (β-blockers) constitute a cornerstone in the treatment of CAD (with the exception of vasospastic angina). β-blockers are the only antiischemic agents providing documented efficacy in preventing recurrence of coronary events, MI, and sudden death following acute MI (14). Most of these agents are satisfactorily absorbed by the gastrointestinal tract with a half-life varying from 9 minutes for esmolol to 26 hours for penbutolol.

Mechanism of Action and Classification

β-blockers are competitive inhibitors of endogenous catecholamines at beta-adrenergic receptors (β-receptors). The β-receptors are divided into β1-receptors (present in the myocardium) and β2-receptors (present in smooth muscle cells, bronchi, and other tissues). The blockage of the postsynaptic beta-1 receptors leads to cardiac inotropic, chronotropic, dromotropic, and bathmotropic negative effects with decrease of cardiac output and oxygen requirement and to a decrease in renin secretion. The blockage of the postsynaptic beta-2 receptors induces vasoconstriction, bronchospasm, metabolic effects, cardiac inotropic, and chronotropic negative effects but less than those which result from beta-1 blockage. The blockage of presynaptic beta-2 receptors decreases noradrenaline release.

β-blockers are classified according to their β-selectivity properties into:

- Non selective (combined β1 β2 blockers): examples are propranolol, nadolol, sotalol, and carvedilol. These agents by blocking β1-receptors slow heart rate, conduction, and decrease contractility. By blocking β2-receptors they may lead to bronchospasm and may worsen diabetes and peripheral vascular disease in predisposed individuals.
- Cardioselective (agents with β1 selectivity): examples are atenolol, bisoprolol, and metoprolol. These agents do not affect glucose metabolism, and are safer when administered in patients with COPD and peripheral vascular disease. However, higher doses attenuate their cardioselective properties.

Focus Box 23.1 The Use of Nitrates in Patients with CAD	
In ACS patients nitrates should be administered for treatment of ongoing ischemia, hypertension or persistent CHF	In patients with stable angina, nitrates increase exercise tolerance
Nitrates should not be administered to patients with hypotension, RV infarction or recent phosphodiesterase inhibitor use	Patients treated with long-acting nitrates should have a "nitrate-free" interval each day to avoid nitrate tolerance

β-blockers are classified according to their lipophilic properties into:

- Lipid soluble, which are subject to hepatic metabolism and penetrate the central nervous system (with the potential to cause insomnia or depression). Examples are propranolol, metoprolol, and carvedilol.
- Lipid insoluble, which are excreted through the kidneys, have longer half-lives, and cause less central nervous system side effects. Examples are atenolol, bisoprolol, and nadolol.

β-blockers with intrinsic sympathomimetic activity (ISA) such as pindolol and acebutalol, are partial β-agonists that have less marked negative chronotropic effects at rest, but prevent stimulation of the heart by catecholamines during emotional stress. Some β-blockers like labetalol and carvedilol have additional vasodilator properties by α-adrenoceptor blocking activity. Table 23.2 summarizes the usual doses of commonly used β-blockers.

Use of β-Blockers in STEMI
A strategy of routine administration of IV β-blockers during the acute phase of MI is not well established. In the COMMIT trial, administration of IV metoprolol followed by oral dosing in 45,852 patients with suspected MI did not improve survival (14). Likewise, a prospectively planned post-hoc analysis of the GUSTO-I dataset, did not provide evidence that early intravenous atenolol administration improved survival (15). A metanalysis of 82 randomized trials assessed the effectiveness of beta-blockers, as a short term treatment after acute MI and in the context of longer term secondary prevention and provided strong evidence for long-term use of b-blockers to reduce morbidity and mortality after STEMI (16). According to the ACC/AHA STEMI guidelines (10) oral beta-blocker therapy should be administered promptly to those patients without a contraindication, irrespective of whether concomitant fibrinolytic therapy or primary PCI is performed. (Class I, level of evidence: A), while it is reasonable to administer IV beta-blockers

to STEMI patients without contraindications, especially if a tachyarrhythmia or hypertension is present. (Class IIa, level of evidence: B). In the presence of moderate LV failure early in the course of STEMI intravenous beta-blockade cannot be given until heart failure has been appropriately treated but is a strong indication for the oral use of beta-blockade prior to discharge from the hospital. All patients after STEMI apart from those at low risk (normal or near-normal ventricular function, successful reperfusion, absence of significant ventricular arrhythmias) and those with contraindications should receive beta-blocker therapy. Treatment should begin within a few days of the event, if not initiated acutely, and continue indefinitely. (Class I, level of evidence: A). Patients with moderate or severe LV failure should receive beta-blocker therapy with a gradual titration scheme. (Class I, level of evidence: B). It is also reasonable to prescribe beta-blockers to low-risk patients after STEMI who have no contraindications. (Class IIa, level of evidence: A).

Use of β-Blockers in UA/NSTEMI
There is no convincing evidence of favorable effects of β-blockers in patients with UA. In a randomized trial comparing metoprolol to placebo in patients with UA, the short-term benefit from metoprolol administration was borderline (17). An analysis of pooled data from five randomized, controlled trials of abciximab during coronary intervention demonstrated lower short-term mortality in patients receiving beta blocker therapy who underwent percutaneous coronary intervention for UA or acute MI (18). B-blockers have shown efficacy in reducing infarct size, reinfarction, and mortality post acute MI, in studies that included both STEMI and NSTEMI patients (19). In patients with LV dysfunction post MI, carvedilol was found to reduce the frequency of all-cause and cardiovascular mortality, and recurrent, non-fatal MI. The ACC/AHA UA/NSTEMI guidelines (3) recommend that oral beta-blocker therapy should be initiated within the first 24 h for patients who do not have 1 or more of the following: (*i*) signs of HF, (*ii*) evidence of a low-output state, (*iii*) increased risk for cardiogenic shock, or (*iv*) other relative contraindications to beta blockade (PR interval greater than 0.24 s, second- or third-degree heart block, active asthma, or reactive airway disease). (Class I, level of evidence: B). It is reasonable to administer intravenous (IV) beta blockers at the time of presentation for hypertension in UA/NSTEMI patients who do not have the abovementioned contraindications (Class IIa, level of evidence: B). Beta blockers are indicated for all patients recovering from UA/NSTEMI unless contraindicated. Treatment should begin within a few days of the event, if not initiated acutely, and should be continued indefinitely. (Class I, level of evidence: B). Patients recovering from UA/NSTEMI with moderate or severe LV failure should receive beta-blocker therapy with a gradual titration scheme (Class I, level of evidence: B). It is also reasonable to prescribe beta blockers to low-risk patients (i.e., normal LV function, revascularized, no high-risk features) recovering from UA/NSTEMI in the absence of absolute contraindications (Class IIa, level of evidence: B).

Table 23.2 Usual Doses of Commonly Used β-blockers

β-blocker	Per os dosing	IV administration
Non cardioselective		
Propranolol	80–160 mg × 2	1 mg/min (up to 6 mg)
Timolol	10 mg × 2	
Cardioselective		
Atenolol	50–200 mg × 1	5 mg over 5 min
Metoprolol	50–200 mg × 2	5 mg × 3 at 2 min intervals
Betaxolol	10–20 mg ×1	
Vasodilatory effect		
Labetalol	100–400 mg × 2	2 mg/min
Pindolol	2.5–7.5 mg × 3	
Carvedilol	12.5–25 mg × 2	
Cardioselective, vasodilatory effect		
Nebivolol	5 mg × 1	

Use of β-Blockers in Stable Angina

Although β-blockers have shown their efficacy in reducing cardiovascular death in patients who have suffered an acute MI, there is a relative lack of evidence of a survival benefit in stable patients with documented CAD without prior MI. In the ASIST trial, a placebo-controlled study of patients with stable CAD and minimal anginal symptoms, treatment with atenolol resulted in a lower incidence of a combined endpoint which included symptoms requiring treatment (20). The larger APSIS and TIBET trials in patients with effort angina were not placebo controlled and showed that β-blockers had equal efficacy to calcium-channel blockers (21,22). The beneficial effect of β-blockers on symptomatic improvement in patients with stable CAD is well documented (23,24). Combining these agents with nitrates controls angina symptoms more effectively than nitrates or beta-blockers alone (25).

The ACC/AHA guidelines for the management of patients with chronic stable angina (13) recommend beta-blockers as initial therapy in the absence of contraindications in patients with prior MI (Class I, level of evidence: A) or without prior MI. (Class I, level of evidence: B).

Side Effects and Interactions with Other Drugs

B-blockers can cause bronchospasm (which may exacerbate dyspnea in COPD patients), erectile dysfunction, worsen peripheral arterial disease, mask hypoglycemic symptoms, and adversely influence lipid profile (by increasing LDL and decreasing HDL cholesterol). Lipid soluble agents are associated with insomnia and depression. Bradycardia and/or hypotension can occur, especially with co-administration of calcium-channel antagonists. Sudden discontinuation of these agents may lead to precipitation of angina symptoms in some patients (rebound phenomenon). The principles of β-blockers use in patients with CAD are summarized in Focus Box 23.2.

CALCIUM CHANNEL BLOCKERS

Mechanism of Action and Classification

Calcium channel blockers (CCBs) inhibit calcium entry into vascular smooth muscle cells and myocardial cells (L-type channels). Some of these agents also inhibit sinoatrial and atrioventricular node conduction (T-type channels).

CCBs are classified into two major classes:

- Dihydropyridines (DHP) include nifedipine, amlodipine, nicardipine, felodipine, nisolidipine, and isradipine.
- Nondihydropyridines (non DHP) include verapamil (phenylalkylamine) and diltiazem (benzothiazepine).

CCBs increase coronary oxygen supply by producing coronary vasodilation and by decreasing coronary spasm. These agents have negative chronotropic effects and reduce afterload by peripheral vasodilation and reduction in blood pressure, leading to decrease in myocardial oxygen demand. They also reduce myocardial contractility, which should be taken into account in patients with reduced LV function. Table 23.3 summarizes the major properties of most commonly used CCBs.

Use of CCBs in STEMI

In general, CCBs have little to offer in the acute phase of STEMI. A meta-analysis of trials involving calcium antagonists early in the course of a STEMI provided weak evidence supporting a benefit on survival or on reduction in reinfarction (26).

The ACC/AHA STEMI guidelines (10) state that it is reasonable to give verapamil or diltiazem to patients in whom beta-blockers are ineffective or contraindicated (e.g., bronchospastic disease) for relief of ongoing ischemia or control of a rapid ventricular response with AF or atrial flutter after STEMI in the absence of CHF, LV dysfunction, or AV block. (Class IIa, level of evidence C). Diltiazem and verapamil are contraindicated in patients with STEMI and associated systolic LV dysfunction and CHF. (Class III, level of evidence: A). Nifedipine (immediate-release form) is contraindicated in the treatment of STEMI because of the reflex sympathetic activation, tachycardia, and hypotension associated with its use. (Class III, level of evidence: B).

Focus Box 23.2 The Use of β-blockers in Patients with CAD

All patients after MI should receive beta-blocker therapy	Beta-blockers improve symptoms in stable angina
They are contraindicated in case of HF, low-output state, increased risk for cardiogenic shock and second or third degree heart block	Sudden discontinuation may precipitate anginal symptoms (rebound phenomenon)

Table 23.3 Major Properties of Most Commonly Used CCBs

	Dose	Onset of action	Vasodilatation	Conduction delay	Negative inotrope effect
Nifedipine SR	30–90 mg × 1	20 min	+++		
Diltiazem	60–90 mg × 3	30–60 min	+	+++	+
Verapamil	40–120 mg × 3	30 min	++	+++	++
Amlodipine	2.5–10 mg × 1	30–60 min	+++		
Felodipine	5–20 mg × 1	120 min	+++		
Isradipine	2.5–10 mg × 1	20 min	+++	+++	

Use of CCBs in UA/NSTEMI

Currently, no strong evidence for a survival benefit of CCBs in UA/NSTEMI exists. A meta-analysis of 19000 patients in 28 randomized trials showed that calcium channel blockers do not reduce the risk of initial or recurrent infarction or death when given routinely to patients with acute MI or UA (27). In a placebo-controlled trial of 576 patients with non-Q wave MI, diltiazem reduced the rates of reinfarction and severe angina (28). In UA/NSTEMI patients with continuing or frequently recurring ischemia and in whom beta blockers are contraindicated, a nondihydropyridine calcium channel blocker (e.g., verapamil or diltiazem) should be given as initial therapy in the absence of clinically significant LV dysfunction or other contraindications. (Class I, level of evidence: B) (3). Oral long-acting nondihydropyridine calcium channel blockers are reasonable for use in UA/NSTEMI patients for recurrent ischemia in the absence of contraindications after beta blockers and nitrates have been fully used. (Class IIa, level of evidence: C). Immediate-release dihydropyridine calcium channel blockers in the presence of adequate beta blockade may be considered in patients with UA/NSTEMI with ongoing ischemic symptoms or hypertension. (Class IIb, level of evidence: B). Finally, medical therapy with nitrates, beta blockers, and calcium channel blockers, alone or in combination, is recommended in patients with cardiovascular syndrome X. (Class I, level of evidence: B).

Use of CCBs in Stable Angina

The ACTION trial, conducted in patients with stable angina, found no reduction in the composite end-point of death, MI, refractory angina, debilitating stroke, and heart failure with long-acting nifedipine compared to placebo (29). In a substudy of the ACTION trial long-acting nifedipine reduced the combined incidence of all-cause mortality, MI, refractory angina, heart failure, stroke, and peripheral revascularization by 13% in hypertensives only (30). In a meta-analysis of 72 trials comparing calcium antagonists and beta-blockers in patients with stable angina pectoris, rates of cardiac death, and MI were not significantly different for treatment with beta-blockers vs calcium antagonists but beta-blockers were discontinued because of adverse events less often than were calcium antagonists (31).

The ACC/AHA guidelines for the management of patients with chronic stable angina (13) recommend calcium antagonists (short-acting dihydropyridine calcium antagonists should be avoided) as initial therapy for reduction of symptoms when beta-blockers are contraindicated, (Class I, level of evidence: B), when initial treatment with beta-blockers is not successful. (Class I, level of evidence: B) or as a substitute for beta-blockers if initial treatment with beta-blockers leads to unacceptable side effects. (Class I, level of evidence: C). Long-acting nondihydropyridine calcium antagonists (short-acting dihydropyridine calcium antagonists should be avoided) instead of beta-blockers as initial therapy (Class IIa, level of evidence: B).

Side-Effects and Interactions with Other Drugs

Calcium channel blockers may cause bilateral edema of ankles and lower limbs (more common with nifedipine and amlodipine), headache, flushing and burning, as well as hypotension and dizziness. Constipation is common with verapamil. Conduction disturbances in predisposed individuals can occur with preparations that block sinoatrial or atrioventricular node. Calcium channel blockers may increase digitalis levels. Verapamil increases the effects of oral anticoagulants.

OTHER ANTIANGINAL AGENTS

Ivabradine

Ivabradine is a selective blocker of the cardiac pacemaker current If with antianginal properties, shown in a placebo-controlled trial (32). In a non-inferiority study of 939 patients with stable angina, ivabradine was proved as effective as atenolol, in terms of exercise capacity (33). This agent has negative chronotropic effect without any negative inotropic one and according to the 2006 ESC guidelines on the management of stable angina pectoris (34) it can be used as an alternative medication in patients with stable angina, who do not tolerate β-blockers (Class IIa, level of evidence: B).

In the BEAUTIFUL trial, a placebo-controlled study of 10, 917 patients with stable CAD and a left-ventricular ejection fraction of less than 40%, ivabradine in addition to appropriate cardiovascular medication did not reduce the primary composite endpoint of cardiovascular death, admission to hospital for acute MI, and admission to hospital for new onset or worsening heart failure. However, in a prespecified subgroup of patients with heart rate of 70 bpm or greater, this agent did reduce admission to hospital for fatal and non-fatal MI and coronary revascularization (35).

Ranolazine

Ranolazine is an inhibitor of the slow inward sodium channel in myocardium, which leads to a reduced calcium entry into the cytosol (36). This reduction in intracellular calcium levels is associated with improved diastolic blood flow with favorable effects on ischemia. As shown in the CARISA trial, a 3-group parallel, placebo-controlled trial of 823 patients with symptomatic chronic stable angina despite taking standard doses of atenolol, amlodipine, or diltiazem, ranolazine increased exercise capacity and provided additional antianginal relief (37). In the ERICA study, which evaluated ranolazine in 565 stable coronary patients with refractory angina despite optimal medical treatment with amlodipine, ranolazine significantly reduced frequency of angina and nitroglycerin consumption compared to placebo (38). This agent has been approved by the U.S. Food and Drug Administration for use in patients with chronic stable angina. Because ranolazine prolongs the QT interval, it should only be used by patients who have not responded to other anti-anginal (long-acting nitrates, calcium channel blockers and beta blockers) drugs. In patients with non-ST elevation acute coronary syndrome, the addition of ranolazine to standard treatment did not reduce the composite end-point of cardiovascular death, MI, or recurrent ischemia. However recurrent ischemia was significantly reduced in the ranolazine group and ranolazine did not adversely affect the risk of all-cause death or symptomatic documented arrhythmia (39).

Nicorandil

Nicorandil is a potassium channel activator and also has a nitrate-like action. In the IONA study, in patients with stable angina, nicorandil resulted in a 17% reduction in the relative risk of nonfatal MI or unplanned hospitalization for angina (40). According to the 2006 ESC guidelines on the management of stable angina pectoris, (34) nicorandil can be used as an alternative medication in patients with stable angina who do not tolerate or do not respond to β-blockers (Class I, level of evidence: C) or as a CCB substitute in case of treatment failure (Class IIa, level of evidence: B).

Trimetazidine and Perhexiline

These agents inhibit fatty acid oxidation and have a favorable effect on ischemia in patients with stable angina without any hemodynamic effect (41). In a placebo-controlled study of 177 patients with stable angina refractory to nitrates or β-blockage, the combination of trimetazidine with beta-blockers or long-acting nitrates significantly improved exercise stress test parameters and relieved anginal symptoms when compared with placebo (42). In the EMIR-FR study, conducted in patients with acute MI who received either thrombolytic therapy or not, trimetazidine (infused intravenously immediately post-MI for 48 hours) showed no benefit on 35-day or long-term mortality (43).

PERSONAL PERSPECTIVE

The management of CAD targets secondary prevention and survival improvement as well as the need to control symptoms and to ameliorate quality of life. This is achieved with a combination of pharmacological therapy and revascularization procedures. Pharmacotherapy has a pivotal role both in acute coronary syndromes where patients are not candidates for revascularization procedures and in patients with stable angina.

Based on available evidence, a β-blocker should be the first-line treatment in patients with prior MI. These agents should be avoided in low output states, in patients at increased risk for cardiogenic shock, in patients with evidence of congestive heart failure, and in vasospastic angina or in patients with MI precipitated by cocaine use. β-blockers are very effective in controlling symptoms for patients with stable angina, alone or in combination with other antianginals.

Nitrates in the form of short-term intravenous treatment, are useful in acute coronary syndromes, in ongoing ischemia, congestive heart failure or hypertension. For patients with stable angina caution should be taken when using long-acting preparations, to preserve a balance between avoidance of tolerance and effective prophylaxis from anginal attacks.

Calcium channel blockers are effective in patients with stable angina, particularly in cases of intolerance or failure of β-blockade. In acute coronary syndromes rate limiting calcium channel blockers should be used if β-blockers are contraindicated or in ongoing ischemia after beta blocker and nitrate use has been maximized. However, immediate-release dihydropyridine calcium channel blockers in the presence of inadequate beta blockade should be avoided.

Newer antianginal agents like ranolazine or ivabradine may be considered in patients with stable angina who do not tolerate β-blockers or experience refractory symptoms after classic antianginals have been used.

Anti-ischemic therapy is a crucial component of the optimal medical therapy in CAD. However, it should be combined with appropriate anti-platelet, lipid-lowering, and arterial pressure-control therapy, and evidence-based indicated revascularization procedures.

REFERENCES

1. Lloyd-Jones D, Adams RJ, Brown TM, et al. Heart disease and stroke statistics–2010 update: a report from the American Heart Association. Circulation 2010; 121: e46–e215.
2. Thygesen K, Alpert JS, White HD, et al. Universal definition of myocardial infarction. Circulation 2007; 116: 2634–53.
3. Wright RS, Anderson JL, Adams CD, et al. 2011 ACCF/AHA focused update incorporated into the ACC/AHA 2007 Guidelines for the Management of Patients with Unstable Angina/Non-ST-Elevation Myocardial Infarction: a report of the American College of Cardiology Foundation/American Heart Association Task Force on Practice Guidelines developed in collaboration with the American Academy of Family Physicians, Society for Cardiovascular Angiography and Interventions, and the Society of Thoracic Surgeons. J Am Coll Cardiol 2011; 57: e215–367.
4. Frye RL, August P, Brooks MM, et al. A randomized trial of therapies for type 2 diabetes and coronary artery disease. N Engl J Med 2009; 360: 2503–15.
5. Boden WE, O'Rourke RA, Teo KK, et al. Optimal medical therapy with or without PCI for stable coronary disease. N Engl J Med 2007; 356: 1503–16.
6. Kelly RP, Gibbs HH, O'Rourke MF, et al. Nitroglycerin has more favourable effects on left ventricular afterload than apparent from measurement of pressure in a peripheral artery. Eur Heart J 1990; 11: 138–44.
7. Harrison DG, Bates JN. The nitrovasodilators. New ideas about old drugs. Circulation 1993; 87: 1461–7.
8. Gruppo Italiano per lo Studio della Sopravvivenza nell'infarto Miocardico. GISSI-3: effects of lisinopril and transdermal glyceryl trinitrate singly and together on 6-week mortality and ventricular function after acute myocardial infarction. Lancet. 1994; 343: 1115–22.
9. ISIS-4 (Fourth International Study of Infarct Survival) Collaborative Group. ISIS-4: a randomised factorial trial assessing early oral captopril, oral mononitrate, and intravenous magnesium sulphate in 58,050 patients with suspected acute myocardial infarction. Lancet. 1995; 345: 669–85.
10. Antman EM, Anbe DT, Armstrong PW, et al. ACC/AHA guidelines for the management of patients with ST-elevation myocardial infarction; A report of the American College of Cardiology/American Heart Association Task Force on Practice Guidelines

(Committee to Revise the 1999 Guidelines for the Management of patients with acute myocardial infarction). J Am Coll Cardiol 2004; 44: E1–E211.

11. Parker JD, Parker JO. Nitrate therapy for stable angina pectoris. N Engl J Med 1998; 338: 520–31.

12. Thadani U, Lipicky RJ. Short and long-acting oral nitrates for stable angina pectoris. Cardiovasc Drugs Ther 1994; 8: 611–23.

13. Gibbons RJ, Abrams J, Chatterjee K, et al. ACC/AHA 2002 guideline update for the management of patients with chronic stable angina–summary article: a report of the American College of Cardiology/American Heart Association Task Force on practice guidelines (Committee on the Management of Patients With Chronic Stable Angina). J Am Coll Cardiol 2003; 41: 159–68.

14. Chen ZM, Pan HC, Chen YP, et al. Early intravenous then oral metoprolol in 45,852 patients with acute myocardial infarction: randomised placebo-controlled trial. Lancet 2005; 366: 1622–32.

15. Pfisterer M, Cox JL, Granger CB, et al. Atenolol use and clinical outcomes after thrombolysis for acute myocardial infarction: the GUSTO-I experience. Global utilization of streptokinase and TPA (alteplase) for occluded coronary arteries. J Am Coll Cardiol 1998; 32: 634–40.

16. Freemantle N, Cleland J, Young P, Mason J, Harrison J. Beta blockade after myocardial infarction: systematic review and meta regression analysis. BMJ 1999; 318: 1730–7.

17. Report of The Holland Interuniversity Nifedipine/Metoprolol Trial (HINT) Research Group. Early treatment of unstable angina in the coronary care unit: a randomised, double blind, placebo controlled comparison of recurrent ischaemia in patients treated with nifedipine or metoprolol or both. Br Heart J 1986; 56: 400–13.

18. Ellis K, Tcheng JE, Sapp S, Topol EJ, Lincoff AM. Mortality benefit of beta blockade in patients with acute coronary syndromes undergoing coronary intervention: pooled results from the Epic, Epilog, Epistent, Capture and Rapport Trials. J Interv Cardiol 2003; 16: 299–305.

19. Yusuf S, Peto R, Lewis J, Collins R, Sleight P. Beta blockade during and after myocardial infarction: an overview of the randomized trials. Prog Cardiovasc Dis 1985; 27: 335–71.

20. Pepine CJ, Cohn PF, Deedwania PC, et al. Effects of treatment on outcome in mildly symptomatic patients with ischemia during daily life. The Atenolol Silent Ischemia Study (ASIST). Circulation 1994; 90: 762–8.

21. Dargie HJ, Ford I, Fox KM. Total Ischaemic Burden European Trial (TIBET). Effects of ischaemia and treatment with atenolol, nifedipine SR and their combination on outcome in patients with chronic stable angina. The TIBET Study Group. Eur Heart J 1996; 17: 104–12.

22. Rehnqvist N, Hjemdahl P, Billing E, et al. Effects of metoprolol vs verapamil in patients with stable angina pectoris. The Angina Prognosis Study in Stockholm (APSIS). Eur Heart J 1996; 17: 76–81.

23. Frishman WH, Heiman M, Soberman J, Greenberg S, Eff J. Comparison of celiprolol and propranolol in stable angina pectoris Celiprolol International Angina Study Group. Am J Cardiol 1991; 67: 665–70.

24. Narahara KA. Double-blind comparison of once daily betaxolol versus propranolol four times daily in stable angina pectoris Betaxolol Investigators Group. Am J Cardiol 1990; 65: 577–82.

25. Krepp HP. Evaluation of the antianginal and anti-ischemic efficacy of slow-release isosorbide-5-mononitrate capsules, bupranolol

26. Yusuf S, Held P, Furberg C. Update of effects of calcium antagonists in myocardial infarction or angina in light of the second Danish Verapamil Infarction Trial (DAVIT-II) and other recent studies. Am J Cardiol 1991; 67: 1295–7.

27. Held PH, Yusuf S, Furberg CD. Calcium channel blockers in acute myocardial infarction and unstable angina: an overview. BMJ 1989; 299: 1187–92.

28. Gibson RS, Boden WE, Theroux P, et al. Diltiazem and reinfarction in patients with non-Q-wave myocardial infarction. Results of a double-blind, randomized, multicenter trial. N Engl J Med 1986; 315: 423–9.

29. Poole-Wilson PA, Lubsen J, Kirwan BA, et al. Effect of long-acting nifedipine on mortality and cardiovascular morbidity in patients with stable angina requiring treatment (ACTION trial): randomised controlled trial. Lancet 2004; 364: 849–57.

30. Lubsen J, Wagener G, Kirwan BA, de Brouwer S, Poole-Wilson PA. Effect of long-acting nifedipine on mortality and cardiovascular morbidity in patients with symptomatic stable angina and hypertension: the ACTION trial. J Hypertens 2005; 23: 641–8.

31. Heidenreich PA, McDonald KM, Hastie T, et al. Meta-analysis of trials comparing beta-blockers, calcium antagonists, and nitrates for stable angina. JAMA 1999; 281: 1927–36.

32. Borer JS, Fox K, Jaillon P, Lerebours G. Antianginal and antiischemic effects of ivabradine, an I(f) inhibitor, in stable angina: a randomized, double-blind, multicentered, placebo-controlled trial. Circulation 2003; 107: 817–23.

33. Tardif JC, Ford I, Tendera M, Bourassa MG, Fox K. Efficacy of ivabradine, a new selective I(f) inhibitor, compared with atenolol in patients with chronic stable angina. Eur Heart J 2005; 26: 25, 29–36.

34. Fox K, Garcia MA, Ardissino D, et al. Guidelines on the management of stable angina pectoris: executive summary: the Task Force on the Management of Stable Angina Pectoris of the European Society of Cardiology. Eur Heart J 2006; 27: 1341–81.

35. Fox K, Ford I, Steg PG, Tendera M,, Ferrari R. Ivabradine for patients with stable coronary artery disease and left-ventricular systolic dysfunction (BEAUTIFUL): a randomised, double-blind, placebo-controlled trial. Lancet 2008; 372: 807–16.

36. Chaitman BR. Ranolazine for the treatment of chronic angina and potential use in other cardiovascular conditions. Circulation 2006; 113: 2462–72.

37. Chaitman BR, Pepine CJ, Parker JO, et al. Effects of ranolazine with atenolol, amlodipine, or diltiazem on exercise tolerance and angina frequency in patients with severe chronic angina: a randomized controlled trial. JAMA 2004; 291: 309–16.

38. Stone PH, Gratsiansky NA, Blokhin A, Huang IZ, Meng L. Antianginal efficacy of ranolazine when added to treatment with amlodipine: the ERICA (Efficacy of Ranolazine in Chronic Angina) trial. J Am Coll Cardiol 2006; 48: 566–75.

39. Morrow DA, Scirica BM, Karwatowska-Prokopczuk E, et al. Effects of ranolazine on recurrent cardiovascular events in patients with non-ST-elevation acute coronary syndromes: the MERLIN-TIMI 36 randomized trial. JAMA 2007; 297: 1775–83.

40. Walker A, McMurray J, Stewart S, et al. Economic evaluation of the impact of nicorandil in angina (IONA) trial. Heart 2006; 92: 619–24.

41. Morrow DA, Givertz MM. Modulation of myocardial energetics: emerging evidence for a therapeutic target in cardiovascular disease. Circulation 2005; 112: 3218–21.

42. Chazov EI, Lepakchin VK, Zharova EA, et al. Trimetazidine in Angina Combination Therapy–the TACT study: trimetazidine versus conventional treatment in patients with stable angina pectoris in a randomized, placebo-controlled, multicenter study. Am J Ther 2005; 12: 35–42.

43. The EMIP-FR Group. European Myocardial Infarction Project–Free Radicals. Effect of 48-h intravenous trimetazidine on short- and long-term outcomes of patients with acute myocardial infarction, with and without thrombolytic therapy; A double-blind, placebo-controlled, randomized trial. Eur Heart J 2000; 21: 1537–46.

24 Antithrombotic pharmacotherapy in patients with established coronary artery disease

Antonio Tello-Montoliu and Dominick J. Angiolillo

OUTLINE

Acute coronary syndromes (ACS), including unstable angina (UA), non–ST-segment elevation myocardial infarction (NSTEMI), and ST-segment elevation myocardial infarction (STEMI) are the clinical expression of non-occlusive and occlusive thrombus formation following plaque rupture and superficial endothelial cell erosion in patients with coronary atherosclerosis. Antithrombotic therapy is pivotal in the management of atherosclerotic coronary disease, as demonstrated by numerous clinical trials whose findings have been incorporated in clinical practice guidelines. Antithrombotic treatment regimens include antiplatelet and anticoagulant agents, used solely or in combination, to overcome the pathological process of intracoronary thrombus formation. This chapter summarizes the currently available antithrombotic therapies used for the acute and long-term management of patients with established coronary artery disease.

BASIC PRINCIPLES OF THROMBOSIS AND RATIONALE FOR ANTITHROMBOTIC THERAPY

In the coronary artery, rupture of an atheromatous plaque and subsequent thrombus formation is the substrate for the majority of acute coronary syndromes (ACS). Plaque rupture or erosion exposes subendothelial collagen which allows platelet adhesion at the site of vessel injury; this is followed by activation and aggregation of platelets (Fig. 24.1) (1,2). The dynamic process of thrombus formation can be summarized in four phases:

1. Initiation and formation of the platelet plug. This phase is composed at the same time of three stages: *initiation phase* involving platelet adhesion, *extension phase* that includes activation, additional recruitment, and aggregation, *perpetuation phase* characterized by platelet stimulation and stabilization of clot.
2. Propagation of the clotting process. Mainly driven from the coagulation cascade which consist in the sequential activation of a series of proenzymes inactive precursor proteins (zymogens) to active enzymes, resulting in significant stepwise response amplification.
3. Termination of clotting by antithrombotic control mechanisms.
4. Removal of the clot by fibrinolysis.

Thrombus formation in acute atherothrombotic events can be either partially or completely occlusive (1,2). The former is composed primarily of platelet aggregates whereas the latter is composed of platelet aggregates and a fibrin-rich clot generated by the coagulation cascade. Platelet-rich, white thrombi are typically not completely occlusive and are often associated with non-ST elevation (NSTE)–ACS. Progression to completely occlusive thrombus mediated by the coagulation cascade involves the formation of a fibrin-rich, red clot superimposed on the underlying platelet-rich, white thrombus, and is usually found in ST elevation myocardial infarction (STEMI) patients (1,2). Advances in the understanding of the complex mechanisms regulating these processes has been pivotal for the development of antithrombotic therapies inhibiting platelets (antiplatelet therapies) and coagulation factors (anticoagulant therapies) used for the prevention of recurrent atherothrombotic events, as described below.

ANTIPLATELET THERAPY

Currently, there are three different classes of antiplatelet agents that are approved for the treatment and/or prevention of recurrent events in patients with coronary artery disease (CAD). These include cyclooxygenase (COX-1) inhibitors, adenosine diphosphate (ADP) $P2Y_{12}$ receptor antagonists, and glycoprotein (GP) IIb/IIIa inhibitors.

Aspirin

Mechanisms of Action

Aspirin exerts its effects by irreversibly inactivating COX activity of prostaglandin H (PGH) synthase 1 and synthase 2, also referred to as COX-1 and COX-2, respectively (Fig. 24.2) (3). Thromboxane A_2 (TXA_2), an amplifier of platelet activation and a vasoconstrictor, is mainly derived from platelet COX-1 and is highly sensitive to inhibition by aspirin, while vascular PGI_2, a platelet inhibitor and a vasodilator, is derived largely from COX-2 and is less susceptible to inhibition by low-doses of aspirin. Therefore, low-dose aspirin ultimately preferentially blocks platelet formation of TXA_2 diminishing platelet activation and aggregation processes mediated by thromboxane (TP) receptor pathways (3). Aspirin is rapidly absorbed in the upper gastrointestinal tract and is associated with detectable platelet inhibition within 60 minutes (3). The plasma half-life of aspirin is approximately 20 minutes and peak plasma levels are achieved within 30–40 minutes. Enteric-coated aspirin delays absorption and peak plasma levels are achieved at 3–4 hours after ingestion. Because platelets have minimal capacity for protein synthesis and since COX-1 blockade induced by aspirin is irreversible, COX-mediated TXA_2 synthesis is prevented for the entire life span of the platelet (~7–10 days) (3).

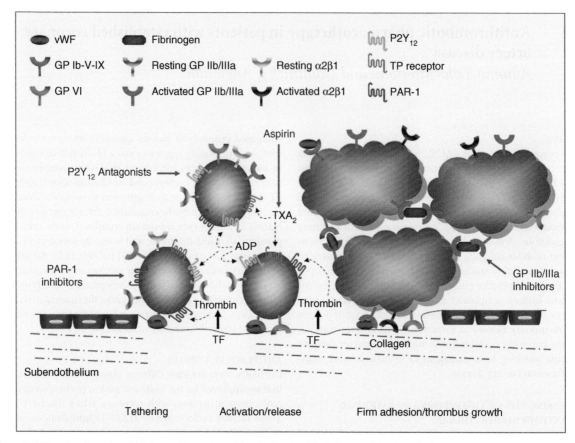

Figure 24.1 Thombus formation: Initiation and formation of the platelet plug. The initiation of the thrombotic response is composed by three stages: platelet adhesion, extension phase, and perpetuation phase. The interaction between glycoprotein (GP) Ib and von Willebrand factor (vWF) mediates platelet tethering, enabling subsequent interaction between GP VI and collagen. This triggers the shift of integrins to a high-affinity state and the release of adenosine diphosphate (ADP) and thromboxane A_2 (TXA_2) which bind to the $P2Y_{12}$ and TP receptors, respectively. Tissue factor (TF) locally triggers thrombin formation, which contributes to platelet activation via binding to the platelet protease activated receptor (PAR-1). *Source*: From Ref. 1.

Dosages, Side Effects, and Contraindications

Pharmacodynamic and in vitro studies have shown that aspirin may be effective in inhibiting COX-1 activity at doses as low as 30 mg/day (3). The Antiplatelet Trialists' Collaboration demonstrated that oral aspirin doses of 75–150 mg/day are as effective as higher doses for long-term prevention of ischemic events; aspirin doses <75 mg have been less widely assessed in clinical trials and thus are not recommended (4). Importantly, higher doses of aspirin (>150 mg) do not offer greater protection from recurrent ischemic events but are associated with a higher incidence of side effects, mainly gastrointestinal, and bleeding (4). In the Antithrombotic Trialists' Collaboration meta-analysis, there was an approximate 60% increase in the risk of a major extracranial bleed with antiplatelet therapy. The proportional increase in fatal bleeds was not significantly different from that for non-fatal bleeds; however, only the excess of non-fatal bleeds was significant (4).

Some non-steroidal anti-inflammatory drugs (NSAIDs), such as naproxen, by competing for the COX-1 active site, may interfere with the action of aspirin when administered concomitantly,

resulting in attenuation of its antiplatelet effects (3). This may contribute to the increased risk of ischemic events in patients treated with NSAID, underscoring the need for careful consideration when prescribing NSAIDs to patients using aspirin. Ultimately, three types of aspirin sensitivity have been described: respiratory sensitivity (asthma and/or rhinitis), cutaneous sensitivity (urticaria and/or angioedema), and systemic sensitivity (anaphylactoid reaction). The prevalence of aspirin-exacerbated respiratory tract disease is approximately 10% and for aspirin-induced urticaria the prevalence varies from 0.07% to 0.2% in the general population. In patients with CAD presenting with allergy or intolerance to aspirin, clopiodogrel is the treatment of choice (5,6). Desensitization using escalating doses of oral aspirin is also a therapeutic option (7).

P2Y12 Inhibitors

Mechanisms of Action

Thienopyridine derivatives (ticlopidine, clopidogrel, prasugrel) are non-direct, orally administered and irreversible P2Y12 receptor inhibitors which selectively and irreversibly inhibit the

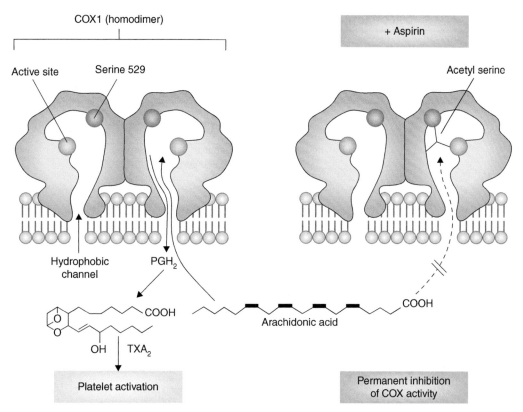

Figure 24.2 Mechanism of aspirin inhibition of cyclo-oxygenase-1. In physiological conditions the substrate of COX1, arachidonic acid, is converted to PGH2, which is consequently converted to TXA2 by thromboxane synthase. Aspirin irreversibly inhibits COX1 through acetylation of a serine residue at position 529 and obstructs the COX1 channel just below the catalytic pocket. preventing its metabolism to the intermediary product, endoperoxide in a irreversible manner. As a result, TXA2 production is inhibited for the platelet's lifespan. *Abbreviations*: COX1, cyclo-oxygenase 1; PGH2, prostaglandin H2; TXA2, thromboxane A2. Acetylation of Ser-529. *Source*: From Sweeny JM, et al. Nat Rev Cardiol 2009; 6: 273–282.

P2Y12 ADP receptor subtype (8,9). When given in combination with aspirin, thienopyridines have a synergistic effect, and therefore achieve greater platelet inhibition than either agent alone (9). Platelet inhibition by thienopyridines is concentration dependent. However, thienopyridines are pro-drugs, thus inactive in vitro and need to be metabolized by the hepatic cytochrome P450 (CYP) system in order to generate an active metabolite which selectively inhibits the P2Y12 receptor (9). Since blockade of P2Y12 is irreversible, platelet inhibitory effects induced by thienopyridines last for the entire life span of the platelet (7–10 days) (Fig. 24.3) (9).

Ticlopidine is a first-generation thienopyridine which has been largely replaced by clopidogrel due to its more favorable safety profile (10). Clopidogrel is a second-generation thienopyridine which requires a two-step oxidation by the hepatic CYP system to generate an active metabolite (9). However, approximately 85% of the prodrug is hydrolyzed by esterases to an inactive carboxylic acid derivative; the remaining 15% is metabolized by the CYP system into an active metabolite. CYP3A4, CYP3A5, CYP2C9, CYP1A2 are involved in one of the oxidation steps; CYP2B6 and CYP2C19 are involved in both steps. Although

clopidogrel has a half-life of only 8 hours, it has an irreversible effect on platelets that lasts for 7–10 days (9).

Prasugrel is a third-generation thienopyridine (9). It is orally administered and, similar to the other thienopyridines, requires hepatic metabolism to generate its active metabolite which irreversibly inhibits the P2Y12 receptor. However, unlike other thienopyridines, prasugrel is more rapidly and effectively converted to an active metabolite through a process involving hydrolysis by carboxyesterases, mainly in the intestine, followed by only a single hepatic CYP-dependent step, involving CYP3A, CYP2B6, CYP2C9 and CYP2C19 isoforms (Fig. 24.3) (9). This more favorable pharmacokinetic profile translates into better pharmacodynamic effects, with more potent platelet inhibition, lower inter-individual variability in platelet response, and a faster onset of activity compared with clopidogrel irrespective of dose (9,11). A 60-mg loading dose of prasugrel achieves 50% platelet inhibition by 30 minutes and 80–90% inhibition by 1–2 hours (9,11).

Ticagrelor is a non-thienopyridine that belongs to a new class of P2Y12 inhibitors called cyclopentyltriazolopyrimidines (CPTP) (12). Ticagrelor is a first-in-class CPTP currently

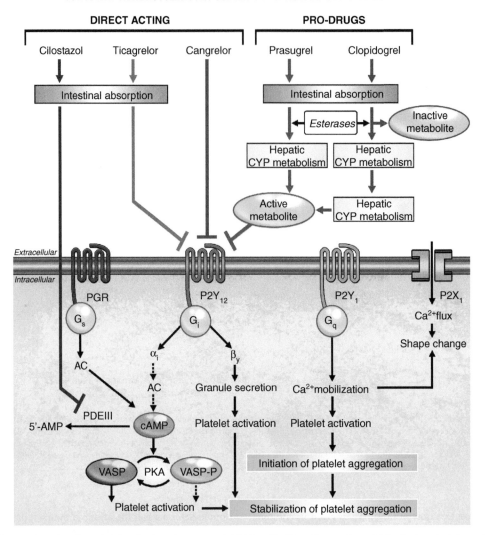

Figure 24.3 Therapeutic options for optimizing platelet P2Y12 receptor inhibition. Clopidogrel is a prodrug, which, after intestinal absorption, undergoes 2-step hepatic oxidation by CYP 2C19 enzymes (CYP3A, CYP2C9, CYP1A2 are involved in 1 step; CYP2B6, CYP2C19 are involved in both steps) to generate an active metabolite that inhibits platelet activation and aggregation processes through irreversible blockade of the P2Y12 receptor. Approximately 85% of clopidogrel is hydrolyzed pre-hepatically by esterases into an inactive compound, thus, only 15% is available for hepatic metabolism. Genetic polymorphisms encoding for proteins/enzymes at various levels modulating clopidogrel metabolism can affect platelet inhibitory effects, intestinal absorption, P-glycoprotein (encoded by ABCB1 gene), hepatic metabolism, CYP enzymes (particularly CYP2C19 loss-of-function alleles), and platelet membrane receptors (e.g., P2 receptors). Increasing the clopidogrel dose is not consistently associated with enhanced platelet inhibition in poor metabolizers, which may be achieved by other strategies. Prasugrel, like clopidogrel, is also an oral prodrug with a similar intestinal absorption process. However, in contrast to clopidogrel, esterases are part of prasugrel's activation pathway, and prasugrel is oxidized more efficiently to its active metabolite via a single CYP-dependent step. Direct-acting antiplatelet agents (cangrelor, ticagrelor, and cilostazol) have reversible effects and do not require hepatic metabolism for pharmacodynamic activity. Ticagrelor and cilostazol are administered orally and, after intestinal absorption, inhibit platelet activation by direct blockade of the P2Y12 receptor and PDE-III, respectively. Cangrelor is administered intravenously, and directly inhibits the P2Y12 receptor, bypassing intestinal absorption. Genetic polymorphisms of target proteins/enzymes (intestine, liver, and platelet membrane) modulating clopidogrel-mediated platelet inhibition do not affect the pharmacodynamic activity of prasugrel, cilostazol, ticagrelor, and cangrelor, which ultimately inhibit platelet activation and aggregation processes by modulating intraplatelet levels of cAMP and VASP-P. *Solid black arrows* indicate activation. *Dotted black arrows* indicate inhibition. *Abbreviations*: AC, adenylyl cyclase; ADP, adenosine diphosphate; ATP, adenosine triphosphate; cAMP, cyclic adenosine monophosphate; PDE-III, phosphodiesterase III (PDEIII); PGE1, prostaglandin E1; PKA, protein kinases; VASP-P, phosphorylation of vasodilator-stimulated phosphoprotein. *Source*: From Angiolillo D, et al. JACC Cardiovasc Interv 2011; 4: 411–14.

approved only in Europe and Canada. Ticagrelor is orally administered and differs in its mechanism of action from thienopyridines due its direct (no metabolism required) and reversible inhibitory effects on the P2Y12 receptor (12). Ticagrelor is rapidly absorbed and has a half-life of 7–12 hours, thus requiring twice daily dosing. However, approximately 5 days are needed after ticagrelor withdrawal to return to baseline function. Compared with clopidogrel, ticagrelor exhibits a higher degree of platelet inhibition, which is achieved more rapidly and with less inter-patient variability (Fig. 24.3) (12).

Dosages, Side Effects, and Contraindications

The approved loading and maintenance doses of clopidogrel are 300 mg and 75 mg, respectively. In the setting of PCI, the recommended loading dose of clopidogrel is 300–600 mg (5,6). A 300-mg loading dose of clopidogrel should be given in patients with STEMI treated with fibrinolytic therapy (6). This should be followed by a maintenance dose of 75 mg daily. No dosage adjustment is necessary for patients with renal impairment, including patients with end-stage renal disease. In patients presenting with an ACS or undergoing PCI, clopidogrel loading dose should be given as early as possible (5,6). Use of a 600-mg clopidogrel load may allow one to reduce the pretreatment period to as short as 2 hours prior to PCI (5,6). In patients presenting with an ACS, clopidogrel 75 mg daily should be given for at least 12 months irrespective of treatment management (medical, PCI, CABG) (5). In patients undergoing PCI, 75 mg daily should be given for at least 12 months regardless of whether the patient was treated with a bare-metal stent (BMS) or drug-eluting stent (DES) (5,6).

Clopidogrel is associated with an increased risk of bleeding which does not differ significantly from that observed with aspirin (13). The incidence of intracranial hemorrhage is 0.4% for clopidogrel compared with 0.5% for aspirin. It is important to note that the combination of both aspirin and clopidogrel, as recommended in the setting of ACS and PCI, has a synergic effect on the occurrence of gastrointestinal bleeding (13). Clopidogrel use is very rarely complicated by neutropenia (0.1%). Thrombotic thrombocytopenic purpura (TTP) is very rare with clopidogrel, but potentially fatal (12). Preoperative clopidogrel exposure increases the risk of reoperation and the requirements for blood and blood product transfusion during and after CABG (13). However, the overall benefits of starting clopidogrel on admission appear to outweigh the risks, even among those who proceed to CABG during the initial hospitalization (14). It is recommended that clopidogrel be discontinued for at least 5 days to allow for dissipation of its antiplatelet effects (5,6). Drug regulatory agencies have recently issued a boxed warning for clopidogrel-treated patients. In particular, this was based on pharmacodynamic studies showing a drug-interaction between proton pump inhibitors (mainly omeprazole and esomeprazole) and clopidogrel, as well as the presence of reduced antiplatelet effects in patients who are carriers of loss-of-function alleles (mainly from CYP2C19) (15).

Prasugrel is currently indicated in patients with ACS in whom PCI is envisaged (5,6,16). These include patients with UA/NSTEMI and patients with STEMI (whether managed with primary or delayed PCI). Treatment with prasugrel should be initiated with a single 60-mg oral loading dose and continued at 10 mg orally once daily. Treatment is recommended for up to 15 months. Prasugrel was also associated with a significantly higher risk of major bleeding, including life-threatening bleeding, compared with clopidogrel (17). The increased risk of bleeding was greater in certain subgroups which limited the net clinical benefit of prasugrel in those subgroups. Patients with prior stroke or TIA had net clinical harm from prasugrel and it should be avoided in these patients. Patients aged ≥75 years and weighing <60 kg had no net benefit from prasugrel (17). One may consider lowering the maintenance dose to 5 mg in the latter settings, although the effectiveness and safety of the 5-mg dose has not been prospectively studied. In patients taking prasugrel in whom CABG is planned and can be delayed, it is recommended that the drug be discontinued for at least 7 days (5,6,16).

Ticagrelor is indicated for the prevention of atherothrombotic events in patients with ACS (UA, NSTEMI, or STEMI), including patients managed medically, and those who are managed with PCI or CABG (16,18). Treatment should be initiated with a single 180 mg loading dose and then continued at 90 mg twice daily. Treatment is recommended for up to 12 months (18). Ticagrelor was not associated in a significant increase in overall bleeding events compared with clopidogrel. However it was associated with a higher rate of major bleeding not related to CABG, including more instances of fatal intracranial bleeding (18). Other non-bleeding adverse events have shown to be higher with ticagrelor versus clopidogrel, including dyspnea, ventricular pauses, and increase in serum uric acid and serum creatinine, which have been associated with higher rates of treatment discontinuation (11,18). In patients taking ticagrelor in whom CABG is planned and can be delayed, it is recommended that the drug be discontinued for at least 7 days (16).

Glycoprotein IIb/IIIa Inhibitors

Mechanisms of Action

There are three parenteral GP IIb/IIIa antagonists approved for clinical use: abciximab, eptifibatide, and tirofiban. Abciximab is a large chimeric monoclonal antibody with a high binding affinity that results in a prolonged pharmacological effect (19). In particular, it is a monoclonal antibody that is a Fab (fragment antigen binding) fragment of a chimeric human-mouse genetic reconstruction of 7E3 (19). Its plasma half-life is biphasic, with an initial half-life of less than 10 minutes and a second-phase half-life of ~30 minutes. However, because of its high affinity for the GP IIb/IIIa receptor, it has a biological half-life of 12–24 hours and because of its slow clearance from the body it has a functional half-life up to 7 days; platelet-associated abciximab can be detected for more than 14 days after treatment discontinuation (19). Eptifibatide is a reversible, and highly selective heptapeptide with a rapid onset and a short plasma half-life of 2–2.5 hours. Recovery of platelet aggregation occurs within 4 hours of infusion discontinuation (19). Tirofiban is a tyrosine-derived non-peptide inhibitor that functions as a mimic of the RGD sequence and is highly specific for the GPIIb/IIIa receptor (19). Tirofiban is associated with a rapid onset and short duration of action, with a plasma half-life of approximately 2 hours. As for eptifibatide, substantial recovery of platelet aggregation is demonstrable within 4 hours of stopping the infusion (19).

Most clinical evidence with the use GP IIb/IIIa inhibitors derives from patients with NSTE–ACS undergoing PCI; these drugs appear to be particularly beneficial in the presence of positive cardiac biomarkers (20). The utility of GP IIb/IIIa inhibitors in patients not undergoing PCI is less clear. Although there is less evidence than in the NSTE–ACS setting, STEMI patients undergoing primary PCI have shown to benefit from GP IIb/IIIa inhibitors in particular abciximab (21).

Dosages, Side Effects, and Contraindications
The recommended dose for abciximab is a bolus dose of 0.25 mg/kg followed by a 12-hour infusion at 0.125 µg/kg/min (to a maximum of 10 µg/min) for patients undergoing PCI (20). In the setting of PCI, a double bolus (10 minutes apart) and infusion regimen of eptifibatide is recommended (180 µg/kg followed by second 180 µg/kg bolus followed by 2 µg/kg/min for a minimum of 12 hours) (6,16,21). Tirofiban is currently not FDA-approved for PCI, although it is both approved and widely used throughout Europe for this indication. Several studies have documented that this approved bolus and infusion regimen for tirofiban (bolus 10 µg/kg followed by infusion 0.15 µg/kg/min for 18–24 hours) achieves suboptimal levels of platelet inhibition for up to 4–6 hours that likely accounted for inferior clinical results in the PCI setting (6,16). For this reason, a high dose bolus regimen (25 µg/kg) achieving more optimal platelet inhibition has been suggested (6,16) . Epifibatide and tirofiban are mostly eliminated through renal mechanism, requiring dose adjustments (epifibatide 1 µg/kg/min in creatinine clearance less than 50 mL/min; tirofiban dose reduction by 50% in creatinine clearance of less than 30 mL/min) (19).

The primary adverse reactions to GP IIb/IIIa receptor antagonists are bleeding and thrombocytopenia. Immune mechanisms responsible for the thrombocytopenia have been identified (19). Although the overall incidence is relatively low, the effects may be life threatening. Thrombocytopenia with abciximab (as defined by a platelet count <100,000/L) occurs in 2.5% to 6% of patients and severe thrombocytopenia (platelet count <50,000/L) occurs in 0.4% to 1.6% of patients in reported clinical trials. Severe thrombocytopenia requires immediate cessation of therapy (19). Thrombocytopenia is less common with eptifibatide and tirofiban. It is important to note that treatment with GP IIb/IIIa inhibitors can also cause pseudo-thrombocytopenia, which occurs as a result of artifactual platelet clumping in vitro, with an incidence be as high as 2.1% with the use of abciximab. A smear to directly examine for the presence of clumped platelets may be required (19).

New Pharmacological Approaches in Antiplatelet Therapy
Cangrelor is a stable ATP analog and a highly selective reversible $P2Y_{12}$ receptor antagonist administered intravenously with a very short half-life (22). Therefore, cangrelor achieves potent platelet inhibition very rapidly (>90% inhibition in a few minutes) with complete restoration of baseline platelet function in less than <60 minutes after treatment discontinuation. However, cangrelor failed to show any clinical benefit in two large-scale phase III trials of patients undergoing PCI (22). Cangrelor is currently being evaluated in another large-scale phase III clinical trial of patients undergoing PCI as well as in a trial in which it is being tested as a bridging strategy for patients undergoing CABG.

Another family of emerging antiplatelet agents is directed toward inhibition of the platelet thrombin receptor or protease activated receptors (PAR) (23). This pathway is of key importance because thrombin is considered to be the most potent activator of platelets. PAR-1 is the principal thrombin receptor on human platelets. PAR-1 antagonists block the binding of thrombin to its receptor thus inhibiting thrombin-induced activation and aggregation of platelets. Pre-clinical observations have shown that inhibition of the platelet PAR-1 receptor selectively interferes with thrombin-induced platelet activation, but not with thrombin-mediated fibrin generation and coagulation that is essential for hemostasis (23). Two PAR-1 antagonists are currently being tested in clinical trials for the prevention of arterial thrombosis: atopaxar (E5555) or vorapaxar (SCH530348).

Other agents are targeted to inhibit TXA2-induced platelet activation mediated by TP receptors (22). The rationale for the development of TP receptor antagonists (e.g. terutroban) is that platelets may continue to be exposed to TXA2 despite complete COX-1 blockade using aspirin. Pre-clinical and clinical studies are currently ongoing for this family of platelet inhibitors as well as for other targets, including serotonin and collagen receptors (Fig. 24.4) (22).

ANTICOAGULANT THERAPY
The role of anticoagulant therapies is to block the activity of coagulation factors. The understanding of the role of coagulation factors in thrombotic processes has led to the development of anticoagulant agents which target specific markers. Factor IIa and factor Xa, are two serine proteases with central roles in the coagulation cascade and have been the target of development of numerous anticoagulant therapies (24).

Unfractionated Heparin
Mechanisms of Action
Unfractionated heparin (UFH) is a heterogeneous mixture of variable molecular weight (2,000–30,000 Daltons) polysaccharide molecules. UFH has two structural components which are pivotal to determine its function: (*i*) a unique pentasaccharide sequence, mainly responsible for factor Xa inhibition and (*ii*) saccharide chain lengths >18 units long, needed to achieve thrombin inhibition (25). The pentasaccharide sequence is

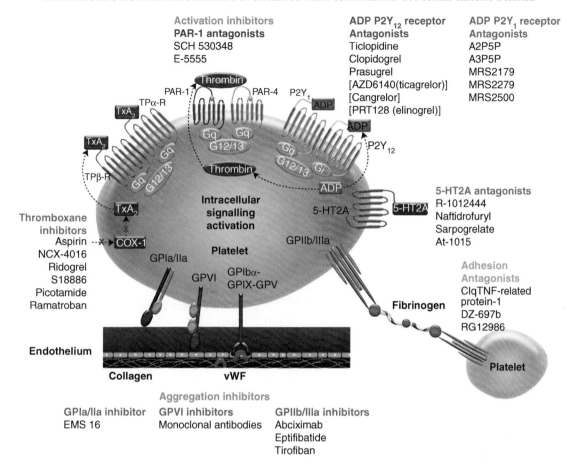

Figure 24.4 Current and emerging antithrombotic drugs and antiplatelet agents. Platelets activation occurs via complex intracellular signaling processes and causes the production and release of multiple agonists, including TXA_2 and ADP, and local production of thrombin. These factors bind to their respective G protein–coupled receptors, mediating paracrine and autocrine platelet activation. Further, they potentiate each other's actions ($P2Y_{12}$ signaling modulates thrombin generation). The major platelet integrin GPIIb/IIIa mediates the final common step of platelet activation by undergoing a conformational shape change and binding fibrinogen and vWF leading to platelet aggregation. The net result of these interactions is thrombus formation mediated by platelet/platelet interactions with fibrin. Current and emerging therapies inhibiting platelet receptors, integrins and proteins involved in platelet activation include the thromboxane inhibitors, the ADP receptor antagonists, the GPIIb/IIIa inhibitors, and the novel PAR antagonists and adhesion antagonists. Reversible-acting agents are indicated by brackets. *Abbreviations*: TP, thromboxane receptor; 5-HT2A, 5-hydroxy tryptamine 2A receptor. *Source*: From Ref. 23.

required for binding of UFH to antithrombin (AT), thereby increasing the potency of AT by up to 1000-fold (Fig. 24.5). This UFH:AT complex inactivates multiple proteases (factors Xa, IXa, XIa, XIIa and IIa). Factor IIa or thrombin and factor Xa are most sensitive to activated AT, but thrombin is ~10 times more susceptible than factor Xa (25).

Dosages, Side Effects, and Contraindications
In patients with ACS, the dose of UFH is usually adjusted to maintain aPTT at an intensity equivalent to a heparin level of 0.2 to 0.4 U/mL as measured by protamine titration or by an anti-factor Xa level of 0.30 to 0.7 U/mL. For many aPTT reagents, this is equivalent to a ratio (patient/control aPTT) of 1.5 to 2.5 (5,6). Treatment with UFH is usually initiated at time of clinical presentation in a patient with ACS. For UA/NSTEMI, an initial IV bolus of 60–70 U per kg (maximum 4,000 U) followed by continuous infusion of 12–15 U/hour (maximum 1,000 U/hour) (5,6). For STEMI patients receiving non-streptokinase fibrinolytic therapy regimens, the dosing of UFH is at the lower end of this range with an initial IV bolus 60 U/kg (maximum 4000 U) followed by continuous infusion of 12 U per kg per hour (maximum 1000 U per hour), adjusted to maintain the aPTT at 1.5–2.0 times control (approximately 50–70 seconds). Monitoring of aPTT should be performed 6 hours after any dosing change or if there is a significant change in the patient's condition. The duration of UFH infusion after fibrinolytic therapy should generally not exceed 48 hours (5,6).

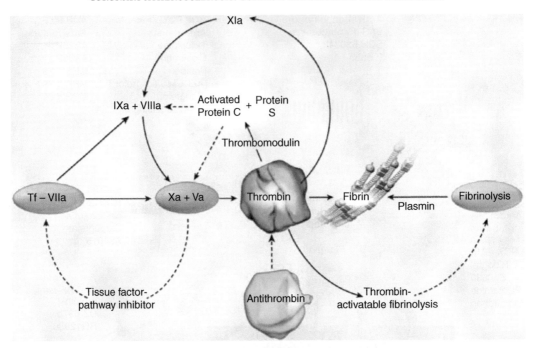

Figure 24.5 Mechanism of thrombin generation. The activation of coagulation proceeds through a stepwise activation of proteases that eventually results in the fibrin framework. After vascular injury, tissue factor expression by endothelial cells is a critical step in the initial formation of fibrin, whereas the activation of factors XI, IX, and VIII is important to continue the formation of fibrin. The molecule of thrombin plays a central role within the coagulation cascade. The formation of the clot is highly regulated by natural anticoagulant mechanisms that confine the hemostatic process to the site of the injury to the vessel. Most of these natural anticoagulants are directed against the generation or action of thrombin and include antithrombin and the protein C system. *Solid lines* denote activation pathways and *dashed lines* denote inhibitory pathway. *Source*: From Ref. 28.

The primary side effect associated with the use of UFH is bleeding. The risk of bleeding with IV unfractionated heparin is <3% in recent trials (25). The bleeding risk increases with higher heparin dosages, concomitant use of antiplatelet drugs, or oral anticoagulants, and with increasing age (>70 years) (25). Reversal of the anticoagulant effect of UFH can be achieved rapidly with an IV bolus of protamine using one milligram of protamine to neutralize 100 U of UFH. Another problem associated with heparin is the development of heparin-induced thrombocytopenia (HIT), usually developing between 5 and 15 days after the initiation of heparin therapy. A more rapid onset form may occur in patients who have previously been exposed to heparin. In the setting of HIT, an alternative antithrombin drug must be selected. Less commonly, long-term use of heparin can be associated with the development of osteoporosis and rare allergic reactions (25).

Low-Molecular Weight Heparin

Mechanisms of Action

Low-molecular weight heparins (LMWHs) are produced through depolymerization of the polysaccharide chains of UFH, producing fragments ranging from 2,000 to 10,000 Da (26). These shorter chain lengths contain the unique pentasaccharide sequence necessary to bind to AT, but are too short (<18 saccharides) to form the ternary complex crosslinking AT

and thrombin. Therefore, the primary effect of LMWHs is limited to AT-dependent factor Xa inhibition. LMWHs are potent inhibitors of both thrombin (anti-IIa effects) and factor Xa (26). LMWHs can be given by subcutaneous administration and do not require monitoring due to their more rapid and predictable absorption. The LMWHs also produce fewer platelet agonist effects and are less often associated with HIT. Following subcuatenous injection, LMWHs have a more predictable anticoagulant response and greater than 90% bioavailability. Anti-Xa levels peak 3–5 hours after a subcutaneous (SC) dose of LMWH (26). The elimination half-life of LMWHs is largely dose-independent and occurs 3–6 hours following a SC dose. However, LMWHs are cleared by the kidney, leading to prolonged anti-Xa effect and linear accumulation of anti-Xa activity in patients with a creatinine clearance <30 ml/min.

Dosages, Side Effects, and Contraindications

The safety and efficacy of LMWHs have been established in patients with UA/NSTEMI and STEMI as well as patients undergoing PCI (5,6). Although many different LMWH preparations have been developed, enoxaparin has been most thoroughly studied. Anticoagulant therapy should be added to antiplatelet therapy in UA/NSTEMI patients as soon as possible after presentation (5,6). Enoxaparin (1 mg/kg subcutaneously twice daily) has established efficacy for patients in whom an invasive or conservative strategy is selected. Careful attention is needed to appropriately adjust LMWH dose in patients with renal insufficiency (1.0 mg/kg subcutaneously every 24 hours for patients with an estimated creatinine clearance of <30 mL/min) (5,6). If LMWH has been started as the upstream anticoagulant it should be continued without **addition** of UFH. If patients undergo PCI, enoxaparin can be administered in several ways: (*i*) the first dosing regimen option is 1 mg/kg subcutaneously twice daily; when this route is used, it is important to ensure that the last dose of subcutaneous LMWH is administered within 8 hours of the procedure and that at least two subcutaneous doses of LMWH are given before the procedure to ensure a steady state; (*ii*) if the last dose of enoxaparin was given 8–12 h before PCI, a 0.3 mg/kg bolus of IV enoxaparin is recommended at the time of PCI; (*iii*) the third dosing regimen option is 1 mg/kg enoxaparin intravenously (if no GP IIb/IIIa inhibitor is used) or 0.75 mg/kg (if a GP IIb/IIIa inhibitor is used) at the time of PCI. For elective PCI, an intravenous dose of 0.5 mg/kg was found to be safe in the STEEPLE (SafeTy and Efficacy of Enoxaparin in PCI patients, an internationaL randomized Evaluation) study (27).

In the setting of patients with STEMI treated with fibrinolysis, in the presence of preserved renal function, the recommended dosing for enoxaparin is: for age < 75 years, 30-mg IV bolus followed by 1 mg/kg SC q12h (maximum of 100 mg for the first two SC doses); and for age >75 years, no IV bolus, 0.75 mg/kg SC q12h (maximum of 75 mg for the first two SC doses) Enoxaparin is preferred over UFH and should be given before fibrinolytic administration (5,6,16).

As with UFH, LMWH should not be given to patients with contraindications to anticoagulant therapy such as active bleeding, significant thrombocytopenia, recent neurosurgery, intracranial bleed, or ocular surgery. Caution should be exercised in patients with bleeding diathesis, brain metastases, recent major trauma, endocarditis, and severe hypertension. LMWH is associated with less major bleeding compared with UFH in acute venous thromboembolism (26). UFH and LMWH are not associated with an increase in major bleeding in ischemic coronary syndromes, but are associated with an increase in major bleeding in ischemic stroke (25,26). Bleeding complications are increased in patients with renal dysfunction, who should have their dose of enoxparin appropriately titrated. The degree to which the anti-Xa activity of LMWH is neutralized by protamine is variable and uncertain. Patients treated with LMWH can develop HIT, and these drugs are not recommended for use in patients with documented or suspected HIT (26).

Direct Thrombin Inhibitors
Direct thrombin inhibitors (DTIs) currently available and approved for use include leprudin, argatroban and bivalirudin (28). All DTIs exert their anticoagulant effects by direct binding to thrombin (Fig. 24.6). In turn, this inhibits thrombin activity and thrombin-mediated activation of other coagulation factors (e.g. fibrin from fibrinogen) as well as thrombin-induced platelet aggregation (28). DTIs inhibit clot-bound as well as free thrombin, thereby providing a potential rationale for clinical use in the setting of ACS and PCI. However, the current indication for lepidurin and agobatran is for the treatment patients with HIT (28), while bivalirudin is indicated in ACS and PCI settings (5,6,16).

Bivalirudin
Mechanisms of Action
Bivalirudin is a 20-amino acid polypeptide and is a synthetic version of hirudin. Its amino-terminal D-Phe-Pro-Arg-Pro domain, which interacts with active site of thrombin, is linked via four Gly residues to a dodecapeptide analogue of the carboxy-terminal of hirudin (thrombin exosite). Bivalirudin forms a 1:1 stoichiometric complex with thrombin, but once bound, the amino terminal of bivalirudin is cleaved by thrombin, thereby restoring thrombin activity (28). Bivalirudin has a half-life of 25 minutes, with proteolysis, hepatic metabolism, and renal excretion contributing to its clearance (28). The half-life of bivalirudin is prolonged with severe renal impairment, and dose adjustment is required for dialysis. In contrast to hirudin, bivalirudin is not immunogenic, although antibodies against hirudin can cross-react with bivalirudin with unknown clinical consequences (28).

Dosages, Side Effects, and Contraindications
Bivalirudin is currently FDA-approved for use during PCI as an alternative to UFH. The recommended dose in PCI is a bolus of 0.75 mg/kg followed by an infusion of 1.75 mg/kg/h for the duration of PCI (5,6,16). There is robust clinical trial experience supporting the use of bivalirudin in patients with UA/NSTEMI and STEMI undergoing PCI as an alternative to UFH plus GP IIb/IIIa inhibitor (29). In particular, bivalirudin has been associated with similar ischemic protection compared with GP IIb/IIIa inhibitors, but with less bleeding complications resulting in a superior net clinical outcome. Importantly, this has also been translated into reduced long-term mortality rates (29).

Patients with moderate renal impairment (30–59 mL/min) should receive an infusion of 1.75 mg/kg/h. If the creatinine clearance is less than 30 mL/min, reduction of the infusion rate to 1 mg/kg/h should be considered. If a patient is on hemodialysis, the infusion rate should be reduced to 0.25 mg/kg/h. The infusion may be continued for 4 hours after the procedure at the discretion of the operator (5,6,16).

Factor Xa Inhibitors
Fondaparinux
Mechanism of Action
Fondaparinux is a synthetic analog of the AT-binding pentasaccharide sequence found in UFH. Fondaparinux is a selective factor Xa inhibitor that binds reversibly to AT producing an irreversible conformational change at the reactive site of AT that enhances its reactivity with factor Xa (30). Once released from AT, fondaparinux is available to activate additional AT molecules. Fonadaparinux has shown to have 100% bioavailability

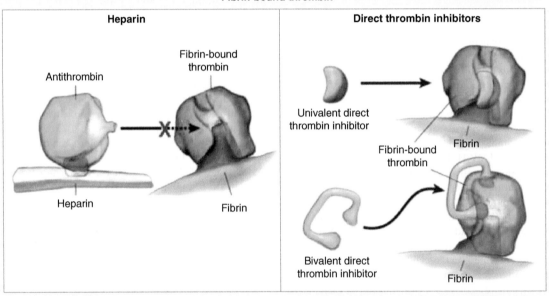

Figure 24.6 Mechanism of action of direct thrombin inhibitors compared with heparin. In the absence of heparin, the rate of thrombin inactivation by antithrombin is relatively low, but after conformational change induced by heparin, antithrombin irreversibly binds to and inhibits the active site of thrombin. Thus, the anticoagulant activity of heparin originates from its ability to generate a ternary heparin–thrombin–antithrombin complex. The activity of DTIs is independent of the presence of antithrombin and is related to the direct interaction of these drugs with the thrombin molecule. Although bivalent DTIs simultaneously bind the exosite 1 and the active site, the univalent drugs in this class interact only with an active site of the enzyme. In the lower panel, the heparin–antithrombin complex cannot bind fibrin-bound thrombin, whereas given their mechanism of action, DTIs can bind to and inhibit the activity of not only soluble thrombin but also thrombin bound to fibrin, as is the case in a blood clot. *Source:* From Ref. 28.

after SC injection with rapid absorption, achieving a steady state after 3–4 daily doses (30). The elimination half-life is 17 hours with clearance that occurs primarily via the kidney and is therefore contraindicated in patients with severe renal impairment. Fondaparinux produces a predictable anticoagulant response and exhibits linear pharmacokinetics when given in SC doses of 2–8 mg or in IV doses ranging from 2–20 mg that result in

anti-Xa activity that is approximately seven times that of LMWHs (30). The anticoagulant effect of fondaparinux can be measured in anti-factor Xa units, although monitoring is not required. Fondaparinux does not affect other parameters of anticoagulation, including aPTT, activated clotting time, or prothrombin time. Fondaparinux has minimal non-specific binding to plasma proteins. Fondaparinux does not induce the formation

Table 24.1 Antiplatelet Therapy

Drug	Mechanism of action	Indication (guidelines)	Dosage Initial	Dosage Maintenance	Side effects/contraindications	Interactions	Level of evidence
Aspirin	Irreversible inhibition COX activity	Secondary prevention ACS (UA, NSTEMI, STEMI)	162–325 mg nonenteric formulation, orally or chewed	75–162 mg After PCI: 162–325 mg nonenteric formulation, orally or chewed[a]	Bleeding complications: gastrointestinal (60% of extracranial bleeding), increase of risk in combination with other antithrombotic therapies Sensitivity: Respiratory, cotaneous and systemic	NSAIDs: attenuation platelet effects	IA
Clopidogrel	Non-direct, and irreversible P2Y12 receptor inhibitor	Secondary prevention (as alternative to aspirin) ACS (UA, NSTEMI, STEMI) PCI (stable patients) with stent	300 mg oral LD[b] In a PCI: 300–600 mg LD In patients already under clopidogrel therapy a second LD of 300 mg could be administered	75 mg oral. At least for 1 year in ACS/PCI with DES. In BMS at least 1 month (in patients without high risk of bleeding)	Bleeding complications. Increase of CABG related bleeding (suspension at least 5 days before if it's possible) Neutropenia, PPT (very rare)	PPIs: Omeprazole and esomeprazole[c] Box warning with carriers of loss-of-function alleles	IA IB (maintenance duration 1 year) IC
Prasugrel	Non-direct, and irreversible P2Y12 receptor inhibitor	ACS who are to be managed with PCI	60 mg oral LD	10 mg oral per day (up to 15 months).	Bleeding Events. It should be avoided in patients with prior stroke or TIA; Increase of CABG related bleeding (suspension at least 7 days) No benefit in >75 years old or weight <60kg	No observed	IB
Ticagrelor	Non-thienopyridine (CPTP), direct acting and reversible P2Y12 receptor inhibitor	ACS (NSTEMI)	180 mg oral LD	90 mg oral twice daily (up to 12 months)	Bleeding events. Increase of major non-CABG related bleeding (contraindicated intracranial hemorrhage history) dyspnea, syncope, ventricular pauses ≥3 s (contraindicated bradicardia or SSS) and increase in serum uric acid and serum creatinine	Caution with concomitant ARB.	Only approved in EU (IB)
Abciximab	Parenteral GP IIb/IIIa antagonist (monoclonal antibody)	ACS with PCI planned	0.25 mg/Kg IV bolus	0.125 μg/Kg/min for 12 hours (max 10 μg/min)	Bleeding events Thrombocytopenia Pseudothrombocytopenia	Re-administration increases slightly the risk of thrombocytopenia	IB
Eptifibatide	Parenteral GP IIb/IIIa antagonist (heptapeptide)	ACS with PCI planned	180 μg/Kg IV bolus	0.2 μg/Kg/min for 18–24 hours	Bleeding events Thrombocytopenia (less risk than abciximab) Pseudothrombocytopenia	None described	IB
Tirofiban	Parenteral GP IIb/IIIa antagonist (tyrosine-derived non-peptide)	ACS with PCI planned	0.4 μg/Kg IV bolus	0.1 μg/Kg/min for 18–24 hours	Bleeding events Thrombocytopenia (less risk than abciximab) Pseudothrombocytopenia	None described	IB

[a]Dosage based in earlier randomized trials. However low-dose aspirin (75–162 mg) should be preferred (see also text). [b]Guidelines usually referred 300–600 mg in ACS, however 600 mg has not shown to be superior to 300 mg if PCI is not planned (results CURRENT-OASIS 7). [c]Pantoprazole is not related with pharmacodynamic interaction with clopidogrel. *Abbreviations:* COX, cyclooxygenase; ACS, acute coronary syndrome; UA, unstable angina; NSTEMI, non ST elevation myocardial infarction; STEMI, ST elevation myocardial infarction; PCI, percutaneous coronary intervention; LD, loading dose; NSAIDs, non-steroidal anti-inflammatory drugs; DES, drug-eluting stent; BMS, bare metal stent; CABG, coronary artery by-pass graft surgery; PPT, Thrombotic thrombocytopenic purpura; PPI, Proton-pump inhibitors; TIA, Transient ischemic attack; CPTP, cyclopentyltriazolopyrimidines; SSS, Sinus-sick syndrome; ARB, Angiotensin recetor blockers; EU, European Union; GP, Glycoprotein. *Source:* Adapted from Refs. 5 and 6.

of UFH:platelet factor-IV complexes and does not cross-react with HIT antibodies, making HIT unlikely to occur (30).

Dosages, Side Effects, and Contraindications
In patients with acute STEMI and not receiving reperfusion therapy, the recommended dosing for fondaparinux is 2.5 mg IV for the first dose and then SC qd up to 9 days (6,29); in patients with acute STEMI receiving fibrinolytic therapy, this fondaparinux regimen could be used as an alternative to heparin (6). In patients with UA/NSTEMI, fondaparinux (2.5 mg SC daily) is also the recommended dose (30) and has been associated with a lower rate of major bleeding events, resulting in superior net clinical benefit with fondaparinux compared with enoxaparin. Importantly, mortality at 6 months was also reduced with fondaparinux compared with enoxaparin. However, in the group of patients who underwent PCI, there was evidence for more catheter-related thrombus formation with fondaparinux, indicating that anticoagulation with fondaparinux alone is insufficient for PCI and adjunctive UFH should be used. Fondaparinux should not be used in patients with acute STEMI undergoing primary PCI. Fondaparinux should be avoided with creatinine clearance of <30 mL/min (5,6,17).

New Pharmacological Approaches in Anticoagulant Therapy
Oral factor IIa and Xa inhibitors are currently under intense clinical investigation for deep venous thrombosis and atrial fibrillation with the hopes of replacing the coumarins for the long-term treatment of thromboembolic disorders. However, they are also under clinical investigation in the setting of ACS

(Fig. 24.7) (24). Dabigatran is a direct oral thrombin inhibitor that has been recently approved for clinical use as a replacement for warfarin in patients with atrial fibrillation based on the RE-LY trial (24). It has a half-life of 12–17 hours and is administered twice daily without need for monitoring. The efficacy and safety of dabigatran in ACS is under investigation; results from phase II clinical trial have been reported showing a low overall increase in major bleeding in comparison with placebo (24). Oral anti-Xa inhibitors, such as apixaban and rivaroxaban, are also under clinical investigation as adjunctive therapies to standard treatment regimens in ACS patients (24). Of note, a phase III clinical investigation with apixaban was interrupted prematurely due to safety concerns. A phase III investigation with rivoroxaban has recently completed enrollment. (24).

GUIDELINES
The current indications, dosage, side effects, and level of recommendation of antithrombotic therapies according to practice guidelines are described in Tables 24.1 and 24.2.

PERSONAL PERSPECTIVE
Antithrombotic therapy is pivotal in the management of CAD manifestations. In particular, antiplatelet and anticoagulant agents used in combination are essential to overcome the pathological process of intracoronary thrombus formation particularly in the early phases of ACS, while prevention of recurrent ischemic events mostly relies on antiplatelet treatment regimens. The continuous advances in our understanding of this process has provided the basis for the development of new

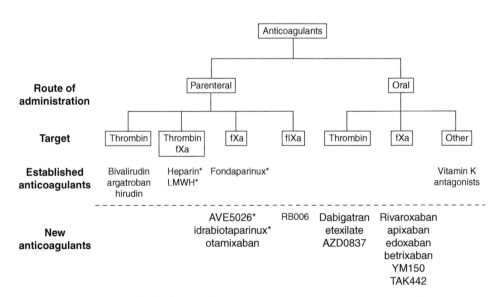

Figure 24.7 Current and new anticoagulants. Classification of established anticoagulants and new anticoagulants, in order of route of administration and target which interacts. fIXa indicates factor IXa. *Indirectly inhibit coagulation by interacting with antithrombin. †AVE5026 is an ultralow-molecular-weight heparin that primarily inhibits fXa and has minimal activity against thrombin. *Source*: From Eikelboom JW, et al. Circulation 2010;121:1523–1532.

Table 24.2 Anticoagulant Therapy

Drug	Mechanism of action	Indication (guidelines)	Dosage initial	Dosage maintenance	Side effects/contraindications	Interactions	Level of evidence
UFH	Factor Xa and IIa inhibition (indirect)	ACS (UA,NSTEMI,STEMI) early treatment PCI (stable patients)	Initial IV bolus of 60–70 U per kg (maximum 4,000 U) pre-fibrinolysis 60 U IV bolus	Continuous infusion of 12–15 U per kg per hour (maximum 1,000 U per hour), 12 U Iv after fibrinolytic therapy[a] Duration: not exceed 48 h	Bleeding complications: <3%. Increases risk: higher dosages, concomitant use of antiplatelet drugs or oral anticoagulants, and increasing age (>70 years) HIT: 5 and 15 days after Osteoporosis and rare allergic reactions (very rare)	Avoid combination with: Corticorelin, and consider modification with Drotrecogin alfa.	IA
LMWHs (enoxaparin)	Factor Xa and IIa inhibition (indirect)	ACS (UA,NSTEMI,STEMI) PCI (stable patients)	30 mg IV bolus	1 mg/kg sc each 12 h 1 mg/kg sc 24 h creatinine clearance of <30 mL/min Duration: up to 8 days	Bleeding complications. Increasing in renal dysfunction HIT.	Same than heparin.	IA Medically managed patient IIa B(no CABG in 24 h)
Bivalirudin	Direct thrombin inhibition	PCI (alternative to UFH) Primary PCI	0.75 mg/kg bolus	1.75 mg/kg/h for the duration of PCI (up to 4 h after) clearance of <30 mL/min: 1 mg/kg/h Hemodialysis: 0.25 mg/kg/h	Bleeding Events	No serious observed	IB
Fondaparinux	Factor Xa inhibition (indirect)	ACS (UA/NSTEMI)		2.5 mg SC daily Avoid with creatinine clearance of <30 mL/min Duration: up to 9 days	Bleeding events. Lower incidence than UFH or LMWHs Increase of catheter-related thrombus formation Should be avoided in STEMI with primary PCI	Same than heparin.	IB IIaB

Abbreviations: ACS, acute coronary syndrome; UA, unstable angina; NSTEMI, non ST elevation myocardial infarction; STEMI, ST elevation myocardial infarction; PCI, percutaneous coronary intervention; UFH, unfractionated heparin; HIT, heparin-induced thrombocytopenia; LMWHs, Low-molecular weight heparin; CABG, coronary artery by-pass graft surgery; IV, intra venous; SC, sub cutaneous.

Source. Adapted from Refs. 5,6.

[a]Adjusted to maintain the APTT at 1.5 to 2.0 times control (approximately 50–70 seconds).

- Aspirin is the mainstay of treatment in patients with CAD manifestations
- Adjunctive P2Y12 receptor inhibiting therapy is associated with enhanced short and long-term ischemic benefit
- Clopidogrel is the most commonly used P2Y12 receptor inhibitor and is approved in all atherosclerotic manifestations
- More novel P2Y12 inhibiting agents, such as prasugrel and ticagrelor, are characterized by more potent platelet inhibition and greater reduction in recurrent atherothrombotic events compared with clopidogrel in ACS patients, albeit at the expense of increased spontaneous bleeding
- Glycoprotein IIb/IIIa inhibitors are associated with a reduction in ischemic events in ACS patients, although they are associated with an increased risk of bleeding. Bivalirudin, a direct thrombin inhibitor, has shown to be associated with similar ischemic benefit, and lower bleeding rates compared with heparin plus glycoprotein IIb/IIIa inhibitors
- Novel antithrombotic strategies are being developed to maximize the fine balance between safety and efficacy of antiplatelet and anticoagulant agents

treatment strategies, which include novel agents, aimed at reducing recurrent atherothrombotic events while minimizing bleeding complications. Ongoing research aimed at defining the thrombotic profile of a given patient will likely set the stage for more tailored antithrombotic treatment regimens. In particular, studies integrating pharmacodynamic and pharmacogenetic data will prove useful in this context. Indeed, integrating this information with the patient's phenotype will hopefully define the optimal balance between safety and efficacy which is the ultimate goal of antithrombotic treatment regimens.

REFERENCES
1. Angiolillo DJ, Ueno M, Goto S. Basic principles of platelet biology and clinical implications. Circ J 2010; 74: 597–607.
2. Davì G Patrono C. Platelet activation and atherothrombosis. N Engl J Med 2007; 357: 2482–94.
3. Patrono C, García Rodríguez LA, Landolfi R, Baigent C. Low-dose aspirin for the prevention of atherothrombosis. N Engl J Med 2005; 353: 2373–83.
4. Baigent C, Blackwell L, Collins R, et al. Antithrombotic Trialists' (ATT) Collaboration. Aspirin in the primary and secondary prevention of vascular disease: collaborative meta-analysis of individual participant data from randomised trials. Lancet 2009; 373: 1849–60.
5. Wright RS, Anderson JL, Adams CD, et al. 2011 ACCF/AHA Focused Update of the Guidelines for the Management of Patients With Unstable Angina/Non-ST-Elevation Myocardial Infarction (Updating the 2007 Guideline) A Report of the American College of Cardiology Foundation/American Heart Association Task Force

on Practice Guidelines Developed in Collaboration With the American College of Emergency Physicians, Society for Cardiovascular Angiography and Interventions, and Society of Thoracic Surgeons. J Am Coll Cardiol 2011; 57: 1920–59.
6. Kushner FG, Hand M, Smith SC Jr, et al. 2009 focused updates: ACC/AHA guidelines for the management of patients with ST-elevation myocardial infarction (updating the 2004 guideline and 2007 focused update) and ACC/AHA/SCAI guidelines on percutaneous coronary intervention (updating the 2005 guideline and 2007 focused update) a report of the American College of Cardiology Foundation/American Heart Association Task Force on Practice Guidelines. J Am Coll Cardiol 2009; 54: 2205–41.
7. Rossini R, Angiolillo DJ, Musumeci G, et al. Aspirin desensitization in patients undergoing percutaneous coronary interventions with stent implantation. Am J Cardiol 2008; 101: 786–9.
8. Hollopeter G, Jantzen HM, Vincent D, et al. Identification of the platelet ADP receptor targeted by antithrombotic drugs. Nature 2001; 409: 202–7.
9. Farid NA, Kurihara A, Wrighton SA. Metabolism and disposition of the thienopyridine antiplatelet drugs ticlopidine, clopidogrel, and prasugrel in humans. J Clin Pharmacol 2010; 50: 126–42.
10. Bertrand ME, Rupprecht HJ, Urban P, Gershlick AH. CLASSICS Investigators. Double-blind study of the safety of clopidogrel with and without a loading dose in combination with aspirin compared with ticlopidine in combination with aspirin after coronary stenting: the clopidogrel aspirin stent international cooperative study (CLASSICS). Circulation 2000; 102: 624–9.
11. Angiolillo DJ, Suryadevara S, Capranzano P, et al. Prasugrel: a novel platelet ADP P2Y12 receptor antagonist. A review on its mechanism of action and clinical development. Expert Opin Pharmacother 2008; 9: 2893–900.
12. Capodanno D, Dharmashankar K, Angiolillo DJ. Mechanism of action and clinical development of ticagrelor, a novel platelet ADP P2Y12 receptor antagonist. Expert Rev Cardiovasc Ther 2010; 8: 151–8.
13. CAPRIE Steering Committee. A randomised, blinded, trial of clopidogrel versus aspirin in patients at risk of ischaemic events (CAPRIE). Lancet 1996; 348: 1329–39.
14. Yusuf S, Zhao F, Mehta SR, et al. Clopidogrel in Unstable Angina to Prevent Recurrent Events Trial Investigators. Effects of clopidogrel in addition to aspirin in patients with acute coronary syndromes without ST-segment elevation. N Engl J Med 2001; 345: 494–502.
15. Holmes DR Jr, Dehmer GJ, Kaul S, et al. ACCF/AHA clopidogrel clinical alert: approaches to the FDA "boxed warning": a report of the American College of Cardiology Foundation Task Force on clinical expert consensus documents and the American Heart Association endorsed by the Society for Cardiovascular Angiography and Interventions and the Society of Thoracic Surgeons. J Am Coll Cardiol 2010; 56: 321–41.
16. Wijns W, Kolh P, Danchin N, et al. European Association for Percutaneous Cardiovascular Interventions. Guidelines on myocardial revascularization: the Task Force on Myocardial Revascularization of the European Society of Cardiology (ESC) and the European Association for Cardio-Thoracic Surgery (EACTS). Eur Heart J 2010; 31: 2501–55.
17. Wiviott SD, Braunwald E, McCabe CH, et al. TRITON-TIMI 38 Investigators. Prasugrel versus clopidogrel in patients with acute coronary syndromes. N Engl J Med 2007; 357: 2001–15.
18. Wallentin L, Becker RC, Budaj A, et al. Ticagrelor versus clopidogrel in patients with acute coronary syndromes. N Engl J Med 2009; 361: 1045–57.

19. Bhatt DL, Topol EJ. Current role of platelet glycoprotein IIb/IIIa inhibitors in acute coronary syndromes. JAMA 2000; 284: 1549–58.

20. Kastrati A, Mehilli J, Neumann FJ, et al. Abciximab in patients with acute coronary syndromes undergoing percutaneous coronary intervention after clopidogrel pretreatment: the ISAR-REACT 2 randomized trial. JAMA 2006; 295: 1531–8.

21. De Luca G, Suryapranata H, Stone GW, et al. Abciximab as adjunctive therapy to reperfusion in acute ST-segment elevation myocardial infarction: a meta-analysis of randomized trials. JAMA 2005; 293: 1759–65.

22. Angiolillo DJ, Bhatt DL, Gurbel PA, et al. Advances in antiplatelet therapy: agents in clinical development. Am J Cardiol 2009; 103(Suppl 3): 40A–51A.

23. Angiolillo DJ, Capodanno D, Goto S. Platelet thrombin receptor antagonism and atherothrombosis. Eur Heart J 2010; 31: 17–28.

24. Ahrens I, Lip GY, Peter K. New oral anticoagulant drugs in cardiovascular disease. Thromb Haemost 2010; 104: 49–60.

25. Hirsh J. Heparin. N Engl J Med 1991; 324: 1565–74.

26. Weitz JI. Low molecular weight heparins. N Engl J Med 1997; 337: 688–98.

27. Montalescot G, White HD, Gallo R, et al. STEEPLE Investigators: Enoxaparin versus unfractionated heparin in elective percutaneous coronary intervention. N Engl J Med 2006; 355: 1058–60.

28. Di Nisio M, Middeldorp S, Buller HR. Direct thrombin inhibitors. N Engl J Med 2005; 353: 1028–40.

29. Mehran R, Pocock S, Nikolsky E, et al. Impact of Bleeding on Mortality After Percutaneous Coronary Intervention: Results from a Patient-Level Pooled Analysis of the REPLACE-2 (Randomized Evaluation of PCI Linking Angiomax to Reduced Clinical Events), ACUITY (Acute Catheterization and Urgent Intervention Triage Strategy), and HORIZONS-AMI (Harmonizing Outcomes With Revascularization and Stents in Acute Myocardial Infarction) trials. J Am Coll Cardiol Interv 2011; 4: 654–64.

30. Yusuf S, Mehta SR, Chrolavicius S, et al. Comparison of fondaparinux and enoxaparin in acute coronary syndromes. N Engl J Med 2006; 354: 1464–76.

Invasive assessment and management of intermediate coronary narrowings
William F. Fearon

OUTLINE

Intermediate coronary narrowings are generally defined as angiographic stenoses narrowed between 40 and 70%. Intermediate coronary disease is extremely prevalent, occurring in a significant proportion of patients undergoing percutaneous coronary interventions (PCI). These lesions are particularly challenging because one third to one half are likely to be responsible for myocardial ischemia, symptoms, and future cardiac events, while the remainder have a more benign prognosis. Furthermore, the coronary angiogram alone cannot distinguish between these two groups (1). In this chapter, we will review adjunctive methods for invasively assessing intermediate coronary lesions in the cardiac catheterization laboratory and how these techniques guide the decision for coronary revascularization versus medical therapy alone.

BACKGROUND

We have known for more than two decades about the limitations of coronary angiography in assessing intermediate coronary lesions (2). Because the angiogram is a two-dimensional representation of a three-dimensional structure, eccentric atherosclerosis which may not have a significant impact on the coronary artery lumen can appear to be causing significant narrowing in some views of the angiogram. Likewise, complex disease which does impact flow can appear as mild narrowing (Fig. 25.1).

We have learned that the ischemic potential of coronary artery disease correlates strongly with adverse outcome. For example, the yearly cardiac death rate in patients with no ischemia on a myocardial perfusion scan is 0.3% and increases to 0.8%, 2.3%, and 4.6% for mild, moderate, or severe ischemia, respectively (3). In a more recent study, the residual burden of myocardial ischemia in patients randomized to either medical therapy alone or to PCI in addition to medical therapy correlated strongly with the occurrence of death and myocardial infarction (Fig. 25.2).(4).

We have also learned that stable coronary disease, not causing myocardial ischemia, can be safely managed with medical therapy (5). Concerns that mild or moderate coronary lesions were more likely to cause myocardial infarction, compared with more severe disease have been shown to be incorrect (6). The concept of the vulnerable plaque has shifted more toward the vulnerable patient and there is greater appreciation of the complex nature of what causes plaque rupture and ultimately myocardial infarction (7). For all of these reasons, there has been a paradigm shift away from anatomy-focused therapy (i.e. anatomic complete revascularization) to an approach based on identifying and reversing myocardial ischemia (i.e. functional complete revascularization) (8).

CORONARY FLOW RESERVE

One of the early invasive techniques for assessing intermediate coronary disease was the measurement of Doppler wire-derived coronary flow reserve (CFR). CFR is defined as the peak flow down a coronary artery divided by the resting flow (9). It can be measured invasively using a Doppler velocity wire and more recently using thermodilution technique. Because coronary velocity is proportional to coronary flow, CFR can be estimated by measuring the coronary velocity at rest and during maximal vasodilation. This can be performed in the catheterization laboratory by using a standard angioplasty guide wire, with a Doppler transducer mounted at its tip, and by administering a vasodilatory agent, such as adenosine or papaverine.

CFR in a patient with normal coronary structure and function should be greater than 2 and can be up to 5. In a patient with a functionally significant coronary stenosis, CFR will be less than 2. Miller et al. compared CFR measured in this manner with nuclear perfusion imaging in 27 patients with intermediate coronary stenoses (30–70% diameter stenosis) (10). They found that among the 14 patients with a CFR less than or equal to two, all had nuclear perfusion imaging studies showing reversible myocardial ischemia. Ten of the 13 patients with a CFR greater than 2 had normal myocardial perfusion studies. The concordance between the two techniques was 89%.

Joye et al. added to these findings by comparing Doppler wire-derived CFR with nuclear perfusion imaging in 30 patients with intermediate coronary stenoses (11). They also found an excellent agreement between the noninvasive and invasive evaluations for ischemia, reporting a sensitivity of 94%, specificity of 95%, and diagnostic accuracy or concordance of 94%. These investigators concluded that the invasive assessment of CFR in a coronary artery with an intermediate lesion can reliably predict the presence of ischemia on nuclear perfusion imaging.

Subsequently, the ability of Doppler wire-derived CFR to detect ischemia producing intermediate coronary lesions has been tested in larger cohorts of patients, as well as in comparison with stress echocardiography (12–14). Unfortunately, these studies have found lower values for concordance between Doppler wire-derived CFR and the noninvasive modality tested, 84%, 79%, and 72%, respectively for the three studies.

Limitations of CFR

CFR interrogates the entire coronary circulation, including both the microvasculature as well as the epicardial artery. For the assessment of intermediate coronary disease, this can be a limitation, as a patient with microvascular disease might have an abnormal CFR, despite normal epicardial physiology.

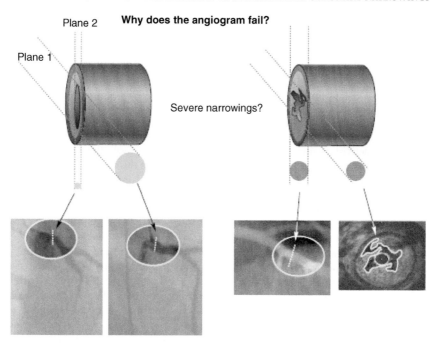

Figure 25.1 Schematic illustrating how an eccentric mild stenosis can appear severe in some views of the angiogram (*left hand panel*) and a complex, severe narrowing can appear mild in multiple views of the angiogram 17.

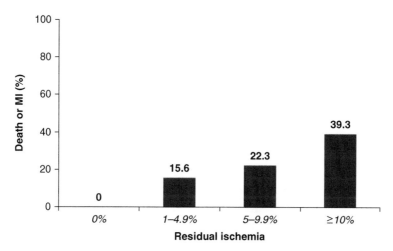

Figure 25.2 Percentage of death or myocardial infarction during follow-up of patients enrolled in the nuclear substudy from the COURAGE trial according to severity of residual myocardial ischemia. *Source*: Adapted from Ref. 4.

To address this limitation, the relative CFR was introduced, which is defined as CFR in a diseased epicardial vessel divided by the CFR in a normal reference vessel. In this manner, the microvascular component, which is assumed to be diffuse will cancel out and the epicardial disease can be more independently interrogated (15).

Another limitation to CFR is that by definition it incorporates resting flow. Unfortunately, resting flow in the catheterization laboratory is quite variable and changes in heart rate, blood pressure, or left ventricular contractility have been shown to significantly impact the reproducibility of CFR (16). In addition, CFR has no absolute normal value. The normal range is between 2 and 5, but in one patient 2.5 may be normal, while in another 4.5 is normal. For all of these reasons, CFR has fallen out of favor for invasively assessing intermediate coronary disease and is no longer performed routinely (17).

INTRAVASCULAR ULTRASOUND

Intravascular ultrasound was introduced in the late 1980s and early 1990s by Yock, Fitzgerald, and others who validated it as a method for obtaining detailed information regarding vessel size, plaque burden and morphology, and lesion length (18). Subsequently, it has been studied as a method for assessing the significance of intermediate coronary disease.

Data Regarding Intravascular Ultrasound

Initial studies compared IVUS-derived minimum lumen area with noninvasive assessment of coronary disease. For example, Nishioka and co-workers compared IVUS parameters measured in 70 de novo coronary lesions (the majority classified as intermediate) to the results of nuclear perfusion imaging (19). The authors found that a minimum lumen crosssectional area defined as $\leq 4\,mm^2$ had a sensitivity of 88% and specificity of 90% for predicting a reversible perfusion defect on the nuclear perfusion imaging study. Others have found that the follow-up event rate is low in patients with intermediate lesions and an IVUS-derived minimum lumen area $\geq 4\,mm^2$ (20).

IVUS has also been compared with other invasive techniques for assessing intermediate coronary disease, such as fractional flow reserve (FFR). Takagi and co-workers performed IVUS in 51 coronary lesions (approximately half were considered intermediate) and compared the, IVUS-derived minimum lumen crosssectional area and percent area stenosis to the FFR result (21). They found a strong positive correlation between the minimum lumen area and FFR ($r = 0.79, p < 0.0001$) and negative correlation between percent area stenosis and FFR ($r = -0.77, p < 0.0001$). Using a cutoff of $<3.0\,mm^2$ to define an abnormal minimum lumen crosssectional area and <0.75 to define an abnormal FFR, the investigators found that IVUS had a sensitivity of 83% and specificity of 92% for detecting ischemia-producing lesions based on FFR.

Other studies comparing IVUS with FFR have identified optimal minimum lumen area cutoff values ranging between 2.4 and $4.0\,mm^2$. For example, Briguori and co-workers found the best cut-point for IVUS minimum lumen area in relation to FFR was $4.0\,mm^2$, yielding a sensitivity and specificity of 92% and 56%, respectively. Presumably the weaker correlation and concordance in this study compared with the study by Takagi et al. can be explained by the inclusion of only intermediate lesions in this study (22). On the other hand, in a more recent study, Kang and co-workers found the best IVUS minimum lumen area cutoff was $2.4\,mm^2$ (23).

Limitations of Intravascular Ultrasound

Because IVUS is inherently an anatomic assessment of coronary disease, it is not ideal for determining the physiologic consequences of intermediate stenoses. The determinants of the ischemic potential of a stenosis relate not only to its minimum lumen area, but also to the lesion length, reference area, entrance and exit angles, and perhaps most importantly, to the flow across the stenosis (Fig. 25.3). For example, a stenosis in a left anterior descending artery, which is anatomically identical to a stenosis in a right coronary artery, may be functionally significant and result in myocardial ischemia because the myocardial territory subtended by the left anterior descending is much larger and hence the flow down the vessel and across the stenosis is much greater. Another scenario resulting in discordance

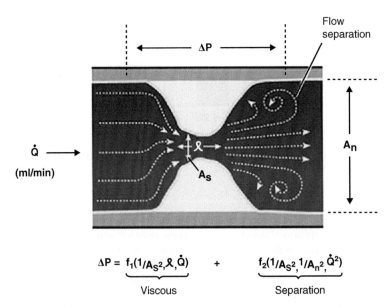

$$\Delta P = \underbrace{f_1(1/A_S^2, \mathcal{l}, \dot{Q})}_{\text{Viscous}} + \underbrace{f_2(1/A_S^2, 1/A_n^2, \dot{Q}^2)}_{\text{Separation}}$$

Figure 25.3 Determinants of a pressure gradient across a stenosis and myocardial ischemia constitute viscous and separation forces due to length (l), area stenosis (A_s), reference area (A_n), flow (Q), and coefficients of viscous friction and laminar separation (F_1 and F_2) 17.

between an anatomic assessment and physiologic assessment of an intermediate narrowing occurs when a vessel with an intermediate lesion supplies collaterals to an occluded vessel. In this case, the flow down of the vessel with the intermediate narrowing is greater than it would be in the usual setting because the vessel is supplying a larger amount of myocardium. This results in a larger gradient across the stenosis and a greater likelihood for myocardial ischemia (Fig. 25.4).

In addition, applying the same absolute cutoff value for the minimum lumen area which identifies ischemia-producing lesions to a small woman and to a large man does not make sense given the different sizes of their hearts and coronary arteries. Along these same lines, it has been shown that the IVUS-derived minimum lumen area best correlates with an abnormal FFR varies depending on whether the lesion is in the proximal, mid, or distal portion of the vessel (24).

One subset of intermediate coronary lesions in which one might expect a better correlation between IVUS and FFR is the intermediate left main lesion. This is because the left main coronary has less variation in its size, length, and the amount of myocardium it supplies. In one study comparing IVUS findings with FFR in 55 patients with angiographically ambiguous left main lesions, an IVUS-derived MLA of 5.9 mm^2 had a sensitivity and specificity of 93% and 95%, respectively, and an IVUS-derived minimum lumen diameter of 2.8 mm had a sensitivity and specificity of 93% and 98%, respectively, for predicting a significant stenosis (25). However, a more recent study found that a cutoff value of 4.5 mm^2 correlated best with FFR (26).

For the reasons mentioned above, when invasively assessing intermediate lesions, fractional flow reserve (FFR) is the preferred method for assessing the physiologic significance of an intermediate coronary lesion, while IVUS can aid in determining plaque morphology, vessel size, lesion length, and optimal stent deployment, all of which can help guide PCI (27).

FRACTIONAL FLOW RESERVE

Fractional flow reserve (FFR) has become the reference standard for invasively assessing the physiologic significance of intermediate coronary disease. First described by Pijls, De Bruyne and co-workers, FFR is defined as the maximum flow down a vessel in the presence of a stenosis compared with the maximum flow in the hypothetical absence of the stenosis (28). It is based on the assumption that at maximal hyperemia microvascular resistance is minimized and constant. Under this condition, resistance is minimized and myocardial flow becomes proportional to pressure. The equation for FFR can be changed to the hyperemic distal coronary pressure in the presence of a stenosis compared with the coronary pressure in the hypothetical absence of the stenosis. In a normal epicardial artery, there is very little loss of pressure from the proximal to distal region. For this reason, in a diseased vessel the proximal pressure is a reflection of what the distal pressure would be if there was no disease. Therefore, FFR can be defined as distal coronary pressure divided by proximal coronary pressure during maximal hyperemia.

In a landmark study, Pijls, De Bruyne, and co-workers validated FFR for the assessment of intermediate coronary narrowings by comparing it with three different noninvasive stress tests (29). If any one of the stress tests was positive for ischemia, then the patient was defined as having ischemia. By using composite information from all three stress tests, the authors were able to increase the accuracy of the noninvasive diagnosis of ischemia. Using a cutpoint of 0.75, they found that 100% of the 21 patients with an FFR below 0.75 had ischemia and 88% of the 24 patients with an FFR of 0.75 or greater did not have ischemia. Importantly, revascularization was not performed in these 24 patients and at an average of 14 month follow-up there were no cardiac events in this group. The overall accuracy of FFR for identifying ischemia-producing lesions in patients with single vessel intermediate disease was 93%.

A number of subsequent studies have confirmed the accuracy of FFR for diagnosing ischemia-producing intermediate lesions in a variety of patient populations, including multivessel coronary disease, in comparison with a variety of noninvasive stress tests, and after myocardial infarction (30). The best cutoff value in most of these studies has been between 0.75 and 0.80. This region has been termed the "gray zone." If the FFR is above 0.80, one can be fairly certain that significant ischemia is not present, and as described in more detail below, the patient will do well with medical therapy alone. If the FFR is below 0.75, one can be certain that ischemia is present and revascularization will improve symptoms and may improve outcomes. When the FFR falls in the "gray zone," clinical judgment is required. If a patient has a proximal left anterior descending coronary lesion and classic symptoms, one might opt for revascularization. If on the other hand, the patient has atypical or no symptoms, an equivocal stress test and/or is undergoing evaluation for noncardiac surgery, one might opt for medical therapy.

Safety of Deferring PCI Based on FFR

The safety of deferring revascularization of intermediate coronary narrowings which are not hemodynamically significant (i.e. FFR ≥0.75) was tested in the deferral study (31). In this multicenter trial, 325 patients with single vessel intermediate coronary disease underwent FFR measurement. If the FFR was below 0.75 then the patient then underwent PCI. If the FFR was ≥0.75, then the patients were randomized to either PCI (with bare-metal stents in approximately 50% and angioplasty alone in the remainder) or to deferral of PCI with medical treatment. At 2-year follow-up, the event-free survival was similar in the defer group as compared with the perform group (89 vs. 83%, $p = 0.27$). More recently, follow-up was extended to 5 years and the event-free survival remained similar between the two groups (80 vs. 73%, $p = 0.52$) and the cardiac death and myocardial infarction rate in the defer group was less than half of what it was in the perform arm (3.3 vs. 7.9%, $p = 0.21$) (32). This study and a number of other retrospective single center studies have confirmed the safety of treating hemodynamically non-significant intermediate coronary disease with medical therapy alone (17).

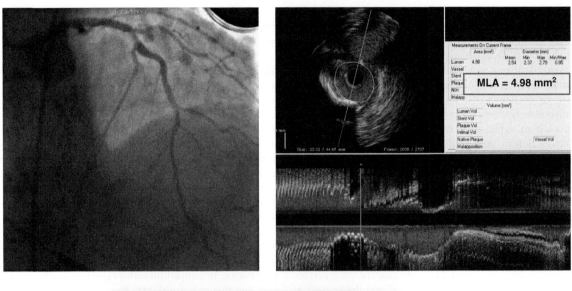

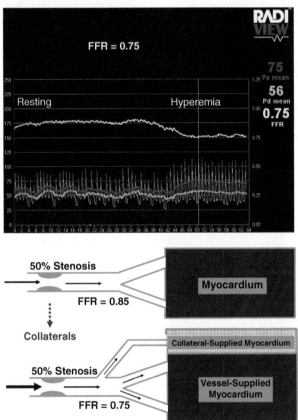

Figure 25.4 A picture of an angiogram with a moderate proximal stenosis in a left anterior descending artery supplying faint collaterals to an occluded vessel (**A**). The IVUS minimum lumen area is 4.98 mm² occurring just distal to the diagonal branch as seen in the crossectional and longitudinal pictures (**B**). The FFR is 0.75, lower than one would expect based on the IVUS and likely a result of the increased flow across the stenosis because the lesion is proximal and in a large vessel supplying a large myocardial territory (**C**). A cartoon illustrating the change in flow and FFR across the same stenosis before and after the vessel develops collateral to a contralateral vessel (**D**). This case example illustrates one of the limitations of IVUS given that it is an anatomic assessment and does not take into account changes in coronary physiology.

FFR and Intermediate Left Main Coronary Disease

An important subset of intermediate coronary lesions in which FFR measurement has been applied is the group with indeterminate left main coronary stenosis. Because of the importance of the left main coronary and the size of the myocardial territory supplied by the left main, there has been concern that FFR, in general, and in particular, a cutoff of 0.75–0.80 may not be valid in this subset. In a recent review of published single center studies evaluating a strategy of deferring revascularization of intermediate left main lesions with an FFR >0.75–0.80 found that in 236 patients the survival at greater than 2 year follow-up was 100% and the event-free survival was excellent and similar, if not better than in patients with an ischemic FFR who underwent revascularization (33).

The largest and most recent study evaluating FFR measurement in patients with moderate left main disease found that in 213 patients with equivocal left main disease, if the FFR was 0.80 or higher, as it was in 138 patients, the five-year survival rate was 90% and compared favorably with the 85% survival rate in the 75 patients with an FFR <0.80 who underwent coronary artery bypass grafting (34). The five year event free survival was 74% in the patients with an FFR of 0.80 or higher and also similar to the revascularization group. This study and the previous smaller studies support the idea that FFR measurement in left main disease is safe and useful in guiding the decision to perform revascularization, just as it is in patients with intermediate coronary disease not involving the left main coronary.

FFR-Guided Management of Intermediate Coronary Disease

If an intermediate coronary narrowing has a non-ischemic FFR then it is unlikely to be responsible for a patient's symptoms and can be safely managed medically. If, however, an intermediate coronary narrowing is responsible for an ischemic FFR, then it is likely contributing to the patient's symptoms and may be more likely to cause future cardiac events. In this setting, if the lesion is amenable to PCI and particularly if the patient continues to have symptoms despite medical therapy, many would advocate revascularization with the aim at relieving symptoms and improving outcome. The data to support this FFR-guided approach come from the FFR versus angiography for multivessel evaluation (FAME) trial (35).

The FAME study was a prospective, multicenter, international, randomized trial comparing two strategies for guiding PCI in patients with multivessel coronary disease, a significant proportion of whom had at least one intermediate lesion. Over 1,000 patients with stenoses ≥50% in two or three vessels which the operator deemed warranted PCI based on the angiographic appearance and clinical data were randomized to either angiography-guided PCI, in which case the identified lesions underwent routine PCI with drug-eluting stents, or to FFR-guided PCI, in which case FFR was measured and PCI was performed on a lesion only if the FFR was <0.80.

Roughly three lesions were identified per patient and 47% of these were between 50 and 70% narrowed. The angiography-guided group received almost three stents per patient, while the FFR-guided group received approximately two stents per patient, a highly significant difference. Importantly, the FFR-guided approach did not take any longer than the angiography-guided one and significantly less contrast media was required in the FFR-guided patients.

The primary endpoint of the study was the one-year major adverse cardiac event rate, a composite of death, myocardial infarction, and the need for repeat revascularization. This occurred in 18.3% of the angiography-guided patients and 13.2% of the FFR-guided patients, a significant difference ($p = 0.02$). The combination of death and myocardial infarction was also significantly reduced by the FFR-guided strategy (11.1 vs. 7.3%, $p = 0.04$) (Fig. 25.5).

These results have been extended out to two years with a persistent significant reduction in death and myocardial infarction (12.9 vs. 8.4%, $p = 0.02$) and a lower rate of major adverse cardiac events (22.4 vs. 7.9, $p = 0.08$) in the FFR-guided patients (36). Importantly, of the 513 lesions in the FFR-guided patients on which PCI was deferred because the FFR was >0.80, only one lesion (0.2%) caused a myocardial infarction and only 16 (3.2%) required revascularization. The percentage of FFR-guided patients free from angina at 2 years was 79.9% compared with 75.8% of the angiography-guided patients ($p = 0.14$).

Another important message from the FAME trial was the limitation of angiography for determining functionally significant lesions (37). Of the intermediate narrowings between 50 and 70% narrowed, 35% had an FFR ≤0.80 and 65% did not. Of those lesions between 71 and 90% narrowed, a group typically deemed significant, 20% had an FFR >0.80, and PCI was safely deferred (Fig. 25.6). Of the patients in the FFR-guided group with angiographic three-vessel coronary disease, only 14% had functional three-vessel coronary disease and the majority had only one or two vessels with FFR ≤0.80. The FAME trial reinforced the safety of deferring PCI on lesions (many of which were intermediate) with an FFR >0.80. It also highlighted a new paradigm of functionally complete revascularization in which ischemia-producing lesions are treated with PCI and non-ischemia-producing lesions are treated medically.

Limitations of Fractional Flow Reserve

FFR assumes that microvascular resistance remains constant. Therefore, in the culprit vessel of a patient with an acute ST segment myocardial infarction, FFR should not be utilized because a variable degree of transient microvascular stunning likely exists. In the acute setting, the maximum achievable hyperemic flow may be lower than it is a week later, after the microvascular stunning has resolved. Therefore, FFR in the culprit vessel might be overestimated. Multiple studies have shown that FFR can be accurately measured in the culprit vessel in the nonacute setting after ST segment myocardial infarction, as long as 3–6 days have passed (17).

It is important to note that FFR can be accurately measured in nonculprit vessels during the acute phase of ST segment elevation myocardial infarction (38). These nonculprit vessels typically

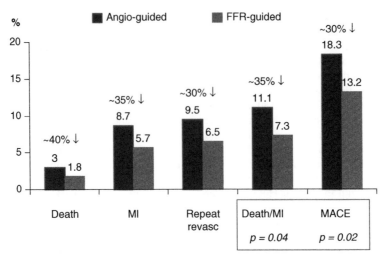

Figure 25.5 One year outcomes in the FFR-guided patients as compared with the angiograph-guided patients enrolled in the FAME trial. *Source*: Adapted from Ref. 36.

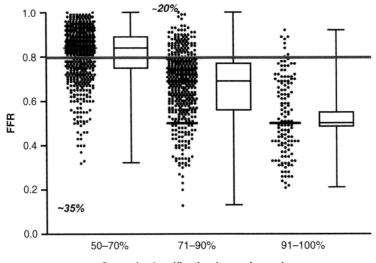

Figure 25.6 Relation between stenosis severity on the angiogram and FFR in the FFR-guided lesions included in the FAME trial. Of the lesions classified as being 50–70% narrowed, 35% resulted in an FFR <0.80. Of the lesions classified as 71–90% narrowed, 20% resulted in an FFR ≥0.80 38.

have intermediate lesions and invasively assessing them at the time of primary PCI can save time and resources and expedite decision making regarding the need for further PCI.

FFR has not been well-studied in patients with severe left ventricular hypertrophy. It is possible that in this setting the myocardium outgrows the microvasculature and requires a larger fraction of flow to avoid ischemia. For this reasons, the usual FFR cutoff value may not apply if there is severe left ventricular hypertrophy.

Another theoretical concern for a false negative FFR is exercise-induced vasoconstriction. A patient may have an intermediate coronary lesion, which itself is not flow-limiting. However, with

exercise there may be vasoconstriction which increases the stenosis and results in myocardial ischemia. In the catheterization laboratory when FFR is measured with pharmacologic vasodilation, this exercise-induced vasoconstriction will be absent and the stenosis may not result in an ischemic FFR.

Personal Perspective
When invasively assessing intermediate coronary narrowings the primary goal should be to determine whether the narrowing is causing a patient's symptoms and whether it is likely to cause future cardiac events (Fig. 25.7). The presence of myocardial ischemia is our best gauge of whether a lesion is responsible for

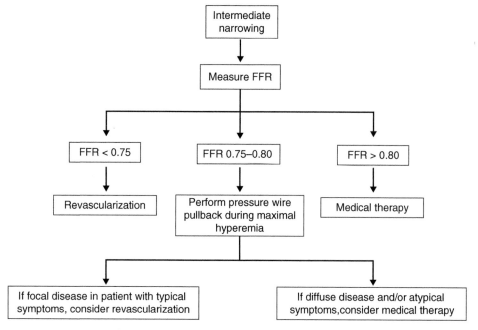

Figure 25.7 Decision tree for intermediate coronary narrowings.

symptoms and likely to result in a future cardiac event. In the catheterization laboratory, FFR is the reference standard for identifying ischemia-producing lesions. Its spatial resolution is unsurpassed being not only vessel- but lesion-specific also. There is now a wealth of data supporting the accuracy of measuring FFR to identify ischemia-producing intermediate lesions. FFR-guided PCI of these lesions results in improved outcomes and saves resources. Non-hemodynamically significant lesions can be safely managed medically with low follow-up cardiac event rates. Whether PCI in the setting of stable coronary disease will be shown to be superior to optimal medical therapy remains an area of active investigation. Most investigators agree that identifying large areas of ischemia and relieving the ischemia should improve patient outcomes. FFR-guided PCI may be the best method for achieving this goal.

Text Boxes:

Limitations of CFR for Assessing Intermediate Narrowings:

1. No absolute normal value
2. Affected by microvascular abnormalities
3. Affected by changes in hemodynamics
4. Unable to account for collaterals

Limitations of IVUS for Assessing Intermediate Narrowings:

1. Multiple criteria for defining a significant lesion depending on vessel size and lesion location
2. Unable to account for the amount of myocardium supplied by a vessel with an intermediate narrowing
3. Unable to account for collaterals

Advantages of FFR for Assessing Intermediate Narrowings:

1. Absolute normal value of 1.0 in every patient and every vessel
2. Discrete cutoff range of <0.75–0.80 for identifying ischemia-producing lesions
3. Takes into account the amount of myocardium supplied by a vessel and for the presence of collaterals
4. Not affected by changes in hemodynamics
5. Wealth of data supporting the safety of treating nonhemodynamically significant lesions medically

REFERENCES

1. White CW, Wright CB, Doty DB, et al. Does visual interpretation of the coronary arteriogram predict the physiologic importance of a coronary stenosis? N Engl J Med 1984; 310: 819–24.
2. Topol EJ, Ellis SG, Cosgrove DM, et al. Analysis of coronary angioplasty practice in the United States with an insurance-claims data base. Circulation 1993; 87: 1489–97.
3. Hachamovitch R, Berman DS, Shaw LJ, et al. Incremental prognostic value of myocardial perfusion single photon emission computed tomography for the prediction of cardiac death: differential stratification for risk of cardiac death and myocardial infarction. Circulation 1998; 97: 535–43.
4. Shaw LJ, Berman DS, Maron DJ, et al. COURAGE Investigators. Optimal medical therapy with or without percutaneous coronary intervention to reduce ischemic burden: results from the Clinical Outcomes Utilizing Revascularization and Aggressive Drug Evaluation (COURAGE) trial nuclear substudy. Circulation 2008; 117: 1283–91.

5. Boden WE, O'Rourke RA, Teo KK, et al. COURAGE Trial Research Group. Optimal medical therapy with or without PCI for stable coronary disease. N Engl J Med 2007; 356: 1503–16.

6. Manoharan G, Ntalianis A, Muller O, et al. Severity of coronary arterial stenoses responsible for acute coronary syndromes. Am J Cardiol 2009; 103: 1183–8.

7. Naghavi M, Libby P, Falk E, et al. From vulnerable plaque to vulnerable patient: a call for new definitions and risk assessment strategies: Part I. Circulation 2003; 108: 1664–72.

8. Park SJ, Ahn JM, Kang SJ. Paradigm shift to functional angioplasty: new insights for fractional flow reserve- and intravascular ultrasound-guided percutaneous coronary intervention. Circulation 2011; 124: 951–7.

9. Gould KL, Lipscomb K, Hamilton GW. Physiologic basis for assessing critical coronary stenosis. Instantaneous flow response and regional distribution during coronary hyperemia as measures of coronary flow reserve. Am J Cardiol 1974; 33: 87–94.

10. Miller DD, Donohue TJ, Younis LT, et al. Correlation of pharmacological 99mTc-sestamibi myocardial perfusion imaging with poststenotic coronary flow reserve in patients with angiographically intermediate coronary artery stenoses. Circulation 1994; 89: 2150–60.

11. Joye JD, Schulman DS, Lasorda D, et al. Intracoronary Doppler guide wire versus stress single-photon emission computed tomographic thallium-201 imaging in assessment of intermediate coronary stenoses. J Am Coll Cardiol 1994; 24: 940–7.

12. Heller LI, Cates C, Popma J, et al. Intracoronary Doppler assessment of moderate coronary artery disease: comparison with 201Tl imaging and coronary angiography. FACTS Study Group. Circulation 1997; 96: 484–90.

13. Verberne HJ, Piek JJ, van Liebergen RA, et al. Functional assessment of coronary artery stenosis by doppler derived absolute and relative coronary blood flow velocity reserve in comparison with (99m)Tc MIBI SPECT. Heart 1999; 82: 509–14.

14. Duffy SJ, Gelman JS, Peverill RE, et al. Agreement between coronary flow velocity reserve and stress echocardiography in intermediate-severity coronary stenoses. Catheter Cardiovasc Interv 2001; 53: 29–38.

15. Kern MJ. Coronary physiology revisited practical insights from the cardiac catheterization laboratory. Circulation 2000; 101: 1344–51.

16. de Bruyne B, Bartunek J, Sys SU, et al. Simultaneous coronary pressure and flow velocity measurements in humans. Feasibility, reproducibility, and hemodynamic dependence of coronary flow velocity reserve, hyperemic flow versus pressure slope index, and fractional flow reserve. Circulation 1996; 94: 1842–9.

17. Kern MJ, Samady H. Current concepts of integrated coronary physiology in the catheterization laboratory. J Am Coll Cardiol 2010; 55: 173–85.

18. Yock PG, Fitzgerald PJ, Linker DT, Angelsen BA. Intravascular ultrasound guidance for catheter-based coronary interventions. J Am Coll Cardiol 1991; 17: 39B–45B.

19. Nishioka T, Amanullah AM, Luo H, et al. Clinical validation of intravascular ultrasound imaging for assessment of coronary stenosis severity: comparison with stress myocardial perfusion imaging. J Am Coll Cardiol 1999; 33: 1870–8.

20. Abizaid AS, Mintz GS, Mehran R, et al. Long-term follow-up after percutaneous transluminal coronary angioplasty was not performed based on intravascular ultrasound findings: importance of lumen dimensions. Circulation 1999; 100: 256–61.

21. Takagi A, Tsurumi Y, Ishii Y, et al. Clinical potential of intravascular ultrasound for physiological assessment of coronary stenosis: relationship between quantitative ultrasound tomography and pressure-derived fractional flow reserve. Circulation 1999; 100: 250–5.

22. Briguori C, Anzuini A, Airoldi F, et al. Intravascular ultrasound criteria for the assessment of the functional significance of intermediate coronary artery stenoses and comparison with fractional flow reserve. Am J Cardiol 2001; 87: 136–41.

23. Kang SJ, Lee JY, Ahn JM, et al. Validation of intravascular ultrasound-derived parameters with fractional flow reserve for assessment of coronary stenosis severity. Circ Cardiovasc Interv 2011; 4: 65–71.

24. Koo BK, Yang HM, Doh JH, et al. Optimal intravascular ultrasound criteria and their accuracy for defining the functional significance of intermediate coronary stenoses of different locations. JACC Cardiovasc Interv 2011; 4: 803–11.

25. Jasti V, Ivan E, Yalamanchili V, Wongpraparut N, Leesar MA. Correlations between fractional flow reserve and intravascular ultrasound in patients with an ambiguous left main coronary artery stenosis. Circulation 2004; 110: 2831–6.

26. Kang SJ, Lee JY, Ahn JM, et al. Intravascular ultrasound derived predictors for fractional flow reserve in intermediate left main disease. JACC Cardiovasc Int 2011; 4: 1168–74.

27. Tobis J, Azarbal B, Slavin L. Assessment of intermediate severity coronary lesions in the catheterization laboratory. J Am Coll Cardiol 2007; 49: 839–48.

28. Pijls NH, van Son JA, Kirkeeide RL, De Bruyne B, Gould KL. Experimental basis of determining maximum coronary, myocardial, and collateral blood flow by pressure measurements for assessing functional stenosis severity before and after percutaneous transluminal coronary angioplasty. Circulation 1993; 87: 1354–67.

29. Pijls NH, De Bruyne B, Peels K, et al. Measurement of fractional flow reserve to assess the functional severity of coronary-artery stenoses. N Engl J Med 1996; 334: 1703–8.

30. Kern MJ, Lerman A, Bech JW, et al. Physiological assessment of coronary artery disease in the cardiac catheterization laboratory. a scientific statement from the American Heart Association Committee on Diagnostic and Interventional Cardiac Catheterization, Council on Clinical Cardiology. Circulation 2006; 114: 1321–41.

31. Bech GJ, De Bruyne B, Pijls NH, et al. Fractional flow reserve to determine the appropriateness of angioplasty in moderate coronary stenosis: a randomized trial. Circulation 2001; 103: 2928–34.

32. Pijls NH, van Schaardenburgh P, Manoharan G, et al. Percutaneous coronary intervention of functionally nonsignificant stenosis: 5-year follow-up of the DEFER Study. J Am Coll Cardiol 2007; 49: 2105–11.

33. Lindstaedt M. Patient stratification in left main coronary artery disease–rationale from a contemporary perspective. Int J Cardiol 2008; 130: 326–34.

34. Hamilos M, Muller O, Cuisset T, et al. Long-term clinical outcome after fractional flow reserve-guided treatment in patients with angiographically equivocal left main coronary artery stenosis. Circulation 2009; 120: 1505–12.

35. Tonino PA, De Bruyne B, Pijls NH, et al. FAME Study Investigators. Fractional flow reserve versus angiography for guiding percutaneous coronary intervention. N Engl J Med 2009; 360: 213–24.

36. Pijls NH, Fearon WF, Tonino PA, et al. FAME Study Investigators. Fractional flow reserve versus angiography for guiding percutaneous

coronary intervention in patients with multivessel coronary artery disease: 2-year follow-up of the FAME (Fractional Flow Reserve Versus Angiography for Multivessel Evaluation) study. J Am Coll Cardiol 2010; 56: 177–84.

37. Tonino PA, Fearon WF, De Bruyne B, et al. Angiographic versus functional severity of coronary artery stenoses in the FAME study fractional flow reserve versus angiography in multivessel evaluation. J Am Coll Cardiol 2010; 55: 2816–21.

38. Ntalianis A, Sels JW, Davidavicius G, et al. Fractional flow reserve for the assessment of nonculprit coronary artery stenoses in patients with acute myocardial infarction. JACC Cardiovasc Interv 2010; 3: 1274–81.

26 Treatment algorithm in patients with stable angina
Andrew Cassar and Bernard J. Gersh

OUTLINE

Stable angina is the clinical manifestation of cardiac ischemia as a result of a mismatch between myocardial oxygen demand and supply. It is highly prevalent in the population, results in decreased quality of life, and has significant implications regarding prognosis of cardiovascular events. Patients with stable angina should be risk stratified to identify the most effective management strategy. Aggressive control of risk factors and optimal medical therapy are the cornerstone of treatment for all patients with stable angina. Persistent symptoms, the magnitude of the ischemic burden, or drug intolerance should drive decision making regarding revascularization. Revascularization is very effective treatment for stable angina when performed on targeted culprit stenoses that are hemodynamically significant or causing ischemia. The method of choice for revascularization depends on the angiographic characteristics of the lesions causing ischemia, left ventricular (LV) dysfunction, and suitability of the patient for surgery in terms of comorbidities, and likelihood of technical success. The ultimate decisions regarding patient care must incorporate evidence based medicine as well as the patient's preference based upon a balanced discussion of the treatment options and realistic expectations of the quality of life.

INTRODUCTION

Stable angina pectoris is characterized by substernal discomfort, heaviness, or a pressure-like feeling, which may radiate to the jaw, shoulder, back, or arm typically lasting minutes; it usually results exertion, emotional stress, cold, or a heavy meal and relieved by rest or nitroglycerin within minutes. Anginal "equivalents" such as epigastric discomfort, dyspnea, fatigue, or faintness may be the dominant symptom in some patients, particularly among the elderly. Symptoms can be classified as typical angina, atypical angina, or non-cardiac chest pain depending on whether the chest pain characteristics meet all three, two, or less than two of the above criteria, respectively (Diamond classification (1). The Canadian Cardiovascular Society's grading for angina severity (2) has gained widespread popularity. (Table 26.1). Stable angina pectoris is due to mismatch between myocardial oxygen demand and supply resulting in myocardial ischemia. This is usually caused by the obstruction of at least one large epicardial coronary artery by atheromatous plaque but may also be due to non-atherosclerotic obstruction such as congenital abnormalities of the coronary arteries, myocardial bridging, coronary arteritis, radiation-induced coronary disease, or coronary spasm. Angina may also occur in patients with non-obstructive epicardial coronary disease such as due to coronary endothelial dysfunction and microvascular disease,

severe left ventricular hypertrophy (hypertrophic cardiomyopathy), or in severe aortic stenosis.

The prevalence of stable angina pectoris in the United States is estimated to be 9 million cases (3). In Europe, about 20,000–40,000 per million of the population have stable angina with 50% having significant limitations in daily life as a consequence (4). The prevalence of angina increases sharply with age in both sexes from 0.1–1% in women and 2–5% in men aged 45–54 to 10–15% in women and 10–20% in men aged 65–74. Angina is the initial manifestation of coronary artery disease (CAD) in approximately 50% of all patients (5). Data from the Framingham Heart Study (5) before the advent of modern optimal medical therapy and revascularization showed that for men and women with an initial clinical presentation of stable angina, the 2-year incidence rates of non-fatal myocardial infarction and cardiac death were 14.3 and 5.5% in men and 6.2 and 3.8% in women, respectively. These sobering figures make the optimal management of stable angina of utmost importance to decrease morbidity and mortality in a large number of patients. Indeed, age-standardized mortality due to CAD has decreased by 40% over the last two decades—half of this decline is due to better risk factor prevention and management and half is due to medical treatment and revascularization (3).

RISK STRATIFICATION OF STABLE ANGINA

The diagnostic approach to coronary atherosclerosis is detailed in Section II of this book. However, once the diagnosis of CAD is made, risk stratification is the fulcrum around which decisions on management in patients with stable angina are taken. The major predictors of survival in patients with stable angina are left ventricular function, anatomical extent and severity of coronary atherosclerosis, severity of ischemia, and the patient's general health and non-coronary co-morbidities.

The history in particular and the physical examination may be helpful in assessing the severity of CAD. Eleven clinical characteristics were identified by Pryor et al. (6)—age, gender, typical angina, chest pain frequency, duration of symptoms, previous myocardial infarction (MI), hypertension, diabetes, hyperlipidemia, smoking and peripheral vascular disease (carotid bruit)—to formulate a model to accurately estimate the likelihood of severe disease in a patient.

The resting electrocardiogram may be normal in up to 50% of patients with stable angina but if normal this is a favorable prognostic finding since this usually implies normal LV function (7). On the other hand, abnormalities such as Q-waves, ST-T changes, LV hypertrophy (8), Left bundle branch block (LBBB), bifascicular block, second and third degree arterio-ventricular (AV) block, atrial fibrillation, and ventricular arrhythmias (9) are associated with a poorer prognosis since they are markers not only of conduction disease but also of significant LV dysfunction.

Left ventricular function is a major predictor of long-term survival in patients with CAD (Fig. 26.1A) (10) and end-systolic LV volume was found to be the best predictor of survival after myocardial infarction (11). Assessment of left ventricular function, usually with echocardiography (but also with magnetic nuclear resonance imaging or nuclear imaging), is appropriate in patients with symptoms or signs of heart failure, a history of prior myocardial infarction, or pathological Q waves on electrocardiogram. In patients with preserved ejection fraction, diastolic dysfunction should be assessed as this may be present in patients with angina (especially in elderly women) and has significant implications for long-term prognosis, in particular in patients with heart failure (12).

Exercise electrocardiographic stress testing is the test of choice for all patients with intermediate or high probability of CAD, except for those patients who are unable to exercise or have resting electrocardiogram (ECG) abnormalities that compromise interpretation and those for whom the information is unlikely to alter management (Focus Box 26.1). Patients with known chronic CAD with a significant change in the severity of cardiac symptoms should also be risk stratified with stress testing. The Duke's

Table 26.1 Modified Canadian Cardiovascular Society Grading for Angina Severity

Class I	Angina occurs with strenuous or rapid or prolonged exertion
Class II	Angina occurs with moderate exertion—walking more than two blocks on the level and climbing more than one flight of ordinary stairs at a normal pace and in normal conditions; or walking uphill; or walking or climbing stairs rapidly, in the cold, in wind, under emotional stress or during the few hours after awakening
Class III	Angina occurs with mild exertion—walking one or two blocks on the level and climbing one flight of stairs in normal conditions and at normal pace
Class IV	Angina occurs with any level of exertion and may be present at rest

Source: Adapted from Ref. 2.

Focus Box 26.1

Exercise electrocardiographic stress testing is the test of choice for all patients with intermediate or high probability of CAD, except for those patients who are unable to exercise or who have resting ECG abnormalities that compromise interpretation

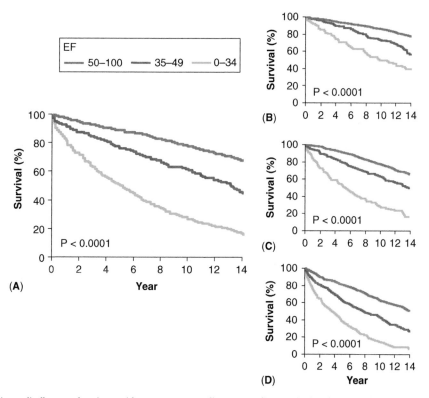

Figure 26.1 Survival in medically treated patients with coronary artery disease according to ejection fraction (EF) and number of diseased vessels. (A) Patients with one, two or three-vessel disease by ejection fraction. (B) Patients with one-vessel disease by ejection fraction. (C) Patients with two-vessel disease by ejection fraction. (D) Patients with three-vessel disease by ejection fraction. *Source*: From Ref. 10.

Table 26.2 Risk Stratification Based on Non-Invasive Testing

High risk (>3% annual mortality rate)
1. Severe resting left ventricular dysfunction (LVEF <0.35)
2. High-risk treadmill score (score ≤−11)
3. Severe exercise left ventricular dysfunction (exercise LVEF <0.35)
4. Stress-induced large perfusion defect (particularly if anterior)
5. Stress-induced multiple perfusion defects of moderate size
6. Large, fixed perfusion defect with LV dilation or increased lung uptake (thallium-201)
7. Stress-induced moderate perfusion defect with LV dilation or increased lung uptake (thallium-201)
8. Echocardiographic wall motion abnormality (involving more than two segments) developing at low dose of dobutamine (≤10 µg/kg/min) or at a low heart rate (<120 beats/min)
9. Stress echocardiographic evidence of extensive ischemia

Intermediate risk (1–3% annual mortality rate)
1. Mild/moderate resting left ventricular dysfunction (LVEF = 0.35–0.49)
2. Intermediate-risk treadmill score (−11 > score < +5)
3. Stress-induced moderate perfusion defect without LV dilation or increased lung intake (thalium-201)
4. Limited stress echocardiographic ischemia with a wall motion abnormality only at higher doses of dobutamine involving two segments or less

Low risk (<1% annual mortality rate)
1. Low-risk treadmill score (score ≥ 5)
2. Normal or small myocardial perfusion defect at rest or with stress
3. Normal stress echocardiographic wall motion or no change of limited resting wall motion abnormalities during stress

Source: From the ACC/AHA guidelines, 18 with permission.

treadmill score (13) is a useful tool to calculate risk incorporating exercise capacity, ST-segment deviation, and angina as major risk determinants. The score is the (exercise time in minutes) − (5× the maximum ST-segment deviation in millimeters) − (4× the angina index), with a value of 0 for no pain, 1 for angina and 2 for angina which was the reason for stopping the test. A score of ≥+5 is considered low risk, −10 to +4 moderate risk, and ≤−11 high risk. The 5-year survival and survival free of death or MI was 97% and 93% in low risk, 91% and 86% in moderate risk and 72% and 63% in high risk score patients. Other risk factor determinants include extensive and prolonged ST segment depression, transient ST elevation, abnormal heart rate recovery, and delayed systolic blood pressure response to exercise (14).

Imaging stress tests are first choice in patients with electrocardiographic abnormalities at rest (paced rhythm, left bundle branch block, Wolf-Parkinson-White or ST depression >1 mm due to left ventricular hypertrophy, digoxin-induced or electrolyte abnormalities) precluding interpretation of the ECG tracing (Focus Box 26.2). Exercise imaging protocols are preferred but pharmacological stressors (such as vasodilator (adenosine or dipyridamole) scintigraphy or dobutamine echocardiography) may be helpful in patients who are unable to exercise. Imaging tests may also provide additional information in regard to the extent, severity, and location of myocardial jeopardy; an estimate of the extent of irreversible scar tissue; and LV function. Stress imaging studies are also indicated for assessment of the functional significance of coronary lesions in planning percutaneous coronary intervention (PCI) (15). Risk stratification based on the results of non-invasive stress testing is shown in Table 26.2.

Coronary angiography helps risk stratify patients based upon the extent and location of atherosclerosis and is indicated in patients who have high-risk criteria on non-invasive testing (Table 26.2) or as a first test in patients with Canadian Cardiovascular Society classes III or IV angina despite medical therapy, patients with angina and signs and symptoms of congestive heart failure, and patients who survived sudden cardiac arrest or serious ventricular arrhythmias. Coronary angiography for patients with class I or II angina who are intolerant to medication, whose lifestyle is still impaired by these symptoms (including occupational reasons such as pilots), who have left ventricular dysfunction, or whose risk status is uncertain after noninvasive testing is acceptable. A low threshold for angiographic evaluation is recommended for patients with angina who have undergone previous revascularization and in patients with a history of prior MI (15). Computed tomography coronary angiography is a non-invasive method for the detection of obstructive CAD in major epicardial arteries but is still limited by a high number of false-positives (especially in calcified or stented arteries), specific patient selection (regular heart rate ≤70 bpm), and high-dose radiation exposure. Its role in the management of stable angina is still not fully elucidated but it may be useful to rule out severe CAD in patients with low to intermediate risk of CAD or in patients with angina in association with other diseases such as hypertrophic cardiomyopathy or aortic stenosis due its high negative predictive value (16).

The extent and severity of coronary atherosclerotic disease and left ventricular dysfunction identified on cardiac catheterization are the most powerful predictors of long-term outcome (Focus Box 26.3; Fig. 26.1B–D;10,17). Several prognostic indices have been used to quantify the extent of severity of CAD but the simplest classification into single-, double-, triple-vessel, or left main CAD is the most widely used and is effective (18). Additional risk stratification is provided by the severity of obstruction and its location, with proximal lesions predicting reduced survival rate (Fig. 26.2) (17). Quantifying the extent of coronary disease including non-obstructive lesions also adds to risk stratification (19).

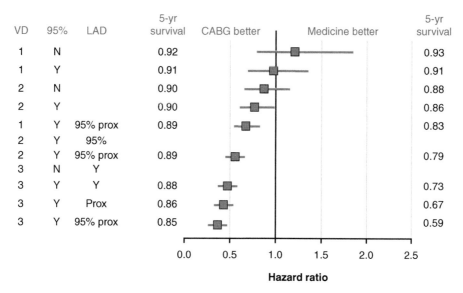

VD	95%	LAD	5-yr survival			5-yr survival
1	N		0.92			0.93
1	Y		0.91			0.91
2	N		0.90			0.88
2	Y		0.90			0.86
1	Y	95% prox	0.89			0.83
2	Y	95%				
2	Y	95% prox	0.89			0.79
3	N	Y				
3	Y	Y	0.88			0.73
3	Y	Prox	0.86			0.67
3	Y	95% prox	0.85			0.59

Figure 26.2 Five-year survival in patients according to severity and proximity of coronary lesions and adjusted hazard ratios for CABG versus medical treatment. *Source:* From Ref. 17.

MANAGEMENT OF STABLE ANGINA

The management of stable angina has two main goals: (*i*) reduce symptoms and ischemia and (*ii*) prevent myocardial infarction and death (Focus Box 26.4). These are modulated by different mechanisms—symptoms and ischemia by the insufficient oxygen supply/demand ratio usually due to coronary atherosclerosis; and myocardial infarction and death usually by unstable coronary artery plaque rupture. The algorithm for the management of patients with stable angina is given in Figure 26.3. After risk stratification, medical management, which includes aggressive risk factor control, is pivotal in all patients with stable angina. The first step is to identify and treat any associated diseases that can precipitate angina by increasing myocardial oxygen demands (such as tachycardia and hypertension) or by decreasing the amount of oxygen delivered to the myocardium (such as heart failure, pulmonary disease, or anemia). The second step is to manage CAD risk factors, symptoms, as well as prevent myocardial infarction with lifestyle changes and pharmacological treatment as detailed in Table 26.3 (20–64). Optimal medical therapy (OMT) remains the cornerstone of the initial management of all patients with stable angina—it is logical, relatively cheap and undeniably effective in improving long-term outcomes. However, many patients remain symptomatic despite OMT or request immediate relief of their symptoms and reduction of their risk for myocardial infarction and death. The impact of coronary revascularization on relief of symptoms, and rates of MI and death in patients with stable angina are discussed below.

INDICATIONS FOR REVASCULARIZATION

In patients with chronic CAD, coronary revascularization is recommended for: (*i*) symptom relief in patients with refractory

Focus Box 26.4

The management of stable angina has two main goals: (*i*) reduce symptoms and ischemia and (*ii*) prevent myocardial infarction and death

Focus Box 26.5

In patients with chronic CAD, coronary revascularization is recommended for: (*i*) symptom relief in patients with refractory symptoms despite optimal medical therapy or (*ii*) for survival benefit in patients at high clinical risk of mortality on non-invasive testing (moderate to large areas of reversible ischemia +/– LV dysfunction) or on angiography (left main stem, three-vessel or two-vessel including proximal LAD disease)

symptoms despite optimal medical therapy or (*ii*) for survival benefit in patients at high clinical risk of mortality on non-invasive testing (moderate to large areas of reversible ischemia +/– LV dysfunction) or on angiography (left main stem, three-vessel or two-vessel including proximal LAD disease) (Focus Box 26.5). It is generally accepted that coronary revascularization is beneficial for symptom relief and indeed, has revolutionized the therapy of CAD over the last 30 years. However, the benefits of revascularization therapy for chronic stable angina in regard to the "hard" endpoints of death and MI are much more controversial unlike the widely accepted benefit in the context of the acute coronary syndromes (ACSs) with ST-elevation MI (65,66) and non-ST elevation MI (66,67). Despite the recent furor over revascularization (and particularly PCI) versus optimal medical therapy generated primarily by the COURAGE trial (68) and

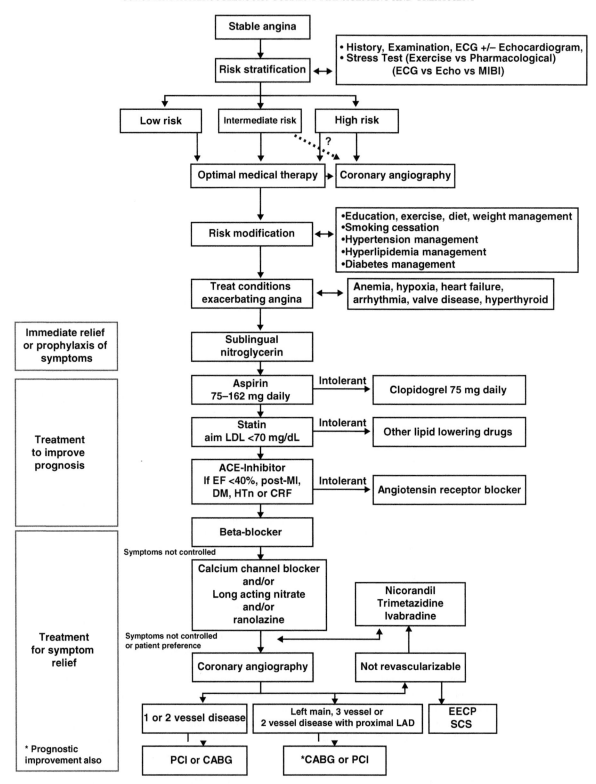

Figure 26.3 Treatment algorithm in patients with stable angina.

Table 26.3 Cardiovascular Risk Reduction for Patients with Coronary Artery Disease

Risk factor or treatment	Recommended management	Benefit of treatment
Physical activity	• 30–45 minutes of physical activity 7 days/week (minimum 5 days/week) • Cardiac rehabilitation for patients at risk (e.g. recent MI or CHF)	• Manages CAD risk factors • Improves exercise tolerance and psychological well-being (22) • Decreases hospitalizations and revascularizations (23) • Decreases mortality rates after MI (24)
Weight management	• Aim for BMI of 18.5–24.9 kg/m^2 • Aim for waist circumference of <35 inches in women and <40 inches in males	• Manages CAD risk factors • Decreases cardiac and all-cause mortality (25)
Smoking cessation	• Complete smoking cessation and avoidance of exposure to tobacco smoke • Counselling, nicotine replacement therapy, buproprion, and varenicline.	• Decreases non-fatal MI and all-cause mortality (26) • Less angina due to slower atherosclerosis progression, less coronary vasoconstriction, less platelet aggregationd and better oxygenation
Blood Pressure Control	• Lifestyle modifications (weight control, physical activity, moderation of alcohol consumption, limited sodium intake and diet high in fresh fruits, vegetables, and low-fat dairy products) • BP control according to Joint National Conference VII guidelines (BP <140/90 mmHg or <130/80 mmHg for patients with diabetes or chronic kidney disease) (27) • Treat initially with beta blockers and/or ACE inhibitors, with addition of other drugs as needed to achieve target BP	• Every 20 mmHg systolic BP increase or 10 mmHg diastolic BP increase above 115/75 mmHg results in a 2 fold increase in CAD (27) • Decreases CAD, CHF, cardiovascular events, stroke, cardiovascular mortality, and all-cause mortality (28) • Regression of LV hypertrophy which is strong risk factor for the development of MI, CHF, and sudden death (29)
Lipid Management	• Diet low in saturated fats (<7% of total calories), trans-fatty acids, and cholesterol (<200 mg/day) • Daily physical activity and weight management • Plant stanol/sterols (2 g/day), viscous fiber (greater than 10 g/day) for LDL-C reduction and Omega-3 fatty acids (1 g/day) for risk reduction • Drug therapy with lipid lowering agents should be used if LDL is ≥100 mg/dL to aim for a 30–40% reduction in LDL-C to a goal of <70 mg/dL • If baseline LDL-C is 70–100 mg/dL, it is reasonable to treat to an LDL-C of <70 mg/dL • Statins (HMG-CoA enzyme inhibitors) are first choice drugs for LDL-C reduction. Ezetimibe, a cholesterol absorption inhibitor, may be used for further LDL lowering to reach goals • If triglycerides are >200 mg/dL, non-HDL-C should be <130 mg/dL (and further reduction to <100 mg/dL is reasonable) with niacin or fibrates (30)	• Decreases cardiac mortality, all-cause mortality, non-fatal MI, stroke and revascularization (31,32) • Improvement in endothelial function and regression of atherosclerosis (33) • Anti-inflammatory effect (34)
Diabetes Management	• Aim for Hemoglobin A1c of <7% with lifestyle and pharmacotherapy	• Possible reduction in non-fatal MI, stroke, and death (35,36)
Anti-platelet agents	• Aspirin 75–162 mg daily should be started and continued indefinitely unless contraindicated • Clopidogrel 75 mg daily may replace aspirin if aspirin is absolutely contraindicated (37) • After acute coronary syndrome, clopidrogrel 75 mg daily should be given for 1 year (38). Alternatives to clopidrogrel include ticlopidine 250 mg twice daily (39), prasugrel 10 mg daily (40), or ticagrelor 90 mg twice daily (41). • After CABG, aspirin 162–325 mg daily should be given for 1 year; then aspirin 75–162 mg daily indefinitely • After PCI, aspirin 162–325 mg daily should be given for at least 1 month after BMS implantation, 3 months after sirolimus-eluting stent implantation, and 6 months after paclitaxel-eluting stent implantation (42); then aspirin 75–162 mg daily indefinitely • For all post-PCI stented patients receiving a DES, clopidogrel 75 mg daily (or alternative antiplatelet as above) should be given for at least 12 months if patients are not at high risk of bleeding. For post-PCI patients receiving a BMS, clopidogrel should be given for a minimum of 1 month and ideally up to 12 months (42)	• Reduce non-fatal MI, stroke and cardiovascular death (43)

(Continued)

Table 26.3 Cardiovascular Risk Reduction for Patients with Coronary Artery Disease (*Continued*)

Risk factor or treatment	Recommended management	Benefit of treatment
Beta Blockers	• Start and continue beta-blocker therapy indefinitely in all patients with a past MI, acute coronary syndrome or LV dysfunction unless contraindicated • Use as needed for angina, hypertension and rhythm management • Contraindicated in severe bradycardia, high grade or second degree atrioventricular block, sick sinus syndrome and severe asthma	• Reduce death and non-fatal MI in patients who have had previous MI (44,45) • Symptomatic improvement of angina (46) by decreasing myocardial oxygen demand (decreased inotropy, chronotropy and hypertension) and increasing myocardial oxygen supply (increased duration of diastole) • Blood pressure control • Anti-arrhythmic
Renin-Angiotensin-Aldosterone System Blockers	• Start ACE-inhibitors and continue indefinitely in all patients with LV ejection fraction ≤40% and in those with hypertension, diabetes, chronic kidney disease (47) or in patients who are not at low risk, unless contraindicated • Consider ACE-inhibitors for all patients with CAD unless contraindicated • Angiotensin receptor blockers may be used in patients who are intolerant to ACE-inhibitors • Aldosterone blockade is recommended in post-MI patients without significant renal dysfunction or hyperkalemia who are already receiving therapeutic doses of ACE inhibitor and beta blocker and who have an LV ejection fraction of ≤40% and have either diabetes or heart failure	• ACE-inhibitors decrease cardiovascular death, all cause death, non-fatal MI and stroke, revascularization procedures and CHF (48,49) • Angiotensin receptor blockers have equal benefits when compared to ACE-inhibitors but the combination of both drugs does not produce increased benefit (50)
Nitrates	• Sublingual nitroglycerin or nitroglycerin spray for the immediate relief of angina or for prophylaxis prior to exercise • Long acting nitrates for symptom relief if beta-blocker treatment alone is unsuccessful or is contraindicated. Nitrate-free interval required to decrease nitrate tolerance	• Symptom relief only by increasing myocardial oxygen supply (coronary artery vasodilatation and redistribution of blood flow to ischemic areas (51)) and decreasing myocardial oxygen demand (decreased preload and afterload) • Additive symptom relief with beta-blocker (52)
Calcium antagonists	• Calcium antagonists for symptom relief if beta-blocker treatment alone is unsuccessful or is contraindicated • Drug of choice for coronary vasospasm (53)	• Symptom relief only by reducing myocardial oxygen demand (decrease afterload +/− decrease inotropy and chronotropy) and increasing myocardial oxygen supply (coronary artery vasodilatation +/− increased duration of diastole) • Additive symptom relief with beta-blocker (54)
Ranolazine	• Consider ranolazine for patients with stable angina for symptom relief (55) • Recently FDA approved as a first line stable angina drug	• Alters the trans-cellular late sodium current resulting in decreased intracellular calcium and less ischemia • Additive symptom relief to beta blockers or calcium antagonists (56,57) but no decrease in MI or death (57) • Does not alter heart rate or BP and may reduce arrhythmias • Reduces HbA1c (58)
Nicorandil	• Consider nicorandil for further symptom relief in addition to the above drugs • Not available in the United States	• Potassium channel opener and a nitrate resulting in coronary vasodilation • Symptom relief equal to calcium antagonists (59) • Possible decrease in coronary events (60)
Trimetazidine	• Consider trimetazidine for further symptom relief in addition to the above drugs • Not available in the United States	• Metabolic agent modulating intracellular calcium and fatty-acid oxidation • Improves symptoms and exercise capacity (61)
Ivabradine	• Consider ivabradine for further symptom relief in addition to the above drugs especially if heart rate is above 70 bpm despite beta-blockers and calcium antagonists • Not available in the United States	• Selective I(f) current inhibitor resulting in decreased heart rate • Equally effective as beta-blockers and further symptom relief when added to beta-blocker (62) but no decrease in MI or death (63)
Influenza vaccine	• Annual vaccine is recommended for all patients with CAD	• Decrease in cardiac events, re-hospitalization and death during the flu season (64)

Abbreviations: ACE, angiotensin-converting enzyme; BMI, body mass index; BMS, bare metal stent; BP, blood pressure; CABG, coronary artery bypass grafting; CHF, congestive heart failure; DES, drug eluting stent; LDL-C, low-density lipoprotein; HDL-C, high-density lipoprotein; HGM-CoA, 3-hydroxy-3-methylglutaryl coenzyme A; LV, left ventricular; MI, myocardial infarction; PCI, percutaneous coronary intervention. *Source*: Adapted from Ref. 20.

two recent meta-analyses (69,70), these basic recommendations remain logical and reasonable (66).

The earliest trials of coronary revascularization, specifically coronary artery bypass grafting (CABG) versus medical therapy in patients with chronic stable angina, were conducted in the 1970s and 1980s (71–73). Despite major advances in medical therapy (especially anti-platelet and lipid lowering therapy) as well as in surgical techniques (including the use of the internal mammary artery), the overall conclusions from these trials and associated registry studies remain valid today. Symptomatic relief was better with CABG but in regard to survival and freedom from MI, there were no overall differences between CABG and medical therapy except in patients considered at higher risk on the basis of left main disease, multi-vessel disease plus LV dysfunction, those with severe angina, and probably in patients with proximal LAD disease in conjunction with multi-vessel disease (74–76). There also appears to be a survival benefit from revascularization in patients with post-infarction angina. The concept of "the greater the risk, the greater benefit" is illustrated in Figure 26.2, which is based on data from the Duke University database—a large, single-center registry study (17). Eighty percent of patients who had CABG in the CASS registry were angina free at 5 years but this decreased to 63% at 10 years and 15% at 15 years. This is most likely due to progression of native CAD as well as vein graft stenosis (60% at 10 years). The use of the left internal mammary graft to the LAD has markedly improved surgical outcomes with about 90% of Left Internal Mammary Artery (LIMA) grafts being patent at 10 years.

The next series of trials performed in the 1990s and 2000s compared revascularization, specifically percutaneous balloon angioplasty with medical therapy in patients with stable CAD. The most important information taken from these studies (77–81) was that balloon angioplasty is associated with further symptomatic relief when compared to medical therapy alone but that it had no significant effect on the hard endpoints of MI and death although cross-over from medical therapy to revascularization was frequent (up to 50%). Subsequent trials comparing medical therapy to PCI with stenting were again neutral for hard endpoints and a recent meta-analysis summarizing 20 years of trials of PCI in patients with non-acute coronary disease concluded that there was no evidence of any benefit on death or MI compared to medical therapy (70). The only two studies showing benefit of revascularization on death or MI included patients with "silent ischemia" —the ACIP pilot study (82) and the SWISSI-2 trial (83) but these included patients who had a prior MI in addition to left main coronary disease and LV dysfunction. Another recent meta-analysis (84) demonstrated a benefit for PCI on mortality but this analysis also included post-MI patients while another metaanalysis showed no benefit on mortality. With regard to current practice, the two most relevant trials attempting to answer the question of whether patients with stable CAD will have better outcomes when treated with OMT and revascularization when compared to OMT alone are the COURAGE (Clinical

Outcomes Utilizing Revascularization and Aggressive Drug Evaluation) trial (68) and the BARI-2D ((Bypass Angioplasty Revascularization Investigation -2D) trial (85).

The COURAGE trial enrolled patients with >70% coronary stenosis in at least one proximal epicardial coronary artery and evidence of myocardial ischemia on stress testing or resting ECG, or patients with at least one coronary stenosis of at least 80% and classic angina without provocative testing. The primary outcome was a composite of death and nonfatal MI and there was no statistical difference between the two groups after a mean follow-up of 4.6 years. Rates of angina were consistently lower in the PCI group than in the medical therapy group during follow-up but were no longer statistically significant at 5 years. Rates of subsequent revascularization were likewise lower in the PCI group. Out of 35,539 patients screened for inclusion to the study, only 2,287 were included, of which 42% had minimal symptoms (Class I or 0) and treatment was randomized only after coronary angiography was done on all patients. We must be cognizant that study trials may have entry and/or selection bias giving results for a study population that may have inherent differences from the general population (86). The recently published BARI-2D trial (85) evaluated 2368 patients with type 2 diabetes and CAD, of which 82% had mild to moderate stable angina and 18% a positive stress test and once again confirmed that there was no significant difference in survival between patients undergoing prompt revascularization (PCI or CABG) and those undergoing OMT. However, diabetic patients who underwent CABG (but not PCI) had significantly fewer major cardiac events, driven mainly by a reduction in nonfatal MI, compared to OMT alone (Fig. 26.4). Patients treated with revascularization had lower rates of new angina, worsening angina or revascularization at 3 years (87). It is important to note that a significant number of patients (32% in COURAGE and 42% in BARI-2D) did cross over from the medical arm to the revascularization arm in these studies. This should not be taken as a weakness of the studies but rather as valuable information for patients who chose a conservative approach—medical therapy is not a 'life sentence' decision since one third to half of patients may require revascularization within 5 years (Fig. 26.5). It should be emphasized that the trial of medical therapy should not be drawn out over many months—the drugs are either effective (as well as tolerated) within approximately 2 months or else a decision regarding revascularization may be taken.

The lack of benefit from PCI in reducing death and MI is most likely due to the fact that PCI is directed at culprit lesions that cause symptoms and/or ischemia. However, there is good evidence that progression of disease and subsequent coronary events may occur from plaque rupture at sites which were at the time of initial angiogram considered to be non-obstructivestenoses and this emphasizes our current inability to predict "future" culprits (19). On the other hand, it is becoming increasingly apparent that OMT including aggressive control of risk factors and lifestyle modification may have a major impact on endothelial function and

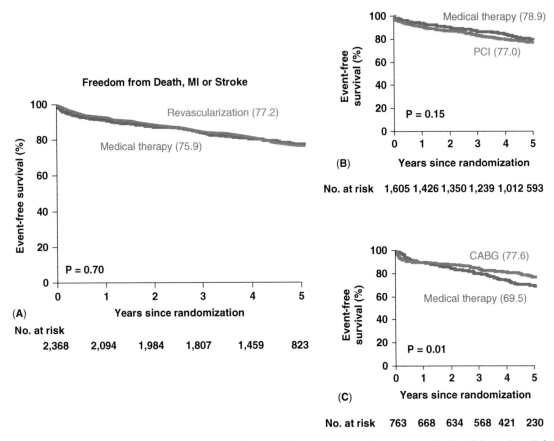

Figure 26.4 Five-year outcomes in diabetic patients treated with medical therapy or revascularization in the BARI-2D trial. *Source:* From Ref. 85.

stability and as such could reduce the incidence of future coronary events. These trials make the point that in a selected subset of patients with stable CAD at low to moderate risk *who underwent angiography prior to randomization,* an initial trial of medical therapy is reasonable with the option of proceeding to revascularization if symptoms and quality of life do not improve on medical therapy alone.

A relatively small nuclear perfusion substudy (88) from COURAGE reinforces the logical precept that the extent of ischemia is an important determinant of long-term outcomes (Fig. 26.6; 89–91). This substudy showed that in patients with ischemia on nuclear perfusion, the percentage reduction in ischemia with PCI was superior to that with OMT and that patients with less ischemia had lower rates of death or MI. Ischemia may be used as an indicator for a more aggressive approach in such patients but this does not negate the overall results and conclusions from the COURAGE trial. The upcoming international randomized controlled ISCHEMIA trial will assess the comparative effectiveness of two initial management strategies for stable patients with moderate-to-severe ischemia on nuclear or echo stress testing: catheterization with revascularization if feasible (PCI or CABG) plus OMT versus OMT alone.

Similarly although retrospective data (92) suggested that revascularization of viable myocardium in patients with LV dysfunction and symptoms of CHF may improve survival, this was debatable in the recently published STICH trial (93). In this trial, patients with ischemic cardiomyopathy (ejection fraction ≤35%) were randomized to medical therapy or medical therapy with CABG. At 6 years of follow-up, the primary outcome of all-cause mortality was equal between the two groups but CABG did reduce cardiovascular mortality and morbidity (re-hospitalization and revascularization). The cross-over rate to CABG was 17% and on per-protocol analysis, there was a decrease in all cause mortality in the CABG arm. In the subgroup study of patients who underwent myocardial viability testing (94), the presence of viability demonstrated greater likelihood of survival. However, there seemed to be no difference in outcomes in the adjusted analysis between patients who were treated with CABG versus those who did not, irrespective of viability. Although this is a subanalysis and could well be underpowered, this is an important although somewhat confusing observation, since many centers routinely perform viability testing prior to considering revascularization in patients with ischemic cardiomyopathy, and patients who do

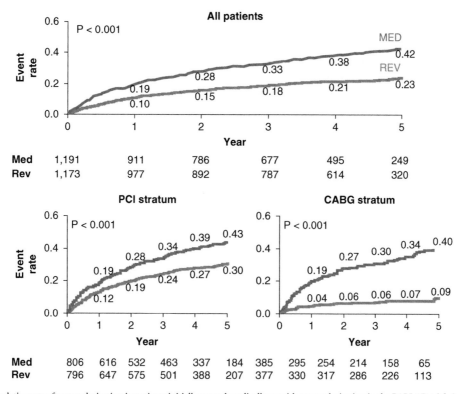

Figure 26.5 Cumulative rate of revascularization in patients initially treated medically or with revascularization in the BARI-2D trial. *Source:* From Ref. 87.

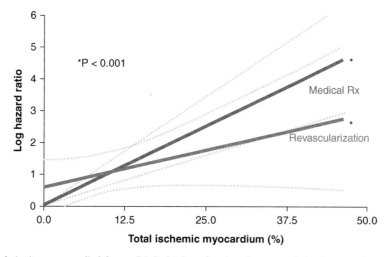

Figure 26.6 Revascularization versus medical therapy (Medical Rx) as a function of percentage ischemic myocardium. *Source:* From Ref. 91.

not demonstrate viability are automatically referred for medical management.

Not all apparently significant stenoses on visual inspection are hemodynamically significant and a recent small trial demonstrated the benefits of targeted revascularization based upon an objective measurement of hemodynamic severity. In this trial (95), fractional flow reserve (FFR) guided (<0.80) PCI was superior compared to angiography-guided PCI for increasing survival free of MI or revascularization (7.3% vs 11.1%). Deferring PCI in patients with stenotic lesions but a normal FFR (≥0.75) was associated with similar 5 year survival free of MI or death (96). In summary, in the absence of symptoms or ischemia, revascularization is not indicated since lesions that may be future "culprits" in regard to subsequent MI or death cannot be identified at this time using current methodologies. The search to find the location of future plaque ruptures or erosions leading to myocardial infarction (so called vulnerable plaques) is an important area of cardiovascular research and could potentially change drastically how CAD is diagnosed and treated.

A valid question arising from the COURAGE and other trials is whether coronary revascularization, and in particular PCI, is currently appropriately or over-utilized. Only 44.5% of patients have non-invasive stress testing prior to PCI in the US with a substantial variation according to geography (22–71%; 97). This is remarkably similar to experience in the UK where 43% of patients have stress testing prior to PCI (98). Furthermore, revascularization rates also vary widely with an 83% higher rate in Florida compared to Oregon. Revascularization rates are dependent on race (28% variation) and cardiac catheterization rates (68% variation), which in turn depends on hospital admission rates for CAD as well as the number of cardiac surgeons and interventionalists in the local population(99). Inappropriate use of PCI may be as high as 43% in stable CAD (100) but underutilization of coronary angiography (57–71%), PCI (34%), and CABG (26%) is also common in clinically indicated cases and not undergoing revascularization is associated with higher coronary events in these patients (101,102). In North New England, there has been a significant 26% decrease in PCI volumes post-COURAGE compared to pre-COURAGE publication (103). Among patients undergoing PCI for stable angina in the UK, coronary angiography is underused in older people, women, South Asians, and people from deprived areas (104). Appropriateness of CABG in Northern New England in 2008 was calculated at being 87.7% (105).

METHOD OF CHOICE FOR REVASCULARIZATION
There are two well-established methods of revascularization for CAD – CABG introduced in 1968 and PCI. PCI includes percutaneous balloon angioplasty introduced in 1977 and stenting with bare metal stents (BMS) since 1995 or drug-eluting stents (DES) since 2003. An estimated 622,000 patients underwent PCI in the USA in 2007, of which 90% had a stent inserted and 76% of these involved using a DES stent (3). CABG was performed on 232,000 patients in the United States in 2007. The mean cost was $56,000 for PCI and $117,000 for CABG (3). In a population-based observational study from Olmsted County, MN, from 1990 to 2004, revascularization utilization increased by 24% but the trends diverged by procedure type, with a sustained increase (69%) for PCI contrasting with a stabilization, then decline (-33%) for CABG (106). CABG procedures continue to decrease at 5% per year and rates of PCI have started to decrease by about 2.5% per year from 2004 to 2009 in the Medicare population in the United States (107).

Over the last 30 years, many trials have compared different methods of revascularization including balloon angioplasty to BMS, BMS to DES, balloon angioplasty to CABG, and BMS to CABG. The common denominator of these trials is that there

was no difference in death or non-fatal MI between these methods of revascularization (70,108). BMS decreased the rate of restenosis and the need for repeat PCI when compared to balloon angioplasty by about 30% (109). DES further decreased the rate of in-stent restenosis and need for target lesion revascularization by 30–70% compared to BMS but there was no improvement in survival or MI up to 4 years after implantation (110). There is no statistical difference in early (≤1 month) and late (>1 month to <1 year) stent thrombosis between BMS and DES but a slight increase in very late (>1 year) stent thrombosis with DES (111) (which is not associated with increased mortality or MI compared to BMS).

Patients with multivessel disease undergoing CABG have been shown to require less additional revascularization compared to those having PCI (108,112) but no survival advantage has been demonstrated with the exception of diabetics in the BARI trial (113). However, recent meta-analyses have had conflicting conclusions regarding this survival advantage in diabetics (108,112). Whether this survival difference in diabetics in favor of CABG still applies in the current era will depend to some extent on the long-term follow-up of the SYNTAX trial and the results of the ongoing NHLBI-sponsored FREEDOM trial. Meta-analysis of the four most important trials of PCI with BMS versus CABG (the ERAC-II trial (114), Stent or surgery trial (115), ARTS trial (116), and MASS-II trial (81)) once again showed similar long term (5-year) safety profiles but increased need for revascularization in the BMS group when compared to CABG (117). The MASS-II trial did show a lower event rate for myocardial infarction in patients treated with CABG between 5 and 10 years of follow-up compared to PCI with BMS, not previously evident in the first 5 years (81).

The SYNTAX (118) trial was recently published in which patients with previously untreated left main stem or three-vessel disease were randomly assigned to undergo state-of-the-art CABG or PCI with DES. At 36 months follow-up, there was no difference between the two groups in the composite endpoint of death, MI, and stroke but the patients in the PCI group needed repeat revascularization more often than the CABG group (Fig. 26.7A–C). The rate of MI was also higher in the PCI group over 3 years most likely due to the fact that PCI targets culprit lesions while CABG bypasses whole segments and thus possibly future culprit lesions. The rate of stroke was higher in the CABG group in the first year but this may be due to the decreased utilization of anti-platelet agents in this group. Furthermore, the investigators used an angiographic grading tool (the SYNTAX score) to determine the complexity of CAD. The SYNTAX score is the sum of the points assigned to each individual lesion identified in the 16 segments of the coronary tree with >50% diameter narrowing in vessels >1.5 mm diameter. The SYNTAX score may help identify patients at low risk who may be appropriately treated with PCI with at least equivalent outcomes as CABG. On the other hand, intermediate- and high-risk patients by SYNTAX score were shown to have decreased major adverse cardiac and cerebrovascular events when assigned to CABG rather than PCI (Fig. 26.7D–F) after 3 years. The final verdict in

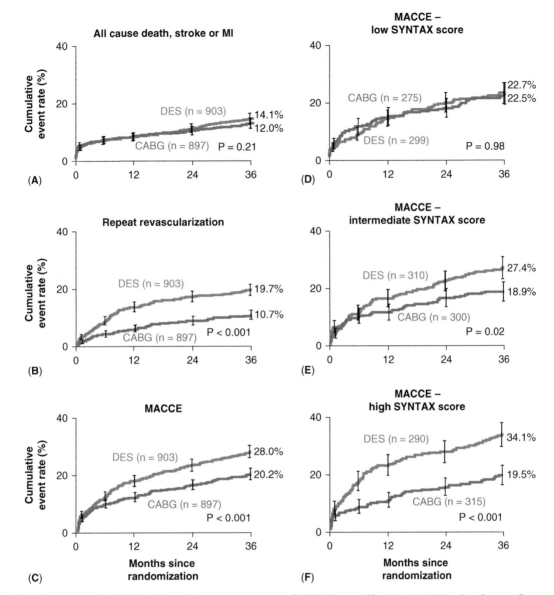

Figure 26.7 Patient outcomes in SYNTAX trial according to treatment group and SYNTAX score. *Abbreviation*: MACCE, major adverse cardiac or cerebrovascular events. *Source*: From the 24th EACTS 2010 meeting SYTNAX 3-year presentation, with permission.

regard to the SYNTAX trial awaits the long-term (5 years) follow-up data but the data do appear to be a following a consistent trend in that among the group of patients with left main or three-vessel disease, there is a subset who do well with PCI but the majority who have more complex and diffuse disease appear to benefit from CABG.

Thus, the method of choice for revascularization depends on the angiographic characteristics of the lesions causing ischemia, LV dysfunction, comorbidities and suitability of the patient for surgery, likelihood of technical success with PCI, quality of life expectations, and patient preference (Focus Box 26.6). The advantages of PCI include lesser invasiveness, no need for general

> *Focus Box 26.6*
>
> The method of choice for revascularization depends on the angiographic characteristics of the lesions causing ischemia, LV dysfunction, comorbidities and suitability of the patient for surgery, likelihood of technical success with PCI, quality of life expectations and patient preference

anesthesia, less post-procedural morbidity, and a shorter hospital stay. CABG surgery has the advantage of bypassing chronic occlusions and complex stenoses as well as a greater ability to achieve complete revascularization by bypassing not only

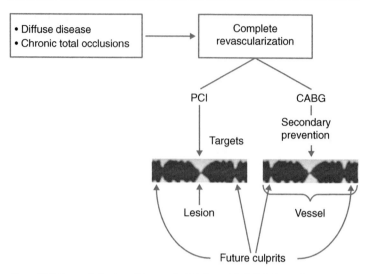

Figure 26.8 Revascularization of future culprit lesions with CABG. *Source*: From Ref. 119.

"culprit lesions" but "future culprits," thus necessitating fewer repeat revascularizations (Fig. 26.8) (119). However, CABG is associated with increased postoperative morbidity including stroke, longer period of hospitalization, and a slower return to normal activities (up to 6 weeks). In current practice, CABG is often the preferred method of revascularization in patients with high-risk left main, triple-vessel, or double-vessel disease with significant (especially proximal) LAD involvement and LV dysfunction particularly in diabetics (66,120). For some patients with left main disease, particularly ostial lesions, there is increasing data to suggest that PCI may be an alternative to CABG with similar risk for the composite of death, MI, or stroke but increased need for revascularization (121,122). A large trial of patients with LMCA disease comparing CABG to DES is currently in progress. CABG is often preferred in patients with chronic total occlusions and multiple complex (Class C) lesions (120). Most patients requiring revascularization with lesions amenable to PCI and who do not fulfill the above criteria undergo PCI rather than CABG. When PCI is the chosen method of revascularization, DES is usually preferred due to the decreased rate of in-stent restenosis and need for target lesion revascularization compared to BMS. However, in patients in whom long-term dual platelet therapy may be problematic (due to bleeding, upcoming noncardiac surgery, or financial issues) BMS may be the stent of choice. The relative indications for PCI versus CABG are part of a changing landscape as technologies of PCI and CABG continue to evolve. A critical issue is the extent to which all forms of therapy are appropriately utilized based on the guidelines and appropriateness criteria, particularly in a changing environment with regard to the costs and affordability of health care.

ALTERNATIVE THERAPIES FOR REFRACTORY STABLE ANGINA
Some patients have CAD with intractable angina despite maximum medical therapy and may not be candidates for revascularization. One option for these patients is spinal cord stimulation (SCS) in which an electrode is inserted into the epidural space at the C7-T1 level. This electrode stimulates axons in the spinal cord that do not transmit pain so as to reduce input to the brain of axons that do transmit pain (gate theory). SCS has been shown to decrease angina frequency by up to 80%, decrease angina severity, and improve quality of life (123). One study showed SCS to be non-inferior to CABG for quality of life and survival after 5 years follow-up in patients with refractory angina (124). Additional trials are needed because all the trials in this area are extremely underpowered.

Another technique used for the treatment of patients with refractory angina is enhanced external counterpulsation (EECP). This involves the use of a series of cuffs wrapped around the patient's legs, which are inflated with compressed air in sequence (distally to proximally) during diastole so as to propel blood back to the heart. EECP is administered as 35 1-hour treatment sessions over 7 weeks. The proposed mechanism of action is reduced myocardial demand, improved myocardial perfusion, and improved endothelial function (125). EECP reduces the frequency and/or severity of angina in up to 80% of patients, extends time to exercise-induced ischemia, and improves quality of life in patients with symptomatic CAD and is generally well tolerated (126).

Transmyocardial laser revascularization is another technique used for refractory angina, which involves the creation of small channels from the epicardial to endocardial surfaces of the heart by laser using a surgical approach. The mechanism of action of laser therapy is incompletely understood and several randomized trials have failed to demonstrate an increase in survival highlighting the important role of the placebo effect in reducing angina with transmyocardial laser revascularization (127), which is now rarely used.

Intramyocardial bone marrow stem cell injection is currently being investigated as a new therapeutic option for patients with chronic ischemia who are ineligible for revascularization. Bone marrow cells are harvested from the iliac crest or by leukapheresis after granulocyte colony-stimulating factor and the mononuclear CD34+ stem cells are isolated and then injected into the ischemic myocardium (128,129). Myocardial injection was found to be safe and a small randomized placebo-controlled study (129) resulted in statistically significant but modest improvement in myocardial perfusion, LVEF as well as exercise capacity and angina severity class compared with placebo. This technique is still in the experimental stages and further studies are required to assess long-term results and efficacy for mortality and morbidity.

CONCLUSION

Patients with stable angina should be risk stratified to identify the most effective management strategy. Aggressive control of risk factors and optimal medical therapy with anti-anginal and anti-ischemic drugs are the cornerstone of treatment for all patients with chronic CAD. Indeed, a conservative trial of medical therapy is reasonable in all patients with stable angina unless they are at high risk for cardiac events. Persistent symptoms, the magnitude of the ischemic burden or drug intolerance should drive decision making regarding revascularization. Ideally, ischemia should be established with a non-invasive stress test prior to angiography. In patients undergoing angiography without a previous non-invasive stress test, FFR may be used to make appropriate decisions regarding revascularization, but the technique requires experience and is not widely used in many catheterization labs. Revascularization, with PCI or CABG, is very effective treatment for stable angina but only when performed on targeted culprit stenoses that are hemodynamically significant or causing ischemia. The method of choice for revascularization depends on the angiographic characteristics of the lesions causing ischemia, LV dysfunction, comorbidities, and suitability of the patient for surgery, and likelihood of technical success. The physician's ultimate decisions regarding patient care must incorporate current evidence-based medicine as well as the patient's preferences and quality of life expectations.

PERSONAL PERSPECTIVE—DR BJ GERSH

The management of chronic stable angina is extremely important from a public health perspective, given the magnitude of the population with stable but severely symptomatic angina.

The symptomatic benefits of medical therapy are well documented, but trials of anti-anginal drugs on mortality have not been performed. The cornerstones of therapy are the beta-blockers and calcium channel blockers plus the use of nitroglycerin during episodes and also prophylactically in addition to a long-acting nitrate, but taking into account the potential for nitrate tolerance. The only new anti-anginal released in the United States in decades has been ranolazine, a drug with potentially interesting application. Hopefully, we will see other new anti-anginal drugs in the future. Aggressive secondary prevention with a concerted attack upon *all* the risk factors is required in each and every patient.

Trials of revascularization versus medical therapy or coronary bypass surgery versus percutaneous coronary intervention are difficult to carry out and always appear to fuel a controversy including some inappropriate criticisms from time to time. One has to realize the trials of two therapies will introduce an "entry bias" and that these trials will be confined to patients in whom there is clinical equipoise and as such are eligible for both therapies. This tends to be a group that is not representative of the majority of patients undergoing angiography. On the other hand, registries are more reflective of practice at large, and the results are generalizable to a wider subset of patients. Nonetheless, registries introduce an unavoidable "selection bias," and although statistical models can adjust for potential confounders they cannot eliminate them entirely. The key to the appropriate interpretation of data is to understand both the strengths and the limitations of registries and randomized trials as they can be complementary to each other.

What have we learned from approximately 30 years of trials of coronary revascularization in chronic stable angina? First, in comparison to medical therapy, the benefits of CABG on survival are in *sicker* patients as defined by the severity of symptoms or ischemia, left ventricular dysfunction, the number of vessels diseased, and the anatomic location of disease. Second, trials of CABG versus PCI have demonstrated similar outcomes in regard to death and myocardial infarction except in sicker patients, for example, diabetes, the BARI trial, and patients with more complex disease in the SYNTAX trial in which CABG is the superior strategy. In patients with left main coronary disease, there may well be a role for PCI based on the SYNTAX data, but we need to await the results of ongoing trials, and I suspect that left main disease in association with complex diffuse disease in other vessels will remain a surgical disease, but in more localized forms of left main coronary disease, PCI may find a niche, particularly in patients who are not good surgical candidates. Two trials of patients with chronic stable angina have not shown a benefit from PCI over optimal medical therapy among angiographically selected patients. The next step is a trial of patients randomized at the time of stress testing and this has recently been initiated.

In conclusion, the benefits of revascularization in high-risk subsets of patients with CAD is not in dispute, for example, patients with severe symptoms or ischemic, left ventricular dysfunction, left main coronary disease, and proximal LAD disease. However, among patients with mild to moderate chronic stable angina, an initial trial of medical therapy, which requires careful follow-up with the option of coronary revascularization if medical therapy fails, remains the most appropriate strategy, and this is reflected in our guidelines. It should be emphasized that the outcome of medical therapy should not be assessed (as in many patients decisions) as the success or lack thereof within a period of four to eight weeks, which allows for drug titration.

Finally, the appropriate utilization of invasive therapies is a subject that must be addressed by the entire profession. It would be a tragedy if after the advances of the last three decades the decision as to who receives coronary revascularization is taken out of the hands of cardiologists and cardiac surgeons, but in order to prevent this the onus of responsibility is on us to use evidence-based strategies to appropriately select patients for invasive versus medical therapy.

CONFLICT OF INTEREST

AC – none. BJG – advisory board member with Boston Scientific and stock shareholder for CV Therapeutics.

REFERENCES

1. Diamond GA. A clinically relevant classification of chest discomfort. J Am Coll Cardiol 1983; 1: 574–5.
2. Campeau L. Letter: grading of angina pectoris. Circulation 1976; 54: 522–3.
3. Roger VL, Go AS, Lloyd-Jones DM, et al. Heart disease and stroke statistics–2011 update: a report from the American Heart Association. Circulation 2011; 123: e18–e209.
4. Fox K, Garcia MA, Ardissino D, et al. Guidelines on the management of stable angina pectoris: executive summary: The Task Force on the Management of Stable Angina Pectoris of the European Society of Cardiology. Eur Heart J 2006; 27: 1341–81.
5. Kannel WB, Feinleib M. Natural history of angina pectoris in the Framingham study. Prognosis and survival. Am J Cardiol 1972; 29: 154–63.
6. Pryor DB, Shaw L, Harrell FE Jr, et al. Estimating the likelihood of severe coronary artery disease. Am J Med 1991; 90: 553–62.
7. Rihal CS, Davis KB, Kennedy JW, et al. The utility of clinical, electrocardiographic, and roentgenographic variables in the prediction of left ventricular function. Am J Cardiol 1995; 75: 220–3.
8. Frank CW, Weinblatt E, Shapiro S. Angina pectoris in men. Prognostic significance of selected medical factors. Circulation 1973; 47: 509–17.
9. Ruberman W, Weinblatt E, Goldberg JD, et al. Ventricular premature complexes in prognosis of angina. Circulation 1980; 61: 1172–82.
10. Emond M, Mock MB, Davis KB, et al. Long-term survival of medically treated patients in the Coronary Artery Surgery Study (CASS) Registry. Circulation 1994; 90: 2645–57.
11. White HD, Norris RM, Brown MA, et al. Left ventricular end-systolic volume as the major determinant of survival after recovery from myocardial infarction. Circulation 1987; 76: 44–51.
12. Senni M, Tribouilloy CM, Rodeheffer RJ, et al. Congestive heart failure in the community: a study of all incident cases in Olmsted County, Minnesota, in 1991. Circulation 1998; 98: 2282–9.
13. Mark DB, Hlatky MA, Harrell FE Jr, et al. Exercise treadmill score for predicting prognosis in coronary artery disease. Ann Intern Med 1987; 106: 793–800.
14. Gibbons RJ, Abrams J, Chatterjee K, et al. ACC/AHA 2002 guideline update for the management of patients with chronic stable angina–summary article: a report of the American College of Cardiology/American Heart Association Task Force on Practice Guidelines (Committee on the Management of Patients With Chronic Stable Angina). Circulation 2003; 107: 149–58.
15. Scanlon PJ, Faxon DP, Audet AM, et al. ACC/AHA guidelines for coronary angiography: executive summary and recommendations. A report of the American College of Cardiology/American Heart Association Task Force on Practice Guidelines (Committee on Coronary Angiography) developed in collaboration with the Society for Cardiac Angiography and Interventions. Circulation 1999; 99: 2345–57.
16. Ovrehus KA, Botker HE, Jensen JM, et al. Influence of coronary computed tomographic angiography on patient treatment and prognosis in patients with suspected stable angina pectoris. Am J Cardiol 2011; 107: 1473–9.
17. Jones RH, Kesler K, Phillips. HR 3rd, et al. Long-term survival benefits of coronary artery bypass grafting and percutaneous transluminal angioplasty in patients with coronary artery disease. J Thorac Cardiovasc Surg 1996; 111: 1013–25.
18. Gersh BJ, Califf RM, Loop FD, et al. Coronary bypass surgery in chronic stable angina. Circulation 1989; 79: I46–59.
19. Bigi R, Cortigiani L, Colombo P, et al. Prognostic and clinical correlates of angiographically diffuse non-obstructive coronary lesions. Heart 2003; 89: 1009–13.
20. Cassar A, Holmes DR Jr, Rihal CS, et al. Chronic coronary artery disease: diagnosis and management. Mayo Clin Proc 2009; 84: 1130–46.
21. Fraker TD Jr, Fihn SD, Gibbons RJ, et al. 2007 chronic angina focused update of the ACC/AHA 2002 Guidelines for the management of patients with chronic stable angina: a report of the American College of Cardiology/American Heart Association Task Force on Practice Guidelines Writing Group to develop the focused update of the 2002 Guidelines for the management of patients with chronic stable angina. Circulation 2007; 116: 2762–72.
22. Thompson PD, Buchner D, Pina IL, et al. Exercise and physical activity in the prevention and treatment of atherosclerotic cardiovascular disease: a statement from the Council on Clinical Cardiology (Subcommittee on Exercise, Rehabilitation, and Prevention) and the Council on Nutrition, Physical Activity, and Metabolism (Subcommittee on Physical Activity). Circulation 2003; 107: 3109–16.
23. Hambrecht R, Walther C, Mobius-Winkler S, et al. Percutaneous coronary angioplasty compared with exercise training in patients with stable coronary artery disease: a randomized trial. Circulation 2004; 109: 1371–8.
24. O'Connor GT, Buring JE, Yusuf S, et al. An overview of randomized trials of rehabilitation with exercise after myocardial infarction. Circulation 1989; 80: 234–44.
25. Kennedy LM, Dickstein K, Anker SD, et al. Weight-change as a prognostic marker in 12 550 patients following acute myocardial infarction or with stable coronary artery disease. Eur Heart J 2006; 27: 2755–62.
26. Critchley JA, Capewell S. Mortality risk reduction associated with smoking cessation in patients with coronary heart disease: a systematic review. JAMA 2003; 290: 86–97.
27. Chobanian AV, Bakris GL, Black HR, et al. Seventh report of the Joint National Committee on prevention, detection, evaluation, and treatment of high blood pressure. Hypertension 2003; 42: 1206–52.
28. Psaty BM, Lumley T, Furberg CD, et al. Health outcomes associated with various antihypertensive therapies used as first-line agents: a network meta-analysis. JAMA 2003; 289: 2534–44.
29. Levy D, Salomon M, D'Agostino RB, et al. Prognostic implications of baseline electrocardiographic features and their serial changes in subjects with left ventricular hypertrophy. Circulation 1994; 90: 1786–93.

30. Grundy SM, Cleeman JI, Merz CN, et al. Implications of recent clinical trials for the National Cholesterol Education Program Adult Treatment Panel III guidelines. Circulation 2004; 110: 227–39.

31. MRC/BHF Heart Protection Study of cholesterol lowering with simvastatin in 20,536 high-risk individuals: a randomised placebo-controlled trial. Lancet 2002; 360: 7–22.

32. LaRosa JC, Grundy SM, Waters DD, et al. Intensive lipid lowering with atorvastatin in patients with stable coronary disease. N Engl J Med 2005; 352: 1425–35.

33. Nissen SE, Nicholls SJ, Sipahi I, et al. Effect of very high-intensity statin therapy on regression of coronary atherosclerosis: the ASTEROID trial. JAMA 2006; 295: 1556–65.

34. Ridker PM, Danielson E, Fonseca FA, et al. Rosuvastatin to prevent vascular events in men and women with elevated C-reactive protein. N Engl J Med 2008; 359: 2195–207.

35. Nathan DM, Cleary PA, Backlund JY, et al. Intensive diabetes treatment and cardiovascular disease in patients with type 1 diabetes. N Engl J Med 2005; 353: 2643–53.

36. Dormandy JA, Charbonnel B, Eckland DJ, et al. Secondary prevention of macrovascular events in patients with type 2 diabetes in the PROactive Study (PROspective pioglitAzone Clinical Trial In macroVascular Events): a randomised controlled trial. Lancet 2005; 366: 1279–89.

37. CAPRIE Steering Committee. A randomised, blinded, trial of clopidogrel versus aspirin in patients at risk of ischaemic events (CAPRIE). Lancet 1996; 348: 1329–39.

38. Yusuf S, Zhao F, Mehta SR, et al. Effects of clopidogrel in addition to aspirin in patients with acute coronary syndromes without ST-segment elevation. N Engl J Med 2001; 345: 494–502.

39. Bhatt DL, Bertrand ME, Berger PB, et al. Meta-analysis of randomized and registry comparisons of ticlopidine with clopidogrel after stenting. J Am Coll Cardiol 2002; 39: 9–14.

40. Wiviott SD, Braunwald E, McCabe CH, et al. Prasugrel versus clopidogrel in patients with acute coronary syndromes. N Engl J Med 2007; 357: 2001–15.

41. Wallentin L, Becker RC, Budaj A, et al. Ticagrelor versus clopidogrel in patients with acute coronary syndromes. N Engl J Med 2009; 361: 1045–57.

42. King SB 3rd, Smith SC Jr, Hirshfeld JW Jr, et al. 2007 Focused Update of the ACC/AHA/SCAI 2005 Guideline Update for Percutaneous Coronary Intervention: a report of the American College of Cardiology/American Heart Association Task Force on Practice Guidelines: 2007 Writing Group to Review New Evidence and Update the ACC/AHA/SCAI 2005 Guideline Update for Percutaneous Coronary Intervention, Writing on Behalf of the 2005 Writing Committee. Circulation 2008; 117: 261–95.

43. Collaborative meta-analysis of randomised trials of antiplatelet therapy for prevention of death, myocardial infarction, and stroke in high risk patients. Bmj 2002; 324: 71–86

44. A randomized trial of propranolol in patients with acute myocardial infarction . I. Mortality results. JAMA 1982; 247: 1707–14

45. A randomized trial of propranolol in patients with acute myocardial infarction. II. Morbidity results. JAMA 1983; 250: 2814–9

46. Quyyumi AA, Crake T, Wright CM, et al. Medical treatment of patients with severe exertional and rest angina: double blind comparison of beta blocker, calcium antagonist, and nitrate. Br Heart J 1987; 57: 505–11.

47. Solomon SD, Rice MM, K AJ, et al. Renal function and effectiveness of angiotensin-converting enzyme inhibitor therapy in patients with chronic stable coronary disease in the Prevention of Events with ACE inhibition (PEACE) trial. Circulation 2006; 114: 26–31.

48. Yusuf S, Sleight P, Pogue J, et al. Effects of an angiotensin-converting-enzyme inhibitor, ramipril, on cardiovascular events in high-risk patients. The Heart Outcomes Prevention Evaluation Study Investigators. N Engl J Med 2000; 342: 145–53.

49. Fox KM. Efficacy of perindopril in reduction of cardiovascular events among patients with stable coronary artery disease: randomised, double-blind, placebo-controlled, multicentre trial (the EUROPA study). Lancet 2003; 362: 782–8.

50. Yusuf S, Teo KK, Pogue J, et al. Telmisartan, ramipril, or both in patients at high risk for vascular events. N Engl J Med 2008; 358: 1547–59.

51. Tadamura E, Mamede M, Kubo S, et al. The effect of nitroglycerin on myocardial blood flow in various segments characterized by rest-redistribution thallium SPECT. J Nucl Med 2003; 44: 745–51.

52. Akhras F, Jackson G. Efficacy of nifedipine and isosorbide mononitrate in combination with atenolol in stable angina. Lancet 1991; 338: 1036–9.

53. Chahine RA, Feldman RL, Giles TD, et al. Randomized placebo-controlled trial of amlodipine in vasospastic angina. Amlodipine Study 160 Group. J Am Coll Cardiol 1993; 21: 1365–70.

54. Savonitto S, Ardissiono D, Egstrup K, et al. Combination therapy with metoprolol and nifedipine versus monotherapy in patients with stable angina pectoris. Results of the International Multicenter Angina Exercise (IMAGE) Study. J Am Coll Cardiol 1996; 27: 311–16.

55. Rousseau MF, Pouleur H, Cocco G, et al. Comparative efficacy of ranolazine versus atenolol for chronic angina pectoris. Am J Cardiol 2005; 95: 311–16.

56. Chaitman BR, Pepine CJ, Parker JO, et al. Effects of ranolazine with atenolol, amlodipine, or diltiazem on exercise tolerance and angina frequency in patients with severe chronic angina: a randomized controlled trial. JAMA 2004; 291: 309–16.

57. Wilson SR, Scirica BM, Braunwald E, et al. Efficacy of ranolazine in patients with chronic angina observations from the randomized, double-blind, placebo-controlled MERLIN-TIMI (Metabolic Efficiency With Ranolazine for Less Ischemia in Non-ST-Segment Elevation Acute Coronary Syndromes) 36 trial. J Am Coll Cardiol 2009; 53: 1510–16.

58. Morrow DA, Scirica BM, Chaitman BR, et al. Evaluation of the glycometabolic effects of ranolazine in patients with and without diabetes mellitus in the MERLIN-TIMI 36 randomized controlled trial. Circulation 2009; 119: 2032–9.

59. Guermonprez JL, Blin P, Peterlongo F. A double-blind comparison of the long-term efficacy of a potassium channel opener and a calcium antagonist in stable angina pectoris. Eur Heart J 1993: 14(Suppl B): 30–4.

60. Effect of nicorandil on coronary events in patients with stable angina: the Impact Of Nicorandil in Angina (IONA) randomised trial. Lancet 2002; 359: 1269–75

61. Detry JM, Leclercq PJ. Trimetazidine European Multicenter Study versus propranolol in stable angina pectoris: contribution of Holter electrocardiographic ambulatory monitoring. Am J Cardiol 1995; 76: 8B–11B.

62. Tardif JC, Ponikowski P, Kahan T. Efficacy of the If current inhibitor ivabradine in patients with chronic stable angina receiving beta-blocker therapy: a 4 month, randomized, placebo-controlled trial. Eur Heart J 2009; 30: 540–8.

63. Fox K, Ford I, Steg PG, et al. Ivabradine for patients with stable coronary artery disease and left-ventricular systolic dysfunction (BEAUTIFUL): a randomised, double-blind, placebo-controlled trial. Lancet 2008; 372: 807–16.

64. Gurfinkel EP, de la Fuente RL, Mendiz O, et al. Influenza vaccine pilot study in acute coronary syndromes and planned percutaneous coronary interventions: the FLU Vaccination Acute Coronary Syndromes (FLUVACS) Study. Circulation 2002; 105: 2143–7.

65. Keeley EC, Boura JA, Grines CL. Primary angioplasty versus intravenous thrombolytic therapy for acute myocardial infarction: a quantitative review of 23 randomised trials. Lancet 2003; 361: 13–20.

66. Patel MR, Dehmer GJ, Hirshfeld JW, et al. ACCF/SCAI/STS/AATS/AHA/ASNC 2009 Appropriateness Criteria for Coronary Revascularization: A Report of the American College of Cardiology Foundation Appropriateness Criteria Task Force, Society for Cardiovascular Angiography and Interventions, Society of Thoracic Surgeons, American Association for Thoracic Surgery, American Heart Association, and the American Society of Nuclear Cardiology: endorsed by the American Society of Echocardiography, the Heart Failure Society of America, and the Society of Cardiovascular Computed Tomography. Circulation 2009; 119: 1330–52.

67. FRagmin and Fast Revascularisation during InStability in Coronary artery disease Investigators. Invasive compared with non-invasive treatment in unstable coronary-artery disease: FRISC II prospective randomised multicentre study. Lancet 1999; 354: 708–15

68. Boden WE, O'Rourke RA, Teo KK, et al. Optimal medical therapy with or without PCI for stable coronary disease. N Engl J Med 2007; 356: 1503–16.

69. Katritsis DG, Ioannidis JP. Percutaneous coronary intervention versus conservative therapy in nonacute coronary artery disease: a meta-analysis. Circulation 2005; 111: 2906–12.

70. Trikalinos TA, Alsheikh-Ali AA, Tatsioni A, et al. Percutaneous coronary interventions for non-acute coronary artery disease: a quantitative 20-year synopsis and a network meta-analysis. Lancet 2009; 373: 911–8.

71. The VA Coronary Artery Bypass Surgery Cooperative Study Group. Eighteen-year follow-up in the veterans affairs cooperative study of coronary artery bypass surgery for stable angina. Circulation 1992; 86: 121–30.

72. Varnauskas E. Twelve-year follow-up of survival in the randomized European Coronary Surgery Study. N Engl J Med 1988; 319: 332–7.

73. Passamani E, Davis KB, Gillespie MJ, et al. A randomized trial of coronary artery bypass surgery. Survival of patients with a low ejection fraction. N Engl J Med 1985; 312: 1665–71.

74. Yusuf S, Zucker D, Peduzzi P, et al. Effect of coronary artery bypass graft surgery on survival: overview of 10-year results from randomised trials by the Coronary Artery Bypass Graft Surgery Trialists Collaboration. Lancet 1994; 344: 563–70.

75. Myers WO, Schaff HV, Gersh BJ, et al. Improved survival of surgically treated patients with triple vessel coronary artery disease and severe angina pectoris. A report from the Coronary Artery Surgery Study (CASS) registry. J Thorac Cardiovasc Surg 1989; 97: 487–95.

76. Eagle KA, Guyton RA, Davidoff R, et al. ACC/AHA 2004 guideline update for coronary artery bypass graft surgery: a report of the American College of Cardiology/American Heart Association Task Force on Practice Guidelines (Committee to Update the 1999 Guidelines for Coronary Artery Bypass Graft Surgery). Circulation 2004; 110: e340–437.

77. Parisi AF, Folland ED, Hartigan P. A comparison of angioplasty with medical therapy in the treatment of single-vessel coronary artery disease. Veterans Affairs ACME Investigators. N Engl J Med 1992; 326: 10–16.

78. Pitt B, Waters D, Brown WV, et al. Aggressive lipid-lowering therapy compared with angioplasty in stable coronary artery disease. Atorvastatin versus Revascularization Treatment Investigators. N Engl J Med 1999; 341: 70–6.

79. Coronary angioplasty versus medical therapy for angina: the second Randomised Intervention Treatment of Angina (RITA-2) trial. RITA-2 trial participants. Lancet 1997; 350: 461–8

80. Trial of invasive versus medical therapy in elderly patients with chronic symptomatic coronary-artery disease (TIME): a randomised trial. Lancet 2001; 358: 951–7

81. Hueb W, Lopes N, Gersh BJ, et al. Ten-year follow-up survival of the Medicine, Angioplasty, or Surgery Study (MASS II): a randomized controlled clinical trial of 3 therapeutic strategies for multivessel coronary artery disease. Circulation 2010; 122: 949–57.

82. Davies RF, Goldberg AD, Forman S, et al. Asymptomatic Cardiac Ischemia Pilot (ACIP) study two-year follow-up: outcomes of patients randomized to initial strategies of medical therapy versus revascularization. Circulation 1997; 95: 2037–43.

83. Erne P, Schoenenberger AW, Burckhardt D, et al. Effects of percutaneous coronary interventions in silent ischemia after myocardial infarction: the SWISSI II randomized controlled trial. JAMA 2007; 297: 1985–91.

84. Schomig A, Mehilli J, de Waha A, et al. A meta-analysis of 17 randomized trials of a percutaneous coronary intervention-based strategy in patients with stable coronary artery disease. J Am Coll Cardiol 2008; 52: 894–904.

85. Frye RL, August P, Brooks MM, et al. A randomized trial of therapies for type 2 diabetes and coronary artery disease. N Engl J Med 2009; 360: 2503–15.

86. Brown ML, Gersh BJ, Holmes DR, et al. From randomized trials to registry studies: translating data into clinical information. Nat Clin Pract Cardiovasc Med 2008; 5: 613–20.

87. Dagenais GR, Lu J, Faxon DP, et al. Effects of optimal medical treatment with or without coronary revascularization on angina and subsequent revascularizations in patients with type 2 diabetes mellitus and stable ischemic heart disease. Circulation 2011.

88. Shaw LJ, Berman DS, Maron DJ, et al. Optimal medical therapy with or without percutaneous coronary intervention to reduce ischemic burden: results from the Clinical Outcomes Utilizing Revascularization and Aggressive Drug Evaluation (COURAGE) trial nuclear substudy. Circulation 2008; 117: 1283–91.

89. Jones RH, Floyd RD, Austin EH, et al. The role of radionuclide angiocardiography in the preoperative prediction of pain relief and prolonged survival following coronary artery bypass grafting. Ann Surg 1983; 197: 743–54.

90. Ladenheim ML, Pollock BH, Rozanski A, et al. Extent and severity of myocardial hypoperfusion as predictors of prognosis in patients with suspected coronary artery disease. J Am Coll Cardiol 1986; 7: 464–71.

91. Hachamovitch R, Hayes SW, Friedman JD, et al. Comparison of the short-term survival benefit associated with revascularization

compared with medical therapy in patients with no prior coronary artery disease undergoing stress myocardial perfusion single photon emission computed tomography. Circulation 2003; 107: 2900–7.

92. Tarakji KG, Brunken R, McCarthy PM. Myocardial viability testing and the effect of early intervention in patients with advanced left ventricular systolic dysfunction. Circulation 2006; 113: 230–7.

93. Velazquez EJ, Lee KL, Deja MA, et al. Coronary-artery bypass surgery in patients with left ventricular dysfunction. N Engl J Med 2011; 364: 1607–16.

94. Bonow RO, Maurer G, Lee KL, et al. Myocardial viability and survival in ischemic left ventricular dysfunction. N Engl J Med 2011; 364: 1617–25.

95. Tonino PA, De Bruyne B, Pijls NH, et al. Fractional flow reserve versus angiography for guiding percutaneous coronary intervention. N Engl J Med 2009; 360: 213–24.

96. Pijls NH, van Schaardenburgh P, Manoharan G, et al. Percutaneous coronary intervention of functionally nonsignificant stenosis: 5-year follow-up of the DEFER Study. J Am Coll Cardiol 2007; 49: 2105–11.

97. Lin GA, Dudley RA, Lucas FL, et al. Frequency of stress testing to document ischemia prior to elective percutaneous coronary intervention. Jama 2008; 300: 1765–73.

98. Fox KA. COURAGE to change practice? Revascularisation in patients with stable coronary artery disease. Heart 2009; 95: 689–92.

99. Hannan EL, Wu C, Chassin MR. Differences in per capita rates of revascularization and in choice of revascularization procedure for eleven states. BMC Health Serv Res 2006; 6: 35.

100. Hemingway H, Crook AM, Dawson JR, et al. Rating the appropriateness of coronary angiography, coronary angioplasty and coronary artery bypass grafting: the ACRE study. Appropriateness of Coronary Revascularisation study. J Public Health Med 1999; 21: 421–9.

101. Hemingway H, Crook AM, Feder G, et al. Underuse of coronary revascularization procedures in patients considered appropriate candidates for revascularization. N Engl J Med 2001; 344: 645–54.

102. Hemingway H, Chen R, Junghans C, et al. Appropriateness criteria for coronary angiography in angina: reliability and validity. Ann Intern Med 2008; 149: 221–31.

103. Ahmed B, Dauerman HL, Piper WD, et al. Recent changes in practice of elective percutaneous coronary intervention for stable angina. Circ Cardiovasc Qual Outcomes 2011; 4: 300–5.

104. Sekhri N, Timmis A, Chen R, et al. Inequity of access to investigation and effect on clinical outcomes: prognostic study of coronary angiography for suspected stable angina pectoris. Bmj 2008; 336: 1058–61.

105. O'Connor GT, Olmstead EM, Nugent WC, et al. Appropriateness of coronary artery bypass graft surgery performed in northern New England. J Am Coll Cardiol 2008; 51: 2323–8.

106. Gerber Y, Rihal CS, Sundt TM 3rd, et al. Coronary revascularization in the community. A population-based study, 1990 to 2004. J Am Coll Cardiol 2007; 50: 1223–9.

107. Riley RF, Don CW, Powell W, et al. Trends in coronary revascularization in the United States from 2001 to 2009: recent declines in percutaneous coronary intervention volumes. Circ Cardiovasc Qual Outcomes 2011; 4: 193–7.

108. Hlatky MA, Boothroyd DB, Bravata DM, et al. Coronary artery bypass surgery compared with percutaneous coronary interventions for multivessel disease: a collaborative analysis of individual patient data from ten randomised trials. Lancet 2009; 373: 1190–7.

109. Brophy JM, Belisle P, Joseph L. Evidence for use of coronary stents. A hierarchical bayesian meta-analysis. Ann Intern Med 2003; 138: 777–86.

110. Kastrati A, Mehilli J, Pache J, et al. Analysis of 14 trials comparing sirolimus-eluting stents with bare-metal stents. N Engl J Med 2007; 356: 1030–9.

111. Morice MC, Serruys PW, Sousa JE, et al. A randomized comparison of a sirolimus-eluting stent with a standard stent for coronary revascularization. N Engl J Med 2002; 346: 1773–80.

112. Bravata DM, Gienger AL, McDonald KM, et al. Systematic review: the comparative effectiveness of percutaneous coronary interventions and coronary artery bypass graft surgery. Ann Intern Med 2007; 147: 703–16.

113. The final 10-year follow-up results from the BARI randomized trial. J Am Coll Cardiol 2007; 49: 1600–6.

114. Rodriguez A, Rodriguez Alemparte M, Baldi J, et al. Coronary stenting versus coronary bypass surgery in patients with multiple vessel disease and significant proximal LAD stenosis: results from the ERACI II study. Heart 2003; 89: 184–8.

115. Coronary artery bypass surgery versus percutaneous coronary intervention with stent implantation in patients with multivessel coronary artery disease (the Stent or Surgery trial): a randomised controlled trial. Lancet 2002; 360: 965–70

116. Serruys PW, Ong AT, van Herwerden LA, et al. Five-year outcomes after coronary stenting versus bypass surgery for the treatment of multivessel disease: the final analysis of the Arterial Revascularization Therapies Study (ARTS) randomized trial. J Am Coll Cardiol 2005; 46: 575–81.

117. Daemen J, Boersma E, Flather M, et al. Long-term safety and efficacy of percutaneous coronary intervention with stenting and coronary artery bypass surgery for multivessel coronary artery disease: a meta-analysis with 5-year patient-level data from the ARTS, ERACI-II, MASS-II, and SoS trials. Circulation 2008; 118: 1146–54.

118. Serruys PW, Morice MC, Kappetein AP, et al. Percutaneous coronary intervention versus coronary-artery bypass grafting for severe coronary artery disease. N Engl J Med 2009; 360: 961–72.

119. Opie LH, Commerford PJ, Gersh BJ. Controversies in stable coronary artery disease. Lancet 2006; 367: 69–78.

120. Kim LJ, King SB 3rd, Kent K, et al. Factors related to the selection of surgical versus percutaneous revascularization in diabetic patients with multivessel coronary artery disease in the BARI 2D (Bypass Angioplasty Revascularization Investigation in Type 2 Diabetes) trial. JACC Cardiovasc Interv 2009; 2: 384–92.

121. Morice MC, Serruys PW, Kappetein AP, et al. Outcomes in patients with de novo left main disease treated with either percutaneous coronary intervention using paclitaxel-eluting stents or coronary artery bypass graft treatment in the synergy between percutaneous coronary intervention with TAXUS and cardiac surgery (SYNTAX) trial. Circulation 2010; 121: 2645–53.

122. Park SJ, Kim YH, Park DW, et al. Randomized trial of stents versus bypass surgery for left main coronary artery disease. N Engl J Med 2011; 364: 1718–27.

123. Hautvast RW, DeJongste MJ, Staal MJ, et al. Spinal cord stimulation in chronic intractable angina pectoris: a randomized, controlled efficacy study. Am Heart J 1998; 136: 1114–20.

124. Ekre O, Eliasson T, Norrsell H, et al. Long-term effects of spinal cord stimulation and coronary artery bypass grafting on quality of life and survival in the ESBY study. Eur Heart J 2002; 23: 1938–45.

125. Bonetti PO, Barsness GW, Keelan PC, et al. Enhanced external counterpulsation improves endothelial function in patients with symptomatic coronary artery disease. J Am Coll Cardiol 2003; 41: 1761–8.

126. Barsness G, Feldman AM, Holmes DR Jr, et al. The International EECP Patient Registry (IEPR): design, methods, baseline characteristics, and acute results. Clin Cardiol 2001; 24: 435–42.

127. Saririan M, Eisenberg MJ. Myocardial laser revascularization for the treatment of end-stage coronary artery disease. J Am Coll Cardiol 2003; 41: 173–83.

128. Losordo DW, Schatz RA, White CJ, et al. Intramyocardial transplantation of autologous CD34+ stem cells for intractable angina: a phase I/IIa double-blind, randomized controlled trial. Circulation 2007; 115: 3165–72.

129. van Ramshorst J, Bax JJ, Beeres SL, et al. Intramyocardial bone marrow cell injection for chronic myocardial ischemia: a randomized controlled trial. Jama 2009; 301: 1997–2004.

27 Treatment algorithm in patients with NSTEMI and unstable angina
Francesco Saia

OUTLINE

Non-ST elevation acute coronary syndrome (NSTE-ACS) comprises a very heterogeneous group of patients with high and durable risk of developing adverse cardiovascular events. Individual (and dynamic) risk stratification based on evaluation of both ischemic and bleeding hazard is mandatory to select the most appropriate pharmacologic and interventional treatment. Recently, a general consensus has been achieved toward an early invasive strategy (i.e., angiography and revascularization when feasible and appropriate) in moderate and high-risk patients, and conservative management and subsequent further risk stratification only in very low-risk patients. Several antithrombotic drugs are recommended by current guidelines. The number of available antiplatelet and anticoagulant drugs, multiple administration routes, and different timing for administration generates a huge spectrum of possible pharmacological combinations. This chapter reviews current guidelines and possible integration derived by most recent clinical trials, in an attempt to provide an evidence-based algorithm of treatment for patients with NSTE-ACS.

INTRODUCTION

The term "acute coronary syndromes" encompasses a spectrum of different conditions that ranges from unstable angina (UA) to non–ST-elevation myocardial infarction (NSTEMI) and ST-elevation myocardial infarction (STEMI), arising from thrombus formation on an atheromatous plaque (Fig. 27.1) (1,2). The major pathophysiologic mechanism is rupture of a "thin cap fibroatheroma," although different types of vulnerable plaque have been described (3). ACS may also arise from other non-atherosclerotic conditions that generate an acute imbalance between myocardial oxygen supply and demand such as dynamic vessel obstruction, coronary artery dissection, tachycardia, hyperadrenergic state, thyrotoxicosis, increased left ventricular afterload, hypotension, anaemia, or hypoxemia (4,5). ACS are associated with increased mortality and morbidity, and their management poses a major clinical challenge both in the acute and in the post-acute phase.

In this chapter, we will focus on the early management of UA and NSTEMI, that is, non-ST-elevation acute coronary syndromes (NSTE-ACS) that share common clinical and diagnostic features. The major difference between these two entities is made by the severity of ischemia, meaning that if the ischemia is severe enough to cause detectable myocardial damage we diagnose NSTEMI, if markers of myocardial injury like troponins or CK-MB are not detectable the diagnosis is UA. A common characteristic of ACS is the early high risk of serious adverse events, which makes mandatory appropriate triage,

risk assessment, and timely use of pharmacological and non-pharmacologic interventions. Differently from STEMI, where most events occur before or shortly after presentation, in NSTE-ACS there is prolonged increased hazard, and long-term follow-up suggests that death rates are actually higher among NSTE-ACS patients (6). Every treatment algorithm should therefore be addressed also to the post-discharge phase.

GUIDELINES AND POTENTIAL INTEGRATION OF NOVEL DATA TO THE GUIDELINES

Management of NSTE-ACS begins with appropriate diagnosis, and comprises a series of clinical "crossroads": the choice between an invasive and a conservative strategy, the timing of an invasive strategy, the choice of the coronary revascularization method (percutaneous coronary intervention, PCI, vs. coronary artery bypass graft, CABG), and selection of the more appropriate antithrombotic pharmacotherapy in the acute phase and after hospital discharge (Focus Box 27.1). All these steps must necessarily be based on rigorous risk stratification (Focus Box 27.2).

It is important to highlight that there are several cardiac and non-cardiac conditions that may mimic NSTE-ACS. Systematic review of differential diagnoses is beyond the scope of this chapter but every clinician should bear in mind that, along with relatively benign diseases, there are life-threatening conditions simulating NSTE-ACS that may require a completely different treatment.

Invasive versus Conservative Strategy

"Better to light a candle than to curse the darkness." ~Chinese Proverb

Once the diagnosis of NSTE-ACS has been made two treatment pathways are possible: an invasive diagnostic evaluation (i.e., coronary angiography with intent to perform revascularization when clinically indicated) without first getting a noninvasive test of ischemia, called "invasive or routinely invasive" strategy, or an initial conservative strategy aimed at patient stabilization with aggressive medical treatment and subsequent risk

---

Focus Box 27.1

Principal Crossroads in the Management of NSTE-ACS
  Invasive vs. conservative strategy
  Timing of the coronary angiography
  Choice of the coronary revascularization method
  Selection of the most appropriate antithrombotic pharmacotherapy

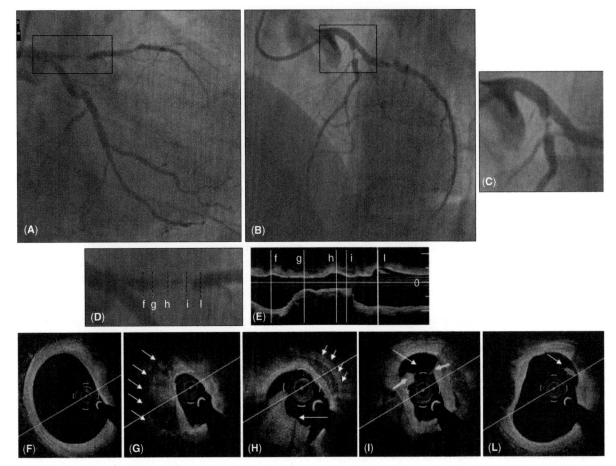

Figure 27.1 Atheromatous plaque rupture causing acute coronary syndrome: angiographic and optical coherence tomography (OCT) appearance. (A and B) Right and left anterior views showing a "complicated" plaque at the level of the proximal left anterior descending coronary artery (magnified in C). A tight stenosis of the left circumflex is also visible. (F to L) OCT images at different levels (as indicated in panels D and E). (F) Normal vessel. (G) Large plaque with mixed composition. (H) Thrombus (*big arrow*) and calcium layer (*small arrows*). (I) Ruptured plaque: *green arrows* indicate the ruptured fibrous cap, *white arrow* indicates the site of prior lipid pool. (L) Distal lesion showing a calcium nodule and some endoluminal thrombus.

Focus Box 27.2

Recommended Scores for Ischemic and Hemorrhagic Risk Stratification in NSTE-ACS

GRACE Risk Score (69)

The GRACE risk score (GRS) provides an estimate of in-hospital mortality based on the following variables: Killip Class, systolic blood pressure, heart rate, age, creatinine level, cardiac arrest at admission, ST-segment deviation, elevated cardiac enzyme levels

Classes of risk (terciles of in-hospital mortality):
  Low (GRS ≤108, in-hospital death <1%)
  Intermediate (GRS 109–140, in-hospital death 1–3%)
  High (GRS >140, in-hospital death >3%)

CRUSADE Bleeding Score (70)

The CRUSADE bleeding score (range 1 to 100 points) quantifies risk for in-hospital major bleeding across NSTE-ACS patients based on the following baseline characteristics: baseline hematocrit, creatinine clearance, heart rate, female gender, signs of heart failure at presentation, systolic blood pressure, prior vascular disease (history of peripheral artery disease or prior stroke), diabetes mellitus

In the derivation cohort, the rates of major bleeding increased by bleeding risk score quintiles:
  Very low (score ≤20, bleeding 3.1%)
  Low (score 21–30, bleeding 5.5%)
  Moderate (score 31–40, bleeding 8.6%)
  High (score 41–50, bleeding 11.9%)
  Very high (score >50, bleeding 19.5%)

stratification for selective use of coronary angiography and revascularization ("conservative" or "selectively invasive" strategy). Several randomized controlled trials (RCTs) have compared these strategies with diverse conclusions (7–13). Taken

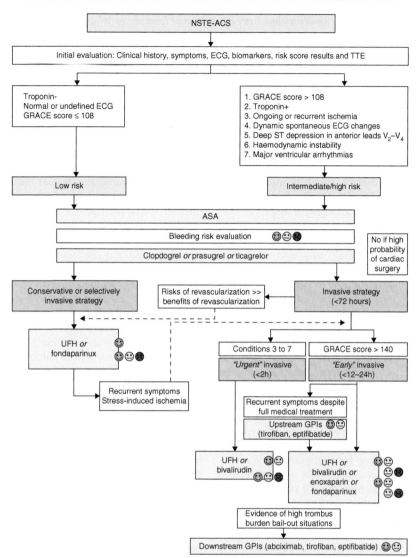

Figure 27.2 Treatment algorithm in patients with NSTEMI and unstable angina. Categorization into low- (score ≤108), intermediate- (score 109–140) and high-risk (score >140) of death is based on the GRACE risk score and other clinical factors. Bleeding risk is estimated based on the CRUSADE bleeding score and represented as follows: green spot (very-low and low-risk, score ≤30), yellow spot (moderate risk, score 31–40), and red spot (high and very-high risk, score >40) (Focus Box 27.2 and Table 27.2). *Abbreviations*: CRUSADE, Can Rapid Risk Stratification of Unstable Angina Patients Suppress Adverse Outcomes With Early Implementation of the American College of Cardiology/American Heart Association Guidelines; GRACE, Global Registry of Acute Coronary Events; TTE, transthoracic echocardiography.

together, RCTs have shown that an invasive strategy is associated with an increased risk of MI ("early hazard") in the peri-procedural phase (14), but reduces ischemic endpoints including mortality and MI up to 5 years of follow-up with the largest absolute effect seen in higher-risk patients (15). Current guidelines recommend risk stratification to lead the choice between invasive and conservative strategy (Fig. 27.2, Focus Box 27.1) (4,5,16). An invasive strategy is indicated in UA/NSTEMI patients who have refractory angina or hemodynamic or electrical instability (without serious comorbidities or contraindications to such procedures),

and in initially stabilized patients who have an intermediate to high risk for clinical events. Different risk score models have been developed, but most recent updates of the European Society of Cardiology (ESC) and of the American Heart Association/ American College of Cardiology (AHA/ACC) guidelines now recommend the Global Registry of Acute Coronary Events (GRACE) risk score as the preferred score to discriminate between an invasive versus a conservative strategy (16–18). A GRACE score >108 (lower threshold for the intermediate risk category) indicates the need of an invasive strategy within

72 hours. Troponin elevation, dynamic ST depression, hemodynamic instability, and major ventricular arrhythmias are other individual predictors of benefit from early invasive treatment.

CT angiography can be used as an alternative to invasive angiography to exclude ACS in patients with a low-to-intermediate likelihood of coronary artery disease when both troponin tests and ECG are inconclusive (16).

Timing of Coronary Angiography

"Festina lente" (Make haste slowly) –Suetonius, Augustus

In close proximity with the conservative versus invasive dispute, another area of uncertainty attracted the interest of the recent clinical research on NSTE-ACS: defining the optimal timing for the execution of coronary angiography and revascularization procedures. The results of the Timing of Intervention in Acute Coronary Syndromes (TIMACS) study have been recently reported (19). In this trial, a routine "early" invasive strategy (i.e., ≤24 h, median time 14 hours) did not offer substantial benefits as compared to a "delayed" invasive strategy (i.e. ≥36 hours, median time 50 hours). Previously, however, the Intracoronary Stenting with Antithrombotic Regimen Cooling off (ISAR-COOL) trial showed that "early" angiography (<6 hours, median time 2.4 hours) was superior to a "delayed" strategy (antithrombotic pretreatment for 3 to 5 days, median 86 hours) (20). The different results of the two studies were probably caused by the different time gap between the study groups within each study: 83 hours in the ISAR-COOL and 36 hours in the TIMACS. In the ISAR-COOL, during this quite extended "delay" many patients in the delayed group experienced adverse events despite optimal antithrombotic therapy, whereas the incidence of post-procedural events was the same between groups. The Angioplasty to Blunt The Rise of Troponin in Acute Coronary Syndromes Randomized for an Immediate or Delayed Intervention (ABOARD) study tested the hypothesis that patients with NSTE-ACS would provide benefit of a more aggressive strategy of very early intervention, analogous to the standards for primary PCI. Patients with NSTE-ACS and a Thrombolysis in Myocardial Infarction (TIMI) score of 3 or more were randomized to receive intervention either immediately (median time 70 min) or on the next working day (between 8 and 60 hours after enrollment, median 21 hours). This strategy was not associated with a reduction of myocardial infarction area defined by the troponin peak (21). Accordingly, a previous exploratory analysis of the TIMACS trial did not reveal any heterogeneity of outcomes among study centers where angiography was performed within 6 hours, from 6 to 12 hours, or after 12 hours in the early-intervention group (19). Nevertheless, both the TIMACS and the ABOARD trial, as well as the ISAR-COOL, demonstrated the safety of an "early" invasive strategy, which can reduce length and costs of hospital stay (21). Hence, current guidelines recommend coronary angiography within 72 hours of admission (4,5,16,17,22). Are there conditions in which an earlier invasive strategy seems advisable? Although there is no clear-cut evidence, it is reasonably assumed that patients at increased risk of adverse events (GRACE score >140) may

benefit from an "early" catheterization (i.e. within 12–24 hours) (17,22). A pre-specified analysis of the TIMACS study, in fact, documented a significant reduction of the primary endpoint in the highest GRACE score tercile (>140) undergoing "early" angiography as compared to a "delayed" invasive strategy. Interestingly, the ABOARD study did not show a benefit of "immediate" catheterization in these patients. "Urgent" (i.e. immediate or as soon as possible) catheterization should be restricted to patients presenting recurrent angina not responding to treatment, hemodynamic instability, major arrhythmias or with ongoing symptoms and marked ST depression in anterior leads (probable posterior transmural ischemia) (Fig. 27.2). Those patients were, in fact, excluded from all clinical trials (17,22). Finally, there are several retrospective studies suggesting that ST-elevation in lead aVR is associated with high-risk coronary lesions and predicts in-hospital and long-term cardiovascular mortality providing additional risk stratification on top of the GRACE score (23). Hence, patients presenting with ST deviation in combination with ST elevation in lead aVR could probably benefit from an "early" (12–24 hours) invasive strategy.

Method of Revascularization

"General propositions do not decide concrete cases. The decision will depend on a judgment or intuition more subtle than any articulate major premise." –Justice Oliver Wendell Holmes Jr.

After coronary angiography, a decision about the type of revascularization must be made. Because no prospective RCT has specifically compared PCI and CABG in stabilized patients after an episode of ACS, general criteria used for other conditions are commonly adopted (16,17,24). The choice of revascularization strategy must integrate angiographic and clinical findings, consider comorbidities, and weight the benefits and risks of each intervention with the help of recommended scoring system. Presently, the most validated score for PCI is the SYNTAX (Synergy between Percutaneous Coronary Intervention with Taxus and Cardiac Surgery) score (25), whilst to evaluate surgical risk both the EuroSCORE (26) and the Society of Thoracic Surgeons score (27) are widely adopted. The SYNTAX score provides information about anatomic suitability (and likelihood of success) for PCI, and is not able to stratify the risk for CABG. Conversely, the EuroSCORE and the STS score are clinical scores to assess the surgical risk for CABG; however, they do not carry information about relevant technical issues for CABG (for example, porcelain aorta or diffusely diseased distal coronary vessel), and they do not have a significant impact on the periprocedural risk of PCI. Clearly, clinical judgment cannot be replaced by any single or combined scoring system and integration of all available information remains a prerogative of the physicians. Approximately one-third of NSTE-ACS patients have single vessel disease, which in most cases is best treated with ad hoc PCI. Conversely, multivessel disease is present in around half of the patients and decision making is more complex. The majority of these patients are treated with PCI, whilst only a minority are referred for bypass surgery during initial hospitalization (13). The risk of bleeding

Table 27.1 Antithrombotic Therapy Changes According to the Method of Revascularization

Recommendations for PCI

	Before-PCI or loading dose	Maintenance dose (daily)	After PCI
Antiplatelet			
ASA	150–325 mg per os or 250–500 mg I.V.	75–162 mg per os	Continue indefinetly
ADP-inhibitors			
Clopidogrel	300–600 mg	75 mg per os	>6–12 months[a]
Prasugrel	60 mg	10 mg per os	>6–12 months[a]
Ticagrelor	180 mg	90 mg twice daily	>6–12 months[a]
GPI			
Abciximab	0.25 mg/kg I.V.	0.125 mcg/kg/min I.V. (max 10 mcg/min)	12 hours
Tirofiban	0.4 mcg/kg/min for 30 min I.V.	0.1 mcg/kg/min I.V.	18–24 hours
Eptifibatide	Double bolus 180 mcg/kg I.V., 10 min apart	2.0 mcg/kg/min I.V.	18–24 hours
Anticoagulants			
UFH	70–100 IU/kg I.V. without GPI, 50–70 IU/kg with GPI	ACT monitoring: target range: 200–250 s with GPI; 250–350 s without GPI.	Stop
Bivalirudin	Before PCI: 0.5 mg/kg I.V. bolus and increase the infusion rate to 1.75 mg/kg/h	0.25 mg/kg/h I.V.	Stop
Enoxaparine	<8 h since last s.c. application: no additional bolus; within 8–12 h of last s.c. application: add 0.30 mg/kg i.v. bolus; >12 h since last s.c. application: 0.75 mg/kg i.v. bolus.	1 mg/kg s.c.	Stop
Fondaparinux	Fondaparinux 2.5 mg s.c. Add UFH 50–100 IU/kg	Fondaparinux 2.5 mg s.c.	Stop

Recommendations for CABG

	Before CABG	During CABG	After CABG
Antiplatelet			
ASA	Continue	–	Continue indefinitely
ADP-inhibitors			
Clopidogrel	Discontinue 5 d before	–	Resumed as soon as possible including a loading dose and continued >6–12 months[a]
Prasugrel	Discontinue ≥7 d before	–	Resumed as soon as possible including a loading dose and continued >6–12 months[a]
Ticagrelor	Discontinue 48–72 h before	–	Resumed as soon as possible including a loading dose and continued >6–12 months[a]
GPI			
Abciximab	Discontinue ≥24 h		Stop
Tirofiban	Discontinue 4 h before		Stop
Eptifibatide	Discontinue 4 h before		Stop
Anticoagulants			
UFH	Continue infusion (ACT guided)	ACT monitoring: target range: 200–250 s with GPI; 250–350 s without GPI.	Stop
Bivalirudin	Discontinue 3 h before and dose with UFH		Stop
Enoxaparin	Discontinue 12–24 h before and dose with UFH		Stop
Fondaparinux	Discontinue 24 h before and dose with UFH		Stop

[a]Depending on the type of stent (bare metal stent vs. drug-eluting stent) and individual bleeding risk. *Abbreviations*: ACT, activated clotting time; ADP, adenosine diphosphate; ASA, acetylsalicylic acid; CABG, coronary artery bypass graft; GPI, glycoprotein IIb/IIIa inhibitors; I.V., intravenous; s.c., subcutaneous; PCI, percutaneous coronary intervention; UFH, unfractioned heparin.

complications in patients undergoing bypass surgery initially treated with aggressive antiplatelet treatments and the higher overall surgical risk of unstable patients are the main reasons for this attitude. Based on the results of the SYNTAX trial, however, there is compelling evidence to discuss the revascularization strategy for a number of patients with intermediate-to-high SYNTAX score within a multidisciplinary heart team (16,17). Antithrombotic therapy should be modified according to the revascularization method chosen (Table 27.1).

Angiography combined with ECG changes is often able to identify the culprit lesion. If PCI is performed, the culprit lesion should be treated first. In the presence of multivessel coronary disease, it is not known if stenting all suitable significant stenoses versus stenting the culprit lesion only is beneficial. The current guidelines basically state that the decision to perform either culprit vessel or complete revascularization (in a single step or with a staged procedure) should be made on an individual basis. Complete functional revascularization should be pursued especially in patients with heart failure, diabetes, and/or reduced left ventricular function. Use of fractional flow reserve evaluation in this setting can be helpful to guide treatment (28). Interesting insights came from the Providing Regional Observations to Study Predictors of Events in the Coronary Tree (PROSPECT) study, a prospective natural history study on ACS (29). All patients enrolled underwent three-vessel coronary angiography and gray-scale and radiofrequency intravascular ultrasonographic imaging after percutaneous coronary intervention. During a median follow-up period of 3.4 years, the incidence of major adverse cardiovascular events related to culprit lesions and those attributable to non-culprit lesions identified at baseline was similar (12.9% and 11.6%, respectively). Most nonculprit lesions responsible for follow-up events, however, were angiographically mild at baseline, although they exhibited specific features of "vulnerability" (a plaque burden ≥70%; a minimal luminal area ≤4.0 mm^2; thin-cap fibroatheromas based on radiofrequency intravascular ultrasonography-virtual histology). These findings further complicated the treatment decision between culprit lesion only versus complete revascularization and support the careful evaluation of the risk and benefit of coronary intervention to each lesion. In addition, the study highlighted the importance of secondary prevention measures and the need of developing new drugs targeting the whole atherosclerotic process.

Antithrombotic Pharmacotherapy

"Incidit in Scyllam cupiens vitare Charybdim" (He ran onto Scylla, wishing to avoid Charybdis) –Virgilio

Patients with ACS have a pro-thrombotic milieu, which derives benefit from potent antithrombotic therapy, with the combination of antiplatelet and anticoagulant drugs. Each one of these drugs, because of their intrinsic properties, increases the hazard of bleeding. A careful evaluation of bleeding versus ischemic risk on an individual basis is therefore mandatory to maximize the net clinical benefit of prescribed therapy (Fig. 27.2, Table 27.2, Focus Box 27.2).

Antiplatelet Therapy

Three classes of drugs will be discussed: aspirin (acetilsalycilic acid, ASA), thienopyridines, glycoprotein IIb/IIIa inhibitors (GPI).

Aspirin

Aspirin should be administrated to NSTE-ACS patients as soon as possible and continued indefinitely unless contraindicated. Despite the fact that ASA has been used for decades in this setting, optimal dose is still uncertain. ESC guidelines recommend 150–300 mg per os or 250 –500 mg i.v. bolus, followed by 75–100 mg daily (16). The latest AHA/ACC guidelines recommend 162 to 325 mg nonenteric formulation, orally or chewed. Then, ASA should be continued indefinitely at a dose of 75 to 162 mg (162 to 325 mg are recommended after stent implantation for at least 1, 3, or 6 months depending on the type of stent) (22). Importantly, a dose-dependent increase in bleeding was observed in patients receiving ASA, whereas there was no difference in the rate of thrombotic events according to dose (30). Very recently, however, the Clopidogrel and Aspirin Optimal Dose Usage to Reduce Recurrent Events–Seventh Organization to Assess Strategies in Ischemic Syndromes (CURRENT–OASIS 7) trial (31) compared, in a 2-by-2 factorial design, double-dose clopidogrel versus standard-dose clopidogrel and either higher-dose aspirin (300 to 325 mg daily) or lower-dose aspirin (75 to 100 mg daily). There was no significant difference between higher-dose and lower-dose aspirin with respect to the primary outcome (death, myocardial infarction, or stroke at 30 days) or major bleeding. A final remark must be made about aspirin "resistance"; a number of studies have correlated this phenomenon with adverse clinical outcomes. It should be emphasized that true aspirin resistance is very rare and the foremost reason for aspirin resistance seems poor patient compliance (32).

Adenosine Diphosphate Receptor Antagonists

Many changes related to the results of important recent clinical trials concern thienopyridines. Ten years ago, the Clopidogrel in Unstable angina to prevent Recurrent Events (CURE) trial demonstrated that, in patients with ACS receiving ASA, a strategy of clopidogrel pretreatment followed by long-term therapy was beneficial in reducing major cardiovascular events compared with placebo (33). Clopidogrel has therefore been recommended in association to ASA with a loading dose of 300–600 mg followed by a 75-mg daily maintenance dose in all patients. Over the years, we have discovered many limitations of clopidogrel, principally related to its metabolism. In fact, clopidogrel is a prodrug that requires biotransformation into an active metabolite. Platelet response to clopidogrel is normally distributed, and patients at the extremes of the distribution curve may be either at risk for ischemia or bleeding (34). A number of studies have shown an association between poor response to clopidogrel (*high on-treatment platelet reactivity*), which interests up to 30% of the patients, and recurrent ischemic events. The mechanisms leading to poor clopidogrel effects are likely multifactorial and comprise genetic, clinical,

Table 27.2 Risk Scores for Ischemic and Bleeding Endpoints

Ischemic events (and mortality)			Bleeding		
TIMI (70)	PURSUIT (71)	GRACE (69,72)	CRUSADE (73)	GRACE[a] (74)	Mehran[a] (75)
Age	Age	Age		Age	Age
	Heart rate	Heart rate	Heart rate		
	Systolic blood pressure	Systolic blood pressure	Systolic blood pressure (≤110 mmHg; ≥180 mmHg)	Systolic blood pressure	
ST-segment deviation	Signs of HF (rales)	Signs of HF (Killip class)	Signs of HF (rales)		
	ST-segment deviation	ST-segment deviation			
		Cardiac arrest during presentation			
		Renal function (serum creatinine level)	Renal function (creatinine clearance)	Renal function (history of renal insufficiency)	Renal function (serum creatinine level)
	Elevated cardiac biomarkers	Elevated cardiac biomarkers			
At least three risk factors for CAD					
Prior documented coronary stenosis >50%					
≥2 anginal events in prior 24 h					
Use of aspirin in prior 7 d					
	Gender (Male)		Gender (Female)	Gender (Female)	Gender (Female)
			Anemia (baseline hematocrit)		Anemia (yes/no)
			Prior vascular disease		
			Diabetes mellitus		
				History of bleeding	
					Presentation (STEMI/NSTEMI/UA)
					White blood cell count

[a]In the analysis of the GRACE study, independent predictors of bleeding were described but no formal risk score was developed. In both the GRACE analysis and the Mehran analysis, treatment variables (both pharmacologic and not) associated with bleeding were included in the model but they have not been reported in the table. *Abbreviations*: HF, heart failure; TIMI, Thrombolysis In Myocardial Infarction; GRACE, Global Registry of Acute Coronary Events; PURSUIT, Platelet Glycoprotein IIb/IIIa in Unstable Angina: Receptor Suppression Using Integrilin Therapy; CRUSADE, Can Rapid Risk Stratification of Unstable Angina Patients Suppress Adverse Outcomes With Early Implementation of the American College of Cardiology/American Heart Association Guidelines.

and cellular factors. Attempts to overcome this limitation have been tested in RCTs and can be summarized as follows: (*i*) increasing doses; (*ii*) tailored treatment guided by bedside platelet response tests; (*iii*) tailored treatment guided by genetic testing; and (*iv*) new drugs (Focus Box 27.3). The CURRENT-OASIS 7 trial randomized NSTE-ACS patients referred for an invasive strategy to either double-dose clopidogrel (a 600-mg loading dose on day 1, followed by 150 mg daily for 6 days and 75 mg daily thereafter) or standard-dose clopidogrel (a 300-mg loading dose and 75 mg daily thereafter). Unfortunately, there was no significant difference between groups with respect to the primary outcome of cardiovascular death, myocardial infarction, or stroke, with increasing rates of major bleedings in the double dose group (31). The hypothesis of tailoring treatment based on measured platelet inhibition was tested in the Gauging Responsiveness with A VerifyNow assay—Impact on Thrombosis and Safety (GRAVITAS) trial (35). Based on the results of the VerifyNow P2Y12 test (Accumetrics, San Diego, CA), patients treated with clopidogrel with P2Y12 reaction units (PRU) ≥230 ("poor responders"), were randomly assigned to a regimen of high-dose or standard-dose clopidogrel. High-dose clopidogrel was given as a total first-day dose of 600 mg followed thereafter by a dose of 150 mg daily for 6 months. Standard-dose clopidogrel was prescribed as a loading dose of placebo followed by a dose of 75 mg and placebo tablet daily. At 6 months, the use of high-dose clopidogrel compared with

Hypotheses to Overcome Clopidogrel Resistence and Relative Principal Clinical Trials

Increasing doses (CURRENT-OASIS 7)

Tailored treatment guided by point-of-care testing (GRAVITAS, TRIGGER-PCI, RECLOSE 2 ACS)

Tailored treatment guided by genetic testing (GIFT, CLOVIS-2, ELEVATE-TIMI 56)

New drugs: prasugrel (TRITON-TIMI 38), ticagrelor (PLATO)

Study Design and Results

CURRENT-OASIS 7: RCT, double dose clopidogrel vs. standard dose clopidogrel – completed – negative

GRAVITAS: RCT, clopidogrel standard dose vs. clopidogrel double dose in non-responders (VerifyNow assay)—completed—negative

TRIGGER PCI: clopidogrel vs. prasugrel based on platelet reactivity test in stable patients after stenting—RCT, trial stopped early due to too few events (Note: ACS patients excluded)

RECLOSE 2 ACS: Prospective, observational cohort study. ACS patients with high on-treatment platelet reactivity received an increased dose of clopidogrel (150–300 mg/day) or switched to ticlopidine (500–1000 mg/day) under adenosine-diphosphate test guidance. High platelet reactivity associated to increased risk of ischemic events at short- and long-term follow-up. Normalization of the platelet test after treatment adjustment was not associated with a better outcome vs a persistent abnormal test result

GIFT: GRAVITAS gene substudy: completed - CYP2C19*2 carriers do not respond to high-dose clopidogrel

CLOVIS-2: Assessment of different loading doses of clopidogrel in herozygous vs. homozygous vs. matched wild type for the CYP2C19*2 genetic variant—completed—clopidogrel resistance can be overcome by increasing the dose in heterozygous carriers but not in homozygous carriers

ELEVATE-TIMI 56: Assessment (in stable patients) of platelet reactivity with different maintenance doses of clopidogrel in relationship with the genotype (noncarriers of a loss-of-function CYP2C19*2 allele vs. heterozygotes vs. homozygotes). Tripling the maintenance dose to 225 mg daily in heterozygotes achieved levels of platelet reactivity similar to 75-mg dose in noncarriers. In homozygotes, doses as high as 300 mg daily did not result in comparable degrees of platelet inhibition

TRITON-TIMI 38: RCT, prasugrel vs. clopidogrel in ACS—completed—prasugrel associated with 19% relative reduction of the primary ischemic endpoint

PLATO: RCT, ticagrelor vs. clopidogrel in ACS—completed—ticagrelor associated with 19% relative reduction of the primary ischemic endpoint

standard-dose clopidogrel provided a 22% absolute reduction in the rate of high on-treatment reactivity at 30 days, but this did not translate into a reduced incidence of the primary endpoint (death from cardiovascular causes, nonfatal myocardial infarction, or stent thrombosis) (35). A subsequent analysis of the GRAVITAS trial investigated the relationship between outcomes and high on-treatment platelet reactivity over the course of the trial. Achievement of a reactivity <208 PRU at 12–24 hours after PCI or during follow-up was associated with a lower risk for cardiovascular events (36). Interestingly, less than half of the patients on the high-dose clopidogrel arm in GRAVITAS reached this threshold, which may explain the negative results of the study. The responsiveness to Clopidogrel and Stent Thrombosis 2–ACS (RECLOSE 2–ACS) study confirmed that, among patients receiving platelet reactivity-guided antithrombotic medication after PCI, high residual platelet reactivity was significantly associated with increased risk of ischemic events at short- and long-term follow-up (37). A puzzling additional result of this study was that normalization of the platelet test after treatment adjustment was not associated with a better outcome versus a persistent abnormal test result.

Cytochrome P450 (CYP) isoenzyme CYP2C19 plays a key role in biotransformation of clopidogrel into its active metabolite, and carriers of reduced function genetic variants in the CYP2C19 gene have lower active clopidogrel metabolite levels and diminished platelet inhibition. A meta-analysis of nine studies suggests that carriers of even one reduced-function CYP2C19 allele have a significantly increased risk of major adverse cardiovascular events and stent thrombosis, and the risk is higher in those in those who harbor two reduced function alleles (38). Indeed, the US Food and Drug Administration issued a boxed warning on clopidogrel addressing the need for pharmacogenomic testing to identify patients' altered clopidogrel metabolism and thus their risk for a suboptimal clinical response to clopidogrel. The Clopidogrel and Response Variability Investigation Study 2 (CLOVIS-2) showed that clopidogrel resistance in carriers of CYP2C19 loss of function gene can be overcome by increasing the dose in heterozygous carriers but not in homozygous carriers (39). The Pharmacogenomics of Antiplatelet Intervention (PAPI) Study demonstrated that CYP2C19*2 genotype accounts for approximately 12% of the variation in clopidogrel response, so the majority of the variation in platelet response to clopidogrel remains unexplained (40). The Genotype Information and Functional Testing (GIFT), the genetic substudy of the GRAVITAS trial, have shown that patients with either one or two CYP2C19 loss-of-function alleles (*2) do not generally respond to double-dose clopidogrel (M. Price, personal communication, American College of Cardiology annual meeting 2011). Recently, two RCTs—the Therapeutic Outcomes by Optimizing Platelet Inhibition with Prasugrel–Thrombolysis in Myocardial Infarction (TRITON–TIMI) 38 trial (41) and the PLATelet inhibition and patient Outcomes (PLATO) trial (42)—compared head-to-head two third-generation thienopyridines with clopidogrel in ACS patients. In these trials, prasugrel and ticagrelor (actually a

Rationale for Tailored Treatment with ADP-Receptor Blockers (clopidogrel to all patients, prasugrel or ticagrelor only to clopidogrel non-responders)

- Resistance to clopidogrel can be easily tested with point-of-care testing
- Genetic tests for most common polymorphisms are commercially available
- Cost saving: Two third of the patients are good responders to clopidogrel and use of new (more expensive) drugs could be limited to clopidogrel non-responders
- Increased safety: use of more powerful agents only in poor responders to clopidogrel will expose less patients to the increased risk of bleeding associated to prasugrel and ticagrelor

Factors Against Tailored Treatment

- Several point-of-care assays for clopidogrel are available, but the optimal test remains undetermined
- Cutoff value for non-responsiveness is uncertain (inhibition of platelet aggregation shows a normal distribution and there is no dichotomous separation between "responders" and "nonresponders")
- Timing of evaluation still not defined (variable response to clopidogrel)
- Several patients show high on-treatment platelet reactivity despite increasing doses of clopidogrel (and correction is more difficult in carriers of a loss-of-function CYP2C19*2 allele and probably not possible in homozygotes)
- Genetic test accounts for only about 12% of variability of platelet inhibition
- In genetic substudies of TRITON-TIMI 38 and PLATO benefits of prasugrel and ticagrelor were observed also in patients without the loss-of-function genotype (CYP2C19*2)

non-thienopyridine ADP receptor blocker), respectively, were found to reduce rates of recurrent ischemic events as compared with clopidogrel. Both drugs increased the rates of non-CABG related bleedings, whereas CABG-related bleedings appeared higher only in prasugrel-treated patients probably because of the longer half-life. Importantly, genetic substudies of both trials have shown that this advantage is independent of CYP2C19 and ABCB1 polymorphisms (43,44), providing further support against a tailored treatment with clopidogrel to most of the patients and prasugrel or ticagrelor to non-responders to clopidogrel. The debate is still open and a number of clinical trials will further clarify these aspects and the correct use of all available P2Y12 inhibitors (Focus Box 27.4). Currently, in patients with ACS both prasugrel and ticagrelor are recommended by European guidelines in alternative to clopidogrel (16,17); differently, the 2011 Focused Update of the ACC/AHA guidelines on UA/NSTEMI gave recommendations only on prasugrel because ticagrelor was not FDA approved or marketed at the time of writing of the update (22). More detailed information about prasugrel and ticagrelor can be found in Chapter 24.

A final remark must be made about the possible interaction between clopidogrel and proton pump inhibitors (PPIs) due to a competitive binding to CYP2C19. The clinical impact of this pharmacodynamic interaction remains controversial, because the results of different registries are conflicting. Furthermore, not all PPIs have the same interaction with the CYP2C19. The only large randomized trial (COGENT [Clopidogrel and the Optimization of Gastrointestinal Events Trial]), that was prematurely interrupted because of financial problems of the sponsor, showed no increased risk of ischemic events with concomitant use of clopidogrel and omeprazole versus clopidogrel alone, whereas gastrointestinal bleedings were significantly reduced (45). Taken together, these results suggest that PPIs should not be withheld when indicated. In high-risk ischemic conditions (for example stenting of the left main), platelet inhibition by clopidogrel should be checked with point-of-care assays. Alternative gastro-protective drugs such as ranitidine can be used when the risk of gastrointestinal bleeding is low.

Glycoprotein IIB/IIIA Inhibitors

For several years glycoprotein IIb/IIIa inhibitors (GPI) represented a mainstay of treatment in NSTE-ACS, especially for high-risk patients undergoing an early invasive strategy. Indeed, thanks to the reduction of periprocedural hazard of PCI associated to their use, they were indicated as the "trump card," which allowed early invasive strategy to be shown advantageous over conservative strategy. Optimization of antithrombotic pharmacotherapy raised serious doubts about the efficacy of GPI in the context of adequate pre-treatment with clopidogrel and in comparison with the direct thrombin inhibitor bivalirudin. A second controversy regarded the timing of administration of GPI, that is, routinely before coronary angiography ("upstream") or selectively in the catheterization laboratory after knowing coronary anatomy ("downstream"). The principal clinical trials addressing these issues were: the Intracoronary Stenting and Antithrombotic Regimen–Rapid Early Action for Coronary Treatment (ISAR-REACT)-2 trial (46), the Acute Catheterization and Urgent Intervention Triage strategy (ACUITY) trial (47), the ACUITY Timing trial (48), and the Early Glycoprotein IIb/IIIa Inhibition in Patients With Non–ST-Segment Elevation Acute Coronary Syndrome (EARLY-ACS) trial (49). Briefly, the ISAR-REACT 2 compared triple-antiplatelet therapy with ASA, clopidogrel, and abciximab to double therapy with ASA and clopidogrel in patients with UA/NSTEMI undergoing PCI. A 600-mg bolus dose of clopidogrel was administered at least 2 hours prior to the procedure. In this setting, abciximab reduced the risk of adverse events, although the benefit appeared to be confined to patients presenting with an elevated troponin level. The ACUITY trial compared three antithrombotic regimens in moderate- and high-risk ACS patients undergoing early invasive therapy: unfractionated heparin or enoxaparin plus a GPI, bivalirudin plus a GPI, or bivalirudin alone. A second randomization between upstream and downstream administration of GPI was performed in the two GPI groups (ACUITY Timing trial). Bivalirudin alone compared with heparin plus GPI resulted in noninferior rates of 30-day composite ischemic endpoint, but significantly reduced major bleeding and was associated to superior net clinical outcomes. No difference was observed between the bivalirudin plus GPI and the heparin plus GPI groups (47). A note of caution came from the subgroup analysis of patients who did not receive a thienopyridine before angiography or PCI in the bivalirudin alone group, showing increased risk of ischemic events as compared to UFH plus GPI. Addressing the issue of "timing," the ACUITY Timing trial did not show noninferiority of deferred selective administration of eptifibatide in the catheterization laboratory as compared to routine upstream administration (48), even if an excess of bleeding was reported in the latter. This trial, however, presented some limitations, including enrollment of patients at moderate, rather than high-risk, and short time between starting of pre-treatment with GPI and angiography (median 4.0 hours). Hence, the results of the EARLY ACS trial were eagerly awaited. In EARLY ACS, high-risk patients were enrolled (at least two of the following: ST-segment depression or transient ST-segment elevation, elevated biomarker levels, or age >60 years), delay before randomization was limited (median 5 h), duration of pre-treatment was appropriate (median 21 h) and consistent with common practice (50). The EARLY ACS trial showed that early routine eptifibatide administration was not superior to the provisional use of eptifibatide after angiography, and was associated with a greater risk of non-life-threatening bleeding and need for transfusion (49). There were no significant interactions with respect to prespecified baseline characteristics, including early clopidogrel administration, and the study endpoints. In a subgroup analysis, early administration of eptifibatide in patients who underwent PCI was associated with numerically fewer ischemic events. Based on these findings, the ESC guidelines on coronary revascularization downgraded upstream GPI treatment to a class III indications (i.e., formally contraindicated) (17). Differently, the last update of ACC/AHA guidelines, subsequently also embraced the 2011 ESC guidelines on NSTE-ACS, made some differentiation: the use of upstream GPI may be considered (class IIb) in patients at high ischemic risk (elevated troponin levels, diabetes, or significant STsegment depression) already receiving ASA and a thienopyridine who are selected for an invasive strategy, provided they have no high risk of bleeding (16,22). A class IIa recommendation was confirmed for UA/NSTEMI patients in whom an initial conservative strategy is selected and who have recurrent ischemia with full antithrombotic treatment. A class I recommendation was also confirmed for patients at medium or high risk and in whom an invasive strategy is planned if not pretreated with dual antiplatelet therapy (16,22).

Limited information is available about the safety and efficacy of GPI in association with novel ADP receptor blockers. In the

---

Focus Box 27.5

General Recommendations for Anticoagulation in NSTE-ACS
- Anticoagulant therapy should be added to antiplatelet therapy as soon as possible after presentation
- Avoid crossover of anticoagulants (especially between UFH and low molecular weight heparin)
- Single institutions should agree on a consistent approach in order to minimize the chance of dosing and administration errors
- Patients at very high ischemic risk (e.g., persistent angina, hemodynamic instability, refractory arrhythmias) who are referred for emergent catheterization should receive UFH. In patients with associated high risk of bleeding, bivalirudin monotherapy should be used
- In medium-to-high ischaemic risk patients (e.g., troponin positive, recurrent angina, dynamic ST changes) for whom an early invasive strategy is planned either UFH 60 IU/kg i.v. bolus followed by infusion until PCI or enoxaparin 1 mg/kg s.c. (reduced doses if renal failure and age >75 years) twice daily until PCI or bivalirudin 0.1 mg/kg i.v. bolus followed by infusion of 0.25 mg/kg/h until PCI or fondaparinux 2.5 mg daily s.c. until PCI with additional bolus of UFH at the time of catheterization
- In low ischaemic risk patients (troponin negative, no ST-segment changes) for whom a primarily conservative strategy is planned, fondaparinux or enoxaparin or UFH can be used. In patients who have an increased risk of bleeding, fondaparinux is preferable
- UFH: reduced targets of activated clotting time seems reasonable in association with GPI (target range: 200–250 s with, 250–350 s without GPI)

TRITON-TIMI 38, 54.5% of the patients received a GPI during the index hospitalization. An analysis of these patients showed that the risk of cardiovascular events and stent thrombosis was significantly reduced by prasugrel as compared to clopidogrel, regardless of whether or not a GPI inhibitor was used (51). Importantly, the use of a GPI did not accentuate the relative risk of bleeding with prasugrel as compared with clopidogrel. In the PLATO trial, GPI were used in around 26% of the patients, but no specific information is available to date (44).

Anticoagulant Therapy

Anticoagulant therapy should be added to antiplatelet therapy in UA/NSTEMI patients as soon as possible after presentation. Four parenteral anticoagulants are currently recommended in NSTE-ACS: UFH, enoxaparin (a low molecular weight heparin), bivalirudin (direct thrombin inhibitor), and fondaparinux (factor Xa inhibitor). The choice of specific agents and doses relies on risk stratification and treatment strategy (Fig. 27.2, Focus Boxes 27.2 and 27.5). In general, bivalirudin and fondaparinux (which have not been yet approved for use in

ACS by the U.S. FDA) are associated with reduced bleeding rates without loss of ischemic protection (47,52), and are therefore appealing especially for patients at increased risk of bleeding. Bivalirudin, however, was not tested in very high-risk patients and in the ACUITY trial patients who did not receive a thienopyridine before angiography or PCI exhibited higher risk of ischemic events (47). Additionally, it should be noted that in this trial there was a short time from study drug to catheterization (median 4 h). Thus, the study results of this trial cannot be extrapolated beyond the group of patients treated in an early invasive fashion (24). Since the major advantage of bivalirudin is reduction of bleeding complications, the question whether or not this advantage is maintained against UFH only (without GPI) remained. Two clinical trials tested bivalirudin versus UFH in the setting of elective PCI (including UA patients but excluding NSTEMI): the Intracoronary Stenting and Antithrombotic Regimen: Rapid Early Action for Coronary Treatment 3 (ISAR-REACT 3) trial (53) and the ARMYDA BIVALVE trial: the former used a non-standard dose of UFH, that is, 140 IU/kg, whilst the latter endorsed a lower dose (75 IU/kg); no routine GPI were used and all patients were pretreated with clopidogrel. Both trials showed that patients randomized to bivalirudin experienced less bleeding and had similar rates of ischemic complications, although in these as well as in some other previous trials the reduction of bleedings appeared in a considerable proportion attributable to access-site complications. Furthermore, in the subsequent ISAR-REACT 3A study, a reduced dose of 100 U/kg UFH compared with the historical control of 140 U/kg UFH reduced bleeding and met the criterion of non-inferiority compared with bivalirudin (54).

Factor Xa inhibitors such as fondaparinux (which is an indirect inhibitor of factor Xa) act more upstream in the coagulation cascade. In the Organization to Assess Strategies for Ischaemic Syndromes-5 (OASIS-5) trial (52), fondaparinux as compared to enoxaparin showed similar combined ischemic events but highly significantly reduced rates of severe bleeding complications, translating into reduced long-term mortality and stroke rates. However, fondaparinux was associated with a higher rate of catheter thrombosis in patients undergoing angiography and PCI. This is probably explained by the fact that factor Xa inhibitors do not have any action against thrombin that is already formed or that is generated. Hence, UFH should be administrated to patients treated with fondaparinux during invasive procedures.

The uncertainty regarding the optimal adjunctive UFH regimen in this setting was addressed by the Fondaparinux with UnfracTionated heparin dUring Revascularization in Acute coronary syndromes (FUTURA/OASIS 8) trial (55). Importantly, the trial showed that low fixed-dose heparin was not superior to standard ACT-guided heparin dosing in terms of preventing bleeding complications. An indirect comparison with the fondaparinux group of the OASIS-5 PCI population suggested that the addition of either dose of unfractionated heparin to fondaparinux does not increase the rate of major bleeding (55).

Enoxaparin is a LMWH that overcomes most of the pharmacokinetic limitations of UFH. Enoxaparin, in fact, presents decreased binding to plasma proteins and endothelial cells and holds a more predictable dose–effect relationship, which does not usually require laboratory monitoring of activity. In addition, enoxaparin is associated with less platelet activation and a lower risk of heparin-induced thrombocytopenia as compared to UFH. Another advantage is the ease of subcutaneous administration. In comparison to UFH, enoxaparin is associated with a reduction in death or MI, which is offset by increased rates of bleeding, leading to an overall neutral effect (56). Some reluctance has been shown by physicians about the substitution of LMWH for UFH during interventional procedures, due to difficult monitoring of anticoagulant therapy. For this reason, it was not uncommon that patients treated with enoxaparin received additional boluses of UFH in the catheterization laboratory. A post-hoc analysis from the Superior Yield of the New Strategy of Enoxaparin, Revascularization and Glycoprotein IIb/IIIa Inhibitors (SYNERGY) trial suggested that in patients already given enoxaparin crossover to UFH at the time of PCI could be associated to excess bleeding (57). Importantly, this hypothesis was recently confirmed in the STACK-on to ENOXaparin (STACKENOX) trial (58), discouraging administration of UFH <10 h after administration of 1 mg/kg enoxaparin, unless factor Xa activity levels are low. Because there are patients who might respond differently to enoxaparin (e.g., patients with marked obesity, severe renal failure and those not yet at steady state—which is achieved after 5–8 subcutaneous doses), it would be desirable to develop a rapid and reliable bedside assessment of anti-Xa activity in patients scheduled for catheterization (50). Alternative strategies based on the timing of enoxaparin pharmacodynamics have been proposed (59).

A small advantage of UFH is that, in the event of bleeding, its effect can be promptly reversed by protamine, whilst enoxaparin is only partially reversed by protamine, and bivalirudin and fondaparinux lack a protamine-binding domain and require transfusion of coagulation factors.

POST-ACUTE CARE

As previously pointed-out, the risk of ischemic events after an ACS remains high for months and after discharge patients with NSTE-ACS have actually higher risk of mortality than patients with STEMI (60). Hence, secondary prevention in this setting is of paramount importance (Fig. 27.3). Aggressive risk factor modifications is recommended (24), but the adherence to behavioral advices on diet, exercise, and smoking cessation after ACS is poor (61), and effective cardiac medications are often under-utilized.

BEYOND THE GUIDELINES

There are a few issues that are either not present or only marginally touched by guidelines because of the lack of clear evidence. Among them, the most important are: (i) the role of ultrasensitive troponin assays; (ii) radial versus femoral access for coronary angiography and PCI; and (iii) the so-called treatment-risk paradox (Focus Box 27.6).

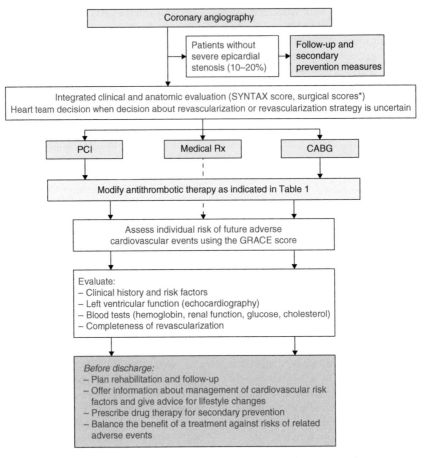

Figure 27.3 Strategy of revascularization and management of the post-acute phase.

Focus Box 27.6

Future Directions
- Understand the role of ultrasensitive troponin assays
- Assess whether N-terminal pro-brain natriuretic peptide (BNP) and C-reactive protein provides additional risk stratification on top of other risk factors and clarify whether and how they should be integrated in clinical decision making
- Address the so-called "treatment-risk paradox"
- Clarify the role of radial vs. femoral access for coronary angiography and PCI
- Increase knowledge on the "vulnerable plaque," its identification in vivo, and possible treatments
- Possible new developments:
  - Biomarkers (e.g., growth-differentiation factor-15, cystatin C, copeptid)
  - Anticoagulants (e.g., otamixaban, a direct intravenous factor Xa inhibitor; rivaroxaban, an oral factor Xa inhibitor; M118, a low-molecular-weight heparin; RB006, an inhibitor of factor IXa)
  - Antiplatelet agents (vorapaxar, oral inhibitor of the platelet receptor for thrombin protease-activated receptor 1)
  - Lipid management drugs (cholesterol ester transfer protein inhibitors that raise HDL like dalcetrapib and anacetrapib)

New higher sensitivity assays for troponin have been recently developed and will enable a more sensitive and rapid diagnosis of myocardial necrosis. However, they will also increase the frequency of false-positive. With these assays, many patients who heretofore were diagnosed with UA will now be reclassified as NSTEMI (62). While the precise role of high sensitivity troponin measurements has yet to be defined, they have been shown to improve risk assessment in ACS and could therefore reveal the need for more aggressive therapies (63,64).

The risk of bleeding is certainly a major issue in ACS patients. Radial artery access for coronary angiography and PCI is associated with a dramatic reduction of access-site bleeding events (65). The AHA/ACC guidelines state only that 'the Writing Committee endorses further research into techniques that could reduce bleeding (e.g., radial access and smaller sheath sizes)'(24), whilst the ESC guidelines give a general recommendation to 'use radial access in patients at high risk of bleeding'(16,17). Indeed, a very recent randomized trial comparing radial versus femoral access in ACS resulted neutral for the primary outcome. Nevertheless, prespecified subgroup analyses revealed a benefit for radial access in highest tertile volume radial centres (HR 0·49, 95% CI 0·28–0·87; $p = 0·015$); radial access was also associated with a lower rate of vascular complications (66).

A number of studies have reported that patients who are at lower risk for ischemic events are more likely to be treated more aggressively than higher-risk patients, including the use of an invasive strategy (67,68). This might be due to the fact that ischemic and hemorrhagic risk increases in parallel, but remains partially unjustified and possibly associated with a worst outcome (60). A conscious approach to these patients with employment of renal protection strategies, careful dosing and dose-adjustment of the drugs based on renal function and body weight, use of trans-radial approach for invasive procedures, might help reducing the gap between guidelines and their implementation into clinical practice.

PERSONAL PERSPECTIVE

The field of ACS is very complex and treatment strategies are always changing based on new research. Over the years, it has clearly emerged that NSTE-ACS is the manifestation of an aggressive disease that must be treated aggressively. Early knowledge of coronary anatomy, leading to revascularization when indicated and using the most appropriate revascularization strategy, that is, adoption of an "early invasive" strategy, is among the most effective measures, and should be used for the vast majority of ACS patients. In general, the greater was the restriction for cardiac catheterization applied in the conservative arm of clinical trials, the greater appeared the benefit for the invasive arm. The timing of coronary angiography must be fast enough to prevent early adverse events but, with very few exceptions, not as fast as in STEMI, in order to allow a precise and dynamic risk stratification for every patient. A wide spectrum of drugs and possible combinations of drugs is now available for tailoring treatment to each single patient, based on careful evaluation of individual ischemic and bleeding risk and depending also upon the selected strategy of treatment. A number of registries suggest that there is a gap between existing guidelines and their implementation into clinical practice, especially regarding risk stratification and its consequences on the whole process of care. Further understanding of the pathophysiobiology of ACS, integration of novel biomarkers into clinical practice, new imaging techniques, new drugs, and improved post-acute management will certainly improve management and outcome of NSTE-ACS in the near future. Management of residual cardiovascular risk after an NSTE-ACS is challenging, especially in some patients subgroups (e.g. elderly patients), and deserves continuous attention, planning of follow-up, and identification of new targets and relative therapeutic agents.

REFERENCES

1. Fuster V, Badimon L, Badimon JJ, Chesebro JH. The pathogenesis of coronary artery disease and the acute coronary syndromes (2). N Engl J Med 1992; 326: 310–18.
2. Fuster V, Badimon L, Badimon JJ, Chesebro JH. The pathogenesis of coronary artery disease and the acute coronary syndromes (1). N Engl J Med 1992; 326: 242–50.
3. Naghavi M, Libby P, Falk E, et al. From vulnerable plaque to vulnerable patient: a call for new definitions and risk assessment strategies: Part I. Circulation 2003; 108: 1664–72.
4. Anderson JL, Adams CD, Antman EM, et al. ACC/AHA 2007 guidelines for the management of patients with unstable angina/non ST-elevation myocardial infarction: a report of the American College of Cardiology/American Heart Association Task Force on Practice Guidelines (Writing Committee to Revise the 2002 Guidelines for the Management of Patients With Unstable Angina/Non ST-Elevation Myocardial Infarction): developed in collaboration with the American College of Emergency Physicians, the Society for Cardiovascular Angiography and Interventions, and the Society of Thoracic Surgeons: endorsed by the American Association of Cardiovascular and Pulmonary Rehabilitation and the Society for Academic Emergency Medicine. Circulation 2007; 116: e148–304.
5. Bassand JP, Hamm CW, Ardissino D, et al. Guidelines for the diagnosis and treatment of non-ST-segment elevation acute coronary syndromes. Eur Heart J 2007; 28: 1598–660.
6. Terkelsen CJ, Lassen JF, Norgaard BL, et al. Mortality rates in patients with ST-elevation vs. non-ST-elevation acute myocardial infarction: observations from an unselected cohort. Eur Heart J 2005; 26: 18–26.
7. The TIMI Investigators. Effects of tissue plasminogen activator and a comparison of early invasive and conservative strategies in unstable angina and non-Q-wave myocardial infarction. Results of the TIMI IIIB Trial. Thrombolysis in Myocardial Ischemia. Circulation 1994; 89: 1545–56.
8. McCullough PA, O'Neill WW, Graham M, et al. A prospective randomized trial of triage angiography in acute coronary syndromes ineligible for thrombolytic therapy. Results of the medicine versus angiography in thrombolytic exclusion (MATE) trial. J Am Coll Cardiol 1998; 32: 596–605.
9. Boden WE, O'Rourke RA, Crawford MH, et al. Outcomes in patients with acute non-Q-wave myocardial infarction randomly assigned to an invasive as compared with a conservative management strategy. Veterans Affairs Non-Q-Wave Infarction Strategies in Hospital (VANQWISH) Trial Investigators. N Engl J Med 1998; 338: 1785–92.
10. Wallentin L, Lagerqvist B, Husted S, et al. Outcome at 1 year after an invasive compared with a non-invasive strategy in unstable coronary-artery disease: the FRISC II invasive randomised trial. FRISC II Investigators. Fast Revascularisation during Instability in Coronary artery disease. Lancet 2000; 356: 9–16.
11. Cannon CP, Weintraub WS, Demopoulos LA, et al. Comparison of early invasive and conservative strategies in patients with unstable coronary syndromes treated with the glycoprotein IIb/IIIa inhibitor tirofiban. N Engl J Med 2001; 344: 1879–87.

12. Fox KA, Poole-Wilson PA, Henderson RA, et al. Interventional versus conservative treatment for patients with unstable angina or non-ST-elevation myocardial infarction: the British Heart Foundation RITA 3 randomised trial. Randomized Intervention Trial of unstable Angina. Lancet 2002; 360: 743–51.

13. de Winter RJ, Windhausen F, Cornel JH, et al. Early invasive versus selectively invasive management for acute coronary syndromes. N Engl J Med 2005; 353: 1095–104.

14. Mehta SR, Cannon CP, Fox KA, et al. Routine vs selective invasive strategies in patients with acute coronary syndromes: a collaborative meta-analysis of randomized trials. JAMA 2005; 293: 2908–17.

15. Fox KA, Clayton TC, Damman P, et al. Long-term outcome of a routine versus selective invasive strategy in patients with non-ST-segment elevation acute coronary syndrome a meta-analysis of individual patient data. J Am Coll Cardiol 2010; 55: 2435–45.

16. Hamm CW, Bassand JP, Agewall S, et al. ESC Guidelines for the management of acute coronary syndromes in patients presenting without persistent ST-segment elevation: The Task Force for the management of acute coronary syndromes (ACS) in patients presenting without persistent ST-segment elevation of the European Society of Cardiology (ESC). Eur Heart J 2011; Epub ahead of print.

17. Wijns W, Kolh P, Danchin N, et al. Guidelines on myocardial revascularization: The Task Force on Myocardial Revascularization of the European Society of Cardiology (ESC) and the European Association for Cardio-Thoracic Surgery (EACTS). Eur Heart J 2010; 31: 2501–55.

18. Kushner FG, Hand M, Smith SC Jr, et al. 2009 focused updates: ACC/AHA guidelines for the management of patients with ST-elevation myocardial infarction (updating the 2004 guideline and 2007 focused update) and ACC/AHA/SCAI guidelines on percutaneous coronary intervention (updating the 2005 guideline and 2007 focused update) a report of the American College of Cardiology Foundation/American Heart Association Task Force on Practice Guidelines. J Am Coll Cardiol 2009; 54: 2205–41.

19. Mehta SR, Granger CB, Boden WE, et al. Early versus delayed invasive intervention in acute coronary syndromes. N Engl J Med 2009; 360: 2165–75.

20. Neumann FJ, Kastrati A, Pogatsa-Murray G, et al. Evaluation of prolonged antithrombotic pretreatment ("cooling-off" strategy) before intervention in patients with unstable coronary syndromes: a randomized controlled trial. JAMA 2003; 290: 1593–9.

21. Montalescot G, Cayla G, Collet JP, et al. Immediate vs delayed intervention for acute coronary syndromes: a randomized clinical trial. JAMA 2009; 302: 947–54.

22. Wright RS, Anderson JL, Adams CD, et al. 2011 ACCF/AHA Focused Update of the Guidelines for the Management of Patients With Unstable Angina/Non-ST-Elevation Myocardial Infarction (Updating the 2007 Guideline) A Report of the American College of Cardiology Foundation/American Heart Association Task Force on Practice Guidelines Developed in Collaboration With the American College of Emergency Physicians, Society for Cardiovascular Angiography and Interventions, and Society of Thoracic Surgeons. J Am Coll Cardiol 2011; 57: 1920–59.

23. Taglieri N, Marzocchi A, Saia F, et al. Short- and Long-term prognostic significance of ST-Segment Elevation in Lead aVR in patients with Non-ST-segment Elevation Acute Coronary Syndrome. Am J Cardiol 2011; 108: 21–8.

24. Anderson JL, Adams CD, Antman EM, et al. 2011 ACCF/AHA Focused Update Incorporated Into the ACC/AHA 2007 Guidelines for the Management of Patients With Unstable Angina/Non-ST-Elevation Myocardial Infarction: a Report of the American College of Cardiology Foundation/American Heart Association Task Force on Practice Guidelines. Circulation 2011; 123: e426–579.

25. Serruys PW, Morice MC, Kappetein AP, et al. Percutaneous coronary intervention versus coronary-artery bypass grafting for severe coronary artery disease. N Engl J Med 2009; 360: 961–72.

26. Roques F, Nashef SA, Michel P, et al. Risk factors and outcome in European cardiac surgery: analysis of the EuroSCORE multinational database of 19030 patients. Eur J Cardiothorac Surg 1999; 15: 816–22; discussion 822–3.

27. Dewey TM, Brown D, Ryan WH, et al. Reliability of risk algorithms in predicting early and late operative outcomes in high-risk patients undergoing aortic valve replacement. J Thorac Cardiovasc Surg 2008; 135: 180–7.

28. Tonino PA, De Bruyne B, Pijls NH, et al. Fractional flow reserve versus angiography for guiding percutaneous coronary intervention. N Engl J Med 2009; 360: 213–24.

29. Stone GW, Maehara A, Lansky AJ, et al. A prospective natural-history study of coronary atherosclerosis. N Engl J Med 2011; 364: 226–35.

30. Yusuf S, Zhao F, Mehta SR, et al. Effects of clopidogrel in addition to aspirin in patients with acute coronary syndromes without ST-segment elevation. N Engl J Med 2001; 345: 494–502.

31. Mehta SR, Bassand JP, Chrolavicius S, et al. Dose comparisons of clopidogrel and aspirin in acute coronary syndromes. N Engl J Med 2010; 363: 930–42.

32. Angiolillo DJ, Suryadevara S, Capranzano P, et al. Antiplatelet drug response variability and the role of platelet function testing: a practical guide for interventional cardiologists. Catheter Cardiovasc Interv 2009; 73: 1–14.

33. Mehta SR, Yusuf S, Peters RJ, et al. Effects of pretreatment with clopidogrel and aspirin followed by long-term therapy in patients undergoing percutaneous coronary intervention: the PCI-CURE study. Lancet 2001; 358: 527–33.

34. Angiolillo DJ, Fernandez-Ortiz A, Bernardo E, et al. Variability in individual responsiveness to clopidogrel: clinical implications, management, and future perspectives. J Am Coll Cardiol 2007; 49: 1505–16.

35. Price MJ, Berger PB, Teirstein PS, et al. Standard- vs high-dose clopidogrel based on platelet function testing after percutaneous coronary intervention: the GRAVITAS randomized trial. JAMA 2011; 305: 1097–105.

36. Price MJ, Angiolillo DJ, Teirstein PS, et al. Platelet reactivity and cardiovascular outcomes after percutaneous coronary intervention. A time-dependent analysis of the Gauging Responsiveness with a VerifyNow P2Y12 Assay: impact on Thrombosis and Safety (GRAVITAS) trial. Circulation 2011; 124: 1132–7.

37. Parodi G, Marcucci R, Valenti R, et al. High residual platelet reactivity after clopidogrel loading and long-term cardiovascular events among patients with acute coronary syndromes undergoing PCI. JAMA 2011; 306: 1215–23.

38. Mega JL, Simon T, Collet JP, et al. Reduced-function CYP2C19 genotype and risk of adverse clinical outcomes among patients treated with clopidogrel predominantly for PCI: a meta-analysis. JAMA 2010; 304: 1821–30.

39. Collet JP, Hulot JS, Anzaha G, et al. High doses of clopidogrel to overcome genetic resistance the randomized crossover CLOVIS-2 (Clopidogrel and Response Variability Investigation Study 2). JACC Cardiovasc Interv 2011; 4: 392–402.

40. Shuldiner AR, O'Connell JR, Bliden KP, et al. Association of cytochrome P450 2C19 genotype with the antiplatelet effect and clinical efficacy of clopidogrel therapy. JAMA 2009; 302: 849–57.

41. Mega JL, Close SL, Wiviott SD, et al. Genetic variants in ABCB1 and CYP2C19 and cardiovascular outcomes after treatment with clopidogrel and prasugrel in the TRITON-TIMI 38 trial: a pharmacogenetic analysis. Lancet 2010; 376: 1312–19.

42. Wallentin L, James S, Storey RF, et al. Effect of CYP2C19 and ABCB1 single nucleotide polymorphisms on outcomes of treatment with ticagrelor versus clopidogrel for acute coronary syndromes: a genetic substudy of the PLATO trial. Lancet 2010; 376: 1320–8.

43. Wiviott SD, Braunwald E, McCabe CH, et al. Prasugrel versus clopidogrel in patients with acute coronary syndromes. N Engl J Med 2007; 357: 2001–15.

44. Wallentin L, Becker RC, Budaj A, et al. Ticagrelor versus clopidogrel in patients with acute coronary syndromes. N Engl J Med 2009; 361: 1045–57.

45. Bhatt DL, Cryer BL, Contant CF, et al. Clopidogrel with or without omeprazole in coronary artery disease. N Engl J Med 2010; 363: 1909–17.

46. Kastrati A, Mehilli J, Neumann FJ, et al. Abciximab in patients with acute coronary syndromes undergoing percutaneous coronary intervention after clopidogrel pretreatment: the ISAR-REACT 2 randomized trial. JAMA 2006; 295: 1531–8.

47. Stone GW, McLaurin BT, Cox DA, et al. Bivalirudin for patients with acute coronary syndromes. N Engl J Med 2006; 355: 2203–16.

48. Stone GW, Bertrand ME, Moses JW, et al. Routine upstream initiation vs deferred selective use of glycoprotein IIb/IIIa inhibitors in acute coronary syndromes: the ACUITY Timing trial. JAMA 2007; 297: 591–602.

49. Giugliano RP, White JA, Bode C, et al. Early versus delayed, provisional eptifibatide in acute coronary syndromes. N Engl J Med 2009; 360: 2176–90.

50. Alexander D, Mann N, Ou FS, et al. Patterns of upstream antiplatelet therapy use before primary percutaneous coronary intervention for acute ST-elevation myocardial infarction (from the CRUSADE National Quality Improvement Initiative). Am J Cardiol 2008; 102: 1335–40.

51. O'Donoghue M, Antman EM, Braunwald E, et al. The efficacy and safety of prasugrel with and without a glycoprotein IIb/IIIa inhibitor in patients with acute coronary syndromes undergoing percutaneous intervention: a TRITON-TIMI 38 (Trial to Assess Improvement in Therapeutic Outcomes by Optimizing Platelet Inhibition With Prasugrel-Thrombolysis In Myocardial Infarction 38) analysis. J Am Coll Cardiol 2009; 54: 678–85.

52. Yusuf S, Mehta SR, Chrolavicius S, et al. Comparison of fondaparinux and enoxaparin in acute coronary syndromes. N Engl J Med 2006; 354: 1464–76.

53. Kastrati A, Neumann FJ, Mehilli J, et al. Bivalirudin versus unfractionated heparin during percutaneous coronary intervention. N Engl J Med 2008; 359: 688–96.

54. Schulz S, Mehilli J, Neumann FJ, et al. ISAR-REACT 3A: a study of reduced dose of unfractionated heparin in biomarker negative patients undergoing percutaneous coronary intervention. Eur Heart J 2010; 31: 2482–91.

55. Steg PG, Jolly SS, Mehta SR, et al. Low-dose vs standard-dose unfractionated heparin for percutaneous coronary intervention in acute coronary syndromes treated with fondaparinux: the FUTURA/OASIS-8 randomized trial. JAMA 2010; 304: 1339–49.

56. Murphy SA, Gibson CM, Morrow DA, et al. Efficacy and safety of the low-molecular weight heparin enoxaparin compared with unfractionated heparin across the acute coronary syndrome spectrum: a meta-analysis. Eur Heart J 2007; 28: 2077–86.

57. Mahaffey KW, Ferguson JJ. Exploring the role of enoxaparin in the management of high-risk patients with non-ST-elevation acute coronary syndromes: the SYNERGY trial. Am Heart J 2005; 149: S81–90.

58. Drouet L, Bal dit Sollier C, Martin J. Adding intravenous unfractionated heparin to standard enoxaparin causes excessive anticoagulation not detected by activated clotting time: results of the STACK-on to ENOXaparin (STACKENOX) study. Am Heart J 2009; 158: 177–84.

59. Martin JL, Slepian M. Use of low-molecular-weight heparins during percutaneous coronary intervention. J Invasive Cardiol 2011; 23: 1–8.

60. McManus DD, Gore J, Yarzebski J, et al. Recent trends in the incidence, treatment, and outcomes of patients with STEMI and NSTEMI. Am J Med 2011; 124: 40–7.

61. Chow CK, Jolly S, Rao-Melacini P, et al. Association of diet, exercise, and smoking modification with risk of early cardiovascular events after acute coronary syndromes. Circulation 2010; 121: 750–8.

62. Goodman SG, Steg PG, Eagle KA, et al. The diagnostic and prognostic impact of the redefinition of acute myocardial infarction: lessons from the Global Registry of Acute Coronary Events (GRACE). Am Heart J 2006; 151: 654–60.

63. Ndrepepa G, Braun S, Mehilli J, et al. Prognostic value of sensitive troponin T in patients with stable and unstable angina and undetectable conventional troponin. Am Heart J 2011; 161: 68–75.

64. Lindahl B, Venge P, James S. The new high-sensitivity cardiac troponin T assay improves risk assessment in acute coronary syndromes. Am Heart J 2011; 160: 224–9.

65. Agostoni P, Biondi-Zoccai GG, de Benedictis ML, et al. Radial versus femoral approach for percutaneous coronary diagnostic and interventional procedures; Systematic overview and meta-analysis of randomized trials. J Am Coll Cardiol 2004; 44: 349–56.

66. Jolly SS, Yusuf S, Cairns J, et al. Radial versus femoral access for coronary angiography and intervention in patients with acute coronary syndromes (RIVAL): a randomised, parallel group, multicentre trial. Lancet 2011; 377: 1409–20.

67. Bhatt DL, Roe MT, Peterson ED, et al. Utilization of early invasive management strategies for high-risk patients with non-ST-segment elevation acute coronary syndromes: results from the CRUSADE Quality Improvement Initiative. JAMA 2004; 292: 2096–104.

68. Fox KA, Anderson FA Jr, Dabbous OH, et al. Intervention in acute coronary syndromes: do patients undergo intervention on the basis of their risk characteristics? The Global Registry of Acute Coronary Events (GRACE). Heart 2007; 93: 177–82.

69. Granger CB, Goldberg RJ, Dabbous O, et al. Predictors of hospital mortality in the global registry of acute coronary events. Arch Intern Med 2003; 163: 2345–53.

70. Antman EM, Cohen M, Bernink PJ, et al. The TIMI risk score for unstable angina/non-ST elevation MI: a method for prognostication and therapeutic decision making. JAMA 2000; 284: 835–42.

71. Boersma E, Pieper KS, Steyerberg EW, et al. Predictors of outcome in patients with acute coronary syndromes without persistent ST-segment elevation. Results from an international trial of 9461 patients. The PURSUIT Investigators. Circulation 2000; 101: 2557–67.

72. Eagle KA, Lim MJ, Dabbous OH, et al. A validated prediction model for all forms of acute coronary syndrome: estimating the risk of 6-month postdischarge death in an international registry. JAMA 2004; 291: 2727–33.

73. Subherwal S, Bach RG, Chen AY, et al. Baseline risk of major bleeding in non-ST-segment-elevation myocardial infarction: the CRUSADE (Can Rapid risk stratification of Unstable angina patients Suppress ADverse outcomes with Early implementation of the ACC/AHA Guidelines) Bleeding Score. Circulation 2009; 119: 1873–82.

74. Moscucci M, Fox KA, Cannon CP, et al. Predictors of major bleeding in acute coronary syndromes: the Global Registry of Acute Coronary Events (GRACE). Eur Heart J 2003; 24: 1815–23.

75. Mehran R, Pocock SJ, Nikolsky E, et al. A risk score to predict bleeding in patients with acute coronary syndromes. J Am Coll Cardiol 2010; 55: 2556–66.

28 Treatment algorithm in patients with STEMI
Luca Golino and Giuseppe De Luca

OUTLINE

ST segment elevation myocardial infarction (STEMI) is the leading cause of mortality in developed countries. When minutes count, and time is muscle, emergency physicians have the opportunity to have a relevant impact on morbidity and mortality by instituting appropriate therapy in a very time-efficient manner in the treatment of STEMI. Guidelines were promulgated to provide recommendations in an effort to standardize and optimize the evaluation, diagnosis, and management of patients with STEMI. These recommendations emphasize the importance of early reperfusion therapy. To achieve this goal, local networks have to be implemented, to promote early in-ambulance treatment, including thrombolysis or immediate transfer of the patient to a primary percutaneous coronary intervention (PPCI) hospital, avoiding delay in vessel reopening. However, even when thrombolysis is the preferred initial therapy, all patients should be transferred to PPCI centers in order to reduce the time to reperfusion where thrombolysis fails or early reocclusion occurs.

Several studies have shown the superiority of PPCI as compared to thrombolysis, which therefore should be the preferred reperfusion therapy when performed by experienced operators and implemented without excessive delays to treatment. Unfortunately, there are wide differences in PPCI centers in terms of geographic distribution, organization and level of competence. The priority should be to obtain a more homogeneous standard of care, based on a consensus triage, efficient regional network, and outcome data auditing. When PPCI is planned, it is important that a strategy be implemented to ensure that optimal early antithmbitic and antiplatelet therapies be administered in order to obtain preprocedural recanalization or at least to guarantee an optimal periprocedural inhibition of the coagulation cascade and of platelet aggregation. Use of thrombus aspiration and of DES should be considered to improve early and late clinical outcome.

INTRODUCTION

STEMI continues to be a significant public health problem in industrialized countries and is becoming an increasingly significant problem in developing countries. Based on the data obtained from the National Registry of Myocardial Infarction-4 (NRMI-4), we may estimate that 500,000 STEMI events per year occur in the United States.

However, several factors have contributed to the significant reduction in mortality observed in the last decades in STEMI patients. These include earlier diagnosis and treatment of the acute event, improved management of complications (such as recurrent ischemia and heart failure), and

more widespread availability of pharmacological therapies such as aspirin, beta-blockers, ACE-inhibitors, and glycoprotein IIb-IIIa inhibitors. Most attention, however, has been focused on therapies that may restore antegrade coronary blood flow in the culprit artery (1,2).

Even though primary angioplasty has certainly contributed to a further reduction in mortality as compared to thrombolysis, it may be unreasonable to mandate the extension of this reperfusion therapy to all STEMI patients. In fact, ischemia time is a major determinant of survival even when mechanical reperfusion is performed (3). Therefore, when minutes count, and time is muscle, emergency physicians have the opportunity to make a crucial impact on morbidity and mortality by applying appropriate therapy in a very time-efficient manner in the treatment of ST segment elevation myocardial infarction (STEMI). Guidelines were promulgated to provide recommendations in an effort to standardize and optimize the evaluation, diagnosis, and management of patients with STEMI and to provide physicians with a framework for clinical and technical advances in mechanical reperfusion and reduce associated complications such as thrombotic re-occlusion, bleeding complications, and cardiogenic shock.

The aim of this chapter is to review current recommendations provided by recent STEMI guidelines, with integration of novel data, and provide an algorithm for the treatment of STEMI patients.

GUIDELINES AND POTENTIAL INTEGRATION OF NOVEL DATA TO THE GUIDELINES

Primary Percutaneous Coronary Intervention

PPCI is defined as percutaneous intervention in the setting of STEMI without previous fibrinolytic treatment. RCTs and meta-analyses comparing primary PCI with in-hospital fibrinolytic therapy in patients presenting within 6–12 h after symptom onset treated in high-volume, experienced centers, have shown more effective restoration of vessel patency, less re-occlusion, improved residual LV function, and better clinical outcome with PPCI. Cities and countries switching from fibrinolysis to PPCI have observed a sharp decrease in mortality after STEMI (4). American College of Cardiology/American Heart Association (ACC/AHA) guidelines specify that PPCI should be performed by operators who perform 75 elective procedures per year and at least 11 procedures for STEMI in institutions with annual volume of 400 elective and 36 PPCI procedures. Such a policy decision is justified by the strong inverse volume-outcome relationship observed in high-risk and emergency PCI (5). Therefore, tolerance of low-volume thresholds for PCI centers for the purpose of providing PPCI is not recommended. It is essential to make every effort to minimize any delay, especially within the first 2 h after onset of the symptoms, by implementation of a system of care network. In fact, time-to-treatment has been shown to be a major determinant of mortality not only for lysis but also for mechanical reperfusion. Therefore, even though we may be able to mechanically recanalize an occluded culprit artery independent of the time of symptom onset, this may remain a cosmetic act, that, despite being esthetically highly pleasing, unfortunately may not overcome the profound necrosis linearly related to the duration of ischemia (6).

Pharmacological Facilitation

Due to the prognostic impact of ischemia time on survival in patients undergoing PPCI, several efforts have been made in order to investigate the advantages of pharmacological recanalization ("Facilitation") during transportation.

The largest trial conducted with full thrombolytic therapy (ASSENT-4) (7) was prematurely stopped due to higher mortality with facilitation. The FINESSE (8) was the largest trial conducted to investigate the benefits from combotherapy or early upstream abciximab. In fact, periprocedural abciximab administration has been shown to reduce mortality (9), and therefore further benefits may be expected by its early administration. This study was prematurely stopped as well, due to slow recruitment, without showing any benefit. However, subsequent subgroup, posthoc analyses, showed benefits in high-risk patients reperfused within the first 4 h from symptoms onset. In fact, the application of this strategy to all STEMI patients would certainly unreasonable from the physiopathologic point of view, since the largest amount of myocardial salvage is mostly expected within the first few hours from symptom onset. An individual patient data meta-analysis of randomized trials on early glycoprotein IIb-IIIa inhibitors (EGYPT cooperation) (10), conducted in well-run networks for PPCI, showed significant benefits in preprocedural recanalization and significant reduction in mortality from early abciximab administration. A major explanation for the different results between these two studies is certainly the shorter time-to-therapy and faster PCI in the EGYPT as compared to the FINESSE trial. In fact, a recent study (11) showed that thrombus composition may significantly change over time, with a greater prevalence of platelets within the first hours from symptom onset, and more fibrin in the later phase.

Similar benefits from early Gp IIb-IIIa inhibitors have been observed in prospective registries and posthoc analyses of trials such as EUROTRANSFER registry, subanalysis of the APEX-MI, the Emilia-Romagna registry, and MISSION registry.

Thus, despite the negative results of the FINESSE trial (8), there is reasonable evidence for a beneficial effect of early Gp IIb-IIIa inhibitor administration that should still be considered a reasonable strategy, especially in high-risk patients and within the first hours from symptom onset. Therefore, the current ESC recommendation on early glycoprotein IIb-IIIa inhibitors (downgrade to class III) is, in our opinion, unjustified. ACC/AHA guidelines still recommend early administration of Gp IIb-IIIa inhibitors (as class IIa).

Oral Antiplatelet Therapies

In addition to acid acetylsalycilic, standard dose clopidogrel (300 mg bolus followed by 75 mg/per day) has been regarded as the gold standard for adjunctive antiplatelet therapy in patients with STEMI treated whether or not they were treated with mechanical reperfusion (Table 28.1). Several limitations of clopidogrel (13) have highlighted attention to the need for new therapies. In fact, due to its complex metabolic pathway, clopidogrel takes 4 h to reach peak platelet aggregation inhibition, and this time may be even longer in the setting of STEMI, where drug absorption may be delayed (14). Since many patients receive the clopidogrel loading dose just before PCI, they are at risk of thrombotic periprocedural events. Furthermore, due to polymorphisms of several enzymes involved in the multistep metabolic pathway of clopidogrel, a large interindividual variability in platelet aggregation inhibition has been observed, with resistance to clopidogrel in between 15 and 30%. Several new therapeutic strategies have been proposed to overcome some of the limitations of standard dose clopidogrel. High-dose clopidogrel has been shown to provide faster and more profound inhibition of platelet aggregation, with a lower percentage of resistance. The CURRENT trial (15) showed that high-dose clopidogrel was associated with a slightly higher risk of bleeding complications but significantly reduced the rate of reinfarction, mainly due to a significant reduction in stent thrombosis. The higher loading dose (600 mg) has been therefore recommended in recent guidelines (Table 28.1).

Prasugrel is a third generation thienopyridine with a faster metabolic activation that hastens the onset of action and increases inhibition of platelet aggregation. Data from the TRITON-TIMI 38 in STEMI patients (16) showed significant benefits in terms of mortality and stent thombosis, without a higher risk of major bleeding complications, as compared to the findings in the overall ACS population. This may be explained by the higher baseline platelet reactivity commonly observed in STEMI patients that may maximize the benefits in terms of thrombotic complications, while containing the risk of bleeding complications. However, based on the results in the overall ACS population, prasugrel is currently contraindicated in elderly patients (>75 years), low body weight (<60 kg), previous stroke, where prasugrel significantly increased the risk of major bleeding complications.

Ticagrelor is a non-thienopiridine with a faster onset of action and significantly higher inhibition of platelet aggregation as compared to 600 mg clopidogrel. One of the important advantages that makes the molecule very appealing is the reversibility of its antiplatelet effects that is implied by twice-a-day administration. Data obtained from the large PLATO trial (17) showed a significant reduction in mortality, in addition to benefits in myocardial infarction and stent thrombosis. No difference was observed in terms of major bleeding complications.

Current ESC PCI guidelines do recommend both prasugrel and ticagrelor as class I (Table 28.1). However, despite the clear superiority of these therapies, guidelines still recommend clopidogrel as class I.

Table 28.1 ESC Recommendations for the treatment of STEMI (Ref. 1,12)

Recommendation	Class	Level
Reperfusion therapy is indicated in all patients with a history of chest pain/discomfort a history of <12 hours and with persistent ST-segment elevation or (presumed) new left bundle-branch block	I	A
Reperfusion therapy should be considered if there is clinical and/or ECG evidence of ongoing ischemia even if, according to the patient, symptoms started >12 hours before	IIa	C
Reperfusion using PCI may be considered in stable patients presenting 12–24 h after symptom onset	IIb	B
PCI of a totally occluded infarct artery 24 h after symptom onset in stable patients without signs of ischemia	III	B
Primary PCI	Preferred treatment if performed by an experienced team as soon as possible after FMC	I
A	Time from FMC to balloon inflation should be, 2 h in any case and 90 min in patients presenting early (e.g., 2 h) with large infarct and low bleeding risk	I
B	Indicated for patients in shock and those with contraindications to fibrinolytic therapy irrespective of time delay	I
B	Antiplatelet co-therapy	
	Aspirin	I
B	NSAID and COX-2 selective inhibitors	III
B	Clopidogrel loading dose (600 mg)	I
C	Prasugrel	I
B	Ticagrelor	I
B	GPIIb/IIIa antagonist	
	Abciximab	IIa
A	Tirofiban	IIb
B	Eptifibatide	IIa
B	Upstream Gp IIb-IIIa inhibitors	III
B	Antithrombin therapy[a]	
	Heparin	I
C	Bivalirudin	I
B	Fondaparinux	III
B	Adjunctive devices	
	Thrombus aspiration	IIa
A	*Rescue PCI*	After failed fibrinolysis
IIa	A	*Fibrinolytic therapy*
In the absence of contraindications (if primary PCI cannot be performed within the recommended time)	I	A
A fibrin-specific agent should be given	I	B
Pre-hospital initiation of fibrinolytic therapy	IIa	A
Antiplatelet co-therapy[a]		
If not already on aspirin oral (soluble or chewable/non-enteric-coated) or i.v. dose of aspirin plus	I	B
Clopidogrel oral loading dose if age 75 years	I	B
If age 75 years start with maintenance dose	IIa	B
Antithrombin co-therapy[a] with alteplase, reteplase, and tenecteplase:		
Enoxaparin i.v. bolus followed 15 min later by first s.c. dose; if age. 75 years no i.v. bolus and start with reduced first s.c. dose	I	A
If enoxaparin is not available: a weight-adjusted bolus of i.v. heparin followed by a weight-adjusted i.v. infusion with first aPTT control after 3 h with streptokinase:	I	A
An i.v. bolus of fondaparinux followed by an s.c. dose 24 h later or	IIa	B
Enoxaparin i.v. bolus followed 15 min later by first s.c. dose; if age. 75 years no i.v. bolus and start with reduced first s.c. dose	IIa	B
Or a weight-adjusted dose of i.v. heparin followed by a weight-adjusted infusion	IIa	C

Anticoagulation

Despite the low costs, several potential disadvantages of unfractionated heparin (UFH) should be highlighted: (*i*) dependency on antithrombin III for inhibition of thrombin activity; (*ii*) sensitivity to platelet factor 4; (*iii*) inability to inhibit clot-bound thrombin; (*iv*) marked inter-individual variability in therapeutic response; (*v*) the need for frequent aPTT monitoring. In order to overcome these limitations, several new antithrombotic therapies have been proposed (18).

Bivalirudin

The process of intracoronary thrombus formation is only partially inhibited by aspirin and heparin. Large amounts of thrombin are generated when the coagulation system is activated by tissue factor exposed at the site of plaque disruption. Fibrin-bound thrombin is protected from inhibition by heparin, and remains enzymatically active, amplifying its own generation and promoting further thrombus formation. Bound thrombin also continues to activate platelets through thromboxane-A2-independent mechanisms that cannot be blocked by aspirin. Direct thrombin inhibitors act on both fluid-phase and clot-bound thrombin, and thus may prevent thrombus formation and its extension by inhibition of both coagulation and platelet aggregation. Several direct thrombin inhibitors have been tested in several randomized trials among STEMI patients treated with thrombolysis, showing negative results.

A large trial has been conducted in the setting of PPCI, the HORIZONS-AMI trial (19). In this trial a total of 3602 STEMI patients undergoing PPCI were randomized to bivalirudin or glycoprotein IIb-IIIa inhibitors (abciximab in 49.9% and eptifibatide in 44.4%) plus UFH. At 3-year follow-up bivalirudin was associated with a significant reduction in mortality, reinfarction, and major bleeding complications, despite a higher risk of early stent thrombosis with bivalirudin. Based on this study, bivalirudin is currently recommended as Class I (Table 28.1).

Low-Molecular-Weight Heparins (LMWHs)

The advantages of LMWHs include: (*i*) a stable and reliable anticoagulation effect that obviates the need for frequent monitoring of coagulation parameters; (*ii*) high bioavailability that allows subcutaneous administration; (*iii*) high anti-Xa: anti-IIa ratio, producing blockade of the coagulation cascade in an upstream location, results in a marked decrement in thrombin generation.

A few studies have investigated the role of LMWHs, mainly enoxaparin, in the setting of PPCI. In a subanalysis from the FINESSE trial, including 759 patients treated with enoxaparin and 1693 patients with UFH, a lower rate of nonintracranial TIMI major bleeding was found with enoxaparin (2.6% vs. UFH 4.4%, adjusted $p = 0.045$), whereas intracranial haemorrhage was similar (0.27% vs. 0.24%, adjusted $p = 0.98$). Lower rates of death, myocardial infarction, urgent revascularization, or refractory ischemia through 30 days was also associated with enoxaparin use (5.3%) versus UFH (8.0%, adjusted $p = 0.0005$) as was all-cause mortality through 90 days (3.8% vs. 5.6%, respectively, adjusted $p = 0.046$).

The only RCT comparing enoxaparin with UFH in PPCI is the ATOLL trial, in which 450 patients were randomized to enoxaparin and 460 patients randomized to UFH. Preliminary results of this study, presented at the 2010 European Society of Cardiology Congress, showed a reduction of the composite survival and ischemic endpoint (death, recurrent MI/ACS or urgent revascularization) with enoxaparin (6.7%) as compared to UFH (11.3%) ($p = 0.001$), without any beneficial effect in terms of bleeding complications. However, the study was underpowered to assess the effect on the individual outcomes.

A recent meta-analysis including observational studies and the ATOLL trial showed that LMWHs were associated with a reduction in mortality (RR [95% CI] = 0.51 [0.41–0.64], $p < 0.001$, ARR = 3%) and major bleeding (RR [95% CI] = 0.68 [0.49–0.94], $p = 0.02$, ARR = 2.0%) as compared to UFH (20).

Current guidelines do not recommend the use of enoxaparin in the setting of STEMI undergoing primary angioplasty. Future randomized trials are certainly needed before definitive conclusions may be reached on this drug.

Radial Approach

It must be recognized that while the use of intense anticoagulation and antiplatelet therapy has proven to reduce short- and long-term ischemic events after PPCI, it also has raised the issue of increased bleeding complications, which occur mostly at the site of vascular access. Despite the miniaturization of catheters, and the advent of hemostatic devices, access-site related bleeding complications occur in up to 10% of cases performed by the conventional transfemoral approach, with a strong negative impact not only on in-hospital morbidity, but also on mid- and long-term survival. Therefore, intense interest has been focused on the trans-radial approach (TRA) in the setting of PPCI. As a matter of fact, the penetration of TRA in clinical practice has been relatively limited, to date far from deep: in the US TRA still accounts for only 10% of the overall PCI procedures; in Europe and Asia this percentage has grown to approximately 30% but with marked geographic variation: while some centers perform TRA as the preferred approach (also for PPCI), others turn to TRA only as a second choice. A recent meta-analysis by Jolly et al. (21), including 23 studies (7020 patients) randomizing patients either to TRA or TFA, highlighted an overwhelming 73% reduction in access-site bleeding complications with TRA (0.05 vs. 2.3%). This also resulted in a lower accomplishment further translated in a lower incidence of MACCE (2.5 vs. 3.8%) and mortality (1.2 vs. 1.8%). Notably, 6 out of 23 randomized studies, included in this meta-analysis, were performed in STEMI patients: when data from this specific sub-cohort of patients were pooled together, the odds ratio for bleeding complications was shown to be 0.13 in favor of TRA. A recent large randomized trial (RIVAL) (22) was conducted in the setting of ACS, including 7021 patients (3507 assigned to TRA and 3514 to TFA). The primary outcome (composite of death, myocardial infarction, stroke, or non-coronary artery bypass graft (non-CABG)-related major bleeding at 30 days) occurred in 3.7% versus 4.0% in the femoral access group ($p = 0.50$). In a prespecified subgroup analysis, TRA in STEMI patients was associated with a significant reduction in mortality as compared to TFA (1.3% vs. 3.2%, $p = 0.006$). Even though hypothesis generating, these data should be incorporated into guidelines to further support the use of TRA in the setting of STEMI.

Thrombectomy
Distal embolization is certainly a major determinant of impaired myocardial reperfusion, occurring with a reported prevalence of 10–20% (23). This has prompted the evaluation of thrombectomy devices in the setting of STEMI. Several mechanisms may account for benefits from thrombus aspiration: (*i*) It may prevent distal embolization and the deleterious effects on microcirculation of vasoactive substances released by platelets. (*ii*) It allows the operator to have a better visualization of the atherosclerotic lesion. It is important to emphasize that we should never stent the thrombus, but limit the stent length to treat the plaque. (*iii*) It allows better evaluation of vessel size. The presence of thrombus and vasoactive substances, may favour vasospasm that may lead to stent undersizing. This is extremely important, especially in the era of DES. (*iv*) It allows direct stenting, a strategy that has been associated with less distal embolization and improved reperfusion. (*v*) It may reduce the incidence of stent malapposition, that is commonly due to disappearance of the residual thrombus potentially trapped between the stent and vessel wall soon after stent implantation. This is quite common in the setting of STEMI and in case of thrombotic lesions treated without thrombectomy.

Clinical Trials with Mechanical Thrombectomy
Several trials have been conducted with different devices resulting with in conflicting results. Negative results have mostly been observed in two large trials. In the AIMI multicenter trial (24), a total of 480 patients were randomized to rheolytic thrombectomy with Angiojet versus conventional primary angioplasty. The primary endpoint was infarct size estimated by technetium-99m Sestamibi. This trial showed a paradoxically larger infarct size and higher mortality in patients treated with thrombectomy in comparison with conventional PPCI. Some factors may have affected the results of this trial, such as the aspiration technique used (retrograde aspiration, from distal to proximal), the inclusion of a low-risk population (mortality rate in the control group of 0.8%), a larger unjustified use of temporary pacemakers in patients randomized to thrombectomy (58% vs. 19%), a larger percentage of preprocedural TIMI 3 flow in the control group (27% vs. 19%), and the fact that evidence of thrombus was not an inclusion criteria (less than 10% of enrolled patients had evidence of a large intracoronary thrombus).

In a Danish single center trial, a total of 215 STEMI patients were randomized to mechanical thrombectomy by the Rescue catheter or conventional PPCI. Also in this study patients were

not selected on the basis of angiographic evidence of thrombus. In accordance with the AIMI trial, enzymatic infarct size (the primary endpoint of the study) was paradoxically larger in patients randomized to thrombectomy. No benefits were observed in terms of ST-segment resolution.

Quite different findings were observed by Antoniucci et al. who conducted a small trial in 100 patients. They found significant benefits in terms of myocardial salvage and epicardial flow in Angiojet treated as compared to control patients. Similar benefits on clinical outcome were observed in the larger JETSTENT trial, a recent multicenter randomized trial leaded by Antoniucci. A total of 500 STEMI undergoing PPCI were randomized to Angiojet or standard therapy. Patients were eligible if they presented within 12 h of symptom onset and had a thrombus grade 3 to 5 detected by angiography. The primary end point of the study was early ST-segment resolution, defined as ≥50% ST-segment-elevation reduction at 30 minutes and infarct size at one month. ST-segment resolution at 30 minutes was significantly improved in patients who underwent thrombectomy prior to direct stenting compared with those who were stented without thrombectomy (85.8% vs. 78.8%, P = 0.043). The infarct size, however, was not different between the two treatment arms. Regarding clinical end points, MACCE, which included death, reinfarction, target lesion revascularization, and stroke, was also significantly improved at one (3.1% vs. 6.9%, $p = 0.05$) and six months (12% vs. 20.7%, $p = 0.012$) with thrombectomy.

Based on these data, mechanical thrombectomy devices may be considered in STEMI patients presenting with a large thrombus burden.

Clinical Trials with Manual Thrombectomy
Several randomized trials have been conducted on manual thrombectomy devices (25). Data from the large TAPAS trial have recently been published (26). In this trial more than 1000 STEMI patients were randomized before angiography to manual thrombectomy (Export catheter) or conventional PPCI. The vast majority of patients received Gp IIb-IIIa inhibitors. This study showed significant benefits on myocardial perfusion (as evaluated by myocardial blush and ST-segment resolution) and significant benefits on 1-year survival. The benefits on myocardial perfusion were confirmed in almost all the analyzed subgroups, greater benefit, as might intuitively be expected, was observed in patients revascularized within 3 hours of symptom onset when the amount of myocardium that can potentially be salvaged is greatest.

A large meta-analysis of randomized trials on manual thrombectomy devices has recently been conducted by De Luca et al. (25), including a total of nine trials, enrolling 2401 patients (1200 patients (50.0%) randomized to manual thrombectomy device and 1201 (50%) to conventional PPCI).

Adjunctive manual thrombectomy was associated with significant benefits in terms of postprocedural TIMI 3 flow (87.2% vs. 81.2%, $p < 0.0001$), postprocedural MBG 3 (52.1% vs. 31.7%, $p < 0.0001$), distal embolization (7.9% vs. 19.5%,

$p < 0.0001$), and 30-day mortality (1.7% vs. 3.1%, $p = 0.04$). Current guidelines do suggest routine manual thrombectomy as class IIa.

Drug-eluting Stents

Coronary stenting has been shown to reduce target vessel revascularization (TVR) in STEMI, without any benefit in terms of death and/or reinfarction, as compared to balloon angioplasty. However, these benefits may be reduced in unselected STEMI patients. Drug-eluting stents (DES) have shown a further significant reduction in restenosis and TVR in elective patients, as compared to bare-metal stents (BMS). Initial meta-analyses showed the safety of DES at shortly-term follow-up in the setting of STEMI. However, recent concerns have emerged regarding the potentially higher risk of stent thrombosis with DES that might be even more pronounced among STEMI patients, as suggested by a prospective registry.

Several randomized trials have been conducted (27). The small PASEO trial showed similar outcome between SES and PES that were both associated with a significant reduction of TVR, without any increased risk in of stent thrombosis and mortality at up to 6 years follow-up. Recent long-term follow-up data from PASSION (5 years), TYPHOON (4 years) and HORIZONS-AMI (3 years) (19), have definitively shown the safety and benefits of DES in the setting of STEMI Figures (28.1–28.3). However,

extreme caution should certainly be exercised in the setting of STEMI, especially in stent size selection (vasospasm is often encountered), careful assessment of the likely compliance with dual antiplatelet therapy, and avoiding their implantation when there is a large thrombus burden prior to stenting as this may carry a high risk of late acquired stent malapposition with the potential for late stent thrombosis. Current guidelines do not provide any recommendation on the use of DES in the setting of STEMI. As suggested in elective patients, due to the higher costs, DES should be considered in STEMI patients at high-risk for in-stent restenosis, such as long-lesions, bifurcations, small vessels, multivessel disease, diabetes, or in case of large ischemic areas, such as proximal LAD or left main.

Fibrinolysis

Despite its frequent contraindications, limited effectiveness in inducing reperfusion, and greater bleeding risk, fibrinolytic therapy, preferably administered as a pre-hospital treatment, remains an important alternative to mechanical revascularization. In Europe, 5–85% of patients with STEMI undergo PPCI, a wide range that reflects the variability or allocation of local resources and capabilities. Even with an optimal network organization, transfer delays may be unacceptably long before PPCI is performed, especially in patients living in mountain or rural areas or presenting to non-PPCI centers. The incremental benefit of

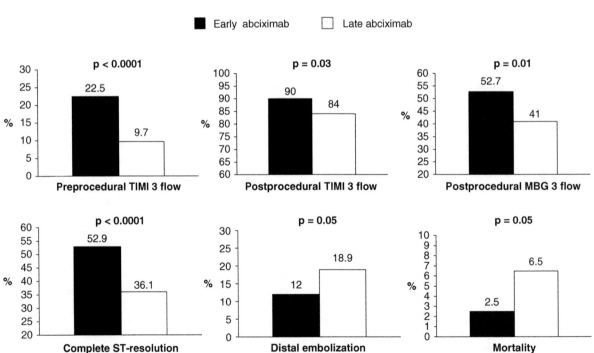

Figure 28.1 Benefits from early abciximab administration in terms of preprocedural recanalization, postprocedural epicardial and myocardial reperfusion, and mortality in the EGYPT cooperation.

PPCI, over timely fibrinolysis, is jeopardized when PCI-related delay exceeds 60–120 min, depending on age, duration of symptoms, and infarct location. Pre-hospital full-dose fibrinolysis has been tested in the CAPTIM trial (28), using an emergency medical service (EMS) able to perform pre-hospital diagnosis and fibrinolysis, with equivalent outcomes to PPCI at 30 days and 5 years. Following pre-hospital fibrinolysis, the ambulance should transport the patient to a 24 h a day/7 days a week PPCI facility. Plans for early pre-hospital administration of lytic therapy should be strongly encouraged in order to further increase the rate of very early reperfusion of myocardial infarction.

Rescue Angioplasty

Rescue PCI is defined as PCI performed to open an artery still occluded despite fibrinolytic therapy. The non-invasive identification of failed fibrinolysis remains a challenging issue, but 50% ST-segment resolution in the lead(s) with the highest ST-segment elevations 60–90 min after start of fibrinolytic therapy has increasingly been used as a surrogate. Rescue PCI has been shown to be feasible and relatively safe. In a randomized study of 427 patients (REACT), the event-free survival at 6 months after failed fibrinolysis was significantly higher with rescue PCI than with repeated administration of a fibrinolytic agent or conservative treatment. A recent meta-analysis (29), showed

that rescue PCI is associated with a significant reduction in heart failure and reinfarction and a trend towards lower all-cause mortality when compared with a conservative strategy, at the cost, however, of an increased risk of stroke and bleeding complications. Rescue PCI should be considered when there is evidence of failed fibrinolysis based on clinical signs and incomplete ST-segment resolution (50%). It is currently recommended as class IIa (Table 28.1).

Delayed Percutaneous Coronary Intervention

Patients presenting between 12 and 24 h, and possibly up to 60 h from symptom onset even if pain free and with stable hemodynamics, may still benefit from early coronary angiography and possibly PCI. Patients without ongoing chest pain or inducible ischemia, presenting between 3 and 28 days with persistent coronary artery occlusion, did not benefit from PCI. Thus, in patients presenting days after the acute event with a fully developed Q-wave MI, only patients with recurrent angina and/or documented residual ischemia and proven viability in a large myocardial territory are candidates for mechanical revascularization.

ALGORITHM

As illustrated in Figure 28.4, the preferred pathway is immediate transportation of STEMI patients to a PCI-capable centre

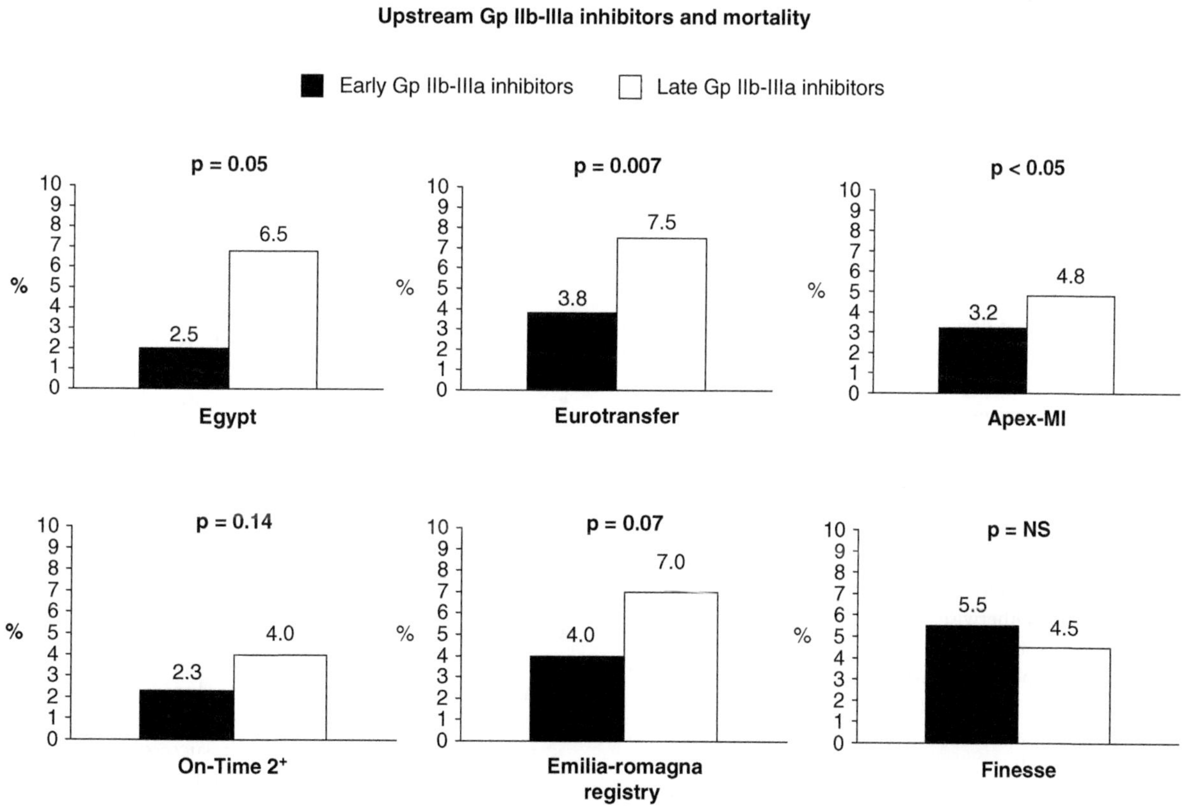

Upstream Gp IIb-IIIa inhibitors and mortality

■ Early Gp IIb-IIIa inhibitors   □ Late Gp IIb-IIIa inhibitors

Figure 28.2 Effects of early Gp IIb-IIIa inhibitors on mortality in several studies.

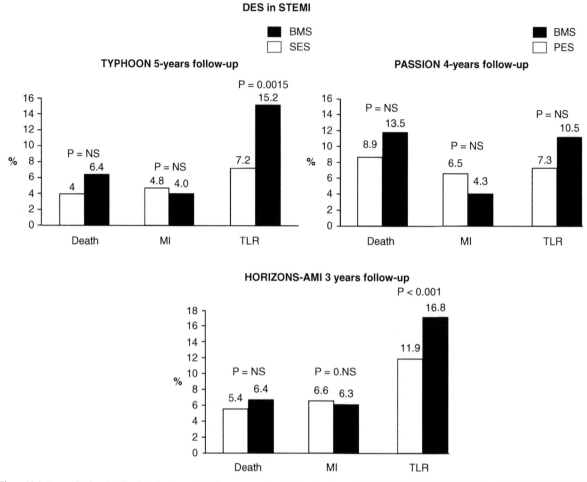

Figure 28.3 Bar graphs showing the clinical outcome of DES as compared to BMS in three large trials: TYPHOON (**A**), PASSION (**B**), and HORIZONS-AMI (**C**).

Focus Box 28.1

- Every minute of delay counts for STEMI patients treated with thrombolysis or primary angioplasty. Therefore, all the efforts should aim at early reperfusion to increase myocardial salvage and the probability of completely aborting of myocardial infarction
- Patients admitted to hospitals without PCI facilities should be transferred for primary PCI if the expected time delay between first medical contact (FMC) and balloon inflation is 2 h (<90 min in patients younger than 75 years old, with large anterior STEMI and recent onset of symptoms, <2 h). Otherwise, lytic therapy should be initiated as early as possible (also in a pre-hospital setting, where initiation of reperfusion therapy is strongly recommended) and then be transferred to a PCI-capable centre where angiography and PCI should be performed in a time window of 3–24 h
- Early, upstream optimal antithrombotic therapy (aspirin, heparin, prasugrel/ticagrelor and abciximab—especially

in high risk patients within the first 4 h) is essential in order to increase the probability of IRA recanalization and minimize the deleteriuos effects of time-delay to treatment in PPCI

- A radial approach is strongly recommended in order to minimize vascular access bleeding complications
- Optimal thrombus removal is essential to improve microvascular perfusion and reduce the risk of late stent malapposition. Manual thrombectomy should be considered in where preprocedural TIMI flow is 0–1 to favor direct stenting. Mechanical thrombectomy should be considered in where there is a case of large thrombus burden
- Postprocedural protamine (or the case of successful procedure) to promote early sheath removal and bivalirudin may be considered to further reduce major bleeding complications. Infusion of Gp IIb-IIIa inhibitors may be stopped after the procedure (if successful), especially where in case of prasugrel or ticagrelor is used

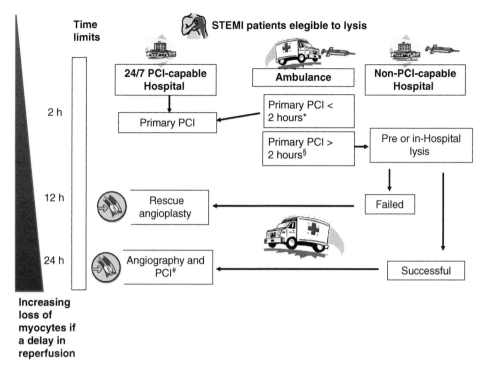

Figure 28.4 Algorithm recommended by guidelines in the treatment of STEMI patients eligible for thrombolysis. *Time from first medical contact to first balloon inflation must be shorter than 90 min in patients presenting early (<2 h after symptom onset), with a large amount of viable myocardium and a low risk of bleeding. §If PCI is not possible within 2 h from first medical contact, thrombolytic therapy should be started as soon as possible. #Not earlier than 3 h after administration of fibinolysis.

offering an uninterrupted PPCI service by a team of high-volume operators. Patients admitted to hospitals without PPCI facilities should be transferred to a PPCI-capable centre and no fibrinolytics should be administered if the expected time delay between first medical contact (FMC) and balloon inflation is 2 h. If the expected delay is longer than 2 h (or 90 min in patients younger than 75 years old, with large anterior STEMI and recent onset of symptoms, <2 h), patients admitted to a non-PPCI centre or with a diagnosis in a pre-hospital setting (where initiation of reperfusion therapy is strongly recommended) should immediately receive fibrinolysis and then be transferred to a PCI-capable centre where angiography and PCI should be performed in a time window of 3–24 h. This is essential to reduce any delay to mechanical reperfusion in case of failed lysis or early reocclusion.

PERSONAL PERSPECTIVE

Network organization is central to offering fast and optimal reperfusion treatment in the individual case. We all know now that "time is muscle". The longer the period of necrosis the higher the chances of heart failure and death. For every 30-min increment in the duration of ischemia there is an 7.5% increase in the relative risk of mortality even in case of PPCI (3). It has been shown repeatedly that early recognition of STEMI and

minimizing time delays is important for the achievement of optimal clinical results. These findings should encourage the building up of regional networks according to specific local constraints, and monitoring their effectiveness by ongoing registries. Financial, regulatory, and political barriers can be resolved and prompt, guideline-recommended care becomes feasible and affordable if stakeholders and participants agree and cooperate.

Independent of the treatment strategy, "aborting" an ongoing myocardial infarction should remain the target in the treatment of STEMI in coming decades. In patients presenting to primary PCI centers, usptream abciximab and prasugrel/ticagrelor, in addition to heparin and aspirin, should remain the key points for optimal antithrombotic therapy. In patients presenting to non-PCI centers or in ambulance, combotherapy (abciximab and half lytic therapy) should be administrated within the first 3 h from symptoms onset, with direct transportation to primary PCI centers, where, based on the success of reperfusion and risk profile, angiography may be performed soon after arrival or within 24 h. After the first 3 h from symptoms onset, the success of lytic therapy significantly decreases, therefore PPCI should be the treatment of choice (Fig. 28.5).

Radial access is our recommended approach in order to minimize the risk of bleeding complications with optimal powerful

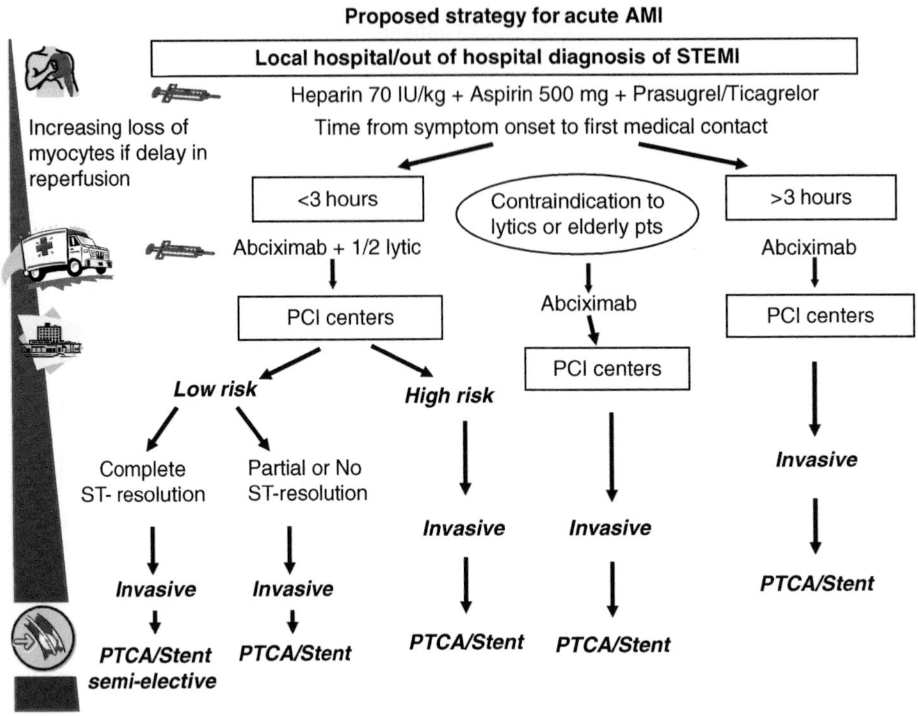

Proposed strategy for acute AMI

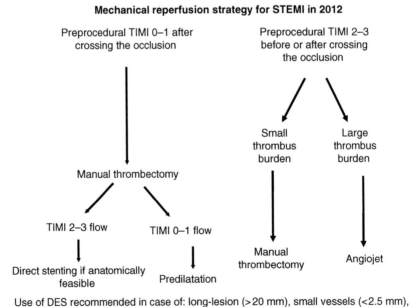

Local hospital/out of hospital diagnosis of STEMI

Heparin 70 IU/kg + Aspirin 500 mg + Prasugrel/Ticagrelor

Time from symptom onset to first medical contact

Increasing loss of myocytes if delay in reperfusion

<3 hours

Abciximab + 1/2 lytic

PCI centers

Contraindication to lytics or elderly pts

Abciximab

PCI centers

>3 hours

Abciximab

PCI centers

Low risk

Complete ST-resolution

Partial or No ST-resolution

High risk

Invasive

Invasive

Invasive

PTCA/Stent semi-elective

PTCA/Stent

PTCA/Stent

PTCA/Stent

Invasive

PTCA/Stent

Figure 28.5 Proposed algorithm for treatment of STEMI patients eligible for thrombolysis.

Mechanical reperfusion strategy for STEMI in 2012

Preprocedural TIMI 0–1 after crossing the occlusion

Preprocedural TIMI 2–3 before or after crossing the occlusion

Small thrombus burden

Large thrombus burden

Manual thrombectomy

TIMI 2–3 flow

TIMI 0–1 flow

Direct stenting if anatomically feasible

Predilatation

Manual thrombectomy

Angiojet

Use of DES recommended in case of: long-lesion (>20 mm), small vessels (<2.5 mm), diabetes, bifurcations, multivessel disease, left main, proximal LAD.

Figure 28.6 Proposed mechanical reperfusion strategy.

antiplatelet therapies. When performing PPCI (Fig. 28.6), if TIMI 0–1 is present manual thrombectomy should be used instead of balloon angioplasty in order to favor direct stenting. If thrombectomy fails, a small balloon (1.5 or 2.0 mm) should be considered with gentle predilatation to obtain recanalization. In cases with a large residual thrombus burden or cases with preprocedural TIMI 2–3 flow and instead of with large thrombus burden, mechanical thrombectomy (Angiojet) should be considered instead of manual aspiration. Direct stenting, when possible, should be the strategy of choice. The use of DES should be considered in patients at high-risk for in-stent restenosis, such as diabetic patients, small vessels (<2.5 mm), long-lesions (>20 mm), or where the area at risk is large such as the proximal LAD or left main.

In order to further reduce the risk of bleeding complications after a successful procedure (optimal myocardial perfusion without any residual dissection or thrombus), we suggest:

1. Protamine administration to reverse the effects of heparin. The safety of this approach has recently been shown (30). In fact, as learned from the HORIZONS-AMI, prolonged anticoagulation is not needed after the procedure, when optimal antiplatelet therapy is the most important factor in the prevention of stent thrombosis.
2. Discontinuation of Gp IIb-IIIa inhibitor infusion at the end of the procedure, especially among patients treated with new oral antiplatelet therapies.

REFERENCES

1. Van de Werf F, Bax J, Betriu A, et al.; ESC Committee for Practice Guidelines (CPG). Management of acute myocardial infarction in patients presenting with persistent ST-segment elevation: the Task Force on the Management of ST-Segment Elevation Acute Myocardial Infarction of the European Society of Cardiology. Eur Heart J 2008; 29: 2909–45.
2. Kushner FG, Hand M, Smith SC Jr, et al. 2009 focused updates: ACC/AHA guidelines for the management of patients with ST-elevation myocardial infarction (updating the 2004 guideline and 2007 focused update) and ACC/AHA/SCAI guidelines on percutaneous coronary intervention (updating the 2005 guideline and 2007 focused update) a report of the American College of Cardiology Foundation/American Heart Association Task Force on Practice Guidelines. J Am Coll Cardiol 2009; 54: 2205–41.
3. De Luca G, Suryapranata H, Ottervanger JP, Antman EM. Time-delay to treatment and mortality in primary angioplasty for acute myocardial infarction: every minute delay counts. Circulation 2004; 109: 1223–5.
4. Saia F, Marrozzini C, Ortolani P, et al. Optimisation of therapeutic strategies for ST-segment elevation acute myocardial infarction: the impact of a territorial network on reperfusion therapy and mortality. Heart 2009; 95: 370–6.
5. Nallamothu BK, Wang Y, Magid DJ, et al. National Registry of Myocardial Infarction Investigators. Relation between hospital specialization with primary percutaneous coronary intervention and clinical outcomes in ST-segment elevation myocardial infarction:

6. De Luca G, van't Hof AW, de Boer MJ, et al. Time-to-treatment significantly affects the extent of ST-segment resolution and myocardial blush in patients with acute myocardial infarction treated by primary angioplasty. Eur Heart J 2004; 25: 1009–13.
7. Assessment of the Safety and Efficacy of a New Treatment Strategy with Percutaneous Coronary Intervention (ASSENT-4 PCI) investigators. Primary versus tenecteplase-facilitated percutaneous coronary intervention in patients with ST-segment elevation acute myocardial infarction (ASSENT-4 PCI): randomised trial. Lancet 2006; 367: 569–78.
8. Ellis SG, Tendera M, de Belder MA, et al. FINESSE Investigators. Facilitated PCI in patients with ST-elevation myocardial infarction. N Engl J Med 2008; 358: 2205–17.
9. De Luca G, Suryapranata H, Stone GW, et al. Abciximab as adjunctive therapy to reperfusion in acute ST-segment elevation myocardial infarction: a meta-analysis of randomized trials. JAMA 2005; 293: 1759–65.
10. De Luca G, Gibson CM, Bellandi F, et al. Early glycoprotein IIb-IIIa inhibitors in primary angioplasty (EGYPT) cooperation: an individual patient data meta-analysis. Heart 2008; 94: 1548–58.
11. Silvain J, Collet JP, Nagaswami C, et al. Composition of coronary thrombus in acute myocardial infarction. J Am Coll Cardiol 2011; 57: 1359–67.
12. Task Force on Myocardial Revascularization of the European Society of Cardiology (ESC) and the European Association for Cardio-Thoracic Surgery (EACTS); European Association for Percutaneous Cardiovascular Intervention (EAPCI). Kolh P, Wijns W, Danchin N, et al. Guidelines on myocardial revascularization. Eur J Cardiothorac Surg 2010; 38(Suppl): S1–S52.
13. Angiolillo DJ, Fernandez-Ortiz A, Bernardo E, et al. Variability in individual responsiveness to clopidogrel: clinical implications, management, and future perspectives. J Am Coll Cardiol 2007; 49: 1505–16.
14. Osmancik P, Jirmar R, Hulikova K, et al. A comparison of the VASP index between patients with hemodynamically complicated and uncomplicated acute myocardial infarction. Catheter Cardiovasc Interv 2010; 75: 158–66.
15. Mehta SR, Tanguay JF, Eikelboom JW, et al.; CURRENT-OASIS 7 trial investigators. Double-dose versus standard-dose clopidogrel and high-dose versus low-dose aspirin in individuals undergoing percutaneous coronary intervention for acute coronary syndromes (CURRENT-OASIS 7): a randomised factorial trial. Lancet 2010; 376: 1233–43.
16. Montalescot G, Wiviott SD, Braunwald E, et al.; TRITON-TIMI 38 investigators. Prasugrel compared with clopidogrel in patients undergoing percutaneous coronary intervention for ST-elevation myocardial infarction (TRITON-TIMI 38): double-blind, randomised controlled trial. Lancet 2009; 373: 723–31.
17. Steg PG, James S, Harrington RA, et al. PLATO Study Group. Ticagrelor versus clopidogrel in patients with ST-elevation acute coronary syndromes intended for reperfusion with primary percutaneous coronary intervention: a Platelet Inhibition and Patient Outcomes (PLATO) trial subgroup analysis. Circulation 2010; 122: 2131–41.
18. De Luca G, Suryapranata H, Chiariello M. Prevention of distal embolization in patients undergoing mechanical revascularization for acute myocardial infarction. A review of current status. Thromb Haemost 2006; 96: 700–10.

National Registry of Myocardial Infarction-4 analysis. Circulation 2006; 113: 222–9.

19. Stone GW, Witzenbichler B, Guagliumi G, et al. HORIZONS-AMI Trial Investigators. Heparin plus a glycoprotein IIb/IIIa inhibitor versus bivalirudin monotherapy and paclitaxel-eluting stents versus bare-metal stents in acute myocardial infarction (HORIZONS-AMI): final 3-year results from a multicentre, randomised controlled trial. Lancet 2011; 377: 2193–204.

20. Navarese EP, De Luca G, Castriota F, et al. Low-molecular-weight Heparins vs. Unfractionated heparin in the setting of percutaneous coronary intervention for ST-elevation myocardial infarction: a meta-analysis. J Thromb Haemost 2011; doi: 10.1111/j.1538-7836.2011.04445.x.

21. Jolly SS, Amlani S, Hamon M, Yusuf S, Mehta SR. Radial versus femoral access for coronary angiography or intervention and the impact on major bleeding and ischemic events: a systematic review and meta-analysis of randomized trials. Am Heart J 2009; 157: 132–40.

22. Jolly SS, Yusuf S, Cairns J, et al. RIVAL trial group. Radial versus femoral access for coronary angiography and intervention in patients with acute coronary syndromes (RIVAL): a randomised, parallel group, multicentre trial. Lancet 2011; 377: 1409–20.

23. De Luca G, Verdoia M, Cassetti E. Thrombectomy during primary angioplasty: methods, devices, and clinical trial data. Curr Cardiol Rep 2010; 12: 422–8.

24. Ali A, Cox D, Dib N, et al.; AIMI Investigators. Rheolytic thrombectomy with percutaneous coronary intervention for infarct size reduction in acute myocardial infarction: 30-day results from a multicenter randomized study. J Am Coll Cardiol 2006; 48: 244–52.

25. De Luca G, Dudek D, Sardella G, et al. Adjunctive manual thrombectomy improves myocardial perfusion and mortality in patients undergoing primary percutaneous coronary intervention for ST-elevation myocardial infarction: a meta-analysis of randomized trials. Eur Heart J 2008; 29: 3002–10.

26. Vlaar PJ, Svilaas T, van der Horst IC, et al. Cardiac death and reinfarction after 1 year in the Thrombus Aspiration during Percutaneous coronary intervention in Acute myocardial infarction Study (TAPAS): a 1-year follow-up study. Lancet 2008; 371: 1915–20.

27. De Luca G, Stone GW, Suryapranata H, et al. Efficacy and safety of drug-eluting stents in ST-segment elevation myocardial infarction: a meta-analysis of randomized trials. Int J Cardiol 2009; 133: 213–22.

28. Steg PG, Bonnefoy E, Chabaud S, et al. Comparison of Angioplasty and Prehospital Thrombolysis In acute Myocardial infarction (CAPTIM) Investigators. Impact of time to treatment on mortality after prehospital fibrinolysis or primary angioplasty: data from the CAPTIM randomized clinical trial. Circulation 2003; 108: 2851–6.

29. Wijeysundera HC, Vijayaraghavan R, Nallamothu BK, et al. Rescue angioplasty or repeat fibrinolysis after failed fibrinolytic therapy for ST-segment myocardial infarction: a meta-analysis of randomized trials. J Am Coll Cardiol 2007; 49: 422–30.

30. Parodi G, De Luca G, Moschi G, et al. Safety of immediate reversal of anticoagulation by protamine to reduce bleeding complications after infarct artery stenting for acute myocardial infarction and adjunctive abciximab therapy. J Thromb Thrombolysis 2010; 30: 446–51.

29   Management of microvascular angina

Juan Carlos Kaski and Peter Ong

OUTLINE

Impaired vasodilation and/or inappropriate vasoconstriction of the coronary microcirculation (i.e. microvascular spasm) can lead to myocardial ischemia and angina (microvascular angina) in patients with normal coronary angiograms. Invasive and non-invasive investigations have documented the occurrence of myocardial ischemia in the absence of epicardial coronary disease in some patients. Myocardial scintigraphy, cardiac MRI perfusion, positron emission tomography, and transthoracic Doppler echocardiography have all been used with characterize blood flow responses in patients with microvascular angina. Microvascular angina is often associated with endothelial dysfunction in the coronary microcirculation caused by traditional cardiovascular risk factors, estrogen deficiency (in women) and chronic inflammation and oxidative stress. Treatment of this condition should aim at improving symptoms (e.g. by the administration of calcium channel blockers or nitrates) and ameliorating endothelial function with the use of ACE-inhibitors and statins. This chapter focuses on the management of microvascular angina in patients without obstructive epicardial coronary artery disease (CAD) or myocardial diseases (Fig. 29.1). Dysfunction of the coronary microvessels (diameter <200 µm, Fig. 29.2) can cause microvascular angina (1). Microvascular dysfunction can occur in patients with stable angina and also in those with acute coronary syndrome.

INTRODUCTION—DEFINITIONS

The widespread use of diagnostic coronary angiography in recent years has shown that a large proportion of patients with typical exertional chest pain have angiographically normal coronary arteries or non-obstructive CAD (2). The presence of normal or near-normal coronary arteriograms often leads the physician to exclude a cardiac cause for the chest pain. However, angina pectoris despite normal coronary angiograms occurs frequently in patients with microvascular dysfunction. Several studies have shown that abnormal coronary microvascular vasodilatory and/or increased coronary vasoconstrictor function (due to endothelial and/or vascular smooth muscle dysfunction) can lead to myocardial ischemia and angina in patients without atherosclerotic coronary artery obstruction (3,4).

The term "microvascular angina" was first used by Cannon et al. in 1988 (4). In a landmark study (5) they showed that in patients without epicardial CAD, angina could be caused by a reduced vasodilator reserve of the small coronary arteries.

Although initially patients with cardiovascular risk factors were excluded from the diagnosis "microvascular angina," it became apparent that traditional cardiovascular risk factors for CAD can affect the coronary microcirculation leading to microvascular dysfunction (6,7). The following features define microvascular angina (8):

- Typical stable angina, exclusively or predominantly induced by effort
- Findings compatible with myocardial ischemia/CMVD on diagnostic investigation
- Completely normal or near normal (<20% diameter reduction) coronary arteries on angiography
- Absence of any other specific cardiac disease (e.g., variant angina, cardiomyopathy, valvular disease)

More recently, it has been recognized that patients with coronary microvascular dysfunction can also present with symptoms compatible with acute coronary syndrome in the absence of epicardial coronary artery obstruction. The following classification according to the clinical presentation has been proposed (2):

- Stable primary microvascular angina
- Unstable primary microvascular angina

We will focus on the management of stable primary microvascular angina in this chapter.

EVALUATION OF THE CORONARY MICROVASCULATURE FOR THE ASSESSMENT OF MICROVASCULAR ANGINA

Currently, no technique allows direct visualization of the coronary microcirculation in vivo in humans. Invasive and non-invasive techniques have been applied to indirectly gain information about the structural and functional status of the coronary microcirculation. Among the invasive techniques, the intracoronary Doppler wire, which measures blood flow ultrasonographically according to the Doppler principle, is commonly used to study the function of the microcirculation. CFR is determined by comparing coronary blood flow at rest (basal flow) and following maximal hyperemia, that is, intracoronary or intravenous infusion of adenosine, intravenous dipyridamole as well as intracoronary infusion of acetylcholine (7,9). In this setting, adenosine and dipyridamole are used as endothelium-independent vasodilators, whereas acetylcholine is used to assess endothelium-dependent vasodilation. Coronary flow reserve (CFR) is expressed as the ratio of blood flow during hyperemia to blood flow at rest. Since flow resistance is primarily determined by the microvasculature, CFR in patients without epicardial coronary disease is a marker of microvascular dysfunction (9). A CFR of less than 2.0 is often considered abnormal. In healthy persons, however, CFR varies

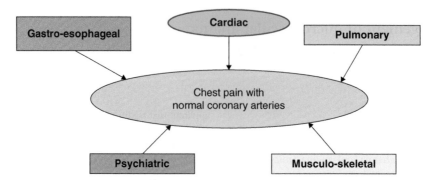

Figure 29.1 Mechanism for chest pain in patients with normal coronary arteries.

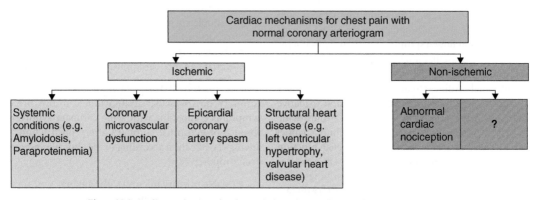

Figure 29.2 Cardiac mechanisms for chest pain in patients with normal coronary arteriogram.

according to age and sex. Therefore, it is essential to compare data on CFR in patients with data obtained in age-matched and sex-matched control subjects.

Reis et al. (10) assessed coronary microvascular function with intracoronary Doppler measurements in 159 women with typical chest pain and unobstructed coronary arteries. Coronary flow velocity reserve (coronary velocity response to intracoronary adenosine) suggestive of microvascular dysfunction was found in as many as 47% of patients. Moreover, Egashira et al. (11) assessed changes in coronary blood flow in response to intracoronary acetylcholine using intracoronary Doppler measurements. Patients with angina despite normal coronary angiograms showed significantly less increase in acetylcholine-induced coronary blood flow compared to controls. Thus, endothelium-dependent dilatation of the resistance coronary arteries is defective in patients with anginal chest pain and normal coronary arteries, and may contribute to the altered regulation of myocardial perfusion in these patients.

Apart from assessing impaired vasodilation, acetylcholine can also be useful to assess whether excessive microvascular constriction can contribute to the pathogenesis of angina in patients with normal coronary angiograms. A recent study from our group showed that among 39 patients with typical angina, positive response to exercise stress testing and normal coronary arteries on angiography, 56% showed reproduction of angina and ischemic ST-shifts in response to ascending doses of intracoronary acetylcholine suggesting that inappropriate microvascular constriction could play a part in the pathogenesis of microvascular angina (illustrative case 1). Structural insights into the microcirculation have been gained by studies performing endomyocardial biopsy in patients with microvascular angina. Apart from arteriolar obliteration and capillary rarefaction as shown by Escaned et al. (Fig. 29.3, Fig. 29.4, (12)), Chimenti et al. (13) found that viral inflammation can frequently be detected in microvascular angina patients, especially those with refractory angina.

Non-invasive techniques have aimed at identifying myocardial ischemia or coronary blood flow abnormalities in patients with microvascular angina. Camici et al. (14) showed that, in patients with chest pain and normal coronary arteries, coronary vasodilator reserve in response to dipyridamole, as assessed with 13N-labeled ammonia and positron emission tomography, was impaired in approximately one third of patients. Panting et al. (15) showed that subendocardial hypoperfusion during intravenous administration of adenosine on perfusion cardiovascular magnetic resonance imaging in

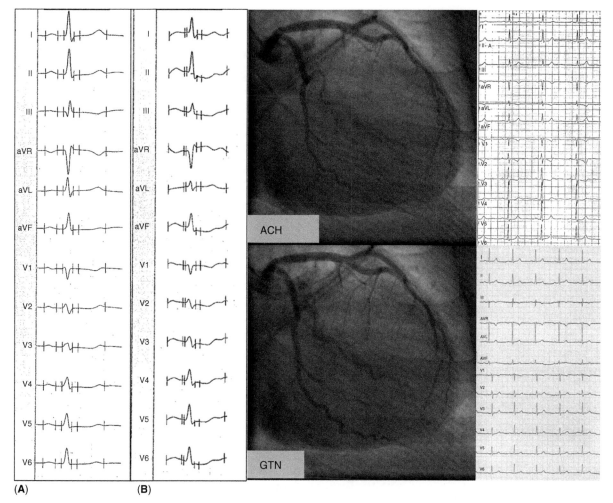

ILLUSTRATIVE CASE 1. A 56-year-old female patient with effort-induced angina and normal 12-lead resting ECG (A). Exercise stress testing showed significant (≥0.1 mV) ST-segment depression (leads II, III, aVF, V3-V6) associated with reproduction of angina at 100 W (B). Coronary angiography revealed no epicardial CAD. Intracoronary acetylcholine administration (ACH) elicited the patient's typical anginal pain with ischemic ECG changes but without significant epicardial diameter reduction at 100 μg ACH indicative of coronary microvascular spasm (*upper right panel*). The symptoms and ECG changes were relieved by glyceryltrinitrate administration (GTN) (*lower right panel*).

patients with microvascular angina was almost always associated with intense chest pain supporting the notion that the chest pain may have an ischemic cause (illustrative case 2). Moreover, Galiuto et al. showed that transthoracic Doppler echocardiography using a dedicated probe can reliably measure CFR in response to adenosine in the LAD territory, which was significantly impaired in microvascular angina patients compared to controls (16). This method has also been shown to correlate with cardiac MRI stress perfusion results in patients with microvascular angina (17). Although these methods have been widely applied to the study of the coronary microcirculation, it should be noted that their sensitivity is limited, as affected areas of microvascular dysfunction can be patchily distributed, thus leading to inconspicuous test results (18).

PATIENT MANAGEMENT (CURRENT STATUS)

Coronary microvascular dysfunction in the absence of obstructive CAD is often the functional counterpart of traditional coronary risk factors (7). Since this type of dysfunction is at least partly reversible, its assessment should be used to guide interventions aimed at both reducing the burden of risk factors and dilating the coronary tree. Apart from traditional cardiovascular risk factors (e.g. smoking, hypercholesterolemia, diabetes, hypertension) life style factors such as obesity have been shown to be associated with microvascular dysfunction (Table 29.1) (19). Furthermore, increased adrenergic activity or abnormal cardiac adrenergic innervation has been shown to be the mechanism for microvascular angina in at least a proportion of patients (20). Microvascular angina in

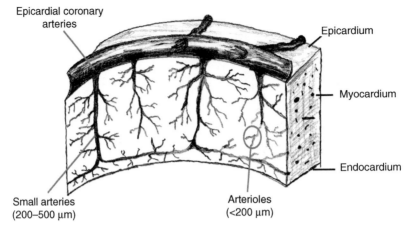

Figure 29.3 Sketch of the coronary vasculature.

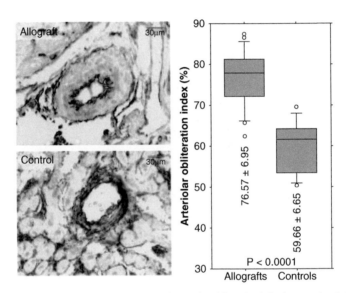

Figure 29.4 Histological examples of myocardial arterioles and box plots of arteriolar obliteration index in control and allograft endomyocardial biopsies. *Source*: From Ref. 12.

Table 29.1 Causes for Coronary Microvascular Dysfunction

Hypercholesterolemia
Smoking
Diabetes mellitus
Hypertension
Obesity
Estrogen deficiency (women)
Chronic systemic inflammatory disorders (e.g. rheumatoid arthritis)
Abnormal cardiac adrenergic innervation

women can be associated with estrogen deficiency (21) and this may represent an explanation for the increased prevalence of cardiac syndrome X or microvascular angina in postmenopausal women.

In addition, chronic systemic inflammation such as that occurs in patients with rheumatoid arthritis can result in microvascular angina, even in the absence of traditional cardiovascular risk factors (22). Understanding the mechanisms underlying microvascular dysfunction may help in identifying appropriate therapy. Management of microvascular angina should be tailored to the individual patient based on their underlying pathophysiology, preference for pharmacotherapy, symptomatology, and motivation to participate in non-pharmacologic programs. A comprehensive treatment approach aimed at risk factor management, including lifestyle counselling regarding smoking cessation, nutrition, and physical activity, has a pivotal role in the management of microvascular angina and should be pursued as the primary therapeutic goal.

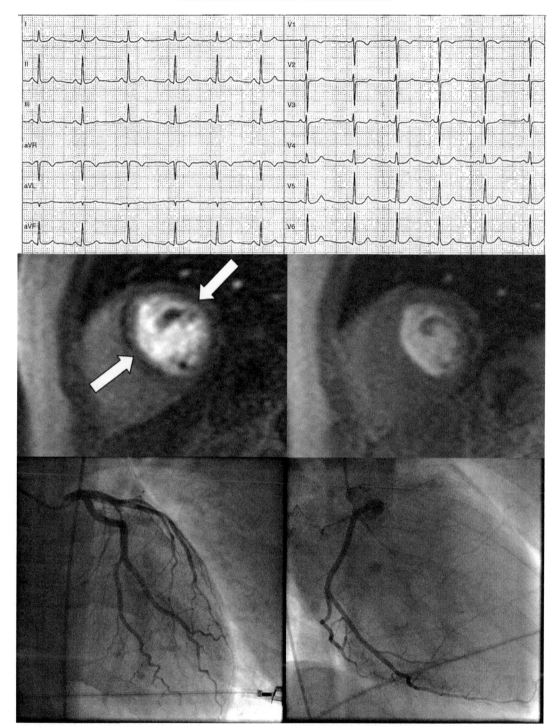

ILLUSTRATIVE CASE 2. A 42-year-old female patient with typical exertional angina and normal resting ECG. Coronary angiography demonstrated no obstructive epicardial coronary disease but perfusion CMR revealed circular subendocardial hypoperfusion suggestive of microvascular coronary dysfunction (*white arrows*).

Table 29.2 Treatment Approaches for Microvascular Angina

Drug	Mechanism of action
Calcium channel blockers (e.g. diltiazem)	Prevention of vasoconstriction, relaxation of vascular smooth muscle
ß-blockers (e.g. atenolol)	Reduction of alpha adrenergic overload, increase of nitric oxide bioavailability (e.g. nebivolol)
Nitrates	Vasodilation
ACE-inhibitor (e.g. ramipril)	Improvement of endothelial dysfunction via angiotensin II blockage and reduction of oxidative stress
Statins (e.g. simvastatin)	Improvement of endothelial dysfunction via reduction cholesterol burden and of inflammatory responses
Nicorandil	Adenosine triphosphate (ATP) sensitive potassium channel opener → dilation of coronary resistance vessels

Focus Box 29.1

1. Microvascular angina can result from functional (impaired dilatation and/or enhanced constriction) and structural abnormalities (e.g. vascular smooth muscle hypertrophy) of the coronary microcirculation (3,4)
2. The prevalence of microvascular dysfunction is relatively high among subjects with chest pain and angiographically normal coronary arteries (49)
3. Traditional cardiovascular risk factors, obesity, chronic inflammation and (in women) estrogen deficiency are among the main causes for coronary microvascular dysfunction (6)
4. Cardiac MRI stress perfusion imaging is a powerful clinical tool to detect transient hypoperfusion (= ischemia) in patients with microvascular angina (15)

Tyni-Lenne, for example, showed that physical activity can significantly improve exercise capacity and quality of life in microvascular angina patients Table 29.2 (23).

Current pharmacotherapy for microvascular angina should include treatment of microvascular (endothelial) dysfunction with statins, angiotensin-converting enzyme (ACE) inhibitors, as well as treatment for angina and myocardial ischemia with β-blockers, calcium channel blockers, or nitrates. Additional pain management techniques may include analgesic therapy with pharmacological agents or spinal cord stimulation (24).

ACE-inhibitors have been shown to have beneficial effects in microvascular angina. In well-characterized patients with microvascular angina, a randomized placebo-controlled trial from our group (25) showed improvement of total exercise duration and time to 1 mm of ST segment depression in patients taking enalapril compared to those on placebo. In addition, Chen et al. (26) showed that long-term ACE-inhibitor treatment with enalapril improved coronary microvascular function as well as myocardial ischemia in patients with microvascular angina. This may be related to the improvement of endothelial nitric oxide bioavailability with the reduction of plasma asymmetric dimethylarginine levels.

HMG-CoA reductase inhibitors (statins) have also shown to be effective for treatment of microvascular angina. Kayikcioglu et al. (27), in a single-blind, randomized, placebo-controlled trial with microvascular angina patients, showed that 3 months treatment with pravastatin (40 mg/d) significantly improved brachial artery flow-mediated dilatation as well as exercise duration, and time to 1-mm ST depression on exercise stress testing, compared to placebo. These findings were reproduced in another study by Fabian et al. using 20 mg of simvastatin daily (28). Moreover, Pizzi et al. (29) demonstrated that six months of therapy with atorvastatin and ramipril improved endothelial function and quality of life in patients with microvascular angina.

Calcium channel blockers have also been shown to be effective in a proportion of patients with microvascular angina. Long-term follow-up observational studies have reported beneficial effects of calcium channel antagonists on chest pain in 31% of patients when given as single agents, and 42% when administered in combination with oral nitrates (30). Two randomized placebo controlled trials have assessed the effect of these agents in patients with chest pain and normal or nearly normal coronary arteries. Cannon et al. (31) reported a reduction in the number of episodes of angina and the consumption of nitroglycerine tablets, as well as an improvement in the exercise capacity of 26 patients with chest pain and reduced coronary vasodilator reserve. Bugiardini et al. (32), however, failed to demonstrate a reduction in the number of episodes of ST segment depression during continuous 48-h electrocardiographic monitoring in 16 patients who fulfilled strict criteria for the diagnosis of microvascular angina and received treatment with verapamil. Differences in patient selection and study design may account for the disparate findings in these small studies.

Controversy exists as to the role of nitrates in the management of microvascular angina patients and there are no large randomized studies on the effects of nitrates in patients with microvascular angina. Although studies in microvascular angina patients failed to show a beneficial effect on time to 1-mm ST segment depression and exercise duration upon exercise stress testing after the administration of nitrates compared to baseline (33,34), observational studies have suggested that nitrates are effective in approximately 40–50% of patients with typical chest pain and normal coronary arteriograms (31,35). The efficacy of oral nitrates for the long-term treatment of microvascular angina patients is perhaps more debatable and large, well-designed studies are necessary to clarify the issue. In our experience, a sizeable proportion of patients respond well to oral nitrates and we therefore prescribe these agents to selected patients with microvascular angina, in particular, to patients who show excellent responses to sublingual nitrates.

β-blockers have also proven useful in subsets of patients with microvascular angina (36), especially those with abnormal cardiac adrenergic innervation, as shown by Romeo et al. (37). In their study, verapamil had a beneficial effect on both exercise tolerance and exercise duration, whilst acebutolol was beneficial exclusively in the patient subgroup showing higher pressure–rate responses to exercise. It appears that patients with increased sympathetic activity and those with typical tachycardia-related chest pain are the ones who benefit the most. More recently, it has been shown that β-blockers with NO-releasing properties such as nebivolol might be particularly effective in microvascular angina patients (38). Sen et al. assessed the effects of 12 weeks of treatment with nebivolol (5 mg/d) compared to metoprolol (50 mg/d) in two equally sized microvascular angina patient groups (total $n = 38$). They demonstrated that after 12 weeks of drug therapy, patients taking nebivolol showed improvement of plasma nitric oxide levels and other circulating endothelial function parameters compared to those of patients taking metoprolol. In addition, exercise duration to 1-mm ST depression and total exercise duration significantly increased after treatment in the nebivolol group compared to the metoprolol group.

Nicorandil, an adenosine triphosphate (ATP) sensitive potassium channel opener which also has nitrate-like effects has been shown in humans to dilate coronary resistance vessels and modulate the vasomotor responses of these vessels to sympathetic stimulation (39). Subsequently, in a randomized placebo-controlled trial in patients with microvascular angina, Chen et al. (40) showed that 2-weeks of oral treatment with nicorandil improved both time to 1-mm of ST segment depression and peak exercise capacity, but failed to significantly improve the magnitude and the incidence of exercise-induced ST segment changes. Therefore, we would recommend nicorandil only in cases where symptoms and ischemia cannot be controlled with other drugs, until more compelling evidence regarding nicorandil is available for treatment of microvascular angina patients.

In women with estrogen deficiency, hormone replacement therapy can be a therapeutic option (41) but this has to be balanced against any potential deleterious effects of estrogen. A recent study by Xiao et al. (42) showed that long-term hormone replacement with 17β-estradiol and progesterone led to marked reduction in vascular tone of arterial resistance vessels underpinning the vasoprotective character of steroid hormones. Nevertheless, hormone replacement therapy should only be initiated after consultation with a gynecologist to evaluate the individual pros and cons as well as side effects of such treatment.

Patients with chronic systemic inflammatory conditions who may develop microvascular angina even in the absence of any cardiovascular risk factors (22) should be considered for treatment with calcium channel blockers, nitrates, statins and ACE-inhibitors, besides standard therapy according to their condition, to improve symptoms and microvascular dysfunction.

Patients with refractory angina unresponsive to conventional drug treatment might benefit from analgesic therapy. This can be achieved through administration of tricyclic antidepressants (e.g. imipramine) (43). Furthermore, spinal cord stimulation via implantation of neurostimulators which is performed in some specialized centres has shown beneficial effects in a number of patients (44). Symptomatic relief of chest pain and improvement of quality of life are achieved through inhibition of sympathetic pain afferences (45).

A novel therapeutic approach suggested for these patients is the use of endothelin-1 antagonists (e.g. atrasentan) to restore the vascular homeostasis between nitric oxide and endothelin-1 which is often shifted toward higher concentrations of the potent vasoconstrictor endothelin-1 (46). In a recent randomized clinical trial, Reriani et al. (47) studied 47 patients without CAD but with coronary microvascular dysfunction. Their study showed that a 6-month treatment with atrasentan significantly improved coronary microvascular dysfunction. Compared to the placebo, atrasentan treatment led to significant improvement in acetylcholine-induced coronary blood flow.

PERSONAL PERSPECTIVE

Microvascular angina due to coronary microvascular dysfunction represents a frequent cause of chest pain in patients with angiographically normal coronary arteries. As such, physicians should consider microvascular angina as a differential diagnosis (48). Routine assessment of coronary microvascular abnormal dilatation and spasm and thorough characterization of its underlying mechanisms is mandatory to initiate appropriate treatment and reassure the patient. Given the substantial number of patients who are unresponsive to conventional treatment, new tailored therapeutic approaches should be evaluated in carefully selected patient groups. In this context the recent evaluation of endothelin-1 receptor antagonists has shown promising results (47). However, more studies are needed to assess the efficacy of this new drug class in microvascular angina patients.

Rational management of this condition should include risk factor control, exercise, pain management, vasodilator agents, and lifestyle modification. Finally, future technical advances should overcome the difficulties posed by the assessment of the coronary microvasculature and enable visualization of the coronary microcirculation. This would surely lead to a better understanding of the disease and the development of patient-specific treatments.

REFERENCES

1. Lanza GA, Crea F. Primary coronary microvascular dysfunction: clinical presentation, pathophysiology, and management. Circulation 2010; 121: 2317–25.
2. Patel MR, Peterson ED, Dai D, et al. Low diagnostic yield of elective coronary angiography. N Engl J Med 2010; 362: 886–95.
3. Cannon RO III, Epstein SE. "Microvascular angina" as a cause of chest pain with angiographically normal coronary arteries. Am J Cardiol 1988; 61: 1338–43.

4. Crea F, Lanza GA. Angina pectoris and normal coronary arteries: cardiac syndrome X. Heart 2004; 90: 457–63.

5. Cannon RO, Watson RM, Rosing DR, Epstein SE. Angina caused by reduced vasodilator reserve of the small coronary arteries. J Am Coll Cardiol 1983; 1: 1359–73.

6. Camici PG, Crea F. Coronary microvascular dysfunction. N Engl J Med 2007; 356: 830–40.

7. Rubinshtein R, Yang EH, Rihal CS, et al. Coronary microcirculatory vasodilator function in relation to risk factors among patients without obstructive coronary disease and low to intermediate Framingham score. Eur Heart J 2010; 31: 936–42.

8. Lanza GA. Cardiac syndrome X: a critical overview and future perspectives. Heart 2007; 93: 159–66.

9. Kaufmann PA, Camici PG. Myocardial blood flow by PET: technical aspects and clinical applications. J Nucl Med 2005; 46: 75–88.

10. Reis SE, Holubkov R, Conrad Smith AJ, WISE Investigators. Coronary microvascular dysfunction is highly prevalent in women with chest pain in the absence of coronary artery disease: results from the NHLBI WISE study. Am Heart J 2001 141: 735–41.

11. Egashira K, Inou T, Hirooka Y, et al. Evidence of impaired endothelium-dependent coronary vasodilatation in patients with angina pectoris and normal coronary angiograms. N Engl J Med 1993; 328: 1659–64.

12. Escaned J, Flores A, García-Pavía P, et al. Assessment of microcirculatory remodeling with intracoronary flow velocity and pressure measurements: validation with endomyocardial sampling in cardiac allografts. Circulation 2009; 120: 1561–8.

13. Chimenti C, Sale P, Verardo R, et al. High prevalence of intramural coronary infection in patients with drug-resistant cardiac syndrome X: comparison with chronic stable angina and normal controls. Heart 2010; 96: 1926–31.

14. Camici PG, Gistri R, Lorenzoni R, et al. Coronary reserve and exercise ECG in patients with chest pain and normal coronary angiograms. Circulation 1992; 86: 179–86.

15. Panting JR, Gatehouse PD, Yang GZ, et al. Abnormal subendocardial perfusion in cardiac syndrome X detected by cardiovascular magnetic resonance imaging. N Engl J Med 2002; 346: 1948–53.

16. Galiuto L, Sestito A, Barchetta S, et al. Noninvasive evaluation of flow reserve in the left anterior descending coronary artery in patients with cardiac syndrome X. Am J Cardiol 2007; 99: 1378–83.

17. Lanza GA, Buffon A, Sestito A, et al. Relation between stress-induced myocardial perfusion defects on cardiovascular magnetic resonance and coronary microvascular dysfunction in patients with cardiac syndrome X. J Am Coll Cardiol 2008; 51: 466–72.

18. Maseri A, Crea F, Kaski JC, Crake T. Mechanisms of angina pectoris in syndrome X. J Am Coll Cardiol 1991; 17: 499–506.

19. Knudson JD, Dincer UD, Bratz IN, et al. Mechanisms of coronary dysfunction in obesity and insulin resistance. Microcirculation 2007; 14: 317–38.

20. Lanza GA, Giordano A, Pristipino C, et al. Abnormal cardiac adrenergic nerve function in patients with syndrome X detected by [123I]metaiodobenzylguanidine myocardial scintigraphy. Circulation 1997; 96: 821–6.

21. Rosano GM, Collins P, Kaski JC, et al. Syndrome X in women is associated with oestrogen deficiency. Eur Heart J 1995; 16: 610–14.

22. Recio-Mayoral A, Mason JC, Kaski JC, et al. Chronic inflammation and coronary microvascular dysfunction in patients without risk factors for coronary artery disease. Eur Heart J 2009; 30: 1837–43.

23. Tyni-Lenne R, Stryjan S, Eriksson B, Col Y. Beneficial therapeutic effects of physical training and relaxation therapy in women with coronary syndrome X. Physiother Res Int 2002; 7:35–43.

24. Kaski JC, Valenzuela Garcia LF. Therapeutic options for the management of patients with cardiac syndrome X. Eur Heart J 2001; 22: 283–93.

25. Kaski JC, Rosano G, Gavrielides S, Chen L. Effects of angiotensin-converting enzyme inhibition on exercise-induced angina and ST segment depression in patients with microvascular angina. J Am Coll Cardiol 1994; 23: 652–7.

26. Chen JW, Hsu NW, Wu TC, et al. Long-term angiotensin-converting enzyme inhibition reduces plasma asymmetric dimethylarginine and improves endothelial nitric oxide bioavailability and coronary microvascular function in patients with syndrome X. Am J Cardiol 2002; 90: 974–82.

27. Kayikcioglu M, Payzin S, et al. Benefits of statin treatment in cardiac syndrome X. Eur Heart J 2003; 24: 1999–2005.

28. Fábián E, Varga A, Picano E, et al. Effect of simvastatin on endothelial function in cardiac syndrome X patients. Am J Cardiol 2004; 94: 652–5.

29. Pizzi C, Manfrini O, Fontana F, Bugiardini R. Angiotensin-converting enzyme inhibitors and 3-hydroxy-3-methylglutaryl coenzyme A reductase in cardiac Syndrome X: role of superoxide dismutase activity. Circulation 2004; 109: 53–8.

30. Kaski JC, Rosano GM, Collins P, et al. Cardiac syndrome X: clinical characteristics and left ventricular function. Long-term follow-up study. J Am Coll Cardiol 1995; 25: 807–14.

31. Cannon R, Watson RM, Rosing DR, Epstein SE. Efficacy of calcium channel blocker therapy for angina pectoris resulting from small-vessel coronary artery disease and abnormal vasodilator reserve. Am J Cardiol 1985; 56: 242–6.

32. Bugiardini R, Borghi A, Biagetti L, Puddu P. Comparison of verapamil versus propanolol therapy in Syndrome X. Am J Cardiol 1989; 63: 286–90.

33. Radice M, Giudici V, Albertini A, Mannarini A. Usefulness of changes in exercise tolerance induced by nitroglycerin in identifying patients with syndrome X. Am Heart J 1994; 127: 531–5.

34. Lanza GA, Manzoli A, Bia E, Crea F, Maseri A. Acute effects of nitrates on exercise testing in patients with syndrome X. Circulation 1994; 90: 2695–700.

35. Kemp HG, Vokonas PS, Cohn PF, Gorlin R. The anginal syndrome associated with normal coronary angiograms. Am J Med 1973; 54: 735–42.

36. Lanza GA, Colonna G, Pasceri V, et al. Atenolol versus amlodipine versus isosorbide-5-mononitrate on anginal symptoms in syndrome X. Am J Cardiol 1999; 84: 854–6.

37. Romeo F, Gaspardone A, Ciavolella M, Gioffre P, Reale A. Verapamil versus acebutolol for syndrome X. Am J Cardiol 1988; 62: 312–13.

38. Sen N, Tavil Y, Erdamar H, et al. Nebivolol therapy improves endothelial function and increases exercise tolerance in patients with cardiac syndrome X. Anadolu Kardiyol Derg 2009; 9: 371–9.

39. Hongo M, Tanenaka H, Uchikawa S, et al. Coronary microvascular response to intracoronary administration of nicorandil. Am J Cardiol 1995; 75: 246–50.

40. Chen JW, Lee WL, Hsu NW, et al. Effect of short-term treatment of nicorandil on exercise-induced myocardial ischemia and abnormal cardiac autonomic activity in microvascular angina. Am J Cardiol 1997; 80: 32–8.

41. Rosano GM, Peters NS, Lefroy D, et al. 17-beta-Estradiol therapy lessens angina in postmenopausal women with syndrome X. J Am Coll Cardiol 1996; 28: 1500–5.

42. Xiao D, Huang X, Yang S, Zhang L. Direct chronic effect of steroid hormones in attenuating uterine arterial myogenic tone: role of protein kinase c/extracellular signal-regulated kinase 1/2. Hypertension 2009; 54: 352–8.

43. Cox I, Hann C, Kaski JC. Low dose imipramine improves chest pain but not quality of life in patients with angina and normal coronary angiograms. Eur Heart J 1998; 19: 250–4.

44. Sestito A, Lanza GA, Le Pera D, et al. Spinal cord stimulation normalizes abnormal cortical pain processing in patients with cardiac syndrome X. Pain 2008; 139: 82–9.

45. Sgueglia GA, Sestito A, Spinelli A, et al. Long-term follow-up of patients with cardiac syndrome X treated by spinal cord stimulation. Heart 2007; 93: 591–7.

46. Cox ID, Bøtker HE, Bagger JP, et al. Elevated endothelin concentrations are associated with reduced coronary vasomotor responses in patients with chest pain and normal coronary arteriograms. J Am Coll Cardiol 1999; 34: 455–60.

47. Reriani M, Raichlin E, Prasad A, et al. Long-term administration of endothelin receptor antagonist improves coronary endothelial function in patients with early atherosclerosis. Circulation 2010; 122: 958–66.

48. Kaski JC. Pathophysiology and management of patients with chest pain and normal coronary arteriograms (cardiac syndrome X). Circulation. 2004; 109: 568–72.

49. Ong P, Athanasiadis A, Borgulya G, et al. High prevalence of a pathological response to acetylcholine testing in patients with stable angina pectoris and unobstructed coronary arteries the ACOVA Study (Abnormal COronary VAsomotion in patients with stable angina and unobstructed coronary arteries). J Am Coll Cardiol. 2012; 59: 655–62.

30 Treatment algorithm in patients with concomitant heart valve disease
Vassilis Voudris and Panagiota Georgiadou

OUTLINE

The incidence of combined coronary and valvular heart disease is increasing as the general population ages. Overall, 40% of patients with valvular heart disease will have concomitant coronary artery disease (CAD) with the combination of calcific aortic stenosis and CAD the most frequently encountered combination. Yet, data regarding optimal strategies for diagnosis and treatment of CAD in such patients are limited. Coronary angiography is recommended in all patients with a primary indication for valve surgery, apart from young patients (men younger than 40 years and pre-menopausal women) with no risk factors for CAD or when the risks of angiography outweigh the benefits. Coronary artery bypass grafting (CABG) should be performed in patients with a primary indication for heart valve surgery for all coronary arteries with stenosis above 70%. Mitral valve surgery is indicated in patients with a primary indication for CABG and severe ischemic mitral regurgitation. Recently published guidelines on combined valve surgery and CABG highlight out the increased mortality risk of a single combined operation. This observation, in conjunction with the higher risk profile of patients currently referred for surgery, has provoked discussion regarding the optimal therapeutic approach in patients with dual pathology. Alternative treatment strategies include "hybrid" percutaneous coronary intervention procedures with scheduled surgery for valve replacement or transcatheter aortic valve implantation with prior percutaneous coronary intervention. At present, however, the data on hybrid procedures are very limited and further studies are warranted to establish the clinical utility of these approaches.

INTRODUCTION

Although valvular heart disease (VHD) is less common than coronary artery disease (CAD), the combination of both pathologies is a frequently encountered problem, which is of great interest for several reasons. First, there is significant overlap between the pathogenesis of atherosclerotic disease of the coronary arteries and the VHD (1). Second, a remarkable evolution has occurred in epidemiology, presentation, and treatment of VHD in recent years. Third, there is limited data avilable for the optimal treatment algorithm and CAD outcomes in such patients (2). Patients with CAD and moderate to severe VHD is an important subgroup which is usually under-represented or even excluded from clinical trials. Management decisions are based on available information that is provided by small randomized studies or registries of CAD treatment, by retrospective, and from comparative evaluations of patients undergoing cardiac surgery for VHD (3,4). Current consensus guidelines raise important questions regarding diagnostic pathways and appropriate management of concomitant CAD and VHD, highlighting the significance of the current gap between existing guidelines and their effective application, and creating issues for future research endeavors.

This chapter summarizes the management of ischemic heart disease in patients with VHD. The discussion focuses on the management of aortic and mitral valve disease, since most frequently these are the valves that get affected in adults. The complex interaction between ventricular function, valvular function, and coronary ischemia requires a good understanding of the pathophysiology, an accurate estimation of the risk and reasonable expectations of the achievable results in order to develop a rational approach and manage these entities successfully.

FREQUENCY AND DIAGNOSIS OF CORONARY ARTERY DISEASE IN PATIENTS WITH VALVULAR HEART DISEASE

The incidence of CAD in patients with VHD can be estimated on the basis of age, gender, and clinical risk factors and should be managed, from the medical viewpoint, in the same way that is recommended for the general population. The Euro Heart Survey programme on VHD confirmed the presence of CAD in 39.4% of the total population: 1-vessel disease in 13.9%, 2-vessel disease in 11.5%, 3-vessel disease in 12.8%, and left main disease in 1.2% (2). The presence of angina alone is a less specific indicator of significant coronary disease in patients with VHD than in The general population. Ischemic symptoms in patients with VHD may have other causes such as left ventricular (LV) chamber enlargement, increased wall stress or wall thickening with subendocardial ischemia and right ventricular hypertrophy (3).

There is a high prevalence of CAD in adults with aortic stenosis (AS), as about 40% of patients undergoing aortic valve (AV) replacement require coronary artery bypass grafting (CABG), (2). The reason for this high prevalence is the presence of common risk factors between these two diseases such as age and gender distribution. Among patients with severe AS, angina has low positive and high negative predictive value for CAD because angina can be induced by AS per se (5). Of the patients with angina pectoris and AS, 40–50% have obstructive CAD while only 20% of patients without chest pain have obstructive CAD. Aortic regurgitation (AR) is less often encountered with CAD because it occurs more frequently in younger populations. Significant CAD is present in 15% to 30% of patients with AR and approximately half of them have typical angina (3).

The coexistence of CAD and mitral stenosis (MS) (an average of 20%) is lower than in AV disease (5,6). The true prevalence of CAD in patients with MS is not yet well known but generally it is considered to be low because this rheumatic disease is predominantly found in young patients. Angina is not a reliable predictor of CAD in patients with concomitant MS and could be attributed to a variety of etiologies, including active rheumatic vasculitis, pulmonary hypertension, pulmonary and coronary emboli (6).

Transient or permanent mitral regurgitation (MR) is often the result of ischemic heart disease. Obstructive coronary atherosclerosis is found in 30% of patients undergoing preoperative angiography to evaluate the cause and severity of MR while 20% of patients undergoing catheterization for acute ischemic syndromes also have associated MR (7). However, the incidence of MR is appreciably higher with echocardiographic evaluation in the latter (up to 50%), (8). Acute ischemic MR is more frequently seen in older patients and women and is found to be associated with extensive wall motion abnormalities, a persistently occluded infarct-related artery, and severe heart failure. Those with chronic CAD and MR usually have lower LV ejection fractions and more extensive CAD than those without MR. The prevalence of significant CAD in patients undergoing mitral valve (MV) prolapse operations is extremely low (1.3%), (7). Various risk-models have been developed in order to estimate the prevalence of obstructive coronary atherosclerosis but their clinical utility remains questionable.

Preoperative detection of CAD in patients undergoing valve surgery is a prerequisite in order to avoid perioperative adverse cardiovascular events and improve long-term postoperative survival. Although the ECG at rest and during exercise is not a specific tool for the accurate diagnosis of concomitant CAD in patients with VHD, exercise testing is often helpful in risk-stratifying such patients, particularly the asymptomatic ones, by unmasking symptoms and abnormal hemodynamic responses (3). Chest X-ray may reveal aortic plaque calcification but its usefulness as a screening tool is extremely limited. The extent of thoracic atherosclerotic plaque, detected by transesophageal echocardiography, is a powerful predictor for the presence of significant CAD; only 10% of VHD patients without thoracic aortic plaque have significant CAD. Combined assessment of thoracic aortic and carotid atherosclerosis could improve its sensitivity.

The sensitivity of perfusion or echocardiographic imaging with exercise or pharmacological stress is below 100% and their specificity is rather low. Regional wall motion abnormalities or abnormal scintigraphy could be related to myocardial hypertrophy, contributing to higher rates of false positive results. Given the importance of the presence of coexisting CAD, caution should be exercised in advocating such non invasive diagnostic techniques as a replacement for cardiac catheterization; non-invasive techniques may have a role in patients with mild to moderate valve stenosis or regurgitation and normal LV cavity size and wall thickness (5). More recent advances in non-invasive visualization of arteriosclerotic coronary arteries, such as computed tomography should be considered as an acceptable alternative, especially in younger patients with risk factors compromising patient outcomes (9).

Coronary angiography is the only method for the definite diagnosis of CAD and the most frequently performed investigation in patients with VHD. Although echocardiography allows an accurate evaluation of VHD, coronary angiography is usually combined with hemodynamic evaluation in approximately 50% of patients.. Cardiac catheterization could be particularly useful for evaluating patients with reduced stroke volumes, mixed valve lesions, or echocardiographically intermediate mean valve gradients (3,4). According to the Euro Heart Survey programme on VHD, the main reason for performing coronary angiography in the global population was the presence of more than one risk factor before surgery (72.1%), (2). This investigation is not recommended in patients with acute endocarditis, aortic dissection, poor hemodynamic condition, and in those undergoing emergency operation because in these cases, it is associated with increased mortality. Coronary angiography is recommended in patients with VHD and symptoms, dysfunction of the left ventricle, objective evidence of ischemia, a history of CAD, or risk factors (including age) (3,4). North American guidelines recommend preoperative coronary angiography in men aged greater than 35 years, premenopausal women aged greater than 35 years with coronary risk factors, and postmenopausal women (10). According to the European recommendations, the most common threshold of age used is 40 years for men and 50 years for women (4). A higher age threshold above 45 years is recommended in patients with MV prolapse in the absence of any symptoms or risk factors.

Focus Box 30.1

Frequency and diagnosis of coronary artery disease associated with heart valve disease: key points
- The frequency of associated VHD varies according to the characteristics of the population involved, such as age, gender, and risk factors for atherosclerosis
- Stress testing has limited sensitivity for detecting significant CAD
- Noninvasive coronary angiography using computed tomography is a possible alternative with high diagnostic accuracy for ruling out the presence of significant CAD in selected patients
- Coronary angiography is the only method for the definite diagnosis of CAD associated with VHD
- Preoperative coronary angiography should be performed in men with VHD above 40 years old and women above 45 years old

---

TREATMENT OF CORONARY ARTERY DISEASE IN PATIENTS WITH CONCOMITANT HEART VALVE DISEASE—GUIDELINES AND POTENTIAL INTEGRATION OF NOVEL DATA TO THE GUIDELINES

Management of Concomitant Aortic Valve Disease and Coronary Artery Disease

Treatment of Coronary Artery Disease at the Time of Aortic Valve Replacement

Over the past years, AV surgery has been increasingly performed in older people with more co-morbidities and a higher incidence of concomitant CAD. Optimal treatment of both pathologies should be tailored according to their severity. There are some conflicting findings in the literature comparing results from studies of aortic valve and coronary surgery with those obtained after isolated AV replacement (AVR) in patients with AS without CAD (5). This limitation arises from the heterogeneity of data in regard to the type of AV disease (AS or mixed AV disease), the severity of coronary disease, and the timing of operation (5).

Although complete revascularization during combined AVR and CABG is associated with longer cross-clamp times and has the potential to increase perioperative myocardial infarction, it seems to improve short- and long-term survival compared to patients with CAD undergoing isolated AVR (11,12). Patients with obstructive CAD who had only AVR tended to have increased rates of perioperative myocardial infarction, operative and late mortality compared to those who had CABG concurrently with AVR (11,12). CAD has a negative impact on postoperative myocardial recovery with less regression of LV mass index and less improvement of ejection fraction (13). The extent of CAD, AS severity, advanced age, worse NYHA class, and depressed LV function, are all significant predictors of postoperative mortality (12). In a multivariate analysis taking into account all these confounding factors, combined AVR and CABG is associated with a relative reduction in operative mortality (12). Even in octogenarians and nonagenarians undergoing AVR, CABG-related risk is lower with careful patient selection despite the higher complication rates in this population. These findings indicate that the negative outcome of such cardiac surgery may be linked to the total atherosclerotic burden and not CABG per se.

Thus, it is recommended that patients undergoing AVR with obstructive stenosis greater than or equal to 70% in major coronary arteries should be treated with CABG (Class I, level of evidence: C), (Fig. 30.1), (3,4). In patients with moderate CAD (stenosis greater than or equal to 50% to 70%), it is reasonable to perform CABG in major coronary arteries (Class IIa, level of evidence: C), (Fig. 30.1), (3,4). The use of the left internal thoracic artery is recommended for grafting left anterior descending coronary artery, particularly in elderly patients (5). Co-existing CAD also appears to be a major determining factor when deciding upon the choice of the type of valve, since porcine heterografts are related to better late survival than mechanical valves after AVR combined with bypass grafting (14). Limited data on patients with AS and significant CAD which cannot be by-passed due to anatomical conditions, strongly support the performance of AVR because of the much worse prognosis of the natural history of AS (4). Future research is warranted to investigate the potential benefit from a combination of laser transmyocardial revascularization and AVR in patients who are unsuitable for CABG although the results of laser techniques, to date, have not been encouraging (5).

Transcatheter aortic valve implantation (TAVI), utilizing stent-based prostheses, is a rapidly evolving field, which should currently be considered only in the elderly high-risk patients (15,16). A logistic EuroSCORE above 20 or Society of Thoracic Surgeons score above 10 have been used to define high operative risk (15). In patients with severe peripheral vascular disease not suitable for valve implantation, it is possible to insert the prosthesis using a minimally invasive, transapical, surgical approach. Mitral regurgitation and non-revascularized CAD are relative contraindications because along with severe LV dysfunction they can predispose to hemodynamic instability during TAVI. However, they are often well-tolerated, once AS is relieved. Because of its negative impact not only on procedural outcomes but also on long-term survival, concomitant CAD is usually pre-treated with percutaneous coronary intervention (PCI) in patients undergoing catheter-based procedures (Fig. 30.2) (13). Recent experiences in minimally invasive and percutaneous approaches have opened the doors to hybrid strategies, which may ultimately prove superior for older patients needing AVR (16).

Aortic Valve Replacement in Patients Undergoing Coronary Artery Bypass Surgery

Patients requiring CABG, who also have severe AV disease or have symptoms, should undergo AVR at the time of revascularization (Class I), (17). The decision whether or not to replace the valve is difficult and remains controversial for asymptomatic patients with mild to moderate AS (18). If no intervention is done at the time of CABG, patients will be exposed to the risks of a redo-operation to replace the valve with additional technical challenges and complications. Conversely, performing combined AVR and CABG is a radical treatment which exposes the patient to a higher operative risk, life long anticoagulation and to prosthesis-related complications long-term. Currently, there are no randomized trials assessing the benefits of prophylactic AVR at the time of initial bypass surgery and decisions have to be guided by non-randomized observational studies (18). These decisions should be made taking into account several clinical factors, including the severity and rate of progression of AS, patient life expectancy, and probability of valve- or operation-related complications.

Studies on the natural history of mild AS showed that 8% of patients developed severe AS by 10 years. A policy of AVR for mild AS at time of initial CABG would result in a cumulative incidence of unnecessary AVR of 91 and excess deaths of 29 at 10 years when compared to a policy of initial isolated CABG and subsequent AVR if necessary (18). Some authors have suggested valve repair and manual or ultrasonic decalcification as options to manage mild AV disease at the time of CABG but with disappointing outcomes; subsequent restenosis and insufficiency may limit their application. A significantly better long-term survival has been reported in patients with mild AV disease undergoing CABG if they have valve replacement rather than repair, inspection, or no procedure at all (19).

AVR for only moderate AS at the time of CABG requires a more complex decision process, that must take into consideration the rate of the disease progression. The mean rate of reduction in valve area is 0.12 cm^2/year and the mean rate of increase in valve velocity is 0.24 ± 0.30 m/sec/year, but the rate

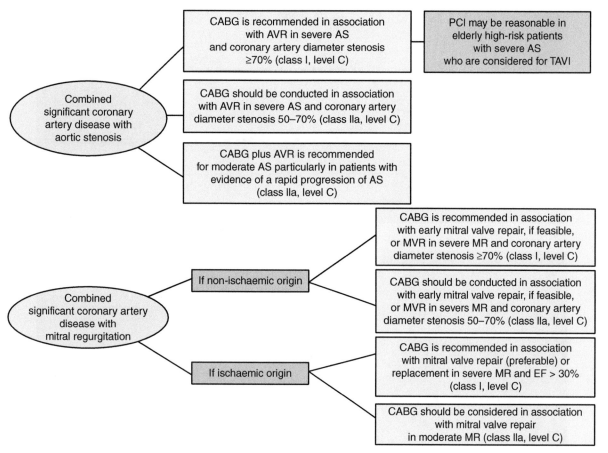

Figure 30.1 Treatment algorithm for combined valve surgery and coronary artery bypass grafting. *Abbreviations:* CABG, coronary artery bypass grafting; AVR, aortic valve replacement; AS, aortic stenosis; TAVI, transcatheter aortic valve implantation; MVR, mitral valve replacement; MR, mitral regurgitation; EF, ejection fraction.

of change in an individual patient is difficult to predict (5). Studies on serial testing of progression of AV disease have identified two groups of patients: one in which there is a decrease in effective valve area of 0.1 to as much as 0.3 cm²/year and the other, comprising the majority of patients, in which there is little or no change over a period of 3–9 years (20). Although, age, concomitant CAD, symptoms, degenerative pathology, and valve calcification has been cited as predictors of AS progression, there is no uniform risk model for progression in clinical use because of inconsistencies in the published data (20).

Retrospective studies of patients have shown that the mean time for reoperation was 5–8 years in patients undergoing AVR after previous CABG. Although definitive data is yet to be available and because of the increased risk of AVR later, patients with intermediate AV gradients (mean gradient 30–50 mmHg or Doppler velocity of 3–4 m/sec) who are undergoing CABG may warrant AVR at the time of revascularization (Class IIa, level of evidence: B), (3,4). In asymptomatic patients with

---

Focus Box 30.2

Combined aortic valve replacement and coronary artery bypass grafting: key points
- All patients with severe AS and severe CAD (>70% stenosis of major coronary arteries) should have AVR and CABG
- CABG is considered reasonable in patients with 50–70% stenosis of major coronary arteries
- The weight of evidence favors the use of a left internal mammary artery graft for ≥50–70% stenosis of the left anterior descending coronary artery
- AVR should not be denied when severe symptomatic AS is associated with non-by-passable CAD
- CABG for severe CAD plus AVR may be reasonable for moderate AS (mean gradient 30–50 mm Hg, Doppler velocity of 3–4 m/sec) , particularly in patients with evidence of rapid progression of AS

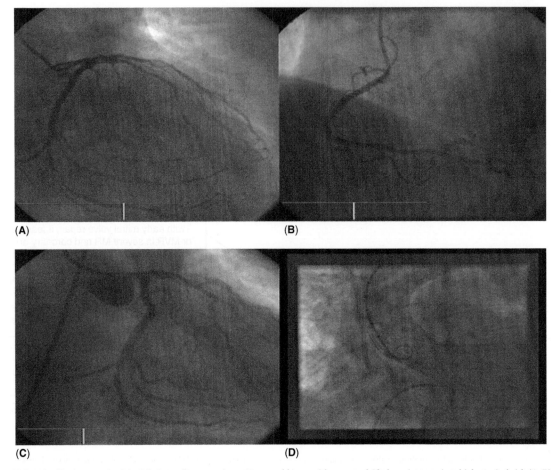

Figure 30.2 A significant stenosis of the left circumflex artery in an 80-year-old man with severe calcified aortic stenosis at high surgical risk (A, B), which was successfully treated with percutaneous coronary intervention before transcatheter aortic valve implantation was performed (C, D).

moderate AS, the degree of mobility and calcification of the AV and/or preexisting evidence of a rapid increase in aortic jet velocity of greater than 0.3 m/sec within one year, should be taken into consideration before making a decision for AVR (Fig. 30.1) (Class IIb, level of evidence: C), (3,4).

Management of Concomitant Mitral Valve Disease and Coronary Artery Disease

Treatment of Coronary Artery Disease Associated with Non-ischemic Mitral Regurgitation

There are few data available in the literature regarding the co-presentation of CAD and MV disease which are not etiologically related. Patients with isolated MV disease and CAD are at higher risk than patients with normal coronary arteries (21,22). Patients undergoing surgery for MVR combined with bypass grafting have had higher in-hospital mortality and worse late survival than patients undergoing AVR combined with bypass grafting (Table 30.1), (21,22). There are three different MV operations, which are currently used for correction of MR: (*i*) MV repair, (*ii*) MV replacement with preservation of part or all of the mitral apparatus, and (*iii*) MV replacement with removal of the mitral apparatus. Each procedure has its own advantages and disadvantages with the type of surgery to be performed is actually established at the time of operation. Valve repair rather than replacement should only be attempted in experienced centers.

The benefit of an early operation for severe MR is particularly pronounced in patients who have concomitant CAD (Fig. 30.1) (23). Although the combination of valve surgery with coronary revascularization generally increases operative risk, complete revascularization is superior to no revascularization in patients with VHD and CAD even if the adverse effect of CAD is not completely ameliorated by bypass grafting. The main factors influencing early and late risk of patients undergoing MVR combined with revascularization are: preoperative LV dysfunction and the number of stenotic coronary arteries (21,23). The advantages of valve repair over valve replacement—namely, lower perioperative mortality

Table 30.1 30-day Mortality in the Euro Heart Survey for Valvular Heart Disease: Comparison with Surgical Registries

	STS	UKCSR	EHS
	2001	1999–2000	2001
Aortic valve replacement no CABG	3.7	3.1	2.7
Aortic valve replacement plus CABG	6.3	7	4.3
Mitral valve repair no CABG	2.2	2.8	0
Mitral valve replacement no CABG	5.8	6.2	1.7
Mitral valve repair or replacement plus CABG	10.1	8.6	8.2
Multiple valve replacement (with or without CABG)	7.2	11.4	6.5

Abbreviations: STS, Society of Thoracic Surgeons (USA); UKCSR, United Kingdom Cardiac Surgical Register; EHS, European Heart Survey; CABG, coronary artery bypass grafting.

and improved event-free late outcome—should be taken into account in this subset of patients.

Treatment of Coronary Artery Disease Associated with Ischemic Mitral Regurgitation

MV dysfunction is a frequent entity, which is overlooked in the setting of acute or chronic ischemic heart disease. In patients with ischemic MR, the coronary artery and valve diseases are not combined; rather the VHD is a direct consequence of the CAD. It results from multiple factors, such as papillary muscle dysfunction, mitral annulus dilatation, and LV remodelling causing papillary muscle migration, restriction in leaflet motion, and excess valvular tenting with loss of systolic contraction (3,4). The incidence of MR is influenced by the size of the infarction and its location—being higher in inferior infarctions than in anterior infarctions of similar size (5). Overall, surgery of ischemic MR remains a challenge and the prognosis of these patients is substantially worse than that for regurgitation from other causes (3).

Acute ischemic MR is caused by papillary muscle rupture occurring at the acute phase of inferior myocardial infarction, has a catastrophic short-term prognosis and is treated by emergent surgical intervention (24,25). Acute, post-myocardial infarction MR with partial or complete papillary muscle rupture requires MV repair or MV replacement with subvalvular preservation, respectively (24,25).

Revascularization therapy should be considered in patients who have ischemic MR associated with an acute myocardial infarction. The favorable impact of thrombolysis or primary PCI on the incidence of ischemic MR has already been documented and has been associated with a reduction of LV remodeling. Late revascularization (percutaneous or surgical) is less likely to have a beneficial effect on MR (26). Preoperative evaluation can help identify patients in which ischemic MR is likely to improve following revascularization. Patients with concomitant presence of viable myocardium and absence of dys-synchrony

between papillary muscles could benefit by isolated coronary revascularization (27).

There are no data to support surgical correction of mild MR due to ischemia when the patient is asymptomatic from the point of view of MR and particularly, when coronary revascularization can be carried out by PCI. However, these patients should be carefully followed up to detect any later change in the degree and the consequences of ischemic MR (4).

Continuing debate exists on the management of mild to moderate ischemic MR (5). In patients with mild to moderate ischemic MR, ischemic symptoms may dictate the need for revascularization, and the MV is rarely repaired or replaced. The disadvantage of performing combined valve and coronary surgery in these patients is that valve surgery increases the likelihood of air embolism and prolongs extracorporeal circulation time, which is likely to increase operative mortality. Such surgery is more likely to be considered in patients with compromised LV function, if myocardial viability is present and if comorbidity and operative risk factors are low, since it yields better survival and improved LV function (28).

Severe ischemic MR should be corrected at the time of bypass surgery, even when there is no definite major organic cause. Although, CABG alone may improve LV function and reduce ischemic MR in selected cases, it is usually insufficient and leaves many patients with significant residual MR, who would benefit from concomitant MV repair (21). Nonrandomized studies have shown that MV surgery at the time of CABG may reduce postoperative MR and improve early symptoms compared with CABG alone but it does not improve long-term functional status or survival in patients with severe functional ischemic MR (29). The clinical decision to perform revascularization and MV repair is based on symptoms, severity of CAD, LV dysfunction and the presence of significant myocardial viability.

MV repair with a tight annuloplasty ring ("ring and run") or MV replacement with subvalvular preservation are the preferred approaches once the decision has been made to proceed with MV surgery (29,30). Even though MV repair carries a higher risk of mortality and of recurrence of MR than in other etiologies, this approach has better results. In the most complex high-risk settings, survival after repair or replacement is similar. Percutaneous MV repair, which involves annuloplasty approaches or the edge-to-edge repair by placing a metal clip on the regurgitant portions of the MV, is increasingly attracting attention since combined with PCI it could be useful for high-risk patients (Fig. 30.3) (31).

Accumulated evidence has led to the following principles for chronic ischemic MR: valve surgery for MR grade 2 to 4 in stable or unstable angina with comcomitant revascularization (Fig. 30.1) (10); the surgical management of chronic, dilated ischemic cardiomyopathy with MR grade 2 to 4 requires the same management whereas in cases with severe MR and presence of dyskinetic or akinetic scars, the same management plus reduction of ventricular volume and restoration of shape with realignment of papillary muscles is a class I recommendation, (Table 30.2) (10).

Percutaneous mitral valve repair

Catheter placement

Mitral valve replacement

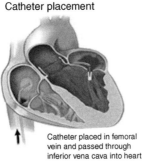

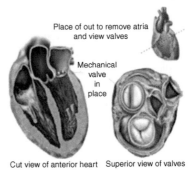

Place of out to remove atria and view valves

Mechanical valve in place

Catheter placed in femoral vein and passed through inferior vena cava into heart

Cut view of anterior heart   Superior view of valves

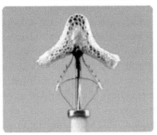

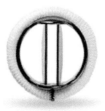

Figure 30.3 Percutaneous mitral valve repair system and surgical mitral valve replacement for the treatment of mitral regurgitation.

Table 30.2 Indications for Surgery in Chronic Ischemic Mitral Regurgitation

Class I-There is evidence and/or general agreement that mitral valve surgery in patients with MR is indicated in the following setting

Patients with severe MR, LVEF >30% undergoing CABG

Class IIa-The weight of evidence or opinion is in favor of the usefulness of mitral valve surgery is indicated in patients with MR in the following settings

Patients with moderate MR undergoing CABG if repair is feasible

Symptomatic patients with severe MR, LVEF <30% and option for revascularization

Class IIb-The weight of evidence or opinion is less well established for the usefulness of mitral valve surgery is indicated in patients with MR in the following settings

Patients with severe MR, LVEF >30%, no option for revascularization, refractory to medical therapy, and low comorbidity

Abbreviations: MR, mitral regurgitation; LVEF, left ventricular ejection fraction; CABG, coronary artery bypass grafting.

Focus Box 30.3

Mitral regurgitation associated with coronary artery disease: key points

- In the preoperative evaluation, it is important to differentiate ischemic MR from non-ischemic regurgitation associated with CAD and the feasibility of valve repair
- Valve repair should be considered early in patients with severe MR, particularly in patients who have concomitant CAD
- Urgent surgery is mandatory for acute ischaemic MR, caused by rupture of the papillary muscle occurring at the acute phase of myocardial infarction
- Combined mitral valve and coronary artery disease surgery is indicated in the case of severe ischemic MR
- Novel catheter-based therapies for MV disease in conjunction with PCI may be an alternative option for selected inoperable cases

Management of Coronary Artery Disease Associated with Other Valve Disease

Aortic Regurgitation

Concomitant AR and CAD generally presents in one of three ways. First, the AR may be detected incidentally during evaluation for symptomatic CAD. Second, a routine clinical examination reveals a murmur of aortic insufficiency in an asymptomatic patient, which leads to cardiac evaluation and detection of

CAD. Finally, patients may present relatively late in the course of VHD with congestive heart failure due to decompensation of the volume overloaded left ventricle or ischemic damage or both.

Most studies of patients undergoing combined AVR and CABG surgery include a relatively small percentage of patients with AR (32,33). While short-term survival after such operation is above 90%, late survival is similar to that for AS and

CAD. Age and LV function have the greatest impact in-hospital mortality death after AVR and CABG (32,33). The co-existence of an incompetent AV and CAD produces different pathophysiological efffects and their specific influence on LV ejection fraction is debatable. Ventricular dilatation and poor ventricular function occurring in the setting of AR are considered irreversible changes whereas revascularization could improve LV function. Yet, AR has not been proven to be an independent risk factor for early or late mortality after combined AVR and CABG. Thus, there is no evidence for using different operative thresholds in patients with or without CAD.

Conventional practice suggests that complete revascularization should be performed at the time of AVR (3,4). Less than complete revascularization may be an acceptable alternative for the elderly patients, particularly in those with no critical coronary lesions or severe angina. In this subset of patients, other possible options include preoperative PCI or off-pump bypass grafting (34). AR is usually associated with an aortic root dilatation, requiring a composite aortic valve and tube replacement with re-implantation of the coronary arteries. Mammary artery grafts should be used in patients also requiring CABG, in order to avoid the anastomosis of the grafts on the pathological ascending thoracic aorta (5).

Mitral Stenosis

Mitral stenosis is usually the primary substrate causing symptoms in patients with MS and CAD. CAD may cause LV dysfunction in few cases. The therapeutic management of CAD does not differ from other valve diseases and it is mainly determined by the severity of MS (5).

Patients with significant heart failure and low cardiac output from severe MS should have a MV operation associated with bypass grafting, if significant CAD is present. It is relatively rare for angina pectoris to be the indication for operation. These patients with significant CAD and MS could be managed with CABG and mitral commissurotomy if this is technically feasible. As an alternative to cardiac surgery, the feasibility of combined percutaneous transvenous mitral commissurotomy and coronary intervention has also been demonstrated in selected cases (35). Early mortality after combined surgery for MS and CAD is approximately 8%, whereas long-term probability of survival is approximately 50% at 7 years. Rheumatic valve pathology, preoperative LV function, and presence of ventricular arrhythmias are risk factors for late death (21,36).

Tricuspid Valve Disease

Tricuspid stenosis (TS), which is almost exclusively of rheumatic origin, is rarely observed in developed countries (3,4). Careful evaluation of such patients almost always leads to the detection of concomitant left-sided valvular lesions, which dominate the presentation (4). CAD is an uncommon finding in patients with pure isolated TS and usually, is the cause of the concomitant left VHD. Intervention on the tricuspid valve is usually carried out at the time of intervention on the other valves in patients who are symptomatic despite medical therapy. Conservative surgery or valve replacement, according to anatomy and surgical expertise in valve repair, is preferred. Percutaneous balloon tricuspid dilatation can be attempted as a first approach in the rare cases of isolated TS and co-existent coronary lesions amenable to percutaneous intervention can be treated as such (3,4).

Tricuspid regurgitation (TR) is only rarely caused by primary abnormalities of the tricuspid leaflets. In most instances it is "functional" in nature and is the consequence of left-sided valvular lesions that is occasionally seen with ischemic heart disease (3,37). TR is often ignored until it is moderate or severe, while it is thought that once the concomitant CAD and left-sided lesions are treated, functional TR would regress spontaneously (38). The timing of surgical intervention and the appropriate technique involved remain controversial, mostly due to inaccurate documentation and their heterogeneous nature. As a general principle, if technically possible, conservative surgery is preferable to valve replacement, and surgery should be carried out early enough to avoid irreversible right ventricular dysfunction (3,4).

REFERENCES

1. Hasdai D, Lev EI, Behar S, et al. Acute coronary syndromes in patients with pre-existing moderate to severe valvular disease of the heart: lessons from the Euro-Heart Survey of acute coronary syndromes. Eur Heart J 2003; 24: 623–9.
2. Iung B, Baron G, Butchart EG, et al. A prospective survey of patients with valvular heart disease in Europe: the Euro Heart Survey on Valvular Heart Disease. Eur Heart J 2003; 24: 1231–43.
3. Bonow RO, Carabello BA, Chatterjee K, et al. 2006 Writing Committee Members; American College of Cardiology/American Heart Association Task Force. 2008 Focused update incorporated into the ACC/AHA 2006 guidelines for the management of patients with valvular heart disease: a report of the American College of Cardiology/American Heart Association Task Force on Practice Guidelines (Writing Committee to Revise the 1998 Guidelines for the Management of Patients With Valvular Heart Disease): endorsed by the Society of Cardiovascular Anesthesiologists, Society for Cardiovascular Angiography and Interventions, and Society of Thoracic Surgeons. Circulation 2008; 118: e523–661.
4. Vahanian A, Baumgartner H, Bax J, et al. Guidelines on the management of valvular heart disease: the Task Force on the Management of Valvular Heart Disease of the European Society of Cardiology. Eur Heart J 2007; 28: 230–68.
5. Iung B. Interface between valve disease and ischaemic heart disease. Heart 2000; 84: 347–52.
6. Mattina C, Green S, Tortolani A, et al. Frequency of angiographically significant coronary arterial narrowing in mitral stenosis. Am J Cardiol 1986; 57: 802–5.
7. Lin SS, Lauer MS, Asher CR, et al. Prediction of coronary artery disease in patients undergoing operations for mitral valve degeneration. J Thorac Cardiovasc Surg 2001; 121: 894–901.
8. Grigioni F, Enriquez-Sarano M, Zehr KJ, Bailey KR, Tajik AJ. Ischemic mitral regurgitation: long-term outcome and prognostic implications with quantitative Doppler assessment. Circulation 2001; 103: 1759–64.

9. Meijboom WB, Mollet NR, Van Mieghem CA, et al. Pre-operative computed tomography coronary angiography to detect significant coronary artery disease in patients referred for cardiac valve surgery. J Am Coll Cardiol 2006; 48: 1658.

10. Jamieson WR, Cartier PC, Allard M, et al. Surgical management of valvular heart disease 2004. Can J Cardiol 2004; 20: 7E–120E.

11. Lund O, Nielsen TT, Pilegaard HK, Magnussen K, Knudsen MA. The influence of coronary artery disease and bypass grafting on early and late survival after valve replacement for aortic stenosis. J Thorac Cardiovasc Surg 1990; 100: 327–37.

12. Kvidal P, Bergström R, Hörte LG, Ståhle E. Observed and relative survival after aortic valve replacement. J Am Coll Cardiol 2000; 35: 747.

13. Grünenfelder J, Kilb I, Plass A, et al. Impact of coronary disease after aortic valve replacement. Asian Cardiovasc Thorac Ann 2009; 17: 248–52.

14. Akins CW, Hilgenberg AD, Vlahakes GJ, et al. Results of bioprosthetic versus mechanical aortic valve replacement performedwith concomitant coronary artery bypass grafting. Ann Thorac Surg 2002; 74: 1098–106.

15. Vahanian A, Alfieri O, Al-Attar N, et al. Transcatheter valve implantation for patients with aortic stenosis: a position statement from the European Association of Cardio-Thoracic Surgery (EACTS) and the European Society of Cardiology (ESC), in collaboration with the European Association of Percutaneous Cardiovascular Interventions (EAPCI). Eur Heart J 2008; 29: 1463–70.

16. Byrne JG, Leacche M, Vaughan DE, Zhao DX. Hybrid cardiovascular procedures. JACC Cardiovasc Interv 2008; 1: 459–68.

17. Wijns W, Kolh P, Danchin N, et al. Guidelines on myocardial revascularization: the Task Force on Myocardial Revascularization of the European Society of Cardiology (ESC) and the European Association for Cardio-Thoracic Surgery (EACTS). Eur Heart J 2010; 31: 2501–55.

18. Rahimtoola SH. Should patients with asymptomatic mild or moderate aortic stenosis undergoing coronary artery bypass surgery also have valve replacement for their aortic stenosis? Heart 2001; 85: 337–41.

19. Ahmed AA, Graham AN, Lovell D, O'Kane HO. Management of mild to moderate aortic valve disease during coronary artery bypass grafting. Eur J Cardiothorac Surg 2003; 24: 535–9.

20. Otto CM. Aortic stenosis: even mild disease is significant. Eur Heart J 2004; 25: 185–7.

21. Lytle BW, Cosgrove DM, Gill CC, et al. Mitral valve replacement combined with myocardial revascularization: early and late results for 300 patients, 1970 to 1983. Circulation 1985; 71: 1179–90.

22. Seipelt RG, Schoendube FA, Vazquez-Jimenez JF, et al. Combined mitral valve and coronary artery surgery: ischemic versus non-ischemic mitral valve disease. Eur J Cardiothorac Surg 2001; 20: 270–5.

23. Dujardin KS, Seward JB, Orszulak TA, et al. Outcome after surgery for mitral regurgitation. Determinants of postoperative morbidity and mortality. J Heart Valve Dis 1997; 6: 17–21.

24. Thompson CR, Buller CE, Sleeper LA, et al. Cardiogenic shock due to acute severe mitral regurgitation complicating acute myocardial infarction: a report from the SHOCK Trial Registry. Should we use emergently revascularize Occluded Coronaries in cardiogenic shocK? J Am Coll Cardiol 2000; 36: 1104–9.

25. Russo A, Suri RM, Grigioni F, et al. Clinical outcome after surgical correction of mitral regurgitation due to papillary muscle rupture. Circulation 2008; 118: 1528–34.

26. Tenenbaum A, Leor J, Motro M, et al. Improved posterobasal segment function after thrombolysis is associated with decreased incidence of significant mitral regurgitation in a first inferior myocardial infarction. J Am Coll Cardiol 1995; 25: 1558–63.

27. Penicka M, Linkova H, Lang O, et al. Predictors of improvement of unrepaired moderate ischemic mitral regurgitation in patients undergoing elective isolated coronary artery bypass graft surgery. Circulation 2009; 120: 1474–81.

28. Prifti E, Bonacchi M, Frati G, et al. Should mild-to-moderate and moderate ischemic mitral regurgitation be corrected in patients with impaired left ventricular function undergoing simultaneous coronary revascularization? J Card Surg 2001; 16: 473–83.

29. Mihaljevic T, Lam BK, Rajeswaran J, et al. Impact of mitral valve annuloplasty combined with revascularization in patients with functional ischemic mitral regurgitation. J Am Coll Cardiol 2007; 49: 2191–201.

30. Vassileva CM, Boley T, Markwell S, Hazelrigg S. Meta-analysis of short-term and long-term survival following repair versus replacement for ischemic mitral regurgitation. Eur J Cardiothorac Surg 2011; 39: 295–303.

31. Feldman T, Cilingiroglu M. Percutaneous leaflet repair and annuloplasty for mitral regurgitation. J Am Coll Cardiol 2011; 57: 529–37.

32. Shahle E, Bergstrom R, Nystrom SO, Hansson HE. Early results of aortic valve replacement with or without concomitant coronary artery bypass grafting. Scand J Thorac Cardiovasc Surg 1991; 25: 29.

33. Flameng W, Szécsi J, Sergeant P, et al. Combined valve and coronary artery bypass surgery: early and late results. Eur J Cardiothorac Surg 1994; 8: 410–19.

34. Kolh P, Kerzmann A, Honore C, Comte L, Limet R. Aortic valve surgery in octogenarians: predictive factors for operative and long-term results. Eur J Cardiothorac Surg 2007; 31: 600–6.

35. Harikrishnan S, Bhat A, Tharakan J. Percutaneous balloon mitral valvotomy and coronary stenting in the same sitting. Heart Vessels 2003; 18: 150–2.

36. Garcia Andrade I, Cartier R, Panisi P, Ennabli K, Grondin CM. Factors influencing early and late survival in patients with combined mitral valve replacement and myocardial revascularization and in those with isolated replacement. Ann Thorac Surg 1987; 44: 607–13.

37. Mascherbauer J, Maurer G. The forgotten valve: lessons to be learned in tricuspid regurgitation. Eur Heart J 2010; 31: 2841–3.

38. Matsunaga A, Duran CM. Progression of tricuspid regurgitation after repaired functional ischemic mitral regurgitation. Circulation 2005; 112: I453–7.

31 Clinical perspectives on the management of advanced stable coronary disease

Ranil de Silva and Kim Fox

OUTLINE

Treatment of stable angina pectoris has two main goals: first, to improve quality of life through symptom reduction, and second, to improve prognosis by preventing death and myocardial infarction. Clinicians are increasingly faced with management of older patients suffering from more advanced and complex coronary disease and multiple co-morbidities, many of whom may have previously undergone multiple coronary revascularizations. Clinical decision-making in these patients is often challenging, and not always directly informed by available literature. In this chapter, we will describe the management of three patients with advanced coronary artery disease (CAD), through which we hope to emphasize the importance of multidisciplinary team involvement as well as describe the use of approved and investigational novel treatment options.

CASE 1

A 58-year-old man was referred with Canadian Cardiovascular Society (CCS)class 3 angina, with an effort tolerance of 100 meter. He was a current smoker with a background of hypertension and type 2 diabetes mellitus (T2D), hyperlipidemia, and a positive family history of premature CAD. Seventeen years previously, following a myocardial infarction, he had undergone coronary artery bypass grafting (CABG) with a pedicled left internal mammary (LIMA) graft to a proximally occluded left anterior descending artery and saphenous vein grafts to the second obtuse marginal and distal right coronary arteries (RCA). Ten years after his CABG, he had percutaneous coronary intervention with drug-eluting stent implantation to the native left circumflex artery and followed four years later by an unsuccessful attempt to open a chronically occluded RCA. On both occasions the LIMA graft was widely patent. The left circumflex stent was patent. Medication at the time of referral included aspirin 75 mg daily, bisoprolol 5 mg daily, amlodipine 10 mg daily, ramipril 10 mg daily, atorvastatin 80 mg, ON and metformin 1 g BD. The results of physical examination was were within normal limits, with a blood pressure of 113/70 mm Hg and heart rate (HR) 55 beats per minute (bpm). Body mass index was 29 kg/m². The patient was in sinus rhythm with QRS duration of 98 msec. Fasting low-density lipoprotein cholesterol was 1.7 mmol/L and HbA1c was 6.7%.

This patient remained significantly limited despite receiving optimal medical therapy for stable angina pectoris. He was on appropriate disease-modifying medications, which are known to improve prognosis in patients with stable coronary disease. Other than continued cigarette smoking, his risk factors were optimally controlled. Our initial approach was to localize and assess the burden of myocardial ischemia and quantify left ventricular function. A stress-gated thallium scan demonstrated apical infarction with mild reversible ischemia in the inferior wall. Cardiac magnetic resonance imaging showed a mildly dilated left ventricle with transmural apical infarction on late gadolinium enhancement imaging, with preserved left ventricular ejection fraction at 53%. Computed tomography (CT) coronary angiography demonstrated patency and excellent run-off of the LIMA graft. Collateral supply to the distal RCA was noted. The proximal left circumflex artery was not well imaged due to stent artifact, though the rest of this vessel appeared unobstructed. The native RCA and vein grafts to the RCA and OM2 were occluded. In summary, this patient had well-preserved left ventricular function with a low burden of myocardial ischemia restricted to the RCA distribution territory, which, combined with the patency of the LIMA graft and current medical therapy, puts the patient at low risk of future cardiovascular death or non-fatal myocardial infarction. Consequently, as an initial approach, we opted to pursue medical therapy, implementation of a supervised domiciliary cognitive behavioral therapy-based regimen (the angina plan), and referral to a smoking cessation clinic rather than attempt to recanalize the occluded RCA. Ranolazine titrated to a dose of 750 mg BD was started, which together with the angina plan, rendered the patient in CCS class 1 and resulted in a significantly improved quality of life and exercise tolerance, which enabled a 5-kg weight reduction. The patient continued to smoke.

Angina pectoris arises from a mismatch between myocardial oxygen supply and myocardial oxygen demand. Conventionally, this is achieved using pharmacologic drugs, which produce vasodilatation, and reduction in HR and ventricular afterload. Contemporary clinical guidelines suggest that optimal medical therapy should consist of drugs that are known to improve prognosis in patients with stable CAD [aspirin, angiotensin-converting enzyme (ACE) inhibitors, and statins] and at least two anti-anginal medications for relief of symptoms. Of the latter, at least one should be a β-blocker, particularly in patients with a history of myocardial infarction, with the aim of achieving a target HR of 60 bpm (1). However, β-blockers at target dose are often poorly tolerated and in many cases the desired dose cannot be achieved (2). In these situations or when a β-blocker is contraindicated, rate-slowing calcium antagonists such as diltiazem or verapamil have been conventionally used as alternatives. More recently, the I_f channel blocker ivabradine, which slows HR through a direct action on the sinoatrial node, has been shown to be an effective anti-anginal agent, either alone (3) or in combination with a β-blocker (4). This agent is particularly useful in patients who are intolerant of other anti-anginals due to low blood pressure. Addition of long-acting nitrates, nicorandil, or dihydropyridine calcium antagonists to β-blocker therapy produces modest improvements in symptoms, objective markers of myocardial ischemia, and exercise duration, though in some patients where HR is not the predominant mechanism, significant clinical benefits may be achieved (1). ACE inhibitors and angiotensin receptor blockers are effective in lowering left ventricular end-diastolic pressure, improving myocardial lusitropy, thereby improving microvascular function, particularly in the subendocardium. These agents may therefore be helpful in relieving symptomatic angina. Notably, in the COURAGE trial, only 59% of the patients were free of angina despite a combination of conventional medical therapy and percutaneous coronary intervention (PCI) (5), and ~70% of the patients remained on at least one anti-anginal drug after CABG (6). These observations highlight the clinical need for development of new well-tolerated treatments to relieve angina pectoris.

To this end, other classes of anti-anginal drug have been developed, which neither lower HR nor produce coronary vasodilatation. Most recently, ranolazine has been approved for treatment of angina pectoris. This drug is proposed to have multiple mechanisms of action, but may reduce myocardial oxygen demand through inhibition of the late sodium current, resulting in reduced ischemia-induced calcium overload and intracellular acidosis, as well as diverting cardiomyocyte metabolism from fatty acid to glucose oxidation, and reduced lactate production (7). In the CARISA trial, compared to placebo, ranolazine was shown to improve significantly the exercise duration (by ~25 second on a Bruce protocol), angina frequency, and short-acting nitrate use in patients with stable angina pectoris already treated with atenolol, diltiazem, or amlodipine (8). In a recent report from a pre-specified subgroup of 3565 patients with known chronic angina participating in the MERLIN-TIMI36 trial (9), ranolazine was shown to reduce recurrent ischemia significantly [(HR: 0.78; 95% confidence interval (CI): 0.67 to 0.91; $p = 0.002$)], worsening symptomatic angina (HR: 0.77; 95% CI: 0.59 to 1.00; $p = 0.048$), and up-titration of anti-anginal therapy (HR: 0.77; 95% CI: 0.64 to 0.92, $p = 0.005$). Ranolazine also reduced severe recurrent ischemia, defined as ischemia associated with new electrocardiographic changes, hospitalization, or revascularization (11.9% vs. 14.4%; HR: 0.81; 95% CI: 0.67 to 0.98; $p = 0.026$). Modulation of metabolism in ischemic myocardium by partial fatty oxidation inhibition using drugs such as trimetazidine has been shown to improve metabolic efficiency in ischemic myocardium and be an effective treatment for angina pectoris (10). Novel approaches to relieve angina pectoris, which are under investigation, include Rho kinase inhibition (11). Interestingly, a preliminary report has also suggested the benefit of allopurinol to reduce angina frequency, sublingual nitrate use, and exercise duration in patients with CCS class 2/3 angina on established β-blocker therapy, potentially through increased myocardial oxygen availability, reduction of oxidative stress, repletion of adenine nucleotides and high-energy phosphates, coronary

vasodilatation, and reduction of ventricular afterload through improved endothelial function (12). If these results are confirmed in larger studies, this may prove to be an extremely cost-effective management approach.

Drugs that are known to improve prognosis in patients with stable angina pectoris include antiplatelet drugs (13,14), ACE inhibitors (15,16), and 3-hydroxy-3-methylglutaryl-coenzyme A (HMGCoA) reductase inhibitors (17,18). Counterintuitively, recent approaches at intensive glycemic control in type 2 diabetic patients (19) and high-density lipoprotein cholesterol elevation using torcetrapib (20) and niacin (AIM-HIGH) have not been associated with improved prognosis, with the latter study being terminated prematurely on grounds of futility. It is increasingly realized that HR is an independent prognostic marker for all cause and cardiovascular death in patients with cardiovascular disease (21–23). The I_f channel blocker ivabradine was evaluated in a placebo-controlled trial to test the hypothesis that HR is a modifiable risk factor, which when lowered, improves prognosis in patients with stable angina pectoris and impaired left ventricular function. Eighty-four percent of the trial participants were already on background β-blocker therapy (24). Participants in the placebo arm of this trial with a resting HR ≥70 bpm were observed to have an increased risk of cardiovascular death (HR 1.34; 95% CI 1.1–1.36, $p = 0.0041$), fatal or non-fatal myocardial infarction (HR 1.46; 95% CI 1.11–1.91, $p = 0.0066$), coronary revascularization (HR 1.38; 95% CI 1.02–1.86, $p = 0.037$), and hospitalization for new or worsening heart failure (HR 1.53; 95% CI 1.25–1.88, $p < 0.0001$), compared to those with a HR <70 bpm. This trial failed to meet the composite primary efficacy endpoint of reduction in cardiovascular death, hospitalization for fatal or non-fatal myocardial infarction, or hospitalization for new-onset or worsening heart failure [17.2% (ivabradine) vs. 18.5% (placebo), HR 0.91 (95% CI 0.81–1.04), $p = 0.17$]. However, in patients with HR ≥70 bpm (pre-specified), ivabradine therapy was associated with significant reductions in hospitalization for myocardial infarction [HR 0.64 (95% CI 0.49–0.84), $p = 0.001$], hospitalization for myocardial infarction or unstable angina [HR 0.78 (95% CI 0.62–0.97), $p = 0.023$] and coronary revascularization by either PCI or CABG [HR 0.70 (95% CI 0.52–0.93), $p = 0.016$). These are intriguing data, which were augmented by the publication of the SHIFT trial; the trial showed that ivabradine therapy was associated with improved prognosis in patients with ischemic cardiomyopathy, principally through a reduction in hospitalization for heart failure (25), and will be informed further by data from the CLARIFY longitudinal registry of patients with stable coronary disease and SIGNIFY trial, which will evaluate the prognostic benefit of HR reduction using ivabradine in patients with stable angina pectoris and preserved left ventricular systolic function. These data lend support to the concept that heart reduction not only improves angina symptoms, but may also improve prognosis in patients with stable CAD.

Optimal medical therapy is the mainstay of management of patients with stable CAD, offering equivalent prognosis to

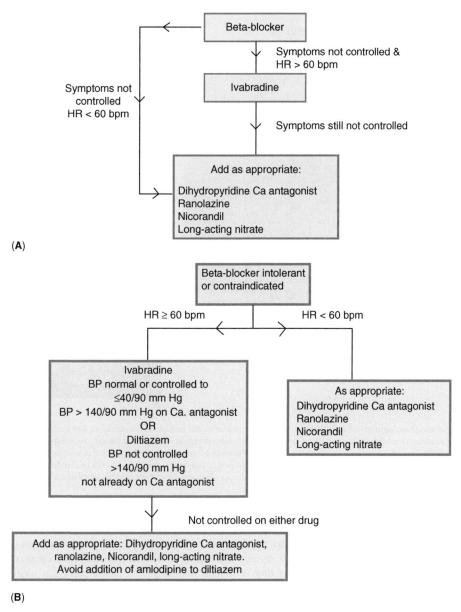

Figure 31.1 Suggested algorithm for medical management of patients with stable angina pectoris: *Panel (A)* for beta-blocker tolerant patients; *panel (B)* for beta-blocker intolerant patients.

revascularization in many patients (26,27). New drugs are available for relief of angina symptoms and some may improve prognosis. A suggested algorithm for pharmacologic management of symptomatic angina is shown in Figure 31.1.

CASE 2

A 75-year-old man was referred for management of refractory angina. Twenty years back, he had CABG, followed by redo surgery five years later with a LIMA graft to the left anterior descending (LAD) and saphenous vein grafts to OM2 and

posterior descending artery (PDA). Eleven years after his redo surgery, he presented with NSTEACS requiring PCI to the vein graft to OM2. Three years later, he experienced increasing angina and presented with an inferior STEACS, which was treated by thrombolysis. Coronary and graft angiography at the referring hospital demonstrated occlusion of the native coronary arteries, with patency of the LIMA and vein graft to OM2. The graft to OM2 was seen to have a filling defect thought to be a thrombus at the site of the previously deployed stent, and the OM2 provided epicardial collaterals to the PDA. The vein graft

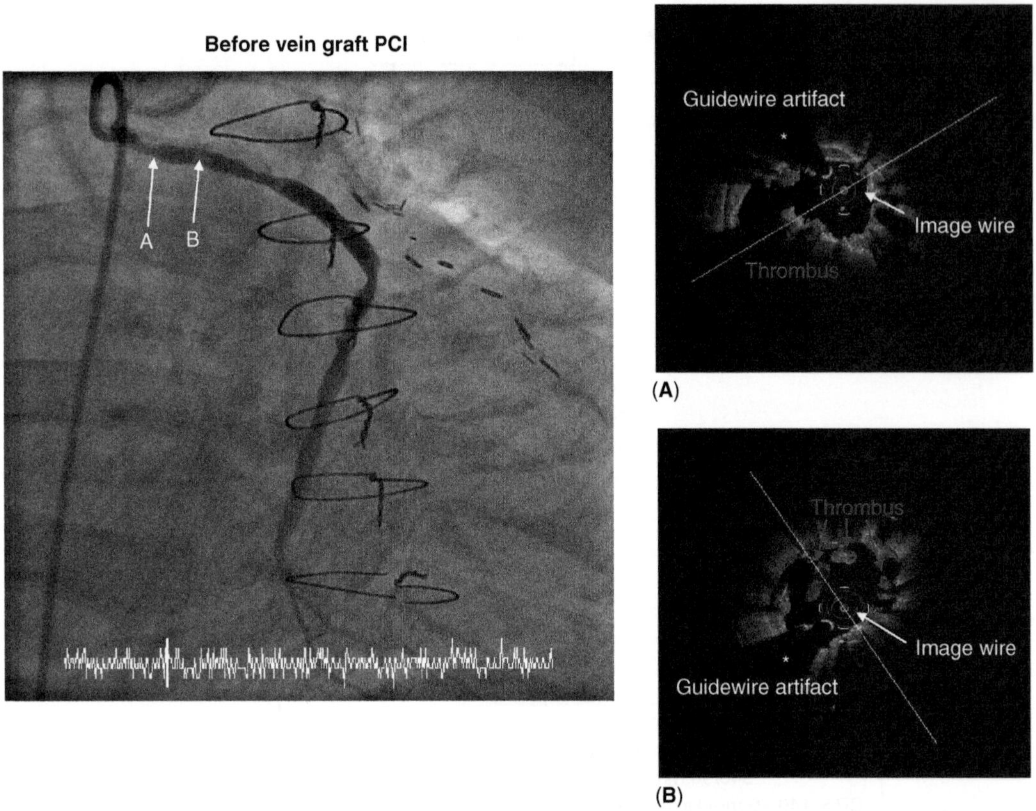

Before vein graft PCI

(A)

(B)

Figure 31.2 Selective contrast angiography of a vein graft to a second obtuse marginal branch shows restenosis and a filling defect within the proximal graft. There is further luminal narrowing at the stent exit. Optical coherence tomography is a light-based imaging technique, which enables intracoronary imaging at 20 micron resolution. This demonstrated under-expansion of the stent proximally (**A**) and organized thrombus within the graft (**A, B**). On the basis of these findings, PCI was undertaken by direct stenting with an equine pericardial stent to minimize the risk of distal embolization of thrombus. This was performed without complication and an excellent angiographic result was obtained, which confirmed patency of collaterals to the distal RCA post-procedure.

to the PDA was occluded. PCI to the OM2 vein graft was considered too high a risk at the referring hospital. The patient had a history of type 2 diabetes, hypertension, hyperlipidemia, previous cigarette smoking, peripheral artery disease, and chronic kidney disease (eGFR 42 ml/min). Medication at the time of referral consisted of aspirin 75 mg daily, clopidogrel 75 mg daily, diltiazem SR 240 mg daily, isosorbide mononitrate 60 mg daily, ramipril 2.5 mg daily, gliclazide MR 30 mg daily, and sublingual GTN as required. He had previously been intolerant of bisoprolol and simvastatin. Resting HR was 56 per minute with blood pressure 118/72 mm Hg. Physical examination results were otherwise within normal limits.

The patient was admitted for investigation. A dobutamine stress echocardiogram showed a resting ejection fraction of 50% with inferoposterior hypokinesis. With dobutamine stress, the patient developed angina with evidence of reversible ischemia in the inferior, posterior, and lateral walls. Repeat coronary angiography was performed, which confirmed the previous anatomy. Only epicardial collaterals from the OM2 to the PDA were seen. In view of the extensive area of ischemia noted on stress echocardiography and the heavy symptom burden despite

medical therapy, we undertook staged PCI to the OM2 vein graft using optical coherence tomography guidance (Fig. 31.2) and deployment of an equine pericardium covered stent; followed six weeks later by retrograde recanalization of the chronically occluded RCA via the previously treated vein graft (Fig. 31.3). The latter procedure was complicated by a coronary perforation and coronary hematoma, which was managed conservatively. The patient was rendered symptom-free as result of these procedures.

Chronic total occlusion (CTO) accounts for ~20% of all coronary lesions found at the time of angiography. In ~30% of cases, CTO is found in the context of multivessel coronary disease and associated left ventricular dysfunction is found in ~50% of the cases. The main objectives of revascularization of chronically occluded arteries are reduction of angina pectoris, improved left ventricular function, and improved event-free survival. Percutaneous treatment of chronic occlusions has presented a significant technical challenge. Historically, the presence of CTO has discouraged the use of PCI, with a greater proportion of patients receiving either continued medical therapy or referral for CABG. However, in the last decade, colleagues in Japan have pioneered

Before CTO PCI

After CTO PCI

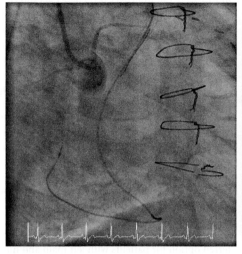 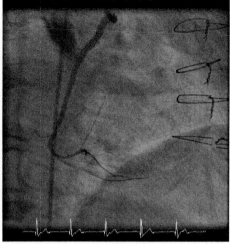

Figure 31.3 Pre- and post-procedure images following successful recanalization of the right coronary artery CTO. The procedure was performed using a retrograde reverse CART technique with externalization of the retrograde wire. The procedure was complicated by a perforation in the proximal RCA (note residual contrast staining on the post-PCI angiogram), which was treated using an equine pericardial covered stent. There was no significant pericardial effusion on echocardiography, though a large hematoma around the RCA was observed by cardiac magnetic resonance imaging. This was managed conservatively, without further complication.

our improved understanding of the pathology of chronic coronary occlusions, development of dedicated CTO wires and devices, as well as the use of the retrograde approach with intracoronary imaging guidance. These developments have resulted in CTO recanalization success rates of ~90% in the most experienced centers (28,29), and potentially enable complete percutaneous revascularization in a greater number of patients. However, percutaneous CTO recanalization can be associated with a number of complications including cutaneous radiation injury from prolonged screening times, contrast-induced nephropathy due to large contrast volumes in high-risk patients, myocardial infarction, tamponade, and coronary perforation. Current recommendations suggest that optimal outcomes may be achieved by careful patient selection and by having the procedures performed by dedicated operators who have been appropriately proctored in advanced CTO-PCI techniques. Furthermore, these procedures should ideally be undertaken in an environment where all the required dedicated CTO wires and devices are readily available and sufficient catheter laboratory time is made available to conduct these lengthy and complex procedures.

Data from several small trials and registries have suggested the clinical benefits of CTO recanalization. In the FACTOR trial, patients with symptomatic angina who had successful CTO recanalization had reduced angina frequency, improved exercise tolerance, and quality of life, as assessed by the Seattle Angina Questionnaire (30). A significant benefit of CTO recanalization in asymptomatic patients was not observed. Improvement of left ventricular function has been reported in patients who have demonstrable pre-procedure evidence of myocardial viability (31). Registry data suggest that successful CTO-PCI is

associated with a reduced risk of major adverse cardiovascular events compared to those with procedural failure, which may in part be accounted for by a deleterious effect of procedural failure (32,33). However, definitive evidence from an appropriately powered randomized trial is currently unavailable, which demonstrates the prognostic benefit and cost-effectiveness of percutaneous CTO recanalization over surgical revascularization and optimal medical therapy. These important data will be provided in part by the EURO-CTO trial, which is a randomized-controlled trial of CTO-PCI and optimal medical therapy versus optimal medical therapy alone. The primary efficacy endpoint is a quality of life score at 12 months, and the primary safety endpoint is the incidence of death and myocardial infarction at 36 months.

Advanced CTO-PCI procedures can significantly reduce angina in patients with complex coronary disease. This should ideally be performed by specialist operators in appropriately staffed and equipped institutions. These procedures are lengthy and complex and should be performed in carefully selected patients who remain symptom limited despite receiving optimal medical therapy, and who have objective evidence of either reversible ischemia or reversible left ventricular systolic dysfunction. The prognostic benefit of CTO-PCI remains undefined and is the subject of ongoing randomized trials.

CASE 3

A 74-year-old woman presented with new onset CCS class 3 angina. She was an ex-smoker with a history of hypertension. There was no other history of note. Her medication on referral consisted of aspirin 75 mg daily and ramipril 5 mg daily.

Physical examination results were within normal limits. Blood pressure was 146/82 mm Hg and HR at 84 bpm. The result of 12-lead electrocardiogram was normal. Transthoracic echocardiography revealed normal biventricular dimensions, excellent LV systolic function, competent valves, and no regional wall motion abnormalities. Treadmill exercise testing by a Bruce protocol was positive in stage 1, with 3-mm ST depression in the precordial leads. She was treated with bisoprolol 5 mg daily and atorvastatin 40 mg nocte, which resolved her angina. Diagnostic angiography revealed a discrete distal left main stem stenosis with significant disease in the ostial LAD and non-flow-limiting plaque in the LCX. The RCA was dominant and unobstructed. The SYNTAX score was 22 and logistic EUROSCORE 1.8%. She was discussed in our multidisciplinary team meeting where there was consensus that revascularization should be offered to improve prognosis. There was clinical equipoise between PCI and CABG. She agreed to participate in the EXCEL trial, and she was randomized to PCI with an everolimus eluting stent. PCI was performed using a single stent from the left mainstem to the LAD with a final kissing inflation and an excellent angiographic result. She was discharged 24 hours post-procedure without complication.

Conventional assessment of the risk of future death and myocardial infarction in patients with stable angina pectoris involves consideration of clinical status (1), response to stress testing (1), left ventricular dysfunction (EF < 0.4) (22,34), and extent of coronary disease (35,36). It is clear that patients with significant stenoses of the left main coronary artery have the worst prognosis and derived the greatest reductions in death and myocardial infarction with surgical revascularization. Recently, there has been increasing debate about the role of PCI for the treatment of left mainstem coronary disease, which traditionally has always been the preserve of the cardiac surgeon.

Recent clinical trials have compared PCI with stent implantation with surgical revascularization for the treatment of complex coronary disease including left mainstem lesions. The recently reported SYNTAX randomized controlled non-inferiority trial compared paclitaxel-eluting stents with surgery in 1800 patients with multi-vessel coronary disease (37). The three-year results of this trial show that all-cause mortality and stroke in the PCI and CABG groups are not significantly different. However, CABG was associated with a significant reduction in repeat revascularization (10.7% vs. 19.7%, $p < 0.001$) and myocardial infarction (3.6% vs. 7.1%, $p = 0.002$). When the data are stratified by the complexity of coronary disease as defined by the SYNTAX score, patients with low scores (<22) achieve identical long-term clinical by both PCI and CABG. Patients with intermediate (23–32) and high (>33) SYNTAX scores have significantly better three-year outcomes with CABG, mainly driven by a reduced need for repeat revascularization. In the CABG and PCI registry, which ran parallel to the randomized study, the primary composite endpoint of death, myocardial infarction, stroke, and repeat revascularization was 16.4% in the CABG group ($N = 649$) and 38.0% in the PCI group ($N = 192$).

Within the SYNTAX trial, 705 patients with left mainstem disease were randomized (38). These data showed no difference in the primary composite endpoint at 12 months [13.7% (CABG) vs. 15.8% (PCI)]. As in the main trial, there was a benefit of CABG in those patients with SYNTAX score >33 [29.7% (PCI) vs. 17.8% (CABG), $p = 0.02$], but no difference in patients with SYNTAX score <32 [20.5% (PCI) vs. 18.3% (CABG), $p = 0.48$]. These data are consistent with the findings of previous small randomized trials (39), registries (39–41), and systematic reviews (42), which have reported favorable results with PCI for the treatment of left mainstem disease. These data have provided the rationale for the EXCEL trial, which is an appropriately powered randomized-controlled non-inferiority trial of PCI with next-generation everolimus-eluting stents against CABG on a background of appropriate contemporary medical therapy in patients with left mainstem disease and SYNTAX score <32, into which our patient was enrolled.

The available data suggest that CABG should remain the preferred option for patients with left main and multivessel coronary disease. PCI is an effective therapy that can be offered to patients who are either ineligible or unwilling to have CABG. In these patients, ad hoc PCI at the time of diagnostic angiography should be avoided, and the clinical case discussed within a multidisciplinary team environment with representation from cardiac surgeons as well as non-invasive and interventional cardiologists. The patient should be provided with the opportunity to consult with both the interventional cardiologist and cardiac surgeon prior to reaching the final treatment decision.

SUMMARY AND CONCLUSIONS

These clinical vignettes highlight recent developments and our multidisciplinary approach to the management of advanced stable CAD. Medical therapy is the mainstay of treatment and should be aggressively uptitrated to achieve the desired heart rate, blood pressure, and lipid targets by using drug classes that have been proven in clinical trials. Coronary revascularization should be offered as an initial strategy to the subset of patients who have prognostically adverse disease, but otherwise be recommended for patients who remain symptomatic despite optimal medical therapy. Of note, ~50% of patients referred for PCI are on suboptimal medical therapy, despite the findings of the COURAGE trial (43). The prognostic benefit of revascularization over contemporary optimal medical therapy in patients without left mainstem disease remains a subject of ongoing debate and will be evaluated in future randomized clinical trials.

Despite aggressive medical therapy and complex revascularization procedures, there is a growing population of patients with refractory angina. We evaluate such patients in our specialist angina service comprising a multidisciplinary team of non-invasive and invasive cardiologists, cardiac surgeons, clinical nurse specialists, cardiac imaging specialists, pain management expertise, and psychologists (44), in order to offer a multi-modality approach for patients, including optimization of medical therapy and prescription of novel anti-anginal drugs, advanced revascularization, cognitive behavioral therapy (e.g., the angina plan), education, counseling, and support (45). Input from a pain management specialist with experience of pharmacologic (e.g., gabapentin, tricyclic antidepressants, and opiates), regional anesthetic (e.g., stellate ganglion blockade), and neuromodulatory interventions (e.g., transcutaneous electrical nerve stimulation and spinal cord stimulation) can produce significant symptomatic relief and improve quality of life for patients with refractory angina. Techniques such as enhanced external counter pulsation can be effective in some patients, though the data demonstrating symptom benefit and reduced ischemic burden are limited (46). Novel interventions such as partial occlusion of the coronary sinus (47) and induction of angiogenesis through extracorporeal shockwave myocardial revascularization (48), as well as growth factor and gene and cell therapy (49) are under evaluation in early-phase clinical trials.

Chronic stable angina pectoris affects ~2–4% of the population in western countries (1,50). The prevalence of angina pectoris increases with age and is estimated at ~10–20% in men aged 65–74 years. A similar pattern is also observed in women, although approximately 10 years later (1). The aging population and increased prevalence of type 2 diabetes mellitus and obesity will likely result in a progressive increase in the burden of patient with stable angina pectoris and increasingly complex CAD. CAD is now the major cause of death in the developing world, and the population of patients with stable coronary disease in these countries is set to increase dramatically. The direct and indirect costs of managing angina pectoris are enormous; therefore, its management represents a major and growing public health and economic concern. The development and implementation of effective, widely applicable, and affordable treatment strategies to address this growing global problem remain major unmet challenges.

REFERENCES

1. Fox K, Garcia MA, Ardissino D, et al. Guidelines on the management of stable angina pectoris: executive summary: the Task Force on the Management of Stable Angina Pectoris of the European Society of Cardiology. Eur Heart J 2006; 27: 1341–81.
2. Gislason GH, Rasmussen JN, Abildstrom SZ, et al. Long-term compliance with beta-blockers, angiotensin-converting enzyme inhibitors, and statins after acute myocardial infarction. Eur Heart J 2006; 27: 1153–8.
3. Borer JS, Fox K, Jaillon P, Lerebours G. Antianginal and antiischemic effects of ivabradine, an I(f) inhibitor, in stable angina: a randomized, double-blind, multicentered, placebo-controlled trial. Circulation 2003; 107: 817–23.
4. Tardif JC, Ponikowski P, Kahan T. Efficacy of the I(f) current inhibitor ivabradine in patients with chronic stable angina receiving beta-blocker therapy: a 4-month, randomized, placebo-controlled trial. Eur Heart J 2009; 30: 540–8.
5. Weintraub WS, Spertus JA, Kolm P, et al. Effect of PCI on quality of life in patients with stable coronary disease. N Engl J Med 2008; 359: 677–87.
6. Serruys PW, Unger F, Sousa JE, et al. Comparison of coronary-artery bypass surgery and stenting for the treatment of multivessel disease. N Engl J Med 2001; 344: 1117–24.
7. Nash DT, Nash SD. Ranolazine for chronic stable angina. Lancet 2008; 372: 1335–41.
8. Chaitman BR, Pepine CJ, Parker JO, et al. Effects of ranolazine with atenolol, amlodipine, or diltiazem on exercise tolerance and angina frequency in patients with severe chronic angina: a randomized controlled trial. JAMA 2004; 291: 309–16.
9. Wilson SR, Scirica BM, Braunwald E, et al. Efficacy of ranolazine in patients with chronic angina observations from the randomized, double-blind, placebo-controlled MERLIN-TIMI (Metabolic Efficiency with Ranolazine for Less Ischemia in Non-ST-Segment Elevation Acute Coronary Syndromes) 36 Trial. J Am Coll Cardiol 2009; 53: 1510–16.
10. Ciapponi A, Pizarro R, Harrison J. Trimetazidine for stable angina. Cochrane Database Syst Rev 2005: CD003614.
11. Vicari RM, Chaitman B, Keefe D, et al. Efficacy and safety of fasudil in patients with stable angina: a double-blind, placebo-controlled, phase 2 trial. J Am Coll Cardiol 2005; 46: 1803–11.
12. Noman A, Ang DS, Ogston S, Lang CC, Struthers AD. Effect of high-dose allopurinol on exercise in patients with chronic stable angina: a randomised, placebo controlled crossover trial. Lancet 2010; 375: 2161–7.
13. CAPRIE Steering Committee. A randomised, blinded, trial of clopidogrel versus aspirin in patients at risk of ischaemic events (CAPRIE). Lancet 1996; 348: 1329–39.
14. Antithrombotic Trialists' Collaboration. Collaborative meta-analysis of randomised trials of antiplatelet therapy for prevention of death, myocardial infarction, and stroke in high risk patients. BMJ 2002; 324: 71–86.
15. Braunwald E, Domanski MJ, Fowler SE, et al. Angiotensin-converting-enzyme inhibition in stable coronary artery disease. N Engl J Med 2004; 351: 2058–68.
16. Fox KM. Efficacy of perindopril in reduction of cardiovascular events among patients with stable coronary artery disease: randomised, double-blind, placebo-controlled, multicentre trial (the EUROPA study). Lancet 2003; 362: 782–8.
17. The Scandinavian Simvastatin Survival Study Group. Randomised trial of cholesterol lowering in 4444 patients with coronary heart disease: the Scandinavian Simvastatin Survival Study (4S). Lancet 1994; 344: 1383–9.
18. LaRosa JC, Grundy SM, Waters DD, et al. Intensive lipid lowering with atorvastatin in patients with stable coronary disease. N Engl J Med 2005; 352: 1425–35.
19. Griffin SJ, Borch-Johnsen K, Davies MJ, et al. Effect of early intensive multifactorial therapy on 5-year cardiovascular outcomes in individuals with type 2 diabetes detected by screening (ADDITION-Europe): a cluster-randomised trial. Lancet 2011; 378: 156–67.
20. Barter PJ, Caulfield M, Eriksson M, et al. Effects of torcetrapib in patients at high risk for coronary events. N Engl J Med 2007; 357: 2109–22.
21. Daly CA, De Stavola B, Sendon JL, et al. Predicting prognosis in stable angina–results from the Euro heart survey of stable angina: prospective observational study. BMJ 2006; 332: 262–7.
22. Emond M, Mock MB, Davis KB, et al. Long-term survival of medically treated patients in the Coronary Artery Surgery Study (CASS) Registry. Circulation 1994; 90: 2645–57.
23. Steg PG, Bhatt DL, Wilson PW, et al. One-year cardiovascular event rates in outpatients with atherothrombosis. JAMA 2007; 297: 1197–206.
24. Fox K, Ford I, Steg PG, Tendera M, Ferrari R. Ivabradine for patients with stable coronary artery disease and left-ventricular

systolic dysfunction (BEAUTIFUL): a randomised, double-blind, placebo-controlled trial. Lancet 2008; 372: 807–16.

25. Swedberg K, Komajda M, Bohm M, et al. Ivabradine and outcomes in chronic heart failure (SHIFT): a randomised placebo-controlled study. Lancet 2010; 376: 875–85.

26. Boden WE, O'Rourke RA, Teo KK, et al. Optimal medical therapy with or without PCI for stable coronary disease. N Engl J Med 2007; 356: 1503–16.

27. Frye RL, August P, Brooks MM, et al. A randomized trial of therapies for type 2 diabetes and coronary artery disease. N Engl J Med 2009; 360: 2503–15.

28. Borgia F, Viceconte N, Ali O, et al. Improved cardiac survival, freedom from mace and angina-related quality of life after successful percutaneous recanalization of coronary artery chronic total occlusions. Int J Cardiol 2011; [Epub ahead of print].

29. Rathore S, Katoh O, Matsuo H, et al. Retrograde percutaneous recanalization of chronic total occlusion of the coronary arteries: procedural outcomes and predictors of success in contemporary practice. Circ Cardiovasc Intervent 2009; 2: 124–32.

30. Grantham JA, Jones PG, Cannon L, Spertus JA. Quantifying the early health status benefits of successful chronic total occlusion recanalization: results from the FlowCardia's Approach to Chronic Total Occlusion Recanalization (FACTOR) trial. Circ Cardiovasc Qual Outcomes 2010; 3: 284–90.

31. Kirschbaum SW, Baks T, van den Ent M, et al. Evaluation of left ventricular function three years after percutaneous recanalization of chronic total coronary occlusions. Am J Cardiol 2008; 101: 179–85.

32. Hoye A, van Domburg RT, Sonnenschein K, Serruys PW. Percutaneous coronary intervention for chronic total occlusions: the thoraxcenter experience 1992–2002. Eur Heart J 2005; 26: 2630–6.

33. Joyal D, Afilalo J, Rinfret S. Effectiveness of recanalization of chronic total occlusions: a systematic review and meta-analysis. Am Heart J 2010; 160: 179–87.

34. Detre KM, Myler RK, Kelsey SF, et al. Baseline characteristics of patients in the National Heart, Lung, and Blood Institute percutaneous transluminal coronary angioplasty registry. Am J Cardiol 1984; 53: 7C–11C.

35. Califf RM, Armstrong PW, Carver JR, D'Agostino RB, Strauss WE. 27th Bethesda Conference: matching the intensity of risk factor management with the hazard for coronary disease events. Task Force 5. Stratification of patients into high, medium and low risk subgroups for purposes of risk factor management. J Am Coll Cardiol 1996; 27: 1007–19.

36. Yusuf S, Zucker D, Peduzzi P, et al. Effect of coronary artery bypass graft surgery on survival: overview of 10-year results from randomised trials by the Coronary Artery Bypass Graft Surgery Trialists Collaboration. Lancet 1994; 344: 563–70.

37. Serruys PW, Morice MC, Kappetein AP, et al. Percutaneous coronary intervention versus coronary-artery bypass grafting for severe coronary artery disease. N Engl J Med 2009; 360: 961–72.

38. Morice MC, Serruys PW, Kappetein AP, et al. Outcomes in patients with de novo left main disease treated with either percutaneous coronary intervention using paclitaxel-eluting stents or coronary artery bypass graft treatment in the Synergy Between Percutaneous Coronary Intervention with TAXUS and Cardiac Surgery (SYNTAX) trial. Circulation 2010; 121: 2645–53.

39. Buszman PE, Kiesz SR, Bochenek A, et al. Acute and late outcomes of unprotected left main stenting in comparison with surgical revascularization. J Am Coll Cardiol 2008; 51: 538–45.

40. Jones RH. Percutaneous intervention vs. coronary-artery bypass grafting in left main coronary disease. N Engl J Med 2008; 358: 1851–3.

41. Mehilli J, Kastrati A, Byrne RA, et al. Paclitaxel- versus sirolimus-eluting stents for unprotected left main coronary artery disease. J Am Coll Cardiol 2009; 53: 1760–8.

42. Naik H, White AJ, Chakravarty T, et al. A meta-analysis of 3,773 patients treated with percutaneous coronary intervention or surgery for unprotected left main coronary artery stenosis. JACC Cardiovasc Intervent 2009; 2: 739–47.

43. Borden WB, Redberg RF, Mushlin AI, et al. Patterns and intensity of medical therapy in patients undergoing percutaneous coronary intervention. JAMA 2011; 305: 1882–9.

44. Wright C, Towlerton G, Fox KM. Optimal treatment for complex coronary artery disease and refractory angina. Br J Cardiol 2006; 13: 306–8.

45. Lewin RJ. Improving quality of life in patients with angina. Heart 1999; 82: 654–5.

46. McKenna C, McDaid C, Suekarran S, et al. Enhanced external counterpulsation for the treatment of stable angina and heart failure: a systematic review and economic analysis. Health Technol Assess 2009; 13: iii–v; ix–xi, 1-90.

47. Banai S, Ben Muvhar S, Parikh KH, et al. Coronary sinus reducer stent for the treatment of chronic refractory angina pectoris: a prospective, open-label, multicenter, safety feasibility first-in-man study. J Am Coll Cardiol 2007; 49: 1783–9.

48. Fukumoto Y, Ito A, Uwatoku T, et al. Extracorporeal cardiac shock wave therapy ameliorates myocardial ischemia in patients with severe coronary artery disease. Coron Artery Dis 2006; 17: 63–70.

49. Losordo DW, Henry TD, Davidson C, et al. Intramyocardial, autologous CD34+ cell therapy for refractory angina. Circ Res 2011; 109: 428–36.

50. Lloyd-Jones D, Adams RJ, Brown TM, et al. Executive summary: heart disease and stroke statistics–2010 update: a report from the American Heart Association. Circulation 2010; 121: 948–54.

32 Interventional perspectives on the management of advanced stable coronary artery disease

Joanne Shannon, Azeem Latib, and Antonio Colombo

OUTLINE

This chapter reviews the evidence base for a percutaneous approach to coronary intervention, and attempts to explain why, contrary to the recommendations of the Clinical Outcomes Utilizing Revascularization and Aggressive Drug Evaluation (COURAGE) trial, percutaneous coronary intervention (PCI) should be the first choice for management of stable angina. Furthermore, and in the aftermath of Synergy between PCI with Taxus® and Cardiac Surgery (SYNTAX), we propose percutaneous coronary intervention as an excellent alternative for the majority of patients with left main and/or triple vessel disease. We provide a critical appraisal of both studies, showing why any conclusions should be interpreted with caution and not necessarily dictate practice. In SYNTAX, the patients received over-aggressive revascularization with an inferior stent in terms of safety and efficacy compared to new-generation stents. COURAGE enrolled a low-risk cohort of patients with minimal anginal symptoms, and used bare metal stents in more than 95% of cases. Neither study is therefore representative of contemporary practice. We describe how, with newer stent technologies, e.g. adjunctive devices such as intravascular ultrasound and pressure wire assessment, complete and optimal revascularization can be achieved that will improve outcomes in the future.

INTRODUCTION

The PCI is an established strategy for acute coronary syndromes (ACS), with top priority for ST elevation acute myocardial infarction (AMI). Several trials have shown primary PCI, when performed expeditiously, to be more effective than thrombolytic therapy in both the short- and long term (1). Furthermore, PCI performed within 6 h of fibrinolysis has been associated with significantly fewer ischemic complications than standard treatment (2,3). In addition, early intervention for non-ST-segment elevation ACS has a clear survival benefit, and it is also considered an acceptable approach in most cases of unstable angina without positive markers for ischemia (4). The publication of the COURAGE study and of the SYNTAX trial has questioned the major role of PCI in the treatment of stable angina. The COURAGE study supports an initial strategy of optimal medical therapy with provisional, as a reasonable alternative to CABG, crossover to PCI (5). While the SYNTAX trial supports PCI in low- and intermediate-risk patients with left main stem (LMS) or triple-vessel disease, it continues to recommend surgery as the optimal revascularization strategy for complex anatomy or in diabetic patients with triple-vessel

or left main disease (6). We seek to challenge the recommendations from both these landmark trials, which lack support from sufficiently robust data.

DISCUSSION

Why Should PCI Should be the First Line of Therapy in Stable Coronary Disease?

Consistent with multiple previous studies comparing PCI to medical therapy for stable angina (Table 32.1) (7), COURAGE merely reaffirms the premise that an initial management strategy of PCI using bare metal stents (BMS), when added to optimal medical therapy (OMT), does not reduce the risk of death, myocardial infarction (MI), or other major cardiovascular events (MACE), compared to a strategy of OMT alone. However, in the context of the design, rationale, and execution of the study, these results are not surprising.

COURAGE is flawed on a number of levels (Focus Box 32.1). Right from the outset, and in the context of existing data (8,9), the trial set an unrealistic goal: to show a 22% reduction in the already low annual rates of death and MI observed on aggressive medical therapy in patients with stable coronary artery disease (CAD) (10). Furthermore, the study was significantly underpowered, reaching only 67% of the projected end-point requirement for death or MI in medically treated patients at three years, despite attempts to liberalize the definition of MI and extend the period of follow-up. The surprisingly 'loose' definition of peri-procedural MI is worth mentioning. 'Symptoms accompanied by *any* creatine kinase-MB enzyme elevation above normal' might well enhance end-point accruement, but probably to the detriment of PCI, and one must question the prognostic relevance.

Patients were only enrolled after angiographic assessment. The exceedingly low, and frankly unrealistic (0.4%), annual cardiac mortality in the entire study cohort must raise questions regarding selection bias toward patients with lower angiographic risk. Indeed, of those screened, only 6.3% were subsequently randomized to the study. In addition, more than three-quarters (78.6%) of the patients had minimal or no anginal symptoms [Canadian Cardiovascular Society (CCS) class II or less, within a median duration of 5 months], and although only severe left ventricular systolic dysfunction with ejection fraction (EF) ≤30% was an exclusion criterion, systolic function in the overall patient cohort was, in fact, preserved (mean EF = 60.9 ± 10.8%). This confirms the 'carefully selected' and 'low risk' nature of the study population.

Table 32.1 Patient Characteristics in Studies Comparing Medical Therapy with PCI

Study	Sample size PCI/MT	Enrolment year	Proportion with MVD (%)	Duration of follow-up (years)
RITA-2	514/502	1992–1996	40	7
ACME-1	115/112	1987–1990	0	5
ACME-2	50/51	1987–1990	100	5
AVERT	164/177	1995–1996	44	1.5
Dakik et al.	22/19	1995–1996	56	1
MASS	73/72	1988–1991	0	5
MASS II	203/205	1995–2000	100	1
ALKK	151/149	1994–1997	0	4.7
Sievers et al.	44/44	ND	0	2
Hambrecht et al.	51/50	1997–2001	42	1
Bech et al.	91/90	ND	34	2

Abbreviations: MT, medical therapy; MVD, multi-vessel disease; ND, no data available; ACME, angioplasty compared to medicine; AVERT, atorvastatin versus revascularization treatment; ALKK, Arbeitsgemeinschaft Leitende Kardiologische Krankenhausärzte.
Source: Adapted from 7.

Focus Box 32.1

Pitfalls of COURAGE
  Underpowered study
  Low risk patient population with minimal symptoms and preserved LVEF
  No angiographic core lab- no assessment/standardization of PCI
  Incomplete revascularization
  Very low DES use (2.7%)
  Unrealistic medical therapy

When examined individually, the implementation of both treatment strategies can be criticized. There was no formal angiographic core laboratory in the COURAGE trial, making it difficult to perform any formal assessment and standardization of PCI strategies, as well as of procedural success rates. Automatically, the validity of PCI outcomes becomes questionable. Furthermore, it is noteworthy that, despite 70% of the patients in the PCI cohort having double-vessel disease, only half of these were completely revascularized and, given that the enrollment period was between 1999 and 2004, drug-eluting stent (DES) usage was extremely low (2.7%). Even among those treated with DES, the Endeavor stent (Medtronic, Santa Rosa, CA, USA) was used exclusively; this stent has since been shown to perform suboptimally when compared with newer DES. With substantive evidence now available demonstrating a 50–70% reduction in restenosis and clinically driven target-vessel revascularization with DES compared with BMS (11–13), these data are already, in effect, outdated. Of further interest is the disparity in PCI outcomes between procedural sites, with patients treated outside of the U.S. Veterans Administration (VA) demonstrating an almost 30% relative reduction in the primary endpoint, which, if consistent across all sites, would have satisfied the primary hypothesis of the study, demonstrating the superiority of PCI over medical therapy. However, despite the limitations of PCI in the COURAGE trial, there was a significant reduction in the requirement for revascularization at follow-up to a median of 4.6 years (21.1% vs. 32.6%; $p < 0.001$), as well as an improvement in quality of life and angina-free status in patients assigned to PCI. Overall, this translated into a 13% relative reduction in mortality out to 4.6 years of follow-up after an initial PCI strategy (10).

With regard to the OMT used in the COURAGE trial, one must question whether it truly reflects the real-world clinical practice, and hence, whether extrapolation of clinical outcomes is feasible. The trial boasts of exemplary compliance with aggressive secondary preventative therapies, with >90% of patients compliant with aspirin, statin, and β-blocker therapies at 1 year, figures that were impressively sustained out to 5 years (86%). This level of compliance differs significantly from published registry data. For example, in the Can Rapid Risk Stratification of Unstable Angina Patients Suppress Adverse Outcomes With Early Implementation of the American College of Cardiology/American Heart Association Guidelines (CRUSADE) registry, compliance with β-blocker therapy alone was less than 50%, falling to 36% when combined with aspirin, and only 21% when a third agent was added (14). Also noteworthy is that almost one-third (32%) of the OMT cohort crossed over to undergo PCI for worsening or severe symptoms. By intention to treat, however, they remained in the 'medically treated' group, thereby skewing the overall analysis in favor of medical therapy. This explains, at least in part, why COURAGE is the only randomized trial comparing PCI with medical therapy that failed to demonstrate long-term symptomatic benefit following a PCI strategy (8,9). Furthermore, although subgroup analysis failed to demonstrate an increased rate of death or MI out to five years in 12% of patients displaying high-risk features (CCS class III angina within 2 months, or stabilized ACS within 2 weeks of enrollment) and treated with OMT compared with PCI, events have been masked by the 42% crossover rate, of which 30% occurred within the first year (15).

Finally, and consistent with previous studies (16), the nuclear substudy of COURAGE provides supportive evidence for an early PCI strategy. When serial rest/stress myocardial perfusion single-

Table 32.2 The Major Trials Comparing PCI with Balloon Angioplasty or Stenting to CABG

Study	Comparison	Year	Number of patients	Disease severity
RITA	PTCA vs CABG	1993	1011	SVD & MVD
ERACI I	PTCA vs CABG	1993	127	MVD
GABI	PTCA vs CABG	1994	323	MVD
CABRI	PTCA vs CABG	1994	1054	MVD
EAST	PTCA vs CABG	1994	392	MVD
BARI	PTCA vs CABG	1996	1829	MVD
ARTS I	Stenting vs CABG	2001	1205	MVD
ERACI II	Stenting vs CABG	2001	450	MVD
AWESOME	PTCA/Stenting vs CABG	2001	454	MVD
SOS	Stenting vs CABG	2002	988	MVD
OCTOSTENT	Stenting vs off-pump CABG	2003	280	SVD/MVD
MASS II	MT vs Stenting vs CABG	2004	408	MVD
ARTS II	Registry of PCI with DES	2005	607	MVD
ERACI III	PCI with DES vs CABG	2007	450	MVD
CARDia	PCI with DES vs CABG	2008	433	MVD in diabetics

Abbreviations: PTCA, percutaneous transluminal coronary angioplasty; CABG, coronary artery bypass graft surgery; MVD, multi-vessel disease; SVD, single vessel disease; DES, drug-eluting stent; MT, medical therapy; RITA, Randomized Intervention Treatment of Angina Trial; ERACI, Argentine Randomized Trial; GABI, German Angioplasty Bypass Surgery Investigation; CABRI, Coronary Angioplasty versus Bypass Revascularization Investigation; EAST, Emory Angioplasty versus Surgery Trial; BARI, Bypass Angioplasty Revascularization Investigation; ARTS, Arterial Revascularization Therapies Study; MASS, Medicine, Angioplasty or Surgery Study; ERACI, Argentine Randomized Trial; AWESOME, Angina with Extremely Serious Operative Mortality Evaluation; SOS, Stent or Surgery; CARDia, Coronary Artery Revascularization in Diabetes.

photon emission computer tomography scans were performed in 314 patients at baseline and again at 6–18 months, the magnitude of residual ischemia was found to be proportional to the risk of MI or death, and even with minimal symptoms, a moderate-to-severe ischemic burden was associated with poor prognosis. Unsurprisingly, more patients derived significant ischemia reduction following PCI and OMT than with OMT alone (33% vs. 19%; $p = 0.0004$), with the greatest reduction seen in patients with moderate-to-severe pre-treatment ischemia ($\geq 10\%$ myocardium at risk) (17). Ischemia reduction by means of PCI should therefore be a goal in itself, even in the presence of OMT.

Overall, and despite the acceptable performance of the conservative arm of the COURAGE study, those patients treated with PCI as a primary strategy had a better quality of life with fewer medications at 4.6 years. We have attempted to explain the rationale behind the failure of COURAGE to meet its unrealistic endpoint, and we believe there is sufficient evidence from the trial data, to at least hypothesize that complete revascularization using newer DES, coupled with effective anti-platelet agents, and in combination with OMT, is the best initial therapy for most patients with stable angina, in order to reduce the short- and long-term risk of death and MI. Importantly, this hypothesis is supported by two recent meta-analyses, which were able to demonstrate a mortality reduction of almost 20% with a PCI- rather than OMT-based strategy (18,19).

Why SYNTAX Has Been Over-Interpreted

Until recently, and based on historical trials conducted in the 1970s and 1980s, coronary artery bypass graft surgery (CABG) has been considered the standard treatment for patients with LMS or three-vessel CAD with left ventricular systolic dysfunction. Two recent meta-analyses of the randomized trials comparing CABG and PCI in almost 9,000 patients (Table 32.2) showed no overall survival advantage with either strategy (20,21), although subgroup analysis of data pooled from six trials did demonstrate improved outcomes in patients with diabetes who underwent CABG (21). While PCI was associated with higher overall major adverse cardiac events (MACE), driven by increased rates of repeat revascularization, this was offset slightly in the CABG group by higher rates of perioperative stroke. It is important to remember that the growth of PCI technology is such that the results of randomized trials are often outdated and invalid at the time of publication, and that the majority of these studies have compared surgery to a PCI strategy of balloon angioplasty or BMS rather than DES usage.

The SYNTAX trial was the first of its kind to compare PCI using DES [albeit the first generation Taxus® Express (Boston Scientific Corporation, Natick, Mass)] with CABG in patients with stable, angiographic 3-vessel CAD, or with LMS disease associated with 1,2, or 3-vessel involvement, and is arguably the most poignant trials in recent years. A major strength of SYNTAX is its all-comer design with few exclusion criteria, allowing 71% of those screened to be enrolled in the study. The significantly higher rates of combined MACE (death from any cause, stroke, myocardial infarction, or repeat revascularization) in the PCI (17.8%, vs. 12.4% for CABG; $p = .002$) group rejected the non-inferiority hypothesis, and led to the generalized and sweeping

Focus Box 32.2

Pitfalls of SYNTAX
  Primary endpoint misleading
  PCI limited by higher rates of repeat revascularization, but
  was comparable to CABG in terms of hard outcomes
  Taxus® Express is an inferior stent in terms of safety and
  efficacy
  Over-aggressive revascularization in the PCI arm to
  include intermediate lesions, increasing the risk of restenosis and stent thrombosis
  Multiple substudies which can only be hypothesis-
  generating

Table 32.3 Syntax Study—Cumulative Event Rates to Three Years

Cumulative event rate	CABG (%)	Taxus DES (%)	P value
MACE	20.2	28.0	<0.001
Death, stroke, MI	12.0	14.1	0.21
All-cause death	6.7	8.6	0.13
Stroke	3.4	2.0	0.07
MI	3.6	7.1	0.002
Repeat revascularization	10.7	19.7	<0.001

conclusions that CABG should remain the gold standard of care for these patients. We wish to challenge this statement, based on a number of limitations leading to over-interpretation of the data (Focus Box 32.2).

First, and most poignantly, the combined endpoint tarnishes the results allowing misinterpretation. It must be highlighted that rates of the important, hard endpoints of death and MI, were comparable in both groups at one year, and that the overall increased rate of MACE in the PCI group was driven by increased rates of repeat revascularization (13.5% vs. 5.9% for CABG; $p < 0.001$). Furthermore, stroke rates were significantly higher with CABG than with PCI (2.2%, vs. 0.6%; $p = 0.003$). There are strong grounds to argue that combined hard endpoints (death, MI, stroke) were almost identical in the two groups (7.6% with PCI vs. 7.7% with CABG), and that with CABG preventing only 76 repeat revascularization procedures in every 1,000 patients treated compared with PCI, the overall conclusions of the study have been based on soft endpoints with questionable clinical relevance (22). In other words, the risk of a second minimally invasive procedure further down the line, necessitating at the most a two-day hospital stay, may be preferable to the trauma of open sternotomy, prolonged hospital stay and rehabilitation, and the risk of neurocognitive decline or catastrophic stroke. It is noteworthy, however, that 'important variables' such as hospital stay, surgical complications, and cognitive decline were all excluded from the SYNTAX analysis.

Supporters of CABG dispute the short duration of follow-up in the SYNTAX study, predicting a divergence of hard outcomes in the longer term. In contrast, the three-year follow-up data showed no significant divergence (Table 32.3), and although there has been a slight increase in the rate of repeat revascularization, we have enough data from meta-analyses comparing PCI with BMS to CABG, to be confident that a divergence in hard outcomes for at least eight years is unlikely (20,21). Indeed, data from the BARI follow-up have shown comparable overall (73.5% for CABG and 71.0% for PCI; $p = 0.18$) and event-free survival (63.6% for CABG and 63.9% for PCI; $p = 0.97$) between CABG and balloon angioplasty for 10 years (23).

More detailed analysis of SYNTAX demonstrates that only those patients with the most complex coronary anatomy (SYNTAX scores ≥33) derive definite benefit from CABG, with PCI at least as efficacious in low and intermediate complexity. However, the sample size encompassing the highest-risk patients is insufficient to draw conclusions regarding MI and death. If anything, we can consider the findings useful to plan a dedicated trial in the future. Furthermore, SYNTAX has provided a long-awaited breakthrough in the interventional therapy of unprotected LMS disease, providing for the first time, in a large number of patients, randomized trial data showing comparable safety and efficacy outcomes with PCI and CABG for at least one year (combined MACE 15.8% for PCI vs. 13.6% for CABG; $p = 0.44$) (24). While overall safety outcomes were independent of the extent of vessel involvement, patients with LMS and two-vessel or three-vessel disease had significantly higher rates of repeat revascularization than those with isolated LMS or single-vessel disease when treated with PCI compared to surgery. While the overall SYNTAX study failed to meet its primary endpoint, making these outcomes only hypothesis-generating, PCI appears to be a safe and effective strategy for many patients with LMS disease. Further, dedicated LMS studies are necessary to confirm this hypothesis.

It is also important to note that all patients in the PCI arm of the SYNTAX trial were treated with the first-generation Taxus® Express DES. The continual improvements in stent technology, with, for example, the recently published SPIRIT III data showing a 45% reduction in MACE and 50% reduction in late loss with the everolimus-eluting Xience V® (Abbott Vascular, Illinois, USA) compared with the Taxus Express DES, gives us confidence that PCI results can only be improved further (25). Given that Taxus is an inferior stent in terms of both safety and efficacy, SYNTAX cannot be considered representative of contemporary outcomes.

Interestingly, over-aggressive revascularization was standard in the PCI arm of SYNTAX, and was driven by an overenthusiastic and non-evidence-based study design advocating the treatment of all stenoses >50% in vessels >1.5 mm. This led to one-third of patients receiving >100 mm of stent length (mean 86.1 ± 47.9 mm), with 4.6 ± 2.3 stents used per patient and almost half of patients receiving a total of five or more stents. Given the wealth of data correlating stent length with the risk of restenosis and stent thrombosis, this may certainly have contributed to the increased rates of revascularization and MI seen in the study and, therefore, reflects another design failure. Had the study used a FAME-guided approach, i.e., hemodynamically driven PCI, the number of stented lesions could have been reduced by 37% (22). Despite the excessive number of stents used in SYNTAX, overall completeness of revascularization was still less in the PCI than the surgical arm, due to a lower rate of successful re-opening of chronic occlusions. But one must ask how complete is complete whether a complete revascularization strategy is always necessary, or whether it should be determined only by the percentage of myocardium at risk. Furthermore, the study design required, where possible, complete revascularization to be performed during the index procedure rather than as a staged approach. This may have influenced some operators against a complete revascularization strategy, and certainly against using adjuncts such as fractional flow reserve (FFR) assessment or intravascular ultrasound (IVUS) to optimize outcomes.

The number of underpowered subgroup analyses of the SYN-TAX data is a source of further confusion and over-interpretation. The diabetic subgroup analysis, for example, reported that among the 452 patients with medically treated diabetes, those with SYN-TAX scores in the third tertile had higher rates of MACE than those without diabetes at one year. This fueled the recommendation that high-risk diabetic patients should be treated surgically. However, when studied further, while they certainly had higher rates of repeat revascularization and death than their non-diabetic counterparts, the composite safety of PCI in diabetic patients (defined by death, stroke, and MI), irrespective of SYNTAX tertile, was comparable to CABG (26). Furthermore, given that repeat revascularization was loosely defined as revascularization of any vessel other than the target lesion or vessel, the aggressive disease progression typically associated with diabetes would undoubtedly have more noticeable impact on the PCI compared to the CABG group. Finally, this substudy fails to provide long-term follow-up data for diabetic patients treated with PCI versus CABG. Further, with SYNTAX failing to meet its primary endpoint, outcomes from any subgroup analysis can only be hypothesis generating, and this should be interpreted with caution and not dictate changes in clinical practice.

It is disappointing that, despite the conclusions and recognized limitations of the SYNTAX study, the latest European Society of Cardiology and European Association for Cardio-Thoracic Surgery guidelines, revised in 2010, continue to recommend CABG as the preferred revascularization modality in all cases (class IA recommendation), with the exception of single-/double-vessel disease not involving the proximal LAD (27). Thereafter, PCI is given a class IIaB recommendation for isolated LMS disease or LMS with multi-vessel involvement, and SYN-TAX scores in the first or second tertile. For high-risk patients with complex multi-vessel ± LMS disease and SYNTAX scores in the third tertile, PCI is not recommended at all (IIIB and IIIA level of evidence, respectively). Therefore, despite comparable outcomes in the PCI cohort with LMS ± multi-vessel disease associated with low or intermediate SYNTAX scores, these

guidelines have failed to incorporate this contemporary data, and continue to recommend CABG based only on historical data. They fail to address PCI as a reasonable, and in many cases, excellent option for the majority of patients in these groups.

As a Primary Revascularization Strategy, How Can We Optimize PCI Outcomes?

With the existing evidence base for PCI in ACS, along with the expanding safety and efficacy data for PCI as a revascularization strategy in stable CAD and multi-vessel/LMS disease, we, as interventional cardiologists, must strive to ensure that we are performing optimally so that outcomes continue to improve. Thus, while managing complex anatomy, we must have a low threshold for the use of IVUS, not only to ensure optimal DES expansion, but also to improve our understanding of vessel size, lesion severity, and plaque morphology. Although we lack robust evidence for IVUS-guided PCI, with most data from underpowered sub-group analyses or retrospective studies (28), there is certainly evidence favoring IVUS to be guiding DES implantation in the unprotected LMS (29). It is our opinion that IVUS guidance should be imperative for unprotected LMS PCI and stent thrombosis, strongly recommended in the treatment of chronic total occlusions and in-stent restenosis, and used liberally in other scenarios such as proximal or bifurcation disease. There are a number of interesting and potentially useful adjuncts to IVUS such as virtual histology to enable plaque characterization. While this is currently a research tool, it could potentially be useful in identifying vulnerable lesions in both stable CAD, and in unstable disease with multi-vessel involvement.

Second, continual improvements in DES technology, ranging from improved anti-proliferative agents to biodegradable polymers and, more recently, bioabsorbable stents, are certainly exciting. With a growing evidence base for a reduction in stent thrombosis, the routine use of new stent systems will reduce the rates of repeat revascularization, the major caveat of PCI in the major randomized trials.

The evaluation and treatment of intermediate lesions (40–70% stenosis angiographically) can often be difficult, and there is sufficient evidence to support the use of an FFR-guided approach (30). It is our opinion, therefore, that FFR should be used liberally for the assessment of angiographically intermediate lesions and lesions with FFR values ≤0.75 in the presence of single-vessel disease, and ≤0.80 with multi-vessel disease should be treated. Importantly, there are occasional scenarios where the FFR is negative, yet subsequent IVUS assessment demonstrates a lesion to be critical. While functional and anatomical assessments independently provide useful information, there is limited evidence supporting the use of IVUS-guided decision making on stent placement. Therefore, while our recommendation at present is to avoid treating such lesions, evidence may soon emerge to suggest otherwise.

Now that we are performing increasingly complex PCI, aiming, where possible, for complete revascularization, we believe that a staged approach to treatment will not only lead to better results, but will also be safer for the patient. Performing complete revascularization in a single procedure increases the risk of contrast nephropathy and radiation exposure, and may also lead to sub-optimal results without, for example, appropriate IVUS or FFR use.

Finally, the issue of anti-platelet therapy must not be overlooked. The current recommendations are for use of aspirin in combination with thienopyridine and clopidogrel, for 12 months following PCI with DES. However, sub-optimal platelet inhibition with clopidogrel has been demonstrated in up to 20% of patients, and as such, a number of alternative agents have emerged. Prasugrel, a novel thienopyridine, was shown in the TRITON-TIMI 38 study to reduce the combined efficacy endpoint of cardiovascular death, MI, and stroke by 19% higher than clopidogrel (9.9% vs. 12.1%; $p < 0.001$), but at a cost of increased bleeding (2.4% vs. 1.8%; $p = 0.03$) in patients with ACS undergoing PCI (31). Among those presenting with stent thrombosis, prasugrel reduced recurrent events by 34% ($p = 0.034$). This benefit was more marked in diabetic patients who saw a 60% risk reduction in subsequent events with prasugrel compared with clopidogrel ($p = 0.003$). In a similar cohort of ACS patients, a second agent, ticagrelor (a direct P2Y12 inhibitor) has been shown to reduce the death rate from vascular causes, MI, and stroke (9.8% vs. 11.7%; $p < 0.001$) without an increase in overall bleeding (11.6% vs. 11.2%; $p = 0.43$) at 12 months (32). Furthermore, ticagrelor was associated with significantly less stent thrombosis at 12 months (2.8% vs. 3.6%; $p = 0.01$). Both prasugrel and ticagrelor have since been included in the revised 2010 European Society of Cardiology and European Association for Cardio-Thoracic Surgery guidelines for revascularization, with a IB recommendation in ST-elevation myocardial infarction, and a IB and IIaB recommendation for ticagrelor and prasugrel, respectively, in patients with non-ST-elevation myocardial infarction (27). Overall, the recommendations for performing optimal PCI are summarized in Focus Box 32.3.

PERSONAL PRESPECTIVE

PCI is already the treatment of choice for acute MI and ACS, and this is supported by a vast evidence-base. In the current era, more than 50% of PCI procedures are acute interventions, and the dramatic decline in cardiovascular mortality supports this development. Although the treatment of patients with stable angina and one- or two-vessel CAD is more controversial, we believe there is enough evidence, through both rapid technological advances in stenting procedures, and the pitfalls of studies such as COURAGE, to support the use of PCI in combination with aggressive medical therapy as the most appropriate early strategy. We also believe that PCI should, for logistical reasons as well as evidence based, be the first-line treatment for patients with three-vessel and/or LMS disease of low or moderate anatomical complexity. For the minority with high SYNTAX scores and favorable anatomy, PCI is a viable option in the hands of experienced operators, capable of complete revascularization using new-generation DES, IVUS, and FFR guidance, as well as contemporary antithrombotic therapy.

Focus Box 32.3

Optimizing PCI Outcomes in LMS ± Multi-vessel Disease
  Aim for complete revascularization, assisted by liberal FFR use for intermediate lesions
  IVUS strongly recommended for LMS disease, CTO, instent restenosis, and stent thrombosis
  Liberal use of IVUS in bifurcation disease
  Staged procedures for revascularization of multi-vessel disease
  Use of novel and contemporary DES systems
  Use of contemporary antithrombotic therapy

Figure 32.1/Video clip 32.1 illustrates an example from our own experience; the patient was a 76-year-old man who presented in 2006 following a positive stress test. Coronary angiography showed complex distal LMS disease involving a trifurcation of the LAD, circumflex (LCx), and ramus intermediate, with further LAD disease at the bifurcation of the first diagonal branch. There was additional disease of the right coronary artery (RCA). LV function was preserved and he was not diabetic. While the SYNTAX score was 39, the presence of significant arteriopathy, including previous abdominal aortic aneurysm repair, severe peripheral vascular, and carotid disease, rendered surgical revascularization as high risk and indeed unattractive. As such, he was successfully revascularized percutaneously using DES, implanted with IVUS guidance, using intra-aortic balloon support, and performed over two procedures staged by six weeks. Angiographic follow-up out to three years has shown no evidence of restenosis, and the patient remains clinically well at five years follow-up. By contrast, Figure 32.2/Video clip 32.2 illustrates an example where the presence of a double occlusion of the LAD makes PCI an unattractive option. The patient, a 66-year-old woman, presented with an episode of ischemic pulmonary edema. LV function was mildly impaired (ejection fraction 45%), she was not diabetic, and had no significant co-morbidity. Again the SYNTAX score was 39. Following a discussion with our surgical colleagues, she underwent successful surgical revascularization with a left internal mammary artery (LIMA) grafted to the LAD, and saphenous vein grafts to the second diagonal branch and RCA.

The first case, in particular, illustrates what we can, and indeed have, been achieving with PCI, even with SYNTAX scores well into the third tertile. Complete revascularization in the second case might well have been achievable by percutaneous means; however, in our experience, the chances of successfully reopening two occlusions in any one vessel are reasonably low. In situations with LAD involvement, an upfront surgical strategy with a LIMA-to-LAD graft remains superior. That said, we believe the future to be exciting, and that, with contemporary practice already surpassing SYNTAX, PCI will emerge as a superior strategy to CABG sooner than we think.

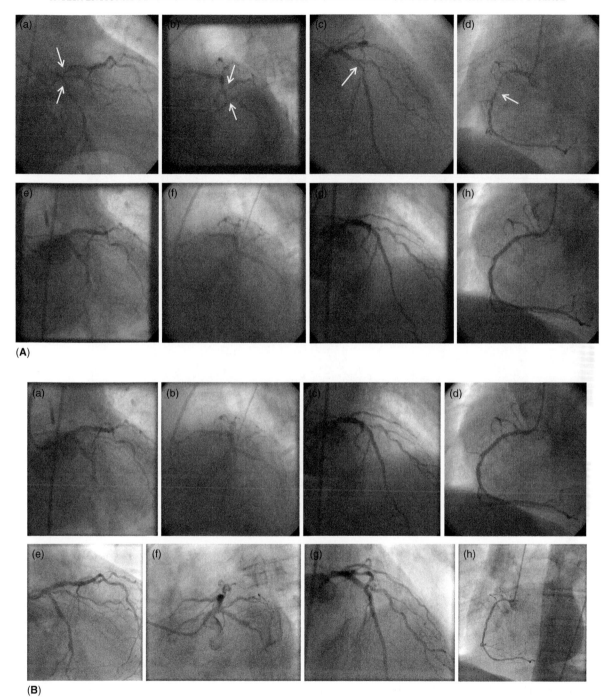

Figure 32.1 (**A**): Example of a complex case treated by PCI. Baseline angiography showing (*a*) and (*b*) complex distal LMS disease, involving the trifurcation of the LAD, LCx, and ramus intermediate (*arrows*); (*c*) additional disease of the mid-LAD (*arrow*); and (*d*) mid-RCA (*arrow*). (*e*)–(*h*) The same angiographic projections following successful multi-vessel PCI using DES. (**B**): Angiographic follow-up at three years. (*a*) –(*d*) Angiographic result following complex PCI. (*e*)–(*h*) The same angiographic projections seen at three years, showing no evidence of instent restenosis.

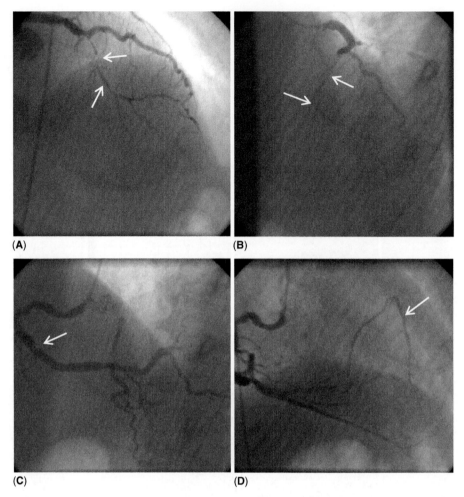

Figure 32.2 Example of a case most suited to CABG. (**A**) and (**B**) double occlusion of LAD (arrows), (**C**) large dominant RCA with focal lesion in the mid-vessel, and (**D**) retrograde filling of the distal LAD indicating a suitable target for LIMA grafting.

VIDEO CLIPS

Video clip 32.1 Example of a complex case successfully treated by PCI with DES.

Video clip 32.2 Example of a case most suited to CABG.

REFERENCES

1. Keeley EC, Boura JA, Grines CL. Primary angioplasty versus intravenous thrombolytic therapy for acute myocardial infarction: a quantitative review of 23 randomized trials. Lancet 2003; 361: 13–20.
2. Cantor WJ, Fitchett D, Borgundvaag B, et al.; For the TRANSFER-AMI trial investigators. Routine early angioplasty after fibrinolysis for acute myocardial infarction. N Engl J Med 2009; 360: 2705–18.
3. Scheller B, Hennen B, Hammer B, et al.; for the SIAM III study group. Beneficial Effects of immediate stenting after thrombolysis in acute myocardial infarction. J Am Coll Cardiol 2003; 42: 634–41.
4. Bavry AA, Kumbhani DJ, Rassi AN, et al. Benefit of early invasive therapy in acute coronary syndromes- a meta-analysis of contemporary randomized clinical trials. J Am Coll Cardiol 2006; 48: 1319–25.
5. Boden WE, O'Rourke RA, Teo KK, et al. Optimal medical therapy with or without PCI for stable coronary disease. N Engl J Med 2007; 356: 1503–16.
6. Serruys PW, Morice M, Kappetein AP, et al.; For the SYNTAX Investigators. Percutaneous coronary intervention versus coronary-artery bypass grafting for severe coronary artery disease. N Engl J Med 2009; 360: 961–72.
7. Katritsis DG Ioannidis, JP. Percutaneous coronary intervention versus conservative therapy in nonacute coronary artery disease: a meta-analysis. Circulation 2005; 111: 2906–12.
8. Henderson RA, Pocock SJ, Clayton TC, et al. Seven-year outcome in the RITA-2 trial: coronary angioplasty versus medical therapy. J Am Coll Cardiol 2003; 42: 1161–70.
9. Hueb W, Lopes NH, Gersh BJ, et al. Five-year follow-up of the Medicine, Angioplasty, or Surgery Study (MASS II)—a randomized controlled clinical trial of 3 therapeutic strategies for multivessel coronary artery disease. Circulation 2007; 115: 1082–9.
10. Kereiakes DJ, Teirstein PS, Sarembock IJ, et al. The truth and consequences of the COURAGE trial. J Am Coll Cardiol 2007; 50: 1598–603.

11. Stone GW, Ellis SG, Cox DA, et al.; TAXUS IV Investigators. A polymer-based, paclitaxel-eluting stent in patients with coronary artery disease. N Engl J Med 2004; 350: 221–31.

12. Moses JW, Leon MB, Popma JJ, et al.; SIRIUS Investigators. Sirolimus-eluting stents versus standard stents in pts with stenosis in a native coronary artery. N Engl J Med 2003; 349: 1315–23.

13. Serruys PW, Kutryk MJ, Ong AT. Coronary artery stents. N Engl J Med 2006; 354: 483–95.

14. Mehta RH, Roe MT, Chen AY, et al. Changing practice for non ST-segment elevation acute coronary syndromes: trends from the CRUSADE luality improvement initiative (abstr). Circulation 2005; 112: II793.

15. Maron DJ, Spertus JA, Mancini J, et al.; For the COURAGE Trial Research Group. Impact of an initial strategy of medical therapy without percutaneous coronary intervention in high-risk patients from the Clinical Outcomes Utilizing Revascularization and Aggressive Drug Evaluation (COURAGE) Trial. Am J Cardiol 2009; 104: 1055–62.

16. Hachamovitch R, Hayes SW, Friedman JD, Cohen I, Berman DS. Comparison of the short-term survival benefit associated with revascularization compared with medical therapy in patients with no prior coronary artery disease undergoing stress myocardial perfusion single photon emission computed tomography. Circulation 2003; 107: 2900–7.

17. Shaw LJ, Berman DS, Maron DJ, et al.; For the COURAGE Investigators. Optimal medical therapy with or without percutaneous coronary intervention to reduce ischemic burden: results from the Clinical Outcomes Utilizing Revascularization and Aggressive Drug Evaluation (COURAGE) trial nuclear substudy. Circulation 2008; 117: 1283–91.

18. Schomig A, Mehilli J, de Waha A, et al. A meta-analysis of 17 randomized trials of a percutaneous coronary intervention-based strategy in patients with stable coronary artery disease. J Am Coll Cardiol 2008; 52: 894–904.

19. Jeremias A, Kaul S, Rosengart TK. The impact of revascularization on mortality in patients with nonacute coronary artery disease. Am J Cardiol 2009; 122: 152–61.

20. Bravata DM, Gienger AL, McDonald KM, et al. Systematic review: the comparative effectiveness of percutaneous coronary interventions and coronary artery bypass graft surgery. Ann Intern Med 2007; 147: 703–16.

21. Hlatky MA, Boothroyd DB, Bravata DM, et al. Coronary artery bypass surgery compared with percutaneous coronary interventions for multivessel disease: a collaborative analysis of individual patient data from ten randomized trials. Lancet 2009; 373: 1190–7.

22. Schächinger V, Herdeg C, Scheller B. Best way to revascularize patients with main stem and three vessel lesions: patients should undergo PCI! Clin Res Cardiol. 2010; 99: 531–9.

23. Brooks MM, Alderman EL, Bates E, et al. The final 10-year follow-up results from the BARI randomized trial. J Am Coll Cardiol 2007; 49: 1600–6.

24. Morice M, Serruys PW, Keppetein AP, et al. Outcomes in patients with de novo left Main Disease treated with either percutaneous coronary intervention using paclitaxel-eluting stents or coronary artery bypass graft treatment in the synergy between percutaneous coronary intervention with TAXUS and cardiac surgery (SYN-TAX) trial. Circulation 2010; 121: 2645–53.

25. Stone GW, Midei M, Newman W, et al.; For the SPIRIT III Investigators. Randomized comparison of everolimus-eluting and paclitaxel-eluting stents: two-year clinical follow-up from the clinical evaluation of the xience v everolimus eluting coronary stent system in the treatment of patients with de novo native coronary artery lesions (SPIRIT) III trial. Circulation 2009; 119: 680–6.

26. Banning AP, Westaby S, Morice M, et al. Diabetic and nondiabetic patients with left main and/or 3-vessel coronary artery disease: comparison of outcomes with cardiac surgery and paclitaxel-eluting stents. J Am Coll Cardiol 2010; 55: 1067–75.

27. Wijns W, Kolh P, Danchin N, et al. Guidelines on myocardial revascularization: the task force on myocardial revascularization of the European Society of Cardiology (ESC) and the European Association for Cardio-Thoracic Surgery (EACTS). Eur Heart J 2010; 31: 2501–55.

28. Mintz GS, Nissen SE, Anderson WD, et al. American College of Cardiology Clinical Expert Consensus Document on Standards for Acquisition, Measurement and Reporting of Intravascular Ultrasound Studies (IVUS). A report of the American College of Cardiology Task Force on Clinical Expert Consensus Documents. J Am Coll Cardiol 2005; 95: 644–7.

29. Park SJ, Kim YH, Park DW, et al. Impact of intravascular ultrasound guidance on long-term mortality for unprotected left main coronary artery stenosis. Circ Cardiovasc Interv 2009; 2: 167–77.

30. Pijls NHJ, van Schaardenburgh P, Manoharan G, et al. Percutaneous coronary intervention of functionally nonsignificant stenosis: 5-year follow-up of the DEFER study. J Am Coll Cardiol 2007; 49: 2105–11.

31. Wiviott SD, Braunwald E, McCabe CH, et al.; Antman EM for the TRITON–TIMI 38 Investigators. Prasugrel versus clopidogrel in patients with acute coronary syndromes. N Engl J Med 2007; 357: 2001–15.

32. Wallentin L, Becker RC, Budaj A, et al.; For the PLATO Investigators. Ticagrelor versus clopidogrel in patients with acute coronary syndromes. N Engl J Med 2009; 361: 1045–57.

33 Surgical perspectives on the management of advanced stable coronary artery disease

Michael Mack, Stuart J. Head, and A. Pieter Kappetein

OUTLINE

Coronary artery bypass grafting (CABG) has historically been regarded as the most appropriate strategy for the management of patient with extensive coronary disease. However, percutaneous coronary intervention (PCI) has emerged as an alternative that has been adopted in increasingly complex patient subsets. Whether PCI or CABG is preferable depends on lesion characteristics and patient co-morbidities. However, PCI and CABG outcomes have converged significantly over the last decade and thus the indication for PCI is expanding. While bypass surgery has seen less spectacular advances than PCI, technical improvements that reduce the invasiveness of the procedure and the advent of off-pump bypass have reinvigorated this field. Off-pump surgery should be performed more often and complete arterial revascularization is encouraged. Further randomized trials, comparing current state of the art surgical techniques with percutaneous intervention, in complex patient subsets, are warranted.

INTRODUCTION

Coronary artery disease (CAD) has historically been treated with CABG, since the Coronary Artery Surgery Study (CASS) trial showed that this was superior to medical management (1). However, after the introduction of PCI with balloon dilatation and, subsequently, stents, interventional cardiologists have increasingly treated patients with this less invasive technique (2–3). The current PCI-to-CABG ratio averages 3.29 in western countries (Fig. 33.1). Whether PCI or CABG should be the preferred treatment in certain patients remains a matter of debate. Indications for PCI have significantly increased over the last decades, but the PCI/CABG tradeoff still depends on specific factors, such as the complexity of coronary disease and co-morbidities. With continuous improvement in stenting, efforts should be made to improve outcomes with bypass surgery even more. This chapter focuses on these aspects and discusses in more detail the advantages of certain CABG techniques.

PCI OR CABG?

Percutaneous intervention was rapidly adopted in the 1980s and subsequently a number of randomized trials were published in the mid-1990s comparing PCI to CABG (3). The effort continued with larger randomized trials, which were pooled in a recent meta-analysis (4). This analysis of nearly 8000 patients showed that PCI and CABG had similar mortality at five years of follow-up. The authors rightfully concluded that especially in more complex patients with diabetes or older age, CABG should be the preferred treatment.

After the era of balloon angioplasty and bare-metal stents, the introduction of drug-eluting stents (DES) raised the expectations that outcomes after PCI may improve and approach those reported with CABG. The Synergy between PCI with TAXus and Cardiac Surgery (SYNTAX) trial was the first to randomize patients with complex coronary disease to PCI with DES or CABG (5). At one year, non-inferiority of PCI was not met for the primary endpoint of major adverse cardiac or cerebrovascular events (MACCE): a composite of death, stroke, myocardial infarction, and repeat revascularization. However, the SYNTAX trial did validate the SYNTAX score, a tool to grade the complexity of coronary disease by combining lesion location and characteristics (6). In the trial, patients with a low complexity (score 0–22) had similar rates of MACCE with PCI and CABG (13.6 vs. 14.7%, respectively), even after three years of follow-up (22.7 vs. 22.5%, respectively) (7). However patients with intermediate (23–32) and high (≥33) complexity scores had better outcome with CABG (Fig. 33.2).

Left Main Disease

Interestingly, subgroup analyses from the SYNTAX trial showed that patients with left main (LM) disease had similar outcomes in the low and intermediate SYNTAX score groups (7). At three years, MACCE occurred less frequently after PCI than CABG in patients with low scores (18.0 vs. 23.0%, respectively). The MACCE rates were identical in the intermediate score patients (23.4%), suggesting that CABG is the preferred treatment only in patients with LM disease and high SYNTAX scores. However, subgroup analyses have low statistical power and these outcomes should, therefore, be labeled as hypothesis-generating (8). Even though a recent meta-analysis showed similar outcomes with PCI and CABG in LM patients, larger trials dedicated to LM patients should be performed (9). An attempt was made with the Premier of Randomized Comparison of Bypass Surgery versus Angioplasty using Sirolimus-Eluting Stent in Patients with Left Main Coronary Artery Disease (PRECOMBAT) trial, but methodological flaws meant the trial data coud not offer any substantiated conclusions (10,11). The currently ongoing Evaluation of XIENCE PRIME or XIENCE V versus Coronary Artery Bypass Surgery for Effectiveness of Left Main Revascularization (EXCEL) trial will determine whether PCI is a legitimate alternative to CABG, and would be a viable treatment option in patients with low or intermediate SYNTAX scores.

Diabetics

Patients with diabetes mellitus have been a challenging subgroup for revascularization ever since the Bypass Angioplasty Revascularization Investigation (BARI) trial showed that this subgroup

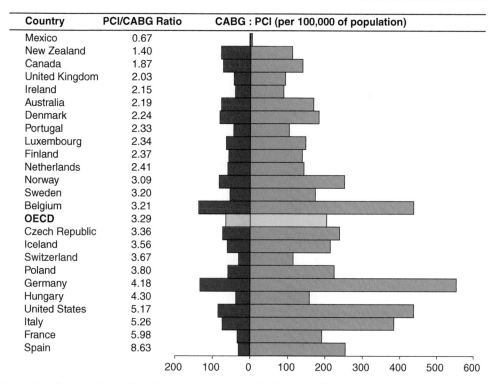

Country	PCI/CABG Ratio
Mexico	0.67
New Zealand	1.40
Canada	1.87
United Kingdom	2.03
Ireland	2.15
Australia	2.19
Denmark	2.24
Portugal	2.33
Luxembourg	2.34
Finland	2.37
Netherlands	2.41
Norway	3.09
Sweden	3.20
Belgium	3.21
OECD	**3.29**
Czech Republic	3.36
Iceland	3.56
Switzerland	3.67
Poland	3.80
Germany	4.18
Hungary	4.30
United States	5.17
Italy	5.26
France	5.98
Spain	8.63

Figure 33.1 Revascularization procedures performed in countries throughout the Western world, showing the PCI-to-CABG ratio. *Source:* From Ref. 48.

had better survival after CABG than PCI (12). At five years, survival was 80.6 versus 65.5% in CABG and PCI patients, respectively ($p = 0.003$). Based on this data, rapid succession of subgroup analyses from other trials followed (13). Again, these were ultimately pooled in a meta-analysis, showing that mortality in non-diabetics was similar with PCI and CABG, but that diabetic patients had significantly better survival with CABG (Fig. 33.3) (4). However, limited results are available from comparisons between CABG and PCI with DES. The SYNTAX trial still showed that results with CABG were better than with PCI. Nevertheless, in patients with a low SYNTAX score, outcomes were nearly identical in non-diabetic and diabetic subgroups (14).

The dedicated Coronary Artery Revascularization in Diabetes (CARDia) trial confirmed that PCI is not non-inferior to CABG in diabetic patients with multivessel coronary disease requiring revascularization (15). Although a trend to significant interaction was found in patients treated with bare-metal or DES compared to CABG, the comparative outcomes of PCI with DES versus CABG should be investigated in other trials dedicated to diabetics. It is expected that the FREEDOM trial will report similar findings in 2012 (16) for diabetic patients.

Decision-making

In general, the current guidelines on myocardial revascularization indicate that patients with stable angina have a class IA indication for CABG, with the exception of patients with single- or two-vessel disease without involvement of the proximal

left anterior descending artery (Fig. 33.4) (17). Despite these and other guidelines, inappropriate use of revascularization procedures remains an issue (18,19). A recent study showed that PCI for stable angina was inappropriate in 11.6%, and in another 38.0%, the indication was uncertain. The Clinical Outcomes Utilizing Revascularization and Aggressive Drug Evaluation (COURAGE) trial reported after a median follow-up of 4.6 years that there was no benefit of PCI on top of optimal medical therapy compared to medical therapy alone, with regard to death and myocardial infarction (20). This suggests that PCI is sometimes performed without a clear indication. Having said this, revascularization can also be underused (21). Studies have shown that approximately 25–30% of patients that needed revascularization were not treated (21–23). This was associated with significantly higher mortality during follow-up over three years, with a hazard ratio of 3.23 [95% confidence interval (CI) 1.96–5.26].

The decision-making process should include a balanced Heart Team, so that patients receive optimal therapy, improving both outcomes of PCI and CABG (24).

Non-randomizable patients

The SYNTAX trial mandated multidisciplinary patient evaluation to judge whether clinical equipoise could be met with PCI and CABG. If so, patients were randomized. Patients in whom either PCI or CABG was favorable were included in nested registries; a PCI-registry for CABG ineligible patients; and a

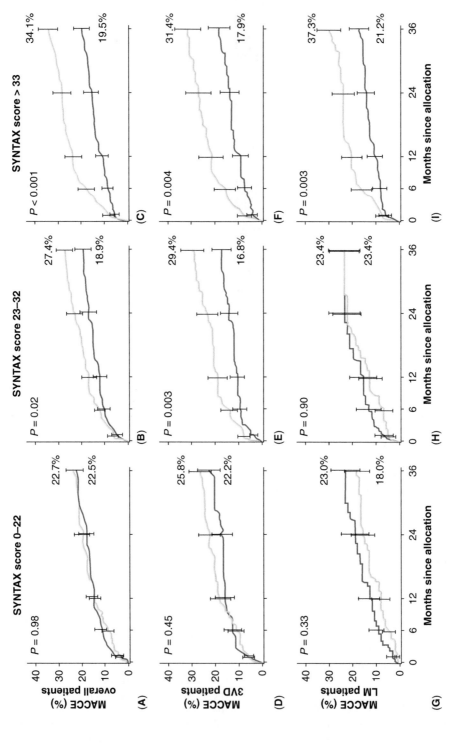

Figure 33.2 Major adverse cardiac or cerebrovascular event rates after PCI (*yellow*) and CABG (*blue*) stratified by lesion and SYNTAX score. *Abbreviations*: 3VD, three-vessel disease; LM, left main; MACCE, major adverse cardiac or cerebrovascular events. *Source*: From Ref. 7.

Number of patients*

CABG no diabetes	3263	3169	3089	2877	2677	2267	1592	1380	1274
CABG diabetes	615	587	575	532	498	421	257	225	200
PCI no diabetes	3298	3217	3148	2918	2725	2281	1608	1393	1288
PCI diabetes	618	574	555	508	475	373	218	179	160

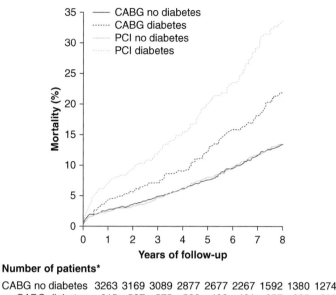

Figure 33.3 Unadjusted mortality in patients assigned to CABG or PCI by diabetic status. *Abbreviations*: CABG, coronary artery bypass grafting; PCI, percutaneous coronary intervention. *Source*: From Ref. 4.

Subset of CAD by anatomy	Favours CABG	Favours PCI
1VD or 2VD – non-proximal LAD	IIb C	I C
1VD or 2VD – proximal LAD	I A	IIa B
3VD simple lesions, full functional revascularization achievable with PCI, SYNTAX score ≤22	I A	IIa B
3VD complex lesions, incomplete revascularization achievable with PCI, SYNTAX score >22	I A	III A
Left main (isolated or 1VD, ostium/shaft)	I A	IIa B
Left main (isolated or 1VD, distal bifurcation)	I A	IIb B
Left main + 2VD or 3VD, SYNTAX score ≤32	I A	IIb B
Left main + 2VD or 3VD, SYNTAX score ≥33	I A	III B

Figure 33.4 Indications for CABG or PCI for patients with stable angina with lesions suitable for both procedures and low predicted surgical mortality. *Abbreviations*: CABG, coronary artery bypass grafting; CAD, coronary artery disease; LAD, left anterior descending; PCI, percutaneous coronary intervention; VD, vessel disease. *Source*: From Ref. 17.

CABG-registry for PCI ineligible patients. Of the 3075 patients treated within SYNTAX, the Heart Team decided that 198 (6.4%) patients could only undergo PCI, while 1075 (35.0%) patients were included in the CABG registry (25). Patients in the PCI registry were generally older and had severe co-morbidities in comparison with the patients in the trial. It was not unexpected that these patients, therefore, had high MACCE rates, but still PCI was feasible in this very high-risk patient population. CABG-registry patients had higher SYNTAX scores compared to patients in the trial, thus were deemed too complex for PCI treatment. A joint analysis of these CABG trial and registry patients showed that contemporary CABG results are excellent (26). Remarkably, the CABG registry patients had better outcomes than in the trial, which was attributed to the achievement of more complete revascularization in the registry arm. This highlights the fact that guidelines propose CABG as the preferred treatment in nearly all indications, and this evidence can even be stronger by the use of specific surgical techniques such as off-pump surgery and improved revascularization by using arterial grafts and pursuing complete revascularization.

CABG

Rapid progression of new technologies caused significant improvements in results with PCI over the last decades. Outcomes after CABG have stagnated relative to PCI. As a result, PCI versus CABG outcomes have converged and many patients who historically were treated with CABG now undergo PCI. However, efforts can be made to furthermore improve perioperative and long-term outcomes of CABG by reducing its invasiveness and ensuring better graft patency over an extended follow-up.

Off-pump CABG

After the initial reports of CABG performed on a beating heart, off-pump surgery was embraced by the community and, in

2001, approximately 25% of CABG procedures were performed off-pump (27). In the SYNTAX trial that enrolled patients between 2005 and 2007, only 15.0% of the procedures were performed off-pump (5). Theoretically, off-pump CABG could reduce rates of morbidity and even mortality by avoiding cardiopulmonary bypass and aortic manipulation. A particular advantage relates to stroke, which would potentially be lower with off-pump than with on-pump CABG.

Initial trials reported similar results for on- and off-pump surgery. Although considerable research has been devoted to the analysis of which revascularization method is superior, there has been no consensus. A recent analysis demonstrated a 30% [95% CI 1–51%] relative risk reduction with pooled data from 49 studies (27). In addition, off-pump surgery was a safe procedure with similar rates of all-cause mortality and myocardial infarction as compared to patients who went on-pump CABG. It can even be suggested that it is much safer than on-pump surgery in patient cohorts at high risk for operative mortality, since off-pump surgery seems to provide significantly better results than on-pump surgery in these patients (28).

Despite the short-term benefit of off-pump surgery over on-pump, concerns were raised about the longevity of the grafts with off-pump surgery. Reports were published of increased rates of mortality and repeat revascularization during follow-up (29). A recent study with 8081 patients and over 48,000 patient-years of follow-up supports this hypothesis and has demonstrated reduced long-term survival in patients that underwent off-pump CABG, with an adjusted hazard ratio of 1.18 [95% CI 1.02–1.38] (Fig. 33.5) (30).

The hypothesis behind the increased incidence of mortality and revascularization is that off-pump CABG does not result in

graft patency as good as on-pump surgery. Data from the largest study to date, the Randomized On/Off Bypass (ROOBY) trial, suggested that even at one year, there was a statistically significant difference in graft patency (31). The relative risk of at least one graft occlusion in a patient was 27% (95% CI 9–48%) with off-pump surgery. Evaluating all grafts, patency was 87.8% in the on-pump group, but only 82.6% in off-pump patients ($p < 0.001$). This was mainly driven by saphenous veins, which showed an overall lower patency of 83.8% and 76.6%, respectively ($p < 0.001$). Left internal thoracic grafts had comparable results (96.2% vs. 95.3%, respectively, $p = 0.46$). The shortcoming of the ROOBY trial was that the operations were performed by surgeons without much experience, although some other trials involving highly experienced surgeons and a meta-analysis confirmed the findings (32–34). Furthermore, off-pump CABG has been associated with increased rates of incomplete revascularization, which could lead to reduced long-term survival (35).

Minimally Invasive CABG

One of the bottlenecks for CABG remains its invasiveness. As some cardiologists refer to CABG as a procedure in which 'the chest is cracked open' patients get scared about the prospect of postoperative pain and extensive rehabilitation, even though CABG might provide a superior outcome over PCI.

Minimally invasive CABG (MIDCAB) surgery has the potential to become a more patient-friendly technique and less of a deterrent procedure. Although MIDCAB has been associated with increased pain postoperatively, length of hospital stay is markedly reduced, and there is a significantly improved quality of life as compared to conventional CABG (36,37). Through a smaller incision, the surgeon can perform bypass surgery without the need for a sternotomy. However, visualization is limited to the left anterior descending (LAD) artery, and therefore, only patients with isolated LAD stenosis can undergo complete revascularization through MIDCAB surgery. Several prospective studies and randomized trials have compared the technique with stenting for patients with isolated LAD disease. A meta-analysis summarized these data and concluded that the two therapies were equivalent for death, stroke, and myocardial infarction (38). As expected, recurrence of angina and repeat revascularization occurred more frequently with PCI.

For patients with multi-vessel disease, the MIDCAB surgery can be combined with PCI to generate a hybrid procedure. In these cases, the LAD will be revascularized with the left internal mammary artery to improve long-term survival, while stents are placed in 'less significant' areas to reduce symptoms and the risk of myocardial infarction.

Arterial Revascularization

The choice of grafts is essential to guarantee excellent long-term results. As alluded to previously, saphenous vein grafts have lower patency than arterial grafts when used for revascularization (39). Therefore, the use of internal mammary artery (IMA) grafts is

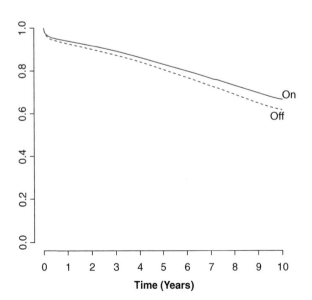

Figure 33.5 Adjusted mortality for on- and off-pump CABG procedures. *Source*: From Ref. 30.

encouraged, especially the left IMA (LIMA), which shows excellent results compared to the right IMA (RIMA), since it remains in situ (40).

Contemporary IMA graft use is still not as high as warranted. Although the rate is increasing, there is some inter hospital-variance in using at least one IMA graft. Some centres only have a rate of 45–65%, failing to provide optimal care to patients that are good candidates (41). In SYNTAX, of the 1541 procedures performed in the trial and registry, the rate of using at least one arterial graft was satisfactory; however, this was still only in 97.1% of cases. More disturbingly, the use of bilateral IMA (BIMA) grafts in the United States was shown to be only 4.0% in an analysis with 541,368 patients (Fig. 33.6) (41). Centers in the SYNTAX trial performed significantly better with a rate of 22.7%.

Bilateral IMA grafting is associated with reduced mortality during the first year post-surgery and during long-term follow-up, and it should be the standard therapy for patients with multivessel coronary disease. An adjusted hazard ratio of 0.76 (95% CI 0.61–0.94) was found after a mean follow-up of 7.1 years, compared to single IMA grafting (42). A meta-analysis had similar results; a pooled analysis of seven studies with 11,269 single and 4693 bilateral IMA grafts demonstrated a hazard ratio for death of 0.81 (95% CI 0.70–0.94) (43). Due to the technically more challenging nature of BIMA grafting, some surgeons might be reticent to use BIMA grafts. In the only randomized trial to date, the ART trial, 16.4% of the patients allocated to BIMA did not receive the allocated treatment (44). It is time-consuming and there are concerns over higher morbidity and mortality rates. The ART trial included 3102 patients and rates of stroke, myocardial, and revascularization at 30 days and one year were similar between single IMA and BIMA groups (45). Indeed, there was an increased risk of sternal wound reconstruction: relative risk 3.24 (95% CI 1.54–6.83), but this did not lead to increased mortality, since the Kaplan-Meier showed a superimposed cumulative incidence. Longer follow-up will determine whether survival is indeed superior with BIMA grafts. Still, surgeons should more often consider using both IMA grafts to improve CABG outcomes.

A patent graft provides an additional advantage over PCI. Stenting directly treats the coronary lesion that causes symptoms. However, other lesions can arise in the same vessel that warrant stenting. A patent graft not only bypasses the current lesion but also protects the myocardium from future lesions. It, therefore, not only functions as treatment but also as prevention.

Complete Revascularization

Incomplete revascularization has been shown to increase the rate of mortality and recurrent symptoms during long-term follow-up. In the SYNTAX trial, patients randomized to PCI had an increased hazard with incomplete revascularization (hazard ratio = 1.55, 95% CI 1.15–2.08), while patients randomized to CABG did not have increased MACCE (Fig. 33.7) (46).

The difference in the effect on outcomes after PCI and CABG can be ascribed to the cause of incomplete revascularization. In CABG patients, this is frequently caused by diffuse disease in distal narrow vessels. However, whether these vessels are actually revascularized only has a minor influence on outcomes. Only a small area of myocardium remains at risk, and this incomplete revascularization is sometimes referred to as appropriate incomplete revascularization. In PCI patients, the cause of incomplete revascularization is most often a chronic total occlusion that cannot be opened. The myocardium at risk can be much larger and incomplete revascularization could result in adverse outcomes. Therefore, this is referred to as inappropriate incomplete revascularization.

The rate of incomplete revascularization has been shown to be higher in patients who underwent off-pump CABG (35,47). In contrast to incomplete revascularization with on-pump surgery, inappropriate incomplete revascularization is more often present in patients that underwent off-pump CABG. A study showed that all-cause mortality was significantly different between complete and incomplete revascularization groups in off-pump patients ($p = 0.02$), while this was not the case in on-pump patients ($p > 0.20$) (47).

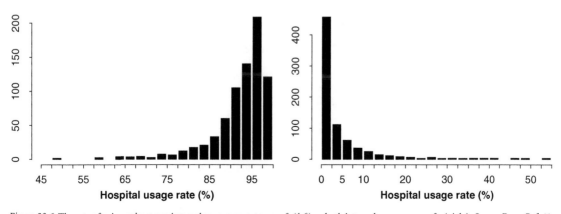

Figure 33.6 The rate of using at least one internal mammary artery graft (*left*) or both internal mammary grafts (*right*). *Source*: From Ref. 41.

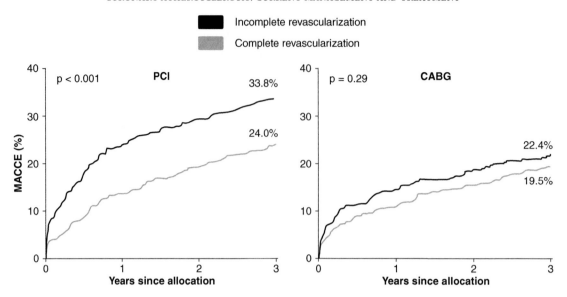

Figure 33.7 The effect of incomplete revascularization on major adverse cardiac or cerebrovascular events (MACCE) in the SYNTAX trial in the PCI (*left*) and CABG (*right*) cohorts. *Abbreviations*: CABG, coronary artery bypass grafting; MACCE, major adverse cardiac or cerebrovascular events; PCI, percutaneous coronary intervention. *Source*: From Ref. 46.

Focus Box 33.1

PCI has emerged as a revascularization strategy to be considered in a large number of patients

The PCI-to-CABG ratio has significantly increased over the last decade

Diabetic patients have been a challenging subgroup for coronary revascularization, but these patients should preferably undergo CABG

In patients with low coronary lesion complexity, PCI can be an alternative to CABG

Inappropriate use of revascularization is not uncommon and introduces unnecessary procedural risk

Underuse of revascularization in good candidates is associated with increased mortality during follow-up

Off-pump surgery reduces the risk of perioperative stroke but may have lower graft patency over follow-up

Off-pump surgery is especially beneficial in patients with a high operative risk

Arterial revascularization is associated with significantly better outcomes than venous grafting and should be performed more

Bilateral internal mammary artery use should be encouraged, since it has been shown to be superior to single internal mammary artery grafting

Completeness of revascularization is especially important in PCI patients, because incomplete revascularization is more often inappropriate in these cases

PERSONAL PERSPECTIVE

Even though PCI is quickly catching up with CABG, for many patients, CABG should still be the preferred revascularization strategy. The 'Achilles heel' of CABG, stroke, can be reduced by performing off-pump surgery, and experienced surgeons should preferably perform off-pump surgery to reduce postoperative complications. Even though graft patency can be slightly reduced after off-pump CABG, the use of at least one IMA graft and preferably both IMAs can eliminate potential late graft occlusion or recurrence of symptoms. Completeness of revascularization remains an issue, but distal small vessels with diffuse disease do not always need revascularization. Nevertheless, one should always avoid incomplete revascularization where this would be inappropriate.

Although CABG already is an excellent therapy with low rates of adverse events postoperatively and during long-term follow-up, efforts should always be made to improve the procedure.

Over the last few years, interventional cardiologists and surgeons have learned to work together as a Heart Team. The complementary nature of PCI and CABG should encourage both specialties even more to combine their efforts so that best care can be given to all patients.

REFERENCES

1. Coronary Artery Surgery Study (CASS) principal investigators and associates. Coronary artery surgery study (CASS): a randomized trial of coronary artery bypass surgery. Survival data. Circulation 1983; 68: 939–50.
2. Epstein AJ, Polsky D, Yang F, Yang L, Groeneveld PW. Coronary revascularization trends in the United States, 2001–2008. JAMA 2011; 305: 1769–76.
3. Yusuf S, Zucker D, Peduzzi P, et al. Effect of coronary artery bypass graft surgery on survival: overview of 10-year results from randomised trials by the Coronary Artery Bypass Graft Surgery Trialists Collaboration. Lancet 1994; 344: 563–70.

4. Hlatky MA, Boothroyd DB, Bravata DM, et al. Coronary artery bypass surgery compared with percutaneous coronary interventions for multivessel disease: a collaborative analysis of individual patient data from ten randomised trials. Lancet 2009; 373: 1190–7.

5. Serruys PW, Morice MC, Kappetein AP, et al. Percutaneous coronary intervention versus coronary-artery bypass grafting for severe coronary artery disease. N Engl J Med 2009; 360: 961–72.

6. Sianos G, Morel MA, Kappetein AP, et al. The SYNTAX Score: an angiographic tool grading the complexity of coronary artery disease. EuroIntervention 2005; 1: 219–27.

7. Kappetein AP, Feldman TE, Mack MJ, et al. Comparison of coronary bypass surgery with drug-eluting stenting for the treatment of left main and/or three-vessel disease: 3-year follow-up of the SYNTAX trial. Eur Heart J 2011; 32: 2125–34.

8. Wang R, Lagakos SW, Ware JH, Hunter DJ, Drazen JM. Statistics in medicine–reporting of subgroup analyses in clinical trials. N Engl J Med 2007; 357: 2189–94.

9. Capodanno D, Stone GW, Morice MC, Bass TA, Tamburino C. Percutaneous coronary intervention versus coronary artery bypass graft surgery in left main coronary artery disease: a meta-analysis of randomized clinical data. J Am Coll Cardiol 2011; 58: 1426–32.

10. Correia LC. Stents versus CABG for left main coronary artery disease. N Engl J Med 2011; 365: 181; author reply-2.

11. Park SJ, Kim YH, Park DW, et al. Randomized trial of stents versus bypass surgery for left main coronary artery disease. N Engl J Med 2011; 364: 1718–27.

12. The Bypass Angioplasty Revascularization Investigation (BARI) Investigators. Comparison of coronary bypass surgery with angioplasty in patients with multivessel disease. N Engl J Med 1996; 335: 217–25.

13. Roffi M, Angiolillo DJ, Kappetein AP. Current concepts on coronary revascularization in diabetic patients. Eur Heart J 2011; 32: 2748–57.

14. Mack MJ, Banning AP, Serruys PW, et al. Bypass versus drug-eluting stents at three years in SYNTAX patients with diabetes mellitus or metabolic syndrome. Ann Thorac Surg 2011; 92: 2140–6.

15. Kapur A, Hall RJ, Malik IS, et al. Randomized comparison of percutaneous coronary intervention with coronary artery bypass grafting in diabetic patients. 1-year results of the CARDia (Coronary Artery Revascularization in Diabetes) trial. J Am Coll Cardiol 2010; 55: 432–40.

16. Farkouh ME, Dangas G, Leon MB, et al. Design of the Future REvascularization Evaluation in patients with Diabetes mellitus: optimal management of Multivessel disease (FREEDOM) Trial. Am Heart J 2008; 155: 215–23.

17. Task Force on Myocardial Revascularization of the European Society of C, the European Association for Cardio-Thoracic S, European Association for Percutaneous Cardiovascular I, et al. Guidelines on myocardial revascularization. Eur J Cardiothorac Surg 2010; 38(Suppl): S1–S52.

18. Chan PS, Patel MR, Klein LW, et al. Appropriateness of percutaneous coronary intervention. JAMA 2011; 306: 53–61.

19. Patel MR, Dehmer GJ, Hirshfeld JW, et al. ACCF/SCAI/STS/AATS/ AHA/ASNC 2009 Appropriateness Criteria for Coronary Revascularization: a report by the American College of Cardiology Foundation Appropriateness Criteria Task Force, Society for Cardiovascular Angiography and Interventions, Society of Thoracic Surgeons, American Association for Thoracic Surgery, American Heart Association, and the American Society of Nuclear Cardiology Endorsed by the American Society of Echocardiography, the Heart Failure Society of America, and the Society of Cardiovascular Computed Tomography. J Am Coll Cardiol 2009; 53: 530–53.

20. Boden WE, O'Rourke RA, Teo KK, et al. Optimal medical therapy with or without PCI for stable coronary disease. N Engl J Med 2007; 356: 1503–16.

21. Filardo G, Maggioni AP, Mura G, et al. The consequences of underuse of coronary revascularization; results of a cohort study in Northern Italy. Eur Heart J 2001; 22: 654–62.

22. Kravitz RL, Laouri M, Kahan JP, et al. Validity of criteria used for detecting underuse of coronary revascularization. JAMA 1995; 274: 632–8.

23. Leape LL, Hilborne LH, Bell R, Kamberg C, Brook RH. Underuse of cardiac procedures: do women, ethnic minorities, and the uninsured fail to receive needed revascularization? Ann Intern Med 1999; 130: 183–92.

24. Head SJ, Bogers AJ, Serruys PW, Takkenberg JJ, Kappetein AP. A crucial factor in shared decision making: the team approach. Lancet 2011; 377: 1836.

25. Head SJ, Holmes DR Jr, Mack MJ, et al. Risk profile and 3-year outcomes from the SYNTAX percutaneous coronary intervention and coronary artery bypass grafting nested registries. JACC Cardiovasc Interv; in press.

26. Mohr FW, Rastan AJ, Serruys PW, et al. Complex coronary anatomy in coronary artery bypass graft surgery: impact of complex coronary anatomy in modern bypass surgery? Lessons learned from the SYNTAX trial after two years. J Thorac Cardiovasc Surg 2011; 141: 130–40.

27. Afilado J, Rasti M, Ohayon SM, Shimony A, Eisenberg MJ. Off-pump vs. on-pump coronary artery bypass surgery: an updated meta-analysis and meta-regression of randomized trials. Eur Heart J; in press.

28. Puskas JD, Thourani VH, Kilgo P, et al. Off-pump coronary artery bypass disproportionately benefits high-risk patients. Ann Thorac Surg 2009; 88: 1142–7.

29. Williams ML, Muhlbaier LH, Schroder JN, et al. Risk-adjusted short- and long-term outcomes for on-pump versus off-pump coronary artery bypass surgery. Circulation 2005; 112: I366–70.

30. Filardo G, Grayburn PA, Hamilton C, et al. Comparing long-term survival between patients undergoing off-pump and on-pump coronary artery bypass graft operations. Ann Thorac Surg 2011; 92: 571–7; discussion 7–8.

31. Shroyer AL, Grover FL, Hattler B, et al. On-pump versus off-pump coronary-artery bypass surgery. N Engl J Med 2009; 361: 1827–37.

32. Sousa Uva M, Cavaco S, Oliveira AG, et al. Early graft patency after off-pump and on-pump coronary bypass surgery: a prospective randomized study. Eur Heart J 2010; 31: 2492–9.

33. Puskas JD, Mack MJ, Smith CR. On-pump versus off-pump CABG. N Engl J Med 2010; 362: 851; author reply 3–4.

34. Takagi H, Matsui M, Umemoto T. Lower graft patency after off-pump than on-pump coronary artery bypass grafting: an updated meta-analysis of randomized trials. J Thorac Cardiovasc Surg 2010; 140: e45–7.

35. Synnergren MJ, Ekroth R, Oden A, Rexius H, Wiklund L. Incomplete revascularization reduces survival benefit of coronary artery bypass grafting: role of off-pump surgery. J Thorac Cardiovasc Surg 2008; 136: 29–36.

36. Groh MA, Sutherland SE, Burton HG 3rd, Johnson AM, Ely SW. Port-access coronary artery bypass grafting: technique and comparative results. Ann Thorac Surg 1999; 68: 1506–8.

37. Diegeler A, Walther T, Metz S, et al. Comparison of MIDCAP versus conventional CABG surgery regarding pain and quality of life. Heart Surg Forum 1999; 2: 290–5; discussion 5–6.

38. Aziz O, Rao C, Panesar SS, et al. Meta-analysis of minimally invasive internal thoracic artery bypass versus percutaneous revascularisation for isolated lesions of the left anterior descending artery. BMJ 2007; 334: 617.

39. Goldman S, Zadina K, Moritz T, et al. Long-term patency of saphenous vein and left internal mammary artery grafts after coronary artery bypass surgery: results from a Department of Veterans Affairs Cooperative Study. J Am Coll Cardiol 2004; 44: 2149–56.

40. Hayward PA, Buxton BF. Contemporary coronary graft patency: 5-year observational data from a randomized trial of conduits. Ann Thorac Surg 2007; 84: 795–9.

41. Tabata M, Grab JD, Khalpey Z, et al. Prevalence and variability of internal mammary artery graft use in contemporary multivessel coronary artery bypass graft surgery: analysis of the Society of Thoracic Surgeons National Cardiac Database. Circulation 2009; 120: 935–40.

42. Kieser TM, Lewin AM, Graham MM, et al. Outcomes associated with bilateral internal thoracic artery grafting: the importance of age. Ann Thorac Surg 2011; 92: 1269–75; discussion 75–6.

43. Taggart DP, D'Amico R, Altman DG. Effect of arterial revascularisation on survival: a systematic review of studies comparing bilateral and single internal mammary arteries. Lancet 2001; 358: 870–5.

44. Kappetein AP. Bilateral mammary artery vs. single mammary artery grafting: promising early results: but will the match finish with enough players? Eur Heart J 2010; 31: 2444–6.

45. Taggart DP, Altman DG, Gray AM, et al. Randomized trial to compare bilateral vs. single internal mammary coronary artery bypass grafting: 1-year results of the Arterial Revascularisation Trial (ART). Eur Heart J 2010; 31: 2470–81.

46. Head SJ, Mack MJ, Holmes DR Jr, et al. Incidence, predictors, and outcomes of incomplete revascularization after stenting and bypass surgery: a 3-year follow-up subgroup analysis of syntax. Eur J Cardiothorac Surg 2012; 41: 535–41.

47. Kleisli T, Cheng W, Jacobs MJ, et al. In the current era, complete revascularization improves survival after coronary artery bypass surgery. J Thorac Cardiovasc Surg 2005; 129: 1283–91.

48. OECD (2009), Health at a Glance 2009: OECD Indicators, OECD Publishing.

34 Hybrid treatments and future perspectives

G. Russell Reiss and Mathew R. Williams

OUTLINE

Hybrid treatments for CAD combine the durability of the LIMA to LAD bypass graft with the limited invasiveness of PCI offering a less morbid yet long-lasting alternative to conventional surgery. Cardiovascular patients today are frail and complex. Many of them will not withstand traditional on-pump bypass surgeries secondary to multiple comorbidities. This fact, coupled with mounting evidence that long-term SVG patency is limited, argues in favor of incorporating DES technology into any definitive myocardial revascularization plan involving non-LAD lesions. Three strategies for HCR include: (*i*) PCI prior to MIDCAB, (*ii*) MIDCAB prior to PCI, and (*iii*) Simultaneous MIDCAB/PCI. Each has its own advantages and disadvantages with no current consensus on best approach. In addition, the economic aspects regarding hospital costs and reimbursement are complicated precluding many hybrid procedures from gaining widespread acceptance. Hybrid procedures are best performed utilizing the Heart Team model involving a multidisciplinary team that includes interventional cardiology, cardiovascular surgery, non-invasive cardiology, and anesthesiology. This team works in concert to assure a seamless operation for the often high-risk hybrid patient. Performing more complex hybrid procedures such as simultaneous MIDCAB/PCI or newer procedures such as TAVR requires a well-designed hybrid operating room.

INTRODUCTION

In the treatment of coronary artery disease (CAD) a "hybrid" approach is one that combines percutaneous revascularization methodology historically only available in the catheterization laboratory with state-of-the-art surgical techniques traditionally only available in the operating room. This combination offers CAD patients the best possible therapeutic option for any given set of cardiovascular lesions (1). Hybrid treatments for CAD are currently in use in several cardiac centers throughout the world with ongoing investigations being performed in an effort to determine safety, efficacy, and cost effectiveness (1–4). Currently, several questions remain in terms of optimal methodology, logistics, and timing of the various stages of hybrid procedures, and whether indeed the hybrid approach imparts both a clinical and economic advantage to both the patient and the hospital (5).

Hybrid Coronary Revascularization

Isolated Coronary Artery Disease

The left internal mammary artery (LIMA) anastamosis to left anterior descending artery (LAD) has a patency rate up to and exceeding 20 years for many patients. Thus, for the foreseeable future, the LIMA–LAD graft remains the most durable method

of target lesion revascularization (TLR) for coronary artery disease (CAD). Unfortunately, the durability of the saphenous vein graft (SVG) has not achieved such status. Current statistics on SVGs to non-LAD targets show that many of these technically well-placed bypasses are no longer in the first few months postoperative with some series reporting a closure rate as high as 30% after year (6,7). The mechanism of premature failure may be related to endothelial activation and injury to the endothelial layer during harvest that promotes leukocyte and platelet adhesion setting up a chronic inflammatory process (8). Along with these data, the advent of the drug-eluting stent (DES) has put the question: what is the best method of reducing TLR for non-LAD targets, SVG or percutaneous coronary intervention (PCI) utilizing DES. In isolated CAD the hybrid approach combines the LIMA-LAD graft, usually through a minimally invasive approach, with PCI using DES to the non-LAD targets. There is currently no consensus on whether this is the best approach for CAD patients and there are few series with enough patients to draw any best practice conclusions.

Concomitant Coronary and Valvular Disease

The morbidity and mortality of adding a concomitant coronary artery bypass graft (CABG) procedure to a heart valve procedure is not insignificant, with data indicating 50–100% increase in predicted risk of mortality in the perioperative period that is especially important in the re-operative setting. However, these studies have also shown that addressing severe CAD at the time of the valve surgery leads to better long-term outcomes despite the higher morbidity risk in the immediate postoperative period (9). Thus, whatever can be done to reduce the immediate perioperative risk associated with TLR for the associated CAD should theoretically bode well for the patient, thus showing a survival benefit over time. Hybrid PCI/valve replacement procedures allow the option of performing a minimally-invasive valve surgery while assuring complete coronary revascularization of coronary target lesions. Hybrid approaches for the patient needing concomitant valve repair or replacement and coronary revascularization usually involves a minimally-invasive valve replacement and PCI to any non-LAD lesions that are clinically significant. As with isolated CAD, there is currently no consensus or long-term data on the hybrid approach and reported series are extremely limited.

CURRENT STATUS

The choice of surgical conduit for coronary artery bypass grafting has remained fairly consistent for several decades with utilization of the SVG and the LIMA being considered the mainstay conduits for revascularization procedures. Techniques utilizing the LIMA–LAD and SVGs to the non-LAD targets are the current gold standard for operative CAD. For patients with multivessel pathology it is currently acceptable to perform these cases with or without cardiopulmonary bypass that is, on- or off-pump. With the increasingly frail surgical population there has been a shift toward minimally-invasive incisions and approaches with the combined use of thorascopic, robotic, and minithoracotomy techniques. The ability to take down the LIMA without a full sternotomy has encouraged many surgeons to perform minimally invasive direct coronary artery bypass (MIDCAB) utilizing a LIMA–LAD through keyhole-like incisions.

Because of the inferior patency rates of the SVG and the increasing durability of DES, hybrid revascularization is now being utilized more frequently in many centers throughout the world. With increasing data to support its use in non-LAD targets, DES may well become a first-line therapy for non-LAD targets in patients previously treated solely with surgical conduit.

Heart Team Approach to CAD

The core of any modern Heart Team is composed of a cardiovascular surgeon, an interventional cardiologist, a non-invasive cardiologist, and an anesthesiologist. There may also be additional members to include radiology and vascular surgeon along with a designated nursing coordinator, depending upon the nature of the intervention. Unlike the traditional patient-care pathway where each practitioner acts as an individual consultant, the Heart Team meets together routinely and functions as a singular unit discussing complex cases at a designated multidisciplinary team (MTD) conference prior to intervention. This core team is also the procedural team that is present in the operating room during the intervention, which promotes open communication throughout the entire hospitalization and treatment course. Depending on case volume, it is wise to convene MTD meetings at least weekly so a set routine becomes incorporated into the schedule of all interested parties. This provides a stable

---

Focus Box 34.1

The hybrid approach to CAD utilizes the LIM-LAD and PCI to the non-LAD lesions. There is currently no consensus on whether the hybrid approach is clinically and economically advantageous for either isolated CAD or combined valvular and coronary artery disease

---

Focus Box 34.2

The Heart Team model takes a multidisciplinary approach to complex coronary artery and valvular heart disease and is the preferred clinical method in centers performing hybrid interventions including HCR and TAVR

---

forum for discussion of all MTD procedures including HCR, transcatheter aortic valve replacement (TAVR) and other complex cases best approached in a hybrid fashion. In addition, this provides a venue for rigid program review with input from multiple viewpoints adding greater levels of quality control as techniques and procedures evolve.

In addition to providing the patient with the best available target vessel revascularization options, HCR is an exceptional example of how utilization of the Heart Team approach can prevent many untoward and adverse events by careful upfront planning and open communication. There is much to be coordinated prior to and during a HCR case including varying intensity levels of anesthetic management, efficient coordination of cross-trained interventional staff, and the ever-present potential need to emergently place a patient on cardiopulmonary bypass. Done well, the Heart Team approach provides the proper preparation for any hybrid procedure by keeping everyone well informed of the clinical plan.

INDICATIONS FOR HCR

Traditionally, the most commonly used conduit for non-LAD targets during conventional CABG has been the SVG. However, several studies employing routine postoperative angiography have demonstrated that the 6–12-month occlusion rates of SVGs range from 13–21% (10–12). The clinical introduction of DES has resulted in significant improvement in restenosis rates compared with bare metal stents (BMS) (13). Although restenosis rates have been quite low in large vessels with short uncomplicated lesions, there has also been an improvement observed in restenosis rates in more challenging target vessels. In a prospective study of 400 diabetic patients undergoing either sirolimus or paclitaxel DES, 6-month angiographic restenosis ranged from 8% in the paclitaxel group to 20% in the sirolimus group (14). In the SYNTAX trial, 226 diabetic patients with triple-vessel disease treated with multivessel stenting with first generation paclitaxel eluting stent had a 14.2% rate of target vessel revascularization at 12 months (15). This near equal short-term patency between DES and SVGs to non-LAD targets provides the fundamental basis for HCR in the treatment of multivessel CAD (16). Indications for HCR are multiple and careful selection and screening should be performed with input from both the surgeon and the cardiologist along with the members of the Heart Team.

One setting for HCR is in that of emergency revascularization of non-LAD lesions where there is isolated but complex LAD disease after successful PCI of the non-LAD culprit lesion with low risk for restenosis. This is commonly seen during ST-elevation myocardial infarction (STEMI) intervention where there is not an indication for complete revascularization during the acute setting but often a decision is made to complete revascularization at a later "staged" setting. The timing of the staged intervention depends on residual disease and type of stent that was used for the primary PCI. Use of minimally-invasive surgical techniques such as MIDCAB or totally endoscopic coronary artery bypass (TECAB) here allows complete revascularization of the complex residual LAD disease in patients who would be poor candidates suited for median sternotomy. The downside to this approach is that patients will be undergoing surgery on dual antiplatelet therapy.

Insufficient native vessel size or absence of venous conduit is another indication for HCR. Many patients have target vessels that are poorly suited for SVG due to size or location. Stenting the native vessel in these situations may provide revascularization without risk of SVG occlusion, which is known to be higher with poor surgical targets. Other patients have limited venous conduits secondary to small caliber native veins, long-standing venous disease, or previous vein-stripping procedures. There are also vessels that are anatomically non-graftable but are stentable such as left circumflex lesions in the atrioventricular groove with small diffuse obtuse marginals; these lesions are excellent candidates for HCR. In addition, PCI is often preferable as an alternative to redo CABG where the surgeon tries to avoid full chest dissection.

Patients with prior mediastinitis, severe obstructive pulmonary disease, previous stroke affecting chest wall expansion, or reduced life expectancy may be have prohibitive risk for sternotomy and should also be considered for HCR. Suitable patients may also include those with concomitant organ dysfunction, extensive MI, or severe atherosclerotic aortic disease. Patients with severe obesity or those with left ventricular systolic dysfunction may also not be ideal candidates for conventional bypass surgery. General contraindications and contraindications to hybrid revascularization are shown in Tables 34.1 and 34.2.

High-risk patients with significant comorbidity, who may benefit most from off-pump coronary bypass (OPCAB), shorter operation times, and avoidance of sternotomy include patients with malignancy, severe calcification of the aorta, prior chest irradiation, obesity with severe diabetes mellitus, or dependence on crutches or wheel chair. There are also with some low-risk patients who should be considered for HCR we have non-stentable LAD lesions but non-LAD lesions suitable for PCI. In these patients minimally-invasive surgery yields shorter recovery times and is also attractive for some younger well-informed

patients who may even request hybrid therapy. However, it is mandatory to educate these patients on the potential risks and benefits of all current revascularization options prior to offering them HCR.

TECHNICAL CONSIDERATIONS

The optimal strategy for HCR remains case specific with three basic approaches, all with specific advantages and disadvantages to be considered prior to intervention. The additional issue of optimal anti-platelet protocol remains unclear with operator preference being the norm over standardization at this time. A proposed set of anti-platelet regimens for the various HCR approaches is outlined in Table 34.3. In the first HCR approach, PCI can be performed initially with surgical revascularization undertaken in a staged manner, usually utilizing a MIDCAB, following a period of stabilization or dual antiplatelet therapy. In the second approach, surgical revascularization can be performed first, followed by a brief postoperative reprieve prior to performing a PCI. And finally, the two interventions can be performed simultaneously during one procedure in a hybrid suite or operating room. All three strategies are currently being performed in many centers but controlled trials

Table 34.2 Contraindications to HCR

Clinical conditions
  Hemodynamically unstable or cardiogenic shock
  Acute MI
  Decompensated congestive heart failure or cardiomyopathy (LVEF <20%)
  Severe chronic lung disease (FEV1 <50%)
  Coagulopathy increasing risk of bleeding
  Malignant ventricular arrhythmias
  Recent "large" myocardial infarction
  History of pericarditis
  Prior left thoracotomy
Exclusions for PCI
  Lesion characteristics indicative of a high–predicted risk of restenosis, such as prior TLR failures
  Creatinine >2.0 mg/dL or eGFR <60 ml/min
  Intolerance to clopidogrel
  Severe peripheral vascular disease precluding safe access for PCI
Exclusions for MIDCAB
  Unusable or previously harvested LIMA
  Previous thoracic surgery involving left pleural space
  Poor quality or diffusely diseased LAD
  Chest wall irradiation
  Left subclavian stenosis

Table 34.1 Indications for HCR

Emergency revascularization of non–LAD lesions
  Successful PCI of a non–LAD culprit lesion with low risk for restenosis
  Residual isolated but complex LAD disease amenable to HCR
Insufficient native vessel size or absence of venous conduits
  LAD lesion suitable caliper for MIDCAB procedure
  Circumflex stenosis without target vessel outside the atrioventricular groove
  Non–LAD lesions located in vessels not ideal for SVG placement
  Absence of suitable venous conduits due to prior vein stripping
"High–risk" comorbidities
  High predicted mortality with conventional CABG
  Older disabled or deconditioned patients
  Limited mobility
  Marked frailty
  Unwilling to undergo median sternotomy despite informed consent

Focus Box 34.3

Careful patient selection with consideration of all appropriate indications for a hybrid procedures and awareness of absolute and relative contraindications is critical to excellent HCR outcomes

are needed to definitively answer which approach is best for individual patients and whether they also make economic sense. Currently, there are no large, prospective, randomized controlled trials under way.

PCI Followed by Surgical Revascularization

The approach that is considered the immediate predecessor to modern HCR is PCI followed by surgical revascularization. For years, patients with complex CAD reporting with STEMI have undergone emergent PCI followed by a "cooling off" period prior to undergoing CABG. In this setting, CABG was most often performed through a midline sternotomy using full cardiopulmonary bypass. Despite advances in stent technology most interventionalists recognize that PCI for multivessel CAD is not the best approach when the LAD is amenable to surgery using the LIMA–LAD. In addition, surgeons are becoming more accustomed to minimally invasive and OPCAB approaches using the MIDCAB. This approach has a few discrete advantages making it attractive for certain lesions. By revascularizing the non-LAD targets first much of the ischemic burden is relieved in the myocardium providing excellent collateral perfusion during MIDCAB in which temporary LAD occlusion is often necessary. This is an added level of safety for the operative team particularly in the depressed myocardium. A second advantage to this approach is that it allows the interventional cardiologist a backup strategy, namely surgical revascularization, if a less than optimal PCI result is attained in the cath lab. Finally, as mentioned previously, in patients presenting with acute myocardial infarction (AMI) where the problematic lesion does not reside within the LAD, PCI can serve to revascularize the non-LAD targets in the immediate setting leaving the LAD for MIDCAB at a later time.

However, this approach has several disadvantages with relation to thrombosis, bleeding, and imaging. With modern DES, dual antiplatelet therapy has become mandatory. This poses a particular dilemma for the surgeon who is now faced with two less-than-optimal surgical-clinical environments for revascularization in the post-PCI setting; one thrombotic and the other hemorrhagic. If one stops the antiplatelet therapy in the post-PCI period the risk of acute stent thrombosis becomes quite real, especially with the additive effects of surgery-induced inflammation. Thus, withholding pharmacologic antiplatelet therapy during MIDCAB is not often an appropriate option with a freshly placed DES. On the other hand, BMS implantation especially in an AMI setting has demonstrated similar efficacy rates to DES implantation. Moreover, large diameter vessels and short lesions treated with BMS have similar restenosis rates with DES. Likewise, AMI patients share a prothrombotic milieu that increases the risk of DES thrombosis. Therefore DES implantation might reasonably be considered only in an AMI patient with an increased risk of restenosis such as a diabetic. The alternative of operating on dual antiplatelet therapy where the risk for significant bleeding is obviously increased is equally unattractive to most surgeons, although many surgeons are becoming accustomed to this scenario secondary to increasing usage of DES with subsequent mandatory dual antiplatelet therapy. Lastly, with increasing availability of hybrid suites and operating rooms, surgeons are increasingly performing completion angiography immediately after the LIMA–LAD anastomosis. This allows immediate revision of the graft in the event of inadequate revascularization or an anastomotic problem. With PCI prior to MIDCAB in a staged setting, the opportunity for post MIDCAB angiography followed by immediate surgical revision, if necessary, is lost.

Surgical Revascularization Followed by PCI

Historically, this approach has been the most common for elective HCR mainly because of the increasingly widespread use of DES, which obligates patients to dual antiplatelet therapy. By performing MIDCAB upfront, aggressive antiplatelet therapy can be instituted following subsequent PCI and can be continued for as long as recommended to maintain stent patency and avoid acute stent thrombosis events. This approach also allows for routine angiography of the LIMA–LAD anastomosis at a time point where the patient is no longer on vasopressors, giving a more accurate visualization of what the mature anastomosis will look like. Probably the greatest advantage of PCI in the post-operative setting is that it allows the interventionists to intervene on high-risk lesions with a greater margin of comfort that they might otherwise not address in the cath lab such as complex left-main and diagonal-bifurcation lesions. Unfortunately if the intervention is unsuccessful it portends a higher morbidity for the patient who may now be faced

---

Table 34.3 Anti-platelet Protocols for HCR

1. PCI prior to MIDCAB
   a. Bare metal stent
      i. Aspirin 80–325 mg per day until OR
      ii. Clopidogrel 75 mg per day for at least 6 weeks after PCI
      iii. Aspirin 250 mg on POD 0 and 80–325 mg once daily thereafter
   b. DES
      i. Aspirin 80–325 mg per day until OR
      ii. Clopidogrel 75 mg per day for at least 12 months after PCI
      iii. Aspirin 250 mg on POD 0 and 80–325 mg once daily thereafter
2. MIDCAB prior to PCI
   a. Bare metal stent
      i. Aspirin 80–325 mg per day until OR
      ii. Clopidogrel 75 mg per day for at least 6 weeks after PCI
      iii. Aspirin 250 mg on POD 0 and 80–325 mg p.o. once daily thereafter
   b. DES
      i. Aspirin 80–325 mg per day until OR
      ii. Clopidogrel 75 mg per day for at least 12 months after PCI
      iii. Aspirin 250 mg on POD 0 and 80–325 mg once daily thereafter
3. Simultaneous MIDCAB and PCI
   i. Preoperative loading with aspirin
   ii. Preoperative loading with Clopidogrel 300–600 mg
   iii. Full heparin reversal using protamine
   iv. Additional heparin with 3–5.000 IU during PCI
   v. Aspirin 250 mg on POD 0 and 80–325 mg once daily thereafter
   vi. Clopidogrel 75 mg per day for 6–52 weeks depending on the type of stent

with long-term residual coronary disease or have to undergo a second CABG procedure possibly through a more conventional approach. Thus, it is extremely important to select patients who have lesion characteristics with the highest probability of successful PCI for the non-LAD targets.

From a surgical perspective, many operators are uncomfortable leaving residual coronary lesions behind at the conclusion of surgery. Sicker patients may struggle immediately postop because of their ongoing ischemic myocardium, depending on the amount of tissue at risk. Intraoperatively, minimally-invasive LIMA–LAD procedures can quickly become complicated secondary to no derived benefit of collateral circulation from would-be-revascularized non-LAD targets. In such cases, appropriate patient selection, liberal use of intracoronary shunting, and attention to intraoperative filling pressures and systemic blood pressure with a low tolerance for partial or full cardiopulmonary bypass are all critical for success.

Currently, the timing of PCI in patients who have recently undergone surgical revascularization, is unclear. Certainly, at least a short period of recovery is reasonable to allow the acute inflammatory state induced by surgery to abate. The range is as early as 3–5 days but many may prefer a longer delay giving the patient more time to prepare for a second procedure. These interventions can be done during the same hospitalization but economics may dictate readmission in order to recoup costs.

Simultaneous Surgery and PCI

With the rapid advancement of transcatheter aortic valve replacement (TAVR) and the already widespread acceptance of endovascular surgery, hybrid operating rooms are becoming more prevalent. Modern hybrid suites allow practitioners to perform conventional surgery and endovascular procedures while simultaneously incorporating coronary angiography and PCI, if needed. The main advantages of this approach are that it is performed in one setting and allows the patient to leave the operating room with confirmation of complete revascularization. By performing completion angiograms, the patency and quality of the LIMA–LAD anastomosis can be investigated with immediate revision if necessary prior to closing the chest. Higher risk non-LAD lesions can be addressed once the LIMA–LAD has been completed. And obviously, conventional surgical revascularization is always immediately available should a less-than-optimal PCI outcome be encountered.

Although the one-stop approach has many advantages including patient satisfaction that they are receiving the best possible intervention for their specific anatomy lesion set; there are distinct concerns that remain, thus mandating further investigation. Among these potential disadvantages and pitfalls are increased operative times, increased hospital costs, and currently inadequate reimbursement; the latter two, which may interfere with patients getting the best possible HCR procedure, are strictly based on medical economics alone. Clinically, increased surgical bleeding secondary to full antiplatelet therapy and incomplete reversal of heparin and acute stent thrombosis secondary to the surgical inflammatory response are of concern. Being the newest of the three approaches leaves simultaneous MIDCAB plus PCI HCR with the most unresolved concerns but it remains attractive nonetheless, as DES technology continues to improve.

Focus Box 34.4

Timing of specific TLR in a hybrid intervention can vary according to the best clinical scenario for an individual patient, available resources, and economic concerns

---

Focus Box 34.5

The three common staging methods for HCR are: PCR prior to MIDCAB, MIDCAB prior to PCI, and simultaneous MDCAB plus PCI during the same operative setting using a hybrid operating room or suite. Each approach has distinct advantages and disadvantages Table 34.4

Table 34.4 Advantages and Disadvantages of HCR Strategies

1. PCI followed by surgical revascularization
   a. Advantages
      i. Lower risk of ischemic myocardium during MIDCAB
      ii. Still have CABG as safety net in case of suboptimal PCI result
      iii. PCI for non-LAD STEMI
   b. Disadvantages
      i. Higher risk for acute stent thrombosis unless antiplatelet therapy is continued
      ii. Increased bleeding with MIDCAB on dual antiplatelet therapy
      iii. Cannot perform completion angiography of LIMA–LAD
2. Surgical revascularization followed by PCI
   a. Advantages
      i. Aggressive antiplatelet therapy not an issue
      ii. High risk PCI can be attempted with LAD protection
      iii. Completion angiography can be performed
   b. Disadvantages
      i. CABG completed leaving residual CAD to be treated
      ii. Ongoing ischemic myocardium without collateral contribution can be an issue during MIDCAB or OPCAB
      iii. If PCI result is suboptimal then fallback CABG portends higher morbidity
3. Simultaneous PCI and surgical revascularization
   a. Advantages
      i. Completion angiography readily available
      ii. High risk PCI can be performed with LAD protection
      iii. Confirm complete revascularization prior to leaving operating room
   b. Disadvantages
      i. Increased risk of bleeding with dual antiplatelet
      ii. Increased risk of acute stent thrombosis secondary to surgical inflammatory response
      iii. Current hospital economic concerns

Results of Hybrid Coronary Revascularization

There are approximately 20 published series pertaining to HCR since its implementation in the mid-1990s with reports published from all over the world (Table 34.5 – Results of HCR Series) (6,17–30). Most series report on less than 50 patients with only two studies enrolling over a 100 participants. These data are mainly uncontrolled series with a heterogeneous cross section of patients and utilization of multiple HCR approaches. The types of procedures performed ranged from traditional on-pump LIMA–LAD via full sternotomy with delayed PCI to simultaneous robotic TECAB with PCI in the same index procedure. Most authors described a variation of the MIDCAB as the main operative approach in combination with PCI in the same or a staged procedure.

The mean follow-up for these series was between 11.5 days and 5 years with most centers reporting between 6 and 24 months. The vast majority of authors reported a 30-day mortality of 0 with only three authors having reporting otherwise; Gilard et al. 1.4% (26), Holzey et al. 1.9% (29), and Zhao et al. 2.6% (6). Lima patency was near 100% overall with a range of 93–100% within individual series. The need for target lesion revascularization, however, was as high as 29.6% in the series reported by Katz et al. (24) and for most series the need for TLR was secondary to restenosis of a coronary stent. Event, free survival throughout the respective follow-up periods was 100% in nearly half of the reported series and above 75% in the remainder that felt the need to report these data. Unfortunately, there are no large, prospective, randomized controlled trials reported to date comparing HCR with total surgical revascularization or 3-vessel PCI intervention. At least six studies are under way worldwide continuing to collect HCR data but again only a few are attempting to truly randomize their enrollees and a blinded prospective fashion.

Antiplatelet Strategy

Striking the ideal balance between aggressive dual, antiplatelet therapy in the setting of a fresh coronary stent and avoiding excessive operative bleeding and transfusion during the perioperative MIDCAB period should be a goal of any HCR strategy. Unfortunately, the optimal antiplatelet regimen for HCR is still under debate. Most surgeons would prefer not to operate on full dual antipatelet therapy under any circumstance, making PCI prior to MIDCAB during the same index hospitalization somewhat unpopular. However, in cases where coronary stenting can follow a MIDCAB or can be performed in the same setting, antiplatelet therapy can be delayed, administered very near anesthetic induction, or even given interoperatively via nasogastric tube. Table 34.3 modified from Bonaros et al. (31) outlines a typical strategy for HCR antiplatelet therapy for the various HCR approaches.

Hybrid Operating Room and Resources

Simultaneous HCR was born out of the increasing popularity of the hybrid operating room. These rooms allow all the safety and security of a traditional OR while permitting interventions traditionally performed in the cath lab environment, such as angiography and PCI. Today such rooms are equipped with state-of-the-art surgical instrumentation and the most

Focus Box 34.6

The timing and dosage of antiplatelet therapy varies depending on which staged approach is undertaken during HCR. It is unwise to withhold antiplatelet therapy in the post-PCI period and therefore meticulous intraoperative hemostasis and awareness of heightened postoperative bleeding potential is key in the early management of HCR patients

Table 34.5 Results of HCR Strategies

Author	Year	(n)	Operative approach	30 day mortality (%)	LIMA patency (%)	TLR/resteosis (%)	Mean follow-up	Event-free survival (%)
Zenati et al.	1999	31	MIDCAB	0	100	9.6	10.8 mos	100
Lloyd et al.	1999	18	MIDCAB	0	100	6	6 mos	89
Wittwer et al.	2000	35	MIDCAB	0	100	7	11.5 days	87
Reiss et al.	2002	57	Hemisternotomy	0	97	24	24 mos	98.3
Stahl et al.	2002	54	MIDCAB	0	100	NA	11.7 mos	100
Cisowski et al.	2002	50	MIDCAB	0	100	10	24 mos	100
Davidavicius et al.	2005	20	MIDCAB	0	100	0	19 mos	100
Katz et al.	2006	27	TECAB	0	96	29.6	9 mos	100
Vassiliades et al.	2006	47	MIDCAB	0	99	6.6	7 mo	100
Gilard et al.	2007	70	MIDCAB	1.4	100	2.3	33 mo	100
Kon et al.	2008	15	MIDCAB	0	100	3	1 yr	100
Kiaii et al.	2008	58	MIDCAB	0	93	10	20 mos	NA
Holzhey et al.	2008	117	MIDCAB/TECAB	1.9	NA	17	1 yr	92.5
Zhao et al.	2009	112	CABG/OPCAB	2.6	NA	NA	5 yr	75
Gao et al.	2009	10	TECAB	0	100	0	5 mos	100

advanced invasive and noninvasive imaging and monitoring equipment. This setting allows complex open and minimally invasive on-or off-pump surgery to be undertaken followed by immediate completion angiography and/or PCI with DES or BMS. These state-of-the-art operating rooms can be quite costly and risk being underutilized if not designed correctly or without proper planning. There are, however, many successful examples where these hybrid operating suites have become quite cost effective through extensive utilization by multiple specialties either individually or convened for shared procedures. A properly outfitted hybrid operating room (Fig. 34.1) should be able to accommodate the needs of the interventional cardiologist, the cardiac surgeon, and the endovascular surgeons while providing monitoring that is familiar and comfortable to the noninvasive imaging specialist (i.e. echocardiographers) and anesthesiologist. These lead-lined rooms are best built with a minimum of 700–1000 square feet of functional space with at least 10-foot ceilings and a separate control room similar to that found in most modern cath labs. Adequate storage space for all the interventional catheters and disposables needs to be provided as well as space for a perfusion team and their equipment.

Focus Box 34.7

Constructing a hybrid operating room should be performed with an eye toward maximal utilization by a multidisciplinary team for complex procedures and use by multiple specialties during non-hybrid cases. The planning stage is the most critical where all persons having a functional role in hybrid procedures can voice input and concerns, thus avoiding critical deficiencies often discovered after the room is completed

---

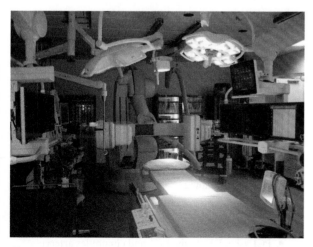

Figure 34.1 Hybrid Operating Room. Hybid operating room fully equipped with floor-mounted image intensifier, permanent anesthesia machine, operating lights, and flat panels on both sides of operating table.

Hybrid operating suites can be either built from scratch or be the product of an operating room or cath lab retrofit. All three approaches can be very successful if a well thought out plan is executed during its construction. This careful planning must include input from the entire Heart Team that will be working in the room including representative staff from cardiology, anesthesia, perfusion, the cath lab, the OR, nursing, and specialist teams.

Case 1: Hybrid Coronary Revascularization: Simultaneous MIDCAB and PCI (http://www.informahealthcare.com/9781841848549/extras)

A 53-year-old female presented with angina and positive stress test suggestive of anterior and lateral wall ischemia. Her past medical history was significant for hypertension, insulin-dependent diabetes mellitus, and obesity. Her mother died of CAD and her father died of cancer. She has a 20-pack-year history of tobacco usage. Her medications included insulin, Simvastatin, Nifedipine, Labatolol, and ASA. Figure 34.2 shows her preoperative coronary angiography and intravascular ultrasound (IVUS) noting severe proximal LAD disease, a tight ostial circumflex lesion, and a right coronary artery (RCA) with only luminal disease.

The patient was taken to the hybrid operating room for a MIDCAB LIMA–LAD and PCI of the circumflex artery. This decision was made based upon: (*i*) the known long-term benefit of the LIMA–LAD, (*ii*) the concern that using BIMAs with a full sternotomy is risky in the morbidly obese diabetic, and (*iii*) the circumflex artery in this case not being an ideal surgical target. The treatment strategy for the single-stage procedure was as follows:

- Plavix 600 mg PO prior to induction
- Small left thoracotomy with direct harvest of LIMA
- Femoral access for PCI
- Off-pump MIDCAB LIMA–LAD
- ½ dose heparin, ACT guided (>300)
- Completion angiogram of LIMA–LAD
- PCI using DES to circumflex artery
- Partial reversal of heparin

The patient underwent an uncomplicated MIDCAB with simultaneous PCI. Figure 34.3 shows postoperative LIMA–LAD completion angiogram and final circumflex PCI result. The patient was extubated within 12 hours, had no significant bleeding with an uneventful postoperative course. She was discharged to home on postoperative day 5.

Case 2: Minimally Invasive Aortic Valve Replacement (AVR) with Simultaneous PCI (http://www.informahealthcare.com/9781841848549/extras)

An 81-year-old female with known aortic stenosis presented with increasing shortness of breath. Her past medical history was significant for hypertension, hypothyroidism, and asthma. Her mother died of an AMI and her father died of CAD. She was a nonsmoker. Her medication included Sythroid, Amlodipine, Atenolol, Singular, ASA, and Lipitor.

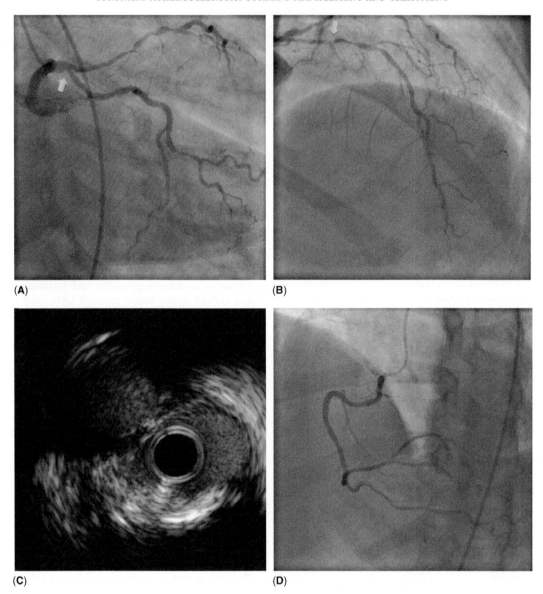

Figure 34.2 Pre-op Angiography Hybrid Case 1: Two-vessel CAD. (A) Angio indicating tight ostial circumflex lesion (B) IVUS proximal circumflex confirming critical stenosis and plaque burden (C) Angiogram LAD (*blue arrow*) indicating tight proximal lesion (D) Angiogram of RCA showing only mild luminal CAD.

Figure 34.4 shows her pre-operative echocardiography and angiography.

The patient was taken to the hybrid operating room for a simultaneous minimally-invasive AVR and IVUS with PCI of the RCA and PCI of the circumflex artery (Fig. 34.5). This decision was supported by the fact that there was a need for a LIMA–LAD and the remaining non-LAD lesions were very conducive to PCI. In addition, our institution routinely performs AVR through a mini-sternotomy avoiding the morbidity

of a full sternotomy. The treatment strategy for this single-stage procedure was as follows:

- Plavix 600 mg PO prior to induction
- Femoral access for PCI and venous return
- PCI using DES to the RCA and circumflex artery
- Minimally-invasive AVR
- Full cardiopulmonary bypass
- Partial reversal of heparin

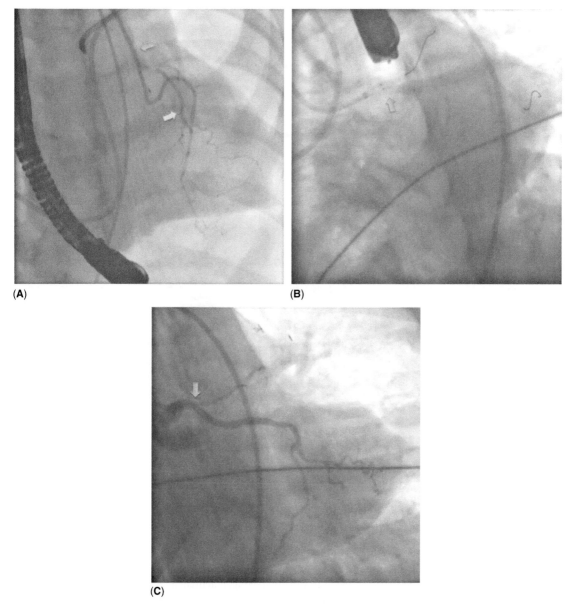

Figure 34.3 Post-op Angiography Hybrid Case 1: Simultaneous MIDCAB plus PCI of circumflex. (**A**) Completion angiogram of LIMA–LAD (*blue arrow*) indicating LIMA and indicating native LAD (*green arrow*) (**B**) PCI of ostial circumflex using "Kissing balloon" technique (*blue arrow*) (**C**) Final angiogram of stented circumflex (*blue arrow*) pointing to DES.

The patient was extubated in 24 hours without significant bleeding or transfusion. She had an uneventful postoperative course and was discharged to home on postoperative day five.

PERSONAL PERSPECTIVE

Currently, several issues remain before HCR can be accepted as a viable alternative to the current popular practices of coronary revascularization, which largely use a singular modality,

surgery, or PCI for the treatment of CAD. First and foremost, more data needs to be collected and these data must come from respected centers with highly-skilled operators adept at both performing these complex procedures and running multi-center trials in a controlled, prospective, randomized fashion. Only with these data, capturing events with a minimum 5-year follow-up, will we begin to tell whether the HCR approach is indeed efficacious for our patients. A more

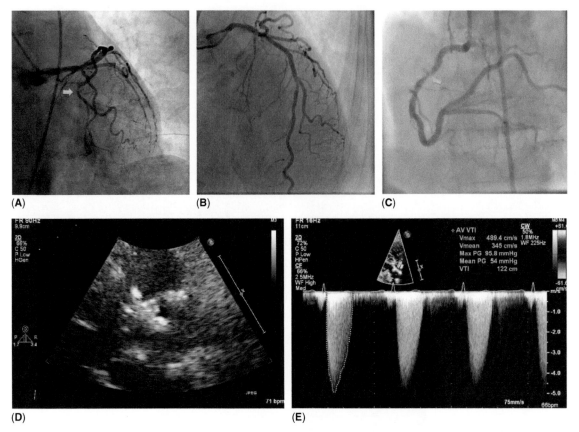

Figure 34.4 Pre-op Angiography and Echocardiogram Hybrid Case 2: Aortic stenosis with two-vessel CAD. (A) Angiogram (*blue arrow*) indicating tight mid-circumflex lesion (B) Angiogram of normal LAD (C) Angiogram (*blue arrow*) indicating significant mid-RCA lesion (D) Echocardiogram of heavily calcified aortic valve (E) Doppler echocardiogram confirming high gradient and velocity across aortic valve consistent with critical aortic stenosis.

sobering issue involves the concern of economics. Regardless of the efficacy results, if the HCR approach cannot be proven to be somewhere close to being "cost effective" for the hospital, it will certainly die a premature death. As of today, third party payers do not provide a mechanism for the individual members of the Heart Team recoup their true costs for services that would have otherwise been provided separately. In other words, there is currently no reimbursement incentive for practitioners to work together in the HCR environment unless it is provided directly by the hospital. This is certainly a major concern as health care reforms looms ominously on the horizon promising to cut deeper into procedure-based revenues. Lastly, the other component holding back the widespread use of HCR is that the vast majority of operators lack access to a hybrid operating room or suite, thus leaving a paucity of current experts with enough experience to conduct well-designed clinical trials. This latter resource issue seems to be changing, albeit slowly, as more new hybrid rooms are

being built throughout the nation and are increasingly being utilized for a greater number of endovascular procedures and peripheral interventions. For the short term, hospitals also see marketing potential in being able to punlicize the hybrid room with its corresponding Heart Team as the latest in technology and expertise related to the treatment of cardiovascular disease. Again, the data here has also yet to be properly validated despite being widely accepted in many centers throughout the world. In summary, setting economics aside, as stent technology and minimally-invasive operative techniques advance in combination with the broader availability of the hybrid suites, HCR stands an excellent chance of becoming standard of care for the treatment of patients with complex constellations of CAD lesions.

ILLUSTRATIVE ON-LINE CASES
Angiography Hybrid CAD
Angiography Hybrid Valve/CABG

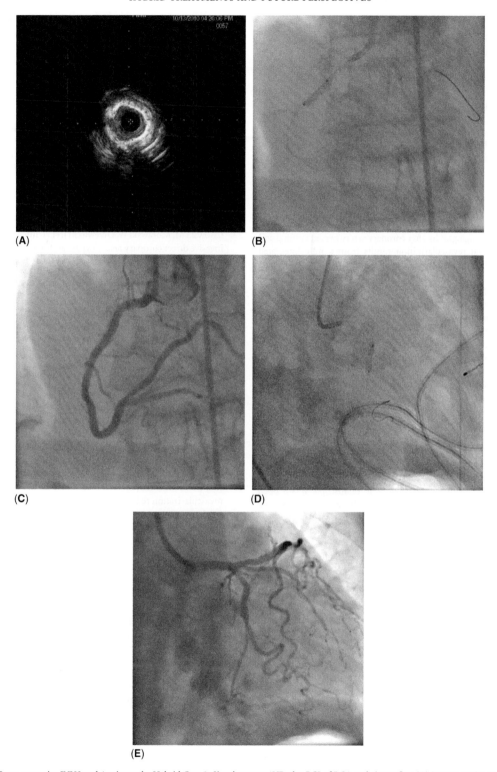

Figure 34.5 Intra-operative IVUS and Angiography Hybrid Case 2: Simultaneous AVR plus PCI of RCA and circumflex. (**A**) Intraoperative IVUS confirming tight mid-RCA lesion (**B**) PCI of RCA (**C**) Final angiogram of stented RCA (**D**) PCI of circumflex (**E**) intraoperative angiogram of circumflex post stenting with DES.

REFERENCES

1. Byrne JG, Leacche M, Vaughan DE, Zhao DX. Hybrid cardiovascular procedures. JACC Cardiovasc Interv 2008; 1: 459–68.

2. Poston RS, Tran R, Collins M, et al. Comparison of economic and patient outcomes with minimally invasive versus traditional off-pump coronary artery bypass grafting techniques. Ann Surg 2008; 248: 638–46.

3. DeRose JJ. Current state of integrated "hybrid" coronary revascularization. Semin Thorac Cardiovasc Surg 2009; 21: 229–36.

4. Popma JJ, Nathan S, Hagberg RC, Khabbaz KR. Hybrid myocardial revascularization: an integrated approach to coronary revascularization. Catheter Cardiovasc Interv 2010; 75(Suppl 1): S28–34.

5. Leacche M, Umakanthan R, Zhao DX, Byrne JG. Surgical update: hybrid procedures, do they have a role? Circulation Cardiovasc Intervent 2010; 3: 511–8.

6. Zhao DX, Leacche M, Balaguer JM, et al. Routine intraoperative completion angiography after coronary artery bypass grafting and 1-stop hybrid revascularization results from a fully integrated hybrid catheterization laboratory/operating room. J Am Coll Cardiol 2009; 53: 232–41.

7. Sarzaeem MR, Mandegar MH, Roshanali F, et al. Scoring system for predicting saphenous vein graft patency in coronary artery bypass grafting. Tex Heart Inst J 2010; 37: 525–30.

8. Wilbring M, Tugtekin SM, Zatschler B, et al. Even short-time storage in physiological saline solution impairs endothelial vascular function of saphenous vein grafts. Eur J Cardiothorac Surg 2011; 40: 811–5.

9. Chikwe J, Croft LB, Goldstone AB, et al. Comparison of the results of aortic valve replacement with or without concomitant coronary artery bypass grafting in patients with left ventricular ejection fraction ≤30% versus patients with ejection fraction >30%. Am J Cardiol 2009; 104: 1717–21.

10. Desai ND, Cohen EA, Naylor CD, Fremes SE; Investigators RAPS. A randomized comparison of radial-artery and saphenous-vein coronary bypass grafts. N Engl J Med 2004; 351: 2302–9.

11. Lopes RD, Hafley GE, Allen KB, et al. Endoscopic versus open vein-graft harvesting in coronary-artery bypass surgery. N Engl J Med 2009; 361: 235–44.

12. Yun KL, Wu Y, Aharonian V, et al. Randomized trial of endoscopic versus open vein harvest for coronary artery bypass grafting: six-month patency rates. J Thorac Cardiovasc Surg 2005; 129: 496–503.

13. Moses JW, Leon MB, Popma JJ, et al. Sirolimus-eluting stents versus standard stents in patients with stenosis in a native coronary artery. N Engl J Med 2003; 349: 1315–23.

14. Lee S-W, Park S-W, Kim Y-H, et al. A randomized comparison of sirolimus- versus paclitaxel-eluting stent implantation in patients with diabetes mellitus 2-year clinical outcomes of the DES-DIABETES trial. J Am Coll Cardiol 2009; 53: 812–3.

15. Serruys PW, Morice M-C, Kappetein AP, et al. Percutaneous coronary intervention versus coronary-artery bypass grafting for severe coronary artery disease. N Engl J Med 2009; 360: 961–72.

16. Narasimhan S, Srinivas VS, DeRose JJ. Hybrid coronary revascularization: a review. Cardiol Rev 2011; 19: 101–7.

17. Zenati M, Cohen HA, Griffith BP. Alternative approach to multivessel coronary disease with integrated coronary revascularization. J Thorac Cardiovasc Surg 1999; 117: 439–44; discussion 44–6.

18. Lloyd CT, Calafiore AM, Wilde P, et al. Integrated left anterior small thoracotomy and angioplasty for coronary artery revascularization. ATS 1999; 68: 908–11; discussion 11–2.

19. Wittwer T, Cremer J, Boonstra P, et al. Myocardial "hybrid" revascularisation with minimally invasive direct coronary artery bypass grafting combined with coronary angioplasty: preliminary results of a multicentre study. Heart 2000; 83: 58–63.

20. Riess F-C, Bader R, Kremer P, et al. Coronary hybrid revascularization from January 1997 to January 2001: a clinical follow-up. ATS 2002; 73: 1849–55.

21. Stahl KD, Boyd WD, Vassiliades TA, Karamanoukian HL. Hybrid robotic coronary artery surgery and angioplasty in multivessel coronaryartery disease. Ann Thorac Surg 2002; 74: S1358.

22. Cisowski M, Morawski W, Drzewiecki J, et al. Integrated minimally invasive direct coronary artery bypass grafting and angioplasty for coronary artery revascularization. Eur J Cardiothorac Surg 2002; 22: 261–5.

23. Davidavicius G, Van Praet F, Mansour S, et al. Hybrid revascularization strategy: a pilot study on the association of robotically enhanced minimally invasive direct coronary artery bypass surgery and fractional-flow-reserve-guided percutaneous coronary intervention. Circulation 2005; 112(9 Suppl): I317–22.

24. Katz MR, Van Praet F, de Canniere D, et al. Integrated coronary revascularization: percutaneous coronary intervention plus robotic totally endoscopic coronary artery bypass. Circulation 2006; 114(1 Suppl): I473–6.

25. Vassiliades TA, Reddy VS, Puskas JD, Guyton RA. Long-term results of the endoscopic atraumatic coronary artery bypass. Ann Thorac Surg 2007; 83:979–84; discussion 84–5.

26. Gilard M, Bezon E, Cornily JC, et al. Same-day combined percutaneous coronary intervention and coronary artery surgery. Cardiology 2007; 108: 363–7.

27. Kon ZN, Brown EN, Tran R, et al. Simultaneous hybrid coronary revascularization reduces postoperative morbidity compared with results from conventional off-pump coronary artery bypass. J Thorac Cardiovasc Surg 2008; 135: 367–75.

28. Kiaii B, McClure RS, Stewart P, et al. Simultaneous integrated coronary artery revascularization with long-term angiographic follow-up. J Thorac Cardiovasc Surg 2008; 136: 702–8.

29. Holzhey DM, Jacobs S, Mochalski M, et al. Minimally invasive hybrid coronary artery revascularization. Ann Thorac Surg 2008; 86: 1856–60.

30. Gao P, Xiong H, Zheng Z, et al. Evaluation of antiplatelet effects of a modified protocol by platelet aggregation in patients undergoing "one-stop" hybrid coronary revascularization. Platelets 2010; 21: 183–90.

31. Bonaros N, Schachner T, Wiedemann D, et al. Closed chest hybrid coronary revascularization for multivessel disease – current concepts and techniques from a two-center experience. Eur J Cardiothorac Surg 2011.

35 Determinants of long-term outcome following percutaneous coronary intervention

Pedro A. Lemos

OUTLINE

The long-term outcomes after coronary angioplasty depend on the interaction between the inherent risks related to the intervention and the potential benefits derived from it, modulated by the aggressiveness of the underlying atherosclerotic disease and other associated co-morbidities. The decision-making process of indicating or deferring a coronary angioplasty procedure is a complex one. Currently, much is known about the factors that influence the results and outcomes after coronary angioplasty, and application of that knowledge in daily practice is the best guide to optimally select the appropriate patients and plan the interventional strategies.

A number of characteristics with prognostic value have been identified for patients treated with percutaneous coronary intervention. Variables at patient level, as well as atherosclerotic disease-related and procedure-related features have been already shown to be important predictors of future events. In this chapter we provide a description and a practical classification of the main factors that influence the outcomes after coronary angioplasty.

INTRODUCTION

As a rule, the purpose of coronary angioplasty in a particular patient is either to alleviate symptoms and improve quality of life or to prevent future adverse events and prolong life expectancy. The final net clinical utility of percutaneous coronary intervention (PCI) is to reflect a balance between its potential harms weighted against its expected benefits. Therefore, a profound understanding of the factors involved in the modulation of the clinical results obtained with the intervention is central when dealing with a possible candidate for angioplasty. Indeed, the final indication for the procedure as well as the choice of the interventional strategy should optimally rely on a meticulous analysis of the clinical subtleties, which vary from patient to patient.

A large number of characteristics have been already described as determinants of the prognosis after PCI. Conditions at patient-level, as well as features of the atherosclerotic disease itself, together with characteristics related to the procedure have all been shown to influence the outcomes following coronary angioplasty.

DISCUSSION

When analysing the whole cohort of patients treated with coronary angioplasty in daily practice (excluding only those with previous revascularization procedures), an overall death rate of 6% and an overall death or myocardial infarction rate of 10% are expected for the first 2 years of follow-up (1). However, the clinical outcomes after coronary intervention vary considerably among different groups of patients. Several characteristics have been shown to directly impact on the outcomes following angioplasty, while a number of other features have been demonstrated to serve as markers of prognosis.

Adverse events occurring during the follow-up after PCI have their genesis mainly related to complications directly associated to the intervention, or caused by the underlying atherosclerotic heart disease, or even linked to other patient-based determinants. Obviously, many of these often occur concomitantly, being the final clinical outcome, a resultant of the interplay among the several features of the patient's risk profile.

PROCEDURE-DERIVED DETERMINANTS

Target Vessel Related Determinants

In the early days of coronary intervention with balloon angioplasty, acute vessel occlusion was perhaps the most feared complication. Although still associated with a high in-hospital mortality rate, the occurrence of peri-procedure acute coronary complications was significantly reduced after the introduction of metallic stents and today is considered to be a rare event, as reflected by the incidence of same-stay coronary bypass surgery of approximately 0.3% (1). Much more frequent, however, is the occurrence of smaller myocardial infarctions caused by intra-procedure reverted/brief coronary occlusion, loss of side branches, distal embolization, or no reflow. Even though peri-procedure myocardial infarctions have a doubtful impact on short-term outcomes, recent evidences suggest that a post-angioplasty increase in cardiac markers is associated with worse prognosis after 2 years (2).

Initially, in the bare metal stent era, coronary stent thrombosis was believed to be a time-limited complication, restricted to the first weeks after implantation. Current evidence, however, clearly show that the risk of stent thrombosis persists long after the index procedure (3,4), especially following drug-eluting stent implantation. Stent thrombosis is an infrequent event, with a 4-year cumulative rate of less than 5% (definite events) in the general population of patients treated with first generation drug-eluting stents (4).

Even though uncommon, stent thrombosis carries a high risk of large myocardial infarction, with a reported short-term mortality of up to 33% (5–7). In addition to being an adverse event *per se*, stent thrombosis appears to be an important marker of future prognosis (8). Patients successfully treated for a first episode of stent thrombosis are at high risk (up to 36%) for recurrent thrombosis (7), which may occur late after the first event (9,10).

Several predictors of stent thrombosis have been already described and indicate that, most probably, the underlying mechanisms of early thrombosis are distinct from those related to thrombotic events occurring later during the follow-up (3,4).

Table 35.1 lists independent predictors of drug-eluting stent thrombosis. To date, numerous studies have been published with a resultant large set of predictors of stent thrombosis already described. However, some risk factors for drug-eluting stent thrombosis appear to be more consistently reported across studies: (*i*) the use of small, undersized, or underexpanded stents; (*ii*) the use of multiple stents with a increased total stent length; (*iii*) bifurcation stenting; (*iv*) residual lesion

Table 35.1 Predictors of Drug-eluting Stent Thrombosis

Stent thrombosis intra-procedure or within the first day
- Decreasing age (39)
- Decreasing baseline MLD (6)
- Increasing stent length per vessel (6)
- Multiple stents in the same lesion (6)
- TIMI flow 0 or I at baseline (39)

Stent thrombosis within the first month
- ACS at baseline (3)
- Angiographic ulceration at baseline (39)
- Baseline TIMI flow 0 or I (39)
- Bifurcation lesion (5,40)
- Decreasing LV function or CHF (5,39,40)
- Diabetes (especially insulin-treated) (3,5,39)
- Increasing number of stents (40)
- Increasing platelet count at baseline (39)
- Increasing stent length (3,5)
- Lack of glycoprotein IIbIIIa use (40)
- Malignancy (40)
- Premature APT discontinuation (5,41)
- Renal failure (3,5)
- Residual lesion distal or proximal (40)
- Stent edge dissection (40)
- Stent undersizing (40)
- Treated vessel LAD (3)

Stent thrombosis after the first month
- ACS at baseline (41)
- Baseline TIMI flow 0 (42)
- Bifurcation lesion (5,40,42)
- Current smoker at baseline (39,42)
- Decreasing age (40,42)
- Decreasing LV function (5)
- Diabetes (especially insulin-treated) (39–41)
- Increasing stent length (40)
- Malignancy (40)
- "Off-label" indication (42)
- Ostial lesion (41)
- Peripheral artery disease (40)
- Premature APT discontinuation (5)
- Previous coronary angioplasty (42)
- Previous myocardial infarction (39)
- Renal failure (41)
- Residual lesion proximal to the stent (40)
- Stent undersizing (40)

Stent thrombosis after the first year
- Bifurcation (43)
- Current smoker at baseline (43)
- Decreasing age (14)
- Decreasing LV function (44)
- Diabetes (especially insulin-treated) (39)
- Multiple stenting (43)
- Previous coronary angioplasty (39)
- Previous coronary bypass surgery (43)
- Prior myocardial infarction (43)
- Renal failure (43)

Stent thrombosis at any time during follow-up
- ACS at baseline (4,45)
- Aneurysm or ulceration at baseline (39)
- Baseline TIMI flow 0 or I (39,45)
- Bifurcation lesion (5,40,48)
- Calcified lesion (49)
- Cardiogenic shock at baseline (45)

- Current smoker at baseline (39,47)
- Decreasing age (4,40)
- Decreasing LV function or CHF (5,8,40,44,45,48,49)
- Decreasing reference vessel diameter (47)
- Decreasing stent diameter (48)
- Diabetes (especially insulin-treated) (4,5,39–41,47,49)
- Final TIMI flow < III (40)
- Increasing platelet count at baseline (39)
- Increasing stent length (4,47,49)
- Large thrombus burden (46)
- Lesion calcification (47)
- Malignancy (40)
- Multiple stenting (45,47)
- Peripheral artery disease (40)
- Premature APT discontinuation (5,40,41,47)
- Previous coronary angioplasty (39)
- Previous stroke (49)
- Renal failure (5,41,49)
- Residual lesion distal or proximal (40)
- Stent edge dissection (40)
- Stent undersizing (40)
- Treated vessel left main (47)
- Use of paclitaxel-eluting stent (4)

Abbreviations: ACS, acute coronary syndrome; APT, antiplatelet therapy; CHF, congestive heart failure; LAD, left anterior descending; LV, left ventricle; MLD, minimal lumen diameter.

or dissection at stent edges; (*v*) acute coronary syndrome at the time of stent implantation; (*vi*) decreased left ventricular function; (*vii*) younger age; (*viii*) renal failure; (*ix*) diabetes (especially insulin dependent); and (*x*) antiplatelet therapy discontinuation.

Several studies pointed out that compliance with dual antiplatelet therapy is one of the most important factors contributing to the occurrence of stent thrombosis. Patients who stop thienopyridine medications before 30 days (between 10% and 15% of the initial population) (8,11) have a 9-fold increase in the risk of dying within the next year (11). The premature withdrawal of thienopyridines appear to be associated with some patients characteristics, such as older age, low education level, unmarried status, avoidance of health care because of cost, pre-existing cardiovascular and renal diseases, prior major bleeding, and deficient discharge instructions (11,12).

Restenosis has been traditionally considered as the major limitation and most important complication of coronary angioplasty. After bare metal stent implantation, restenosis-related events are the predominant type of complications during the first year of follow-up, occurring in approximately 12–17% of patients (13,14). Conversely, between the second and the fifth year after bare metal stenting, target-lesion revascularization is infrequent, only occurring at a rate of 1.5–2.0% per year, mostly in conjunction with another procedure in a non-related vessel (13,14). Undoubtedly, the introduction of drug-eluting stents led to a marked reduction in the risk of future restenosis (14,15). Even though restenosis-motivated re-intervention affects <10% of the overall patient population, it is still the most common adverse event during the first year following drug-eluting stent implantation, and remain an important factor hampering the durability of PCI (14,15). Despite some angiographic studies showing very late lumen re-narrowing after drug-eluting stenting (16) in clinical practice the timing of restenosis-related complications appears to be similar to bare stents, with most events occurring during the first year after implantation (14,15).

Risk factors for restenosis after drug-eluting stent implantation (Table 35.2) are similar to those previously described for

Table 35.2 Predictors of Restenosis or Target Lesion Revascularization after DES Implantation

Treatment of bare metal stent restenosis(50,51)
Ostial location(50,51)
Diabetes(50)
Increasing stent length(50,52)
Decreasing stent diameter(50,51)
Treated vessel left anterior descending(50,51) or bypass graft(53)
Decreasing minimal stent area by IVUS(52)
Decreasing vessel size(54)
Increasing final diameter stenosis(54)
Multi-lesion stenting or multi-vessel disease(51,53)
Increasing age(51)
Renal failure(51)

Abbreviation: DES, drug-eluting stent.

bare metal stenting. Overall, the "complexity" of the case is proportional to the risk of restenosis. Indeed, it is in the scenario of complex patients that restenosis of drug-eluting stents still poses a substantial and challenging clinical problem. The recent SYNTAX trial allocated patients with triple-vessel disease or left main stenosis to angioplasty with paclitaxel-eluting stents or surgery (17). After 3 years, both strategies were similar regarding the occurrence of death, myocardial infarction, or stroke, but patients treated with stenting had a significantly worse outcome in terms of the risk for repeat revascularization (11.0% vs. 21.0%; *p* < 0.001) (17).

In an attempt to quantify the morphological complexity of the coronary disease and aiming to predict the outcomes after multivessel stenting, the SYNTAX score was created as a multi-level scoring system that integrates numerous angiographic characteristics of the coronary bed and lesions (18). It has been shown that such morphological analysis has a predictive value as it was able to identify a subgroup of patients of low complexity (one third of the population), for whom coronary surgery and drug-eluting stenting appeared similar after 3 years (17). Conversely, the population with higher scores had a significant benefit after surgery, especially for patients with triple-vessel disease (17).

Also for patients with multivessel disease, the impact of the completeness of revascularization has been much debated over the last few years, with conflicting results. Large population-based studies have suggested that incomplete revascularization procedures may increase the risk of late adverse events (19), even though this concept has been challenged by other reports (20). Mostly, those studies have used only angiographic data to evaluate the completeness of revascularization. It is possible that a more functional, ischemia-driven concept of completeness of revascularization may improve the ability to select the best candidate lesions to be treated, ultimately improving clinical outcomes (21).

In addition to "traditional" procedure-derived adverse events (i.e. stent thrombosis, restenosis etc.), a new clinical entity has been recently described after PCI. Recent studies using intra-vascular imaging and histopathology have suggested that drug-eluting stents may predispose to accelerated atherosclerosis inside the stented segment (22,23), even though the risk factors as well as the clinical impact of this novel phenomenon is currently unknown.

Much of the above mentioned data regarding the late-term safety and efficacy of contemporary PCI are derived from studies that used first generation drug-eluting stents. Recently introduced drug-eluting stents, however, have consistently shown a clinical performance that equalled or improved the outcomes achieved with early drug-eluting stents. The rates of 2-year stent thrombosis, myocardial infarction (both Q-wave and non-Q-wave), and re-intervention (both percutaneous and surgical) were significantly reduced with everolimus-eluting stents, compared with paclitaxel stents (24,25). Increasing evidence therefore suggest that the type of drug-eluting stent used might be an important determinant of future outcomes.

Non-target Vessel Related Determinants

The occurrence of bleeding complications has long been identified as an important potential issue after PCI. Bleeding events may be related to access-site complications as well as non-access site haemorrhages (e.g. gastrointestinal), especially in patients receiving potent anti-thrombotic medications (26). The risk for post-angioplasty bleeding appears to be diminishing over time (27,28). Among 17,901 consecutive patients treated between 1994 and 2005, the incidence of major femoral access site bleeding decreased progressively from 8.4% to 3.5% ($p < 0.001$), as did the need for large-volume (i.e. three or more units) blood transfusions (4.5–1.8%; $p < 0.001$) (27). Indeed, a number of bleeding avoidance strategies have been introduced and are currently available in practice. These may, at least partially, explain the observed temporal reduction in bleeding (28). In particular, the modern use of bivalirudin, fondaparinux, or enoxaparin, smaller catheters, as well as the radial approach may have resulted in the decreased bleeding tendency seen with contemporary coronary procedures (26,28). Nevertheless, regardless of the trend despite the reduction in post-intervention bleeding, the occurrence of hemorrhagic complications remains an important predictor of poor outcomes. Previous reports have described a 14-fold increase of in 30-day mortality (27) and a 3-fold increase in one-year mortality (26) after a peri-procedure bleeding event.

Transient as well as persistent renal dysfunction after PCI occurs in 2–25% of patients and have been shown to be independent predictors of late mortality (29,30). Data from 7,856 consecutive patients undergoing PCI between 2000 and 2006 have shown that late survival was significantly worse in patients with renal dysfunction (either transient or persistent) compared with those with no renal impairment after the procedure (approximately 60% vs. 95% at 1 year and 45% vs. 88% at 3 years; $p < 0.01$ for all) (30). Pre-procedure creatinine, hypotension or the need for intra-aortic balloon pump, urgent priority, congestive heart failure, previous chronic kidney disease, diabetes, older age, and higher volume of contrast have been identified as predictors of any contrast-induced nephropathy (0.5 ml/dl increase in creatinine) and of serious post-procedure renal dysfunction (new dialysis, ≥2.0 mg/dl increase in creatinine, or ≥50% increase in creatinine (30,31). Even though a list of protective measures has been proposed described (e.g. sodium bicarbonate hydration, N-acetylcysteine, statins, iso-osmolar contrast agents, RenalGuard system), their capacity of preventing contrast-induced nephropathy is conflicting across several reports. More importantly, it is totally unclear whether those strategies are efficacious in reversing the deleterious effects of post-intervention renal function loss on late term prognosis.

ATHEROSCLEROTIC DISEASE-RELATED DETERMINANTS

PCI is, by its own nature, a localized treatment primarily aimed to the dilatation of lumen-narrowed coronary segments. Therefore, it is not expected that the procedure will alter the natural history of the atherosclerotic disease outside the target segment. Indeed, after the first year, non-target lesion events dominate as the most common complications (13–15), as shown in Table 35.3. Accordingly, during years 2 through 5 after the procedure, the multivariate predictors that increase the incidence of non-target lesion events are well-known risk factors for atherosclerosis progression (i.e. diabetes, hypertension, and atherosclerotic burden) (13,14). Importantly, the type of stent used, either bare stent or drug-eluting stent, do not seem to change the natural course of the disease (Table 35.3).

The concept that non-target lesion events are fundamentally influenced by the basic patient's atherosclerotic risk profile is supported by the recent PROSPECT trial that examined the

Table 35.3 Non-TL Adverse Events during the Follow-up

	Year 1		Annualized rates from 2 to 5 years		Cumulative 5-year	
	BMS%	DES%	BMS%	DES%	BMS%	DES%
Cutlip et al. (13)						
Non-TL target vessel revasc.	3.2	–	1.2	–	7.6	–
Non-target vessel revasc.	8.9	–	3.5	–	21.7	–
Non-target lesion event[a]	12.4	–	6.3	–	37.4	–
Leon et al. (14)						
Non-TL target vessel revasc.	4.5	4.3	2.1	1.8	–	–
Non-target vessel Q wave MI	0.1	0.2	0.1	0.1	–	–
Chacko et al. (15)						
Non-TL target vessel revasc.	–	–	–	–	15.0	11.7
Non-target vessel revasc.	–	–	–	–	22.9	22.3
Non-target vessel MI	–	–	–	–	2.5	3.6

[a]Composite of re-intervention involving the target vessel outside the target lesion, non-target vessel revascularization, and any death, myocardial infarction, acute coronary syndrome, or congestive heart failure clearly not attributable to the target lesion.
Abbreviations: BMS, bare metal stent; DES, drug-eluting stent; MI, myocardial infarction; TL, target lesion.

influence of patient-level and coronary-level factors on 3-year outcomes (32). In that study, approximately 700 patients with acute coronary syndromes were treated with coronary angioplasty and evaluated with 3-vessel intravascular ultrasound with plaque tissue composition analysis (32). After 3 years, the cumulative rate of major adverse cardiovascular events related to non-culprit lesions was 11.6% (the rate of events related to culprit lesions was 12.9%). At multivariate analysis, the only predictors of non-culprit events were insulin-treated and previous coronary angioplasty, together with the following findings at the baseline intravascular ultrasound of the non-culprit lesion: plaque burden >70%, minimal lumen area <4.0 mm^2, or a thin-cap fibroatheroma morphology (32). Such results reinforces the importance of strategies for secondary prevention after percutaneous coronary intervention, which is in line with a previous randomized study that demonstrated the beneficial effects of statins in reducing 4-year non-restenosis adverse events in patients treated with coronary intervention (33).

Several patient-level risk factors have been described as potential factors influencing the outcomes after percutaneous coronary disease. As mentioned above, diabetes is a major risk factor for virtually every coronary adverse event, including stent thrombosis, restenosis, and non-target lesion complications. Also, baseline impaired renal function is a well-established risk factor for future events (34,35), increasing 7-year mortality by 2-fold, regardless of the type of stent utilized (34). More recently, resistance to the anti-platelet effect of clopidogrel has been shown an important determinant of the prognosis after coronary intervention (36).

LONG-TERM SURVIVAL AFTER PCI
As highlighted above, the outcomes after PCI are modulated by numerous factors that eventually converge to shape the global patient prognosis. A fatal event is the obvious final endpoint to be avoided. Commonly, in clinical studies in the field of interventional cardiology, deaths are classified into cardiac or non-cardiac, being are defined latter as those caused by an unequivocally non-cardiac cause (and the former not rarely ascertained as of cardiac origin only by exclusion). This definition, although widely applied, has several obvious limitations related to the well-known difficulty in diagnosing the cause(s) and contributor(s) to death for many patients. Accordingly, some authors have suggested that total death should be utilized as the metric of choice for evaluating the survival status in clinical studies (37).

The long-term risk of all-cause death after angioplasty varies considerably among different subsets, ranging from stable patients with very low mortality rates (38) to extreme-risk patients with acute myocardial infarction and cardiogenic shock. A number of studies have already validated a list of risk factors for short- and long-term death after coronary angioplasty. Table 35.4 summarizes the determinants of late survival after coronary interventions, according to the clinical syndrome at presentation.

PERSONAL PERSPECTIVE
Solid scientific knowledge about the epidemiology, pathophysiology, and clinical aspects of the coronary heart disease is a central pre-requisite for physicians dedicated to interventional cardiology. In addition to a full-range and objective education on the specific technical issues of the specialty, the interventional cardiologist should also acquire the capacity to estimate the risks and potential benefits related to the percutaneous procedure, not in the short-term but also long after the intervention. Thus far, several determinants have been described that serve well to the assessment of the effectiveness of a coronary intervention, as well as its durability. Variables at patient level (such as diabetes and baseline renal impairment) or related to the atherosclerotic disease (such as plaque progression at a non-culprit vessel during follow-up) or even related to the procedure itself (such as stent restenosis or thrombosis) have been shown to predict the final results obtained with the procedure. For patients undergoing coronary percutaneous interventions, non-modifiable risk factors must be dealt with clinical measures aiming to indirectly minimize their effects. Concomitantly, modifiable determinants are treated with actions that counterbalance or abolish their negative impact.

Table 35.4 Determinants of Long-term Survival for Patients Treated with Percutaneous Coronary Angioplasty

Stable CAD(38)	Stable CAD and low-risk ACS(24)	General population including high risk ACS[a](55)	STEMI without cardiogenic shock(56)
Age	Age	Age	Age
Triple-vessel disease	Current smoking	Triple-vessel disease	Triple-vessel disease
PAD	Diabetes	Diabetes	Hypercholesterolemia
Congestive heart failure		Left ventricular function	Left ventricular function
Procedural success		STEMI/NSTEMI	LAD infarction
		Cardiogenic shock	Baseline TIMI 0/1
		Renal failure	

[a]Predictors of death or myocardial infarction.
Abbreviations: ACS, acute coronary syndrome; CAD, coronary artery disease; LAD, left anterior descending; NSTEMI, non-ST elevation myocardial infarction; PAD, peripheral arterial disease; STEMI, ST elevation myocardial infarction.

Focus Box 35.1

As a rule, coronary angioplasty is indicated only for alleviating symptoms and/or preventing future adverse events

The final net clinical utility of PCI derives from the balance between its potential harms weighted against its expected benefits.

A large number of characteristics have been described as determinants of the prognosis after PCI

Adverse events occurring during follow-up after PCI are mainly related to (*i*) complications directly associated with the intervention, or (*ii*) caused by the underlying atherosclerotic heart disease, or (*iii*) linked to other patient-based determinants

Procedure-derived determinants would include target-vessel complications (e.g. restenosis, thrombosis, in-stent accelerated atherosclerosis) and non-target vessel related complications (e.g bleeding, renal failure).

Atherosclerotic disease-related determinants are mainly related to distant-site disease progression, and

Patient-level risk factors include characteristics such as diabetes, impaired renal function, resistance to clopidogrel

REFERENCES

1. Hannan EL, Racz M, Holmes DR, et al. Comparison of coronary artery stenting outcomes in the eras before and after the introduction of drug-eluting stents. Circulation 2008; 117: 2071–8.

2. Feldman DN, Minutello RM, Bergman G, Moussa I, Wong SC. Relation of troponin I levels following nonemergent percutaneous coronary intervention to short- and long-term outcomes. Am J Cardiol 2009; 104: 1210–5.

3. de la Torre-Hernandez JM, Alfonso F, Hernandez F, et al. Drug-eluting stent thrombosis: results from the multicenter Spanish registry ESTROFA (Estudio ESpanol sobre TROmbosis de stents FArmacoactivos). J Am Coll Cardiol 2008; 51: 986–90.

4. Wenaweser P, Daemen J, Zwahlen M, et al. Incidence and correlates of drug-eluting stent thrombosis in routine clinical practice. 4-year results from a large 2-institutional cohort study. J Am Coll Cardiol 2008; 52: 1134–40.

5. Iakovou I, Schmidt T, Bonizzoni E, et al. Incidence, predictors, and outcome of thrombosis after successful implantation of drug-eluting stents. JAMA 2005; 293: 2126–30.

6. Biondi-Zoccai GG, Sangiorgi GM, Chieffo A, et al. Validation of predictors of intraprocedural stent thrombosis in the drug-eluting stent era. Am J Cardiol 2005; 95: 1466–8.

7. Lemesle G, Sudre A, Modine T, et al. High incidence of recurrent in stent thrombosis after successful treatment of a first in stent thrombosis. Catheter Cardiovasc Interv 2008; 72: 470–8.

8. Roy P, Bonello L, Torguson R, et al. Temporal relation between Clopidogrel cessation and stent thrombosis after drug-eluting stent implantation. Am J Cardiol 2009; 103: 801–5.

9. van Werkum JW, Heestermans AA, de Korte FI, et al. Long-term clinical outcome after a first angiographically confirmed coronary stent thrombosis: an analysis of 431 cases. Circulation 2009; 119: 828–34.

10. Porto I, Burzotta F, Parma A, et al. Angiographic predictors of recurrent stent thrombosis (from the Outcome of PCI for stent-ThrombosIs MultIcentre STudy [OPTIMIST]). Am J Cardiol 2010; 105: 1710–5.

11. Spertus JA, Kettelkamp R, Vance C, et al. Prevalence, predictors, and outcomes of premature discontinuation of thienopyridine therapy after drug-eluting stent placement: results from the PREMIER registry. Circulation 2006; 113: 2803–9.

12. Ferreira-Gonzalez I, Marsal JR, Ribera A, et al. Background, incidence, and predictors of antiplatelet therapy discontinuation during the first year after drug-eluting stent implantation. Circulation 2010; 122: 1017–25.

13. Cutlip DE, Chhabra AG, Baim DS, et al. Beyond restenosis: five-year clinical outcomes from second-generation coronary stent trials. Circulation 2004; 110: 1226–30.

14. Leon MB, Allocco DJ, Dawkins KD, Baim DS. Late clinical events after drug-eluting stents: the interplay between stent-related and natural history-driven events. JACC Cardiovasc Intervent 2009; 2: 504–12.

15. Chacko R, Mulhearn M, Novack V, et al. Impact of target lesion and nontarget lesion cardiac events on 5-year clinical outcomes after sirolimus-eluting or bare-metal stenting. JACC Cardiovasc Intervent 2009; 2: 498–503.

16. Park KW, Kim CH, Lee HY, et al. Does "late catch-up" exist in drug-eluting stents: Insights from a serial quantitative coronary angiography analysis of sirolimus versus paclitaxel-eluting stents. Am Heart J 2010; 159: 446–53; e443.

17. Kappetein AP, Feldman TE, Mack MJ, et al. Comparison of coronary bypass surgery with drug-eluting stenting for the treatment of left main and/or three-vessel disease: 3-year follow-up of the SYNTAX trial. Eur Heart J 2011.

18. Sianos G, Morel MA, Kappetein AP, et al. The SYNTAX Score: an angiographic tool grading the complexity of coronary artery disease. EuroIntervention 2005; 1: 219–27.

19. Hannan EL, Racz M, Holmes DR, et al. Impact of completeness of percutaneous coronary intervention revascularization on long-term outcomes in the stent era. Circulation 2006; 113: 2406–12.

20. Kim YH, Park DW, Lee JY, et al. Impact of angiographic complete revascularization after drug-eluting stent implantation or coronary artery bypass graft surgery for multivessel coronary artery disease. Circulation 2011; 123: 2373–81.

21. Pijls NH, Fearon WF, Tonino PA, et al. Fractional flow reserve versus angiography for guiding percutaneous coronary intervention in patients with multivessel coronary artery disease: 2-year follow-up of the FAME (Fractional Flow Reserve Versus Angiography for Multivessel Evaluation) study. J Am Coll Cardiol 2010; 56: 177–84.

22. Higo T, Ueda Y, Oyabu J, et al. Atherosclerotic and thrombogenic neointima formed over sirolimus drug-eluting stent: an angioscopic study. JACC Cardiovasc Imaging 2009; 2: 616–24.

23. Nakazawa G, Vorpahl M, Finn AV, Narula J, Virmani R. One step forward and two steps back with drug-eluting-stents: from preventing restenosis to causing late thrombosis and nouveau atherosclerosis. JACC Cardiovasc Imaging 2009; 2: 625–8.

24. Kereiakes DJ, Smits PC, Kedhi E, et al. Predictors of death or myocardial infarction, ischaemic-driven revascularisation, and major adverse cardiovascular events following everolimus-eluting or paclitaxel-eluting stent deployment: pooled analysis from the SPIRIT II, III, IV and COMPARE trials. EuroIntervention 2011; 7: 74–83.

25. Smits PC, Kedhi E, Royaards KJ, et al. 2-year Follow-Up of a Randomized Controlled Trial of Everolimus- and Paclitaxel-Eluting

Stents for Coronary Revascularization in Daily Practice COM-PARE (Comparison of the everolimus eluting XIENCE-V stent with the paclitaxel eluting TAXUS LIBERTE stent in all-comers: a randomized open label trial). J Am Coll Cardiol 2011; 58: 11–8.

26. Verheugt FW, Steinhubl SR, Hamon M, et al. Incidence, prognostic impact, and influence of antithrombotic therapy on access and nonaccess site bleeding in percutaneous coronary intervention. JACC Cardiovasc Intervent 2011; 4: 191–7.

27. Doyle BJ, Ting HH, Bell MR, et al. Major femoral bleeding complications after percutaneous coronary intervention: incidence, predictors, and impact on long-term survival among 17,901 patients treated at the Mayo Clinic from 1994 to 2005. JACC Cardiovasc Interv 2008; 1: 202–9.

28. Dauerman HL, Rao SV, Resnic FS, Applegate RJ. Bleeding avoidance strategies consensus and controversy. J Am Coll Cardiol 2011; 58: 1–10.

29. Solomon R, Dauerman HL. Contrast-induced acute kidney injury. Circulation 2010; 122: 2451–5.

30. Brown JR, Malenka DJ, DeVries JT, et al. Transient and persistent renal dysfunction are predictors of survival after percutaneous coronary intervention: insights from the Dartmouth Dynamic Registry. Catheter Cardiovasc Interv 2008; 72: 347–54.

31. Brown JR, DeVries JT, Piper WD, et al. Serious renal dysfunction after percutaneous coronary interventions can be predicted. Am Heart J 2008; 155: 260–6.

32. Stone GW, Maehara A, Lansky AJ, et al. A prospective natural-history study of coronary atherosclerosis. N Engl J Med 2011; 364: 226–35.

33. Serruys PW, de Feyter P, Macaya C, et al. Fluvastatin for prevention of cardiac events following successful first percutaneous coronary intervention: a randomized controlled trial. JAMA 2002; 287: 3215–22.

34. Appleby CE, Ivanov J, Lavi S, et al. The adverse long-term impact of renal impairment in patients undergoing percutaneous coronary intervention in the drug-eluting stent era. Circ Cardiovasc Interv 2009; 2: 309–16.

35. Lemos PA, Arampatzis CA, Hoye A, et al. Impact of baseline renal function on mortality after percutaneous coronary intervention with sirolimus-eluting stents or bare metal stents. Am J Cardiol 2005; 95: 167–72.

36. Sofi F, Marcucci R, Gori AM, et al. Clopidogrel non-responsiveness and risk of cardiovascular morbidity. An updated meta-analysis. Thromb Haemost 2010; 103: 841–8.

37. Gottlieb SS. Dead is dead–artificial definitions are no substitute. Lancet 1997; 349: 662–3.

38. Lemos PA, Campos CA, Falcao JL, et al. Prognostic heterogeneity among patients with chronic stable coronary disease: determinants of long-term mortality after treatment with percutaneous intervention. EuroIntervention 2009; 5: 239–43.

39. Dangas GD, Caixeta A, Mehran R, et al. Frequency and predictors of stent thrombosis after percutaneous coronary intervention in acute myocardial infarction. Circulation 2011; 123: 1745–56.

40. van Werkum JW, Heestermans AA, Zomer AC, et al. Predictors of coronary stent thrombosis: the Dutch Stent Thrombosis Registry. J Am Coll Cardiol 2009; 53: 1399–409.

41. Yan BP, Duffy SJ, Clark DJ, et al. Rates of stent thrombosis in bare-metal versus drug-eluting stents (from a Large Australian Multicenter Registry). Am J Cardiol 2008; 101: 1716–22.

42. Mishkel GJ, Moore AL, Markwell S, Shelton ME. Correlates of late and very late thrombosis of drug eluting stents. Am Heart J 2008; 156: 141–7.

43. Baran KW, Lasala JM, Cox DA, et al. A clinical risk score for the prediction of very late stent thrombosis in drug eluting stent patients. EuroIntervention 2011; 6: 949–54.

44. Voudris V, Kariofillis P, Thomopoulou S, et al. Predictors for very late stent thrombosis after drug-eluting stent implantation in diabetic patients. EuroIntervention 2009; 4: 485–91.

45. Tin-Hay EL, Poh KK, Lim YT, et al. Clinical predictors of stent thrombosis in the "real world" drug-eluting stent era. Int J Cardiol 2010; 145: 422–5.

46. Sianos G, Papafaklis MI, Daemen J, et al. Angiographic stent thrombosis after routine use of drug-eluting stents in ST-segment elevation myocardial infarction: the importance of thrombus burden. J Am Coll Cardiol 2007; 50: 573–83.

47. Baran KW, Lasala JM, Cox DA, et al. A clinical risk score for prediction of stent thrombosis. Am J Cardiol 2008; 102: 541–5.

48. de la Torre Hernandez JM, Alfonso F, Gimeno F, et al. Thrombosis of second-generation drug-eluting stents in real practice results from the multicenter Spanish registry ESTROFA-2 (Estudio Espanol Sobre Trombosis de Stents Farmacoactivos de Segunda Generacion-2). JACC Cardiovasc Interv 2010; 3: 911–9.

49. Machecourt J, Danchin N, Lablanche JM, et al. Risk factors for stent thrombosis after implantation of sirolimus-eluting stents in diabetic and nondiabetic patients: the EVASTENT Matched-Cohort Registry. J Am Coll Cardiol 2007; 50: 501–8.

50. Lemos PA, Hoye A, Goedhart D, et al. Clinical, angiographic, and procedural predictors of angiographic restenosis after sirolimus-eluting stent implantation in complex patients: an evaluation from the Rapamycin-Eluting Stent Evaluated At Rotterdam Cardiology Hospital (RESEARCH) study. Circulation 2004; 109: 1366–70.

51. Zahn R, Hamm CW, Schneider S, et al. Coronary stenting with the sirolimus-eluting stent in clinical practice: final results from the prospective multicenter German Cypher Stent Registry. J Interv Cardiol 2010; 23: 18–25.

52. Hong MK, Mintz GS, Lee CW, et al. Intravascular ultrasound predictors of angiographic restenosis after sirolimus-eluting stent implantation. Eur Heart J 2006; 27: 1305–10.

53. Zahn R, Hamm CW, Schneider S, et al. Incidence and predictors of target vessel revascularization and clinical event rates of the sirolimus-eluting coronary stent (results from the prospective multicenter German Cypher Stent Registry). Am J Cardiol 2005; 95: 1302–8.

54. Kastrati A, Dibra A, Mehilli J, et al. Predictive factors of restenosis after coronary implantation of sirolimus- or paclitaxel-eluting stents. Circulation 2006; 113: 2293–300.

55. Zahn R, Hamm CW, Schneider S, et al. Predictors of death or myocardial infarction during follow-up after coronary stenting with the sirolimus-eluting stent. Results from the prospective multicenter German Cypher Stent Registry. Am Heart J 2006; 152: 1146–52.

56. Kandzari DE, Tcheng JE, Gersh BJ, et al. Relationship between infarct artery location, epicardial flow, and myocardial perfusion after primary percutaneous revascularization in acute myocardial infarction. Am Heart J 2006; 151: 1288–95.

A. Pieter Kappetein and Stuart J. Head

OUTLINE

Coronary artery bypass grafting (CABG) is a well-established therapy for patients with extensive and diffuse coronary artery disease (CAD) and is arguably the most intensively studied surgical procedure ever undertaken with excellent short- and medium-term results. The long-term outcome is determined by both procedural and patient-related factors. This chapter provides a perspective on the determinants of the long-term follow-up.

INTRODUCTION

Revascularization with either coronary artery bypass grafting (CABG) surgery or percutaneous coronary intervention (PCI) is the choice of therapy in many patients who present with angina pectoris. During the last decade the introduction of drug-eluting stents, together with antiplatelet and antithrombotic treatments has improved the outcome of PCI by reducing the number of repeat revascularizations. Coronary bypass surgery has improved as well by using more arterial grafts, better perioperative care, and optimizing medical treatment postoperatively. CABG surgery remains superior to PCI and medical treatment for the long-term relief of angina for patients with complex coronary artery disease (CAD) with little difference in overall costs between PCI (with the need for repeat procedures) and CABG (1). This chapter will discuss the elements that may play a role in optimizing the outcome of coronary bypass surgery.

The long-term outcome of coronary surgery depends on factors associated with the procedure and on patient-related factors. Procedure-related factors that influence long-term outcomes include graft patency, completeness of revascularization, and myocardial injury during surgery. Post-operative complications such as stroke and renal dysfunction will also negatively influence the long-term outcome. Patient factors relate to a large extent to the severity of CAD and the physiologic impact of ischemia on ventricular function at the time of the operation. During screening for coronary bypass surgery it is also important to consider the overall health status, age, gender, and presence of peripheral vascular disease, cerebrovascular events history, and other comorbidities (2).

DIFFERENT GRAFTS AND GRAFT PATENCY

Graft patency is a major determinant of long-term outcome following CABG surgery. The efficacy of different conduits is measured by their long-term patency. Failure of coronary artery grafts is multifactorial, and may be influenced by the choice of conduit, degree of competitive flow from the native

vessels, extent of the vascular bed for run-off, and technical errors at distal or proximal anastomoses (3).

Left Internal Thoracic Artery Grafts

The patency of the left internal thoracic artery (LITA) graft is better than that of venous grafts, and it has also been demonstrated that the usage of the LITA to the anterior wall coronary artery leads to an improved survival (4). The patency of the LITA graft is highest when it is anastomosed to the left anterior descending (LAD) resulting in 96% patency at 5 years (3) and 85% at 10 years (5). The majority of patients therefore receive LITA grafts to the LAD coronary artery and saphenous vein grafts to the remaining vessels. Left internal mammary artery (LIMA) grafting not only provides a better long-term outcome but it is also associated with an almost 50% lower perioperative mortality (6). Because of the survival advantage of a LITA to the LAD this is considered a clinical standard in all patient groups.

It is not surprising that the improved patency of the in situ left internal mammary has led researchers to explore the use of other arterial grafts, such as the right internal thoracic artery (RITA), or free internal thoracic artery, the gastroepiploic artery (GEA), and the radial artery (RA), as second or third arterial grafts in coronary bypass surgery (7).

Right Internal Mammary Artery Graft

The right ITA is anatomically the same as the LITA and the patency of the RITA graft is comparable to the LITA if the RITA is used as an in situ graft to the LAD artery (8). If the RITA is used as a free arterial conduit the RITA patency is lower than the patency of a LIMA in situ graft (3). The RITA patency at 5 years is 96%, at 10 years 81%, and at 15 years it is 65% (9).

Bilateral Mammary Artery Grafts

A single internal mammary artery graft (SIMA) rather than a vein graft to the LAD coronary artery is the standard therapy in coronary bypass surgery. Surprisingly, the usage of bilateral mammary arteries (BIMA) has not been accepted as the standard of care and the benefits and disadvantages have been a matter of debate for years. A systematic review of observational studies including 15,962 patients showed a survival benefit for BIMA grafts (10).

Although non-randomized studies suggested that the use of BIMA grafts improves outcome, there is some concern is that the short-term perioperative risk of using a BIMA does not outweigh the long-term benefits. The operation is technically more challenging, and the operation time longer; this may increase the risk of early mortality. The usage of two internal thoracic arteries may result in more perioperative wound infections and the incidence of mediastinitis is higher especially in elderly, obese, or diabetic patients, characteristics common to CABG patients (11). The adoption, in clinical practice of the use of two mammary grafts is therefore low; around 4% in the United States and around 12% in Europe.

The concerns regarding an increased rate of wound infections might not be entirely true. In the Arterial Revascularisation Trial (ART) trial patients were randomized to receive a single mammary artery graft versus bilateral mammary artery grafts and the one year results demonstrated similar mortality and major morbidity rates for SIMA and BIMA groups at 30 days and one year. There was only a small increase in sternal wound reconstruction in the BIMA group (12). Skeletonization of the internal thoracic arteries may reduce the risk of sternal wound complications particularly in those with diabetes (13).

Radial Artery

The RA has gained popularity over the last few years as the second or third arterial graft. Preoperative assessment of the RA and collateral hand circulation is mandatory to avoid hand ischemia in patients with an inadequate collateral circulation. The RA may be proximally anastomosed to the LITA, forming a composite graft, or to the ascending aorta to bypass all coronary territories. The drawback of the RA is that it has a much thicker muscular wall which is prone to spasm. To minimize spasm the artery should be harvested as a pedicle, pharmacological dilatation with papaverine should be applied locally, and vasodilator therapy with calcium channel blockers prescribed postoperatively. The more muscular structure of the RA makes the graft also more sensitive to vasoconstricting agents such as norepinephrine sometimes used in the postoperative period. The internal diameter of the radial artery is larger than that of the ITA making it less suitable as a composite graft.

One of the most important factors determining radial artery graft patency and development of string sign is the degree of stenosis in the native target vessel which should exceed at least 70%. The Radial Artery Patency Study investigators performed a prospective randomized trial which compared the patency rate of the radial artery to the saphenous vein graft (SVG). at 1 year. In this study, complete graft occlusion occurred less frequently with RA grafts than with SVGs (8.2 versus 13.6%); however, string signs occur more commonly with RA grafts than with SVGs (7% versus 0.9%). More severe target coronary lesions were associated with a lower rate of occlusion (5.9% for >90% stenosis versus 11.8% for 70–89% stenosis). The authors concluded that radial artery grafts should preferentially be used for target vessels with high-grade lesions (14).

Right GEA

The right GEA is primarily used as an in situ graft to bypass the right coronary artery and its branches and provides a reasonable long-term survival and freedom from angina of almost 90% up to 5 years postoperatively (15). The artery is, however, fragile and often has a small diameter at the site of the anastomosis. Vessel twisting, limited length of the conduit, increased perioperative time, and ileus are other concerns in the usage of this conduit.

Saphenous Vein Graft

The greater saphenous veins (SV) from the leg are still widely utilized, primarily to bypass vessels other than the LAD. It is has a large diameter, is plentiful, readily accessed, long, and easily harvested. The drawback is that the occlusion rate is up to 12% within the first 4 weeks, and upto 15% at one year. Furthermore, by 10 years postoperatively at least 50% demonstrate significant disease (14). Factors that predispose to saphenous vein graft disease are target vessel diameter less than 2.0 mm, smoking, hypertension, and lipid abnormalities. Aspirin and statin therapy provide a better graft patency.

There are three phases and distinct disease processes that influence the early, intermediate, or late failure of saphenous vein grafts. During the first 30 postoperative days, up to 12% of grafts may become occluded; this is referred to as early graft failure and might be related to small vessel size, the degree of stenosis of the native vessel, technical factors, and thrombosis. Ischemia during vein harvesting by transient loss of luminal blood and vasa vasorum, nonphysiologic pH of the distending fluid when a fluid other than blood is used to support and dilate the vein before implantation, and exposure to the high pressures in the arterial circulation may lead to damage of the endothelium and predispose veins to thrombosis (16). Mural thrombus in grafts is found in 75% of patients dying in the first months after surgery and platelet activation related to cardiopulmonary bypass and vascular injury play a major role (17).

Technical errors promote thrombus formation and occur due to inaccuracy in performing the distal anastomosis, kinks from excessive or insufficient graft length, and mismatched sizes of graft and recipient artery, which can compromise flow, promote turbulence, or both (16). Between 1 month and 1 year, fibrointimal hyperplasia (the accumulation of smooth muscle cells and extracellular matrix in the intimal compartment) with or without superimposed thrombosis can occur. In the media there is fibrous scarring with replacement of smooth muscle cells by thick collagen bundles that may extend into the adventitia. At the end of the first year the diameter of the graft is reduced by 25%. Although this condition rarely leads to a clinically significant stenosis, it could provide the foundation for the development of graft atheroma (17).

The 30-year outcome of patients who underwent venous CABG between 1971 and 1980 showed a median life expectancy of 18 years and 94% of patients needed a repeat intervention (18).

INCOMPLETE REVASCULARIZATION

The usual goal of coronary bypass surgery is complete revascularization as incomplete revascularization could lead to persistent angina, repeat revascularization, myocardial infarction, and potentially death. There is no universal definition for what is meant by "complete" revascularization. Different studies employ different definitions, and for that reason, comparisons between studies must be interpreted with caution. In a post hoc analysis from the ARTS trial, complete revascularization was not associated with a difference in mortality or in major adverse cerebral or cardiac events (MACCE) compared with patients with incomplete revascularization at 1 year. The respective freedom from MACCE was 89.9% versus 87.8% (19). In a study with an angiographic definition of complete revascularization the 5-year major adverse cardiovascular event rate was slightly elevated for patients with multivessel disease and incomplete revascularization (20). Where there is a mammary artery conduit to the LAD reasonable incomplete revascularization, usually related to the presence of small distal or severely calcified coronary vessels, seems to be well tolerated (21). Only extensive incomplete revascularization is likely to be hazardous and associated with significant residual angina burden, myocardium at risk, and adverse cardiovascular events (22).

TECHNIQUE OF GRAFTING: SEQUENTIAL OR COMPOSITE
Several modifications to CABG surgery have been proposed to improve graft patency including the sequential anastomotic technique. With this technique more than one distal anastomosis is constructed per segment of conduit used resulting in two or more distal anastomoses per single proximal anastomosis. It is believed that by sequencing multiple small coronary arteries with poor run-off bypass graft blood flow can be maximized, resulting in a bypass graft that is more likely than individual grafts to remain open. The safety of this strategy has been demonstrated in observational studies and allows performance of coronary bypass surgery in patients with advanced coronary artery disease or with limited available conduits who are likely to require sequential grafting.

Data from the Prevent IV trial however suggests that patients who received a SV graft with multiple distal anastomoses were more likely to experience graft failure and had a trend toward higher mortality, myocardial infarction, or repeat revascularization (23). Although the angiographic results in this study came from patients enrolled in a randomized trial it remains an observational study as patients were not randomly assigned to receive SV grafts with either single or multiple distal anastomoses (24).

A composite technique can also be used for arterial grafts whereby the proximal free RIMA, the right gastroepiploic artery GEA, or the radial artery is connected end-to-side to an in situ LIMA. The safety and efficacy of total arterial composite grafts have been demonstrated in randomized and observational studies resulting in a 94% freedom from reintervention as long as 8.5 years after operation. Another advantage of composite arterial grafts is that this technique avoids manipulation of the aorta and thereby reduces the incidence of stroke secondary to manipulation of the aorta (25).

OFF-PUMP SURGERY
There is still an ongoing debate as to whether the benefits of off-pump CABG versus on-pump surgery lead to a better outcome. There was a hope that off-pump surgery would decrease perioperative morbidity and possibly mortality by eliminating cardiopulmonary bypass (on-pump surgery). The concern with off-pump surgery is that the difficulty of operating with the heart beating would lead to less complete and less effective revascularization at the time of surgery and worse long-term outcomes. Several prospective randomized controlled trials and a meta-analysis suggest that grafts performed during off-pump surgery have a significantly lower patency rate and result in less complete revascularization than grafts constructed on pump (26). A review of patients undergoing coronary bypass surgery in the state of New York during 2001 to 2004 examined 30-day mortality and complication rates and the occurrence over 3 years after surgery of death and repeat revascularization. This study showed that off-pump surgery is associated with lower in-hospital mortality and complication rates than on-pump CABG, but long-term outcomes are comparable, except for freedom from revascularization, which favors on-pump CABG (27). A randomized study between on- and off-pump in patients at higher risk, defined as an Euroscore of 5 or greater, showed no significant difference in the primary outcome of MACCE at a median of 3.7 years follow-up and mortality seemed higher after off-pump CABG (28).The identification of patient subsets that may benefit from off-pump surgery will allow for a tailored therapy. Observational data suggests that patients with a high risk of stroke, particularly in the presence of known aortic atherosclerosis or cerebrovascular disease, derive the most benefit from off-pump surgery in regard to the avoidance of perioperative complications. This type of information will allow us to select the best strategy for each patient and to maximize the advantages and minimize the disadvantages of both techniques (29).

PERIOPERATIVE MYOCARDIAL INJURY
Perioperative myocardial infarction with new Q-waves and elevations in creatine kinase (CK-MB) are associated with adverse outcomes an increase in short- and long-term mortality. Increases in CK-MB or troponin levels following CABG are common, occur even in the absence of graft occlusion, and are ascribed to a number of causes including, though not limited to, cell death resulting from insufficient myocardial protection during cardiopulmonary bypass or with off-pump techniques, air embolism, and regional and global ischemia during the procedure (30). Myocardial enzyme elevation within 24 hours after undergoing CABG surgery continues to be prognostically important for 30 days and 1 year mortality with a hazard ratio of 1.12 and 1.17, respectively, per five fold increase in 5-peak CK-MB ratio (30).

MEDICAL THERAPY TO OPTIMIZE LONG-TERM OUTCOME
Medical interventions to lower cardiovascular complications and improve long-term outcome include antiplatelet therapy, statins, β-blockers, and angiotensin-converting enzyme (ACE) inhibitors. The Prevent IV trial showed that secondary prevention medications are associated with a lower incidence of death

or myocardial infarction after coronary bypass surgery (31). Avoidance of smoking, treatment of hypertension, and control of glucose levels in patients with diabetes are essential.

Antiplatelet Agents

Thrombosis accounts for graft failure within the first month after CABG and may be related to endothelial injury and technical errors. Treatment with agents to prevent platelet activation and aggregation decreases the vein graft occlusion rate.

Normally ASA is stopped 3–7 days before surgery but acetylsalicylic acid (ASA) should not be discontinued after ST-elevation myocardial infarction. Some studies suggest that administration of ASA prior to CABG even improves graft patency but this needs to be balanced against excess bleeding rates (32). ASA should be administered 6 hours after operation to reduce early and late graft occlusion (33).

Combination antiplatelet therapy with ASA and clopidogrel in patients with stable CAD is controversial as it is associated with higher postoperative bleeding and there is regarding whether or not it improves graft patency (34,35).

Antiplatelet therapy with the combination of ASA and clopidogrel or ticagrelor reduces recurrent ischemic events more than ASA alone in patients with acute coronary syndromes. Approximately 10% of these patients require CABG surgery during the index admission. Randomized clinical trials suggest that patients undergoing CABG after receiving clopidogrel or ticagrelor benefit from the anti-ischemic effects of the antiplatelet agent and it is recommended that patients who receive clopidogrel or ticagrelor pre-CABG for a recent acute coronary syndrome indication should have clopidogrel or ticagrelor restarted after surgery to decrease the risk of recurrent ACS (36). The PLATO trial showed that the composite end point of vascular death, myocardial infarction, and stroke was reduced by 16% with ticagrelor compared to clopidogrel treatment with no difference in major bleeding rates in the two groups (37).

β-Blockers

While β-adrenergic blockade has been demonstrated to improve acute outcomes and long-term prognosis in ischemic heart disease there have been no randomized trials evaluating preoperative β-blockade in CABG patients. In an observational analysis, however, preoperative β-blocker therapy was associated with a small but consistent survival benefit for patients undergoing CABG, except among patients with a left ventricular ejection fraction of less than 30% (38). Another observational study showed that β-blocker usage lowered mortality across all examined subgroups, including patients without prior myocardial infarction or without heart failure (39).

Statin

Aggressive lowering of lipid levels may reduce the progression of atherosclerosis in SV grafts and reduce the rates of clinical events (40). A 30% reduction in revascularization procedures and a 24% reduction in cardiovascular death, myocardial infarction (MI),

stroke, CABG, or angioplasty were seen during 7.5 years of follow-up after CABG (41). Progression of atherosclerosis in the native coronary arteries also continues as well after CABG and is associated with deterioration in left ventricular function. Aggressive secondary prevention to diminish the progression of native coronary atherosclerosis may also be important.

ACE Inhibitors

ACE inhibitors have been shown to prolong survival and to decrease infarct size in patients after acute coronary syndromes. ACE inhibitors may also provide cardiovascular protection during CABG surgery and reduce the number of ischemic events in the years after surgery. The cardio-protective effect of ACE-inhibitors is particularly marked in patients with hypertension, diabetes, decreased left ventricular function end with or who present with an acute coronary syndrome (42).

NEUROLOGIC COMPLICATIONS FOLLOWING CARDIAC SURGERY

Neurologic injury is a devastating complication following cardiac surgery and is subject to great variability depending on patient disease, age, sex, and overall illness. The incidence of stroke after CABG ranges from 1.6 to 3%. Symptoms of stroke may even underestimate the incidence of stroke as the rate of cerebral infarction is significantly higher if postoperative magnetic resonance imaging data with diffusion-weighted imaging is performed (43). Some patients develop stroke intraoperatively, with a neurologic deficit apparent immediately after awakening from anesthesia. These strokes are attributed to surgical activity in the mediastinum, usually aortic manipulation. Half of the strokes however, occur postoperatively with a peak at postoperative day 2 and atherosclerosis of the ascending aorta and brachiocephalic vessels and atrial arrhythmias are thought to cause brain damage through embolization in this period (43,44). The 5- and 10-year survival rates for patients without a neurological events are 5–30% lower than others (45,46).

Neurocognitive Dysfunction

Disturbances in memory, executive function, motor speed, attention, and other cognitive functions can be detected in 3–34% of patients in the first several weeks after CABG depending on the specific criteria used. These short-term changes appear to be reversible by 3 months after surgery for most patients. Late cognitive decline between 1 and 5 years after surgery also occurs but appears to be mild and may be secondary to high rates of cerebrovascular disease among candidates for CABG (47).

PERSONAL PERSPECTIVE

Coronary artery bypass surgery is not in competition with PCI. The two methods of treatment are complementary (48,49). In patients with severe three-vessel CAD and left main disease coronary bypass surgery with at least one arterial graft and

Focus Box 36.1

Single ITA grafting to the LAD is the standard of care with improved long-term outcome compared to venous grafting

Bilateral mammary artery grafting carries a slightly higher incidence of wound complications but may offer a better long-term outcome in patients with a reasonable overall life expectancy

The benefits of multiple arterial grafts are mainly related to the use of BIMAs and not to the usage of other arterial conduits

Graft patency is better in on-pump surgery but patients with atherosclerotic disease of the aorta may benefit from off-pump surgery. Identification of patient subsets in which major differences in outcomes exist based on surgical strategy is highly important

Perioperative cerebral injury decreases the quality of life and affects the long-term survival

preferably two, is still the most effective treatment at this moment and the therapy of choice. In patients with less severe CAD PCI is the more attractive therapy due to its limited invasiveness. Improvements in stent technology and anti-platelet therapy, however, will also make PCI a very attractive option in patients with more complex disease. Coronary surgery can also be further developed and research should be directed toward more use of arterial grafts, modified vein grafts, less invasive approaches, better perioperative care, and postoperative medical therapy, and reduction of neurological events to achieve a more effective and less morbid operation (50,51). Hybrid coronary revascularization is also an option but the comparative effectiveness to both conventional CABG and multivessel stenting should be evaluated.

REFERENCES

1. Serruys PW, Morice MC, Kappetein AP, et al. Percutaneous coronary intervention versus coronary-artery bypass grafting for severe coronary artery disease. N Engl J Med 2009; 360: 961–72.
2. Shahian DM, O'Brien SM, Filardo G, et al. The society of thoracic surgeons 2008 cardiac surgery risk models: Part 1–coronary artery bypass grafting surgery. Ann Thorac Surg 2009; 88: S2–22.
3. Hayward PAR, Buxton BF. Contemporary coronary graft patency: 5-year observational data from a randomized trial of conduits. Ann Thora Surg 2007; 84: 795–9.
4. Loop FD, Lytle BW, Cosgrove DM, et al. Influence of the internal-mammary-artery graft on 10-year survival and other cardiac events. N Engl J Med 1986; 314: 1–6.
5. Goldman S, Zadina K, Moritz T, et al. Long-term patency of saphenous vein and left internal mammary artery grafts after coronary artery bypass surgery: Results from a department of veterans affairs cooperative study. J Am Coll Cardiol 2004; 44: 2149–56.
6. Leavitt BJ, O'Connor GT, Olmstead EM, et al. Use of the internal mammary artery graft and in-hospital mortality and other adverse outcomes associated with coronary artery bypass surgery. Circulation 2001; 103: 507–12.
7. Goldman S, Sethi GK, Holman W, et al. Radial artery grafts vs saphenous vein grafts in coronary artery bypass surgery: A randomized trial. JAMA 2011; 305: 167–74.
8. Fukui T, Tabata M, Manabe S, et al. Angiographic outcomes of right internal thoracic artery grafts in situ or as free grafts in coronary artery bypass grafting. J Thorac Cardiovasc Surg 2010; 139: 868–73.
9. Tatoulis J, Buxton BF, Fuller JA. Patencies of 2,127 arterial to coronary conduits over 15 years. Ann Thorac Surg 2004; 77: 93–101.
10. Taggart DP, D'Amico R, Altman DG. Effect of arterial revascularisation on survival: a systematic review of studies comparing bilateral and single internal mammary arteries. Lancet 2001; 358: 870–5.
11. Toumpoulis IK, Theakos N, Dunning J. Does bilateral internal thoracic artery harvest increase the risk of mediastinitis? Interact Cardiovasc Thorac Surg 2007; 6: 787–91.
12. Taggart DP, Altman DG, Gray AM, et al. Randomized trial to compare bilateral vs. Single internal mammary coronary artery bypass grafting: 1-year results of the arterial revascularisation trial (art). Eur Heart J 2010; 31: 2470–81.
13. Saso S, James D, Vecht JA, et al. Effect of skeletonization of the internal thoracic artery for coronary revascularization on the incidence of sternal wound infection. Ann Thorac Surg 2010; 89: 661–70.
14. Desai ND, Cohen EA, Naylor CD, Fremes SE. A randomized comparison of radial-artery and saphenous-vein coronary bypass grafts. N Engl J Med 2004; 351: 2302–9.
15. Tavilla G, Kappetein AP, Braun J, et al. Long-term follow-up of coronary artery bypass grafting in three-vessel disease using exclusively pedicled bilateral internal thoracic and right gastroepiploic arteries. Ann Thorac Surg 2004; 77: 794–9; discussion 799.
16. Nwasokwa ON. Coronary artery bypass graft disease. Ann Intern Med 1995; 123: 528–45.
17. Cox JL, Chiasson DA, Gotlieb AI. Stranger in a strange land: the pathogenesis of saphenous vein graft stenosis with emphasis on structural and functional differences between veins and arteries. Prog Cardiovasc Dis 1991; 34: 45–68.
18. van Domburg RT, Kappetein AP, Bogers AJ. The clinical outcome after coronary bypass surgery: a 30-year follow-up study. Eur Heart J 2009; 30: 453–8.
19. van den Brand MJBM, Rensing BJWM, Morel M-aM, et al. The effect of completeness of revascularization on event-free survival at one year in the arts trial. J Am Coll Cardiol 2002; 39: 559–64.
20. Kim Y-H, Park D-W, Lee J-Y, et al. Impact of angiographic complete revascularization after drug-eluting stent implantation or coronary artery bypass graft surgery for multivessel coronary artery disease/ clinical perspective. Circulation 2011; 123: 2373–81.
21. Rastan AJ, Walther T, Falk V, et al. Does reasonable incomplete surgical revascularization affect early or long-term survival in patients with multivessel coronary artery disease receiving left internal mammary artery bypass to left anterior descending artery? Circulation 2009; 120: S70–7.
22. Dauerman HL. Reasonable incomplete revascularization. Circulation 2011; 123: 2337–40.
23. Mehta RH, Ferguson TB, Lopes RD, et al. Saphenous vein grafts with multiple versus single distal targets in patients undergoing coronary artery bypass surgery: one-year graft failure and five-year outcomes from the project of ex-vivo vein graft engineering via transfection (prevent) iv trial. Circulation 2011; 124: 280–8.

24. Sabik JF 3rd. Understanding saphenous vein graft patency. Circulation 2011; 124: 273–5.

25. Raja SG. Composite arterial grafting. Expert Rev Cardiovasc Ther 2006; 4: 523–33.

26. Khan NE, De Souza A, Mister R, et al. A randomized comparison of off-pump and on-pump multivessel coronary-artery bypass surgery. N Engl J Med 2004; 350: 21–8.

27. Hannan EL, Wu C, Smith CR, et al. Off-pump versus on-pump coronary artery bypass graft surgery. Circulation 2007; 116: 1145–52.

28. Møller CH, Perko MJ, Lund JT, et al. Three-year follow-up in a subset of high-risk patients randomly assigned to off-pump versus on-pump coronary artery bypass surgery: the best bypass surgery trial. Heart 2011; 97: 907–13.

29. Lytle BW. On-pump and off-pump coronary bypass surgery. Circulation 2007; 116: 1108–9.

30. Domanski MJ, Mahaffey K, Hasselblad V, et al. Association of myocardial enzyme elevation and survival following coronary artery bypass graft surgery. JAMA 2011; 305: 585–91.

31. Goyal A, Alexander JH, Hafley GE, et al. Outcomes associated with the use of secondary prevention medications after coronary artery bypass graft surgery. Ann Thorac Surg 2007; 83: 993–1001.

32. Sethi GK, Copeland JG, Goldman S, et al. Implications of preoperative administration of aspirin in patients undergoing coronary artery bypass grafting. Department of veterans affairs cooperative study on antiplatelet therapy. J Am Coll Cardiol 1990; 15: 15–20.

33. Goldman S, Copeland J, Moritz T, et al. Starting aspirin therapy after operation. Effects on early graft patency. Department of veterans affairs cooperative study group. Circulation 1991; 84: 520–6.

34. Kulik A, Le May MR, Voisine P, et al. Aspirin plus clopidogrel versus aspirin alone after coronary artery bypass grafting: the clopidogrel after surgery for coronary artery disease (cascade) trial. Circulation 2010; 122: 2680–7.

35. Gao G, Zheng Z, Pi Y, et al. Aspirin plus clopidogrel therapy increases early venous graft patency after coronary artery bypass surgery a single-center, randomized, controlled trial. J Am Coll Cardiol 2010; 56: 1639–43.

36. Fitchett D, Eikelboom J, Fremes S, et al. Dual antiplatelet therapy in patients requiring urgent coronary artery bypass grafting surgery: a position statement of the canadian cardiovascular society. Can J Cardiol 2009; 25: 683–9.

37. Held C, Asenblad N, Bassand JP, et al. Ticagrelor versus clopidogrel in patients with acute coronary syndromes undergoing coronary artery bypass surgery: results from the plato (platelet inhibition and patient outcomes) trial. J Am Coll Cardiol 2011; 57: 672–84.

38. Ferguson TB Jr, Coombs LP, Peterson ED. Preoperative beta-blocker use and mortality and morbidity following cabg surgery in North America. JAMA 2002; 287: 2221–7.

39. Chan AYM, McAlister FA, Norris CM, Alberta Provincial Program for Outcome Assessment in Coronary Heart Disease Investigators. Effect of {beta}-blocker use on outcomes after discharge in patients who underwent cardiac surgery. J Thorac Cardiovasc Surg 2010; 140: 182–7.

40. The post coronary artery bypass graft trial investigators. The effect of aggressive lowering of low-density lipoprotein cholesterol levels and low-dose anticoagulation on obstructive changes in saphenous-vein coronary-artery bypass grafts. N Engl J Med 1997; 336: 153–62.

41. Knatterud GL, Rosenberg Y, Campeau L, et al. Long-term effects on clinical outcomes of aggressive lowering of low-density lipoprotein cholesterol levels and low-dose anticoagulation in the post coronary artery bypass graft trial. Post cabg investigators. Circulation 2000; 102: 157–65.

42. Lazar HL. All coronary artery bypass graft surgery patients will benefit from angiotensin-converting enzyme inhibitors. Circulation 2008; 117: 6–8.

43. Hammon JW, Stump DA. Editorial comment does the time of onset of postoperative stroke determine outcome? Eur J Cardiothorac Surg 2011; 40: 387–8.

44. Tarakji KG, Sabik JF, Bhudia SK, Batizy LH, Blackstone EH. Temporal onset, risk factors, and outcomes associated with stroke after coronary artery bypass grafting. JAMA 2011; 305: 381–90.

45. Ngaage DL, Dickson J, Chaudhry M, Cale AR, Cowen ME. Early and late prognostic significance of remote and reversible preoperative neurological events in patients undergoing coronary artery bypass grafting. Eur J Cardiothorac Surg 2010; 37: 1075–80.

46. Hedberg M, Boivie P, Engstrom KG. Early and delayed stroke after coronary surgery - an analysis of risk factors and the impact on short- and long-term survival. Eur J Cardiothorac Surg 2011; 40: 379–87.

47. Selnes OA, McKhann GM. Neurocognitive complications after coronary artery bypass surgery. Ann Neurol 2005; 57: 615–21.

48. Kolh P, Wijns W, Danchin N, et al. Guidelines on myocardial revascularization. Eur J Cardiothoracic Surg 2010; 38(Suppl): S1–S52.

49. Kappetein AP, Feldman TE, Mack MJ, et al. Comparison of coronary bypass surgery with drug-eluting stenting for the treatment of left main and/or three-vessel disease: 3-year follow-up of the syntax trial. Eur Heart J 2011; 32: 2125–34.

50. Uva MS, Cavaco S, Oliveira AG, et al. Early graft patency after off-pump and on-pump coronary bypass surgery: a prospective randomized study. Eur Heart J 2010; 31: 2492–9.

51. Elghobary T, Légaré J-F. What has happened to multiple arterial grafting in coronary artery bypass grafting surgery? Expert Rev Cardiovasc Ther 2010; 8: 1099–105.

37 Novel therapeutic approaches to prevention and regression of atherosclerosis
Kuang-Yuh Chyu and Prediman K. Shah

OUTLINE

The conventional therapeutic approach for atherosclerotic vascular disease focuses on the adoption and maintenance of a healthy life style coupled with management of modifiable risk factors such as hypertension, diabetes mellitus, cigarette smoking, and dyslipidemia. Reducing low density lipoprotein (LDL)-cholesterol levels using statins and other agents serves as the primary pharmacological approach to stabilize atherosclerotic vascular disease but a large residual risk burden remains which has stimulated research into additional novel therapies for atherosclerosis management. This chapter will focus on new and emerging therapeutic strategies targeting atherosclerosis.

INTRODUCTION

Atherosclerosis is currently viewed as a chronic inflammatory disease of the arterial wall. At the center of this inflammatory process are atherogenic lipoproteins, activation of immune responses toward atherogenic antigens with subsequent activation of inflammatory signaling molecules and the cytokine cascade (1–4). Since retention and deposition of atherogenic lipoproteins in the arterial wall is essential for development of plaque, lowering circulating levels of atherogenic lipoproteins has been the major target for current management of atherosclerotic cardiovascular diseases. Statins, based on substantial body of evidence supporting their clinical efficacy, have emerged as the mainstay of atherosclerosis management (5,6). However, atherosclerotic cardiovascular disease continues to be highly prevalent despite the use of statins.

Many reasons such as underutilization of statins, lack of long-term compliance, intolerance of statins due to adverse effects, inability to achieve target cholesterol levels at tolerable doses, global epidemic trends in obesity, metabolic syndrome, and diabetes may partially account for the continuing epidemic of cardiovascular disease. Additionally statins, which upregulate hepatic LDL receptors by inhibiting 3-hydroxy-3-methyl-glutaryl-CoA reductase (HMG-COA) reductase and cholesterol synthesis, are often used later in life when atherosclerotic cardiovascular disease or its complication has been already well established leading to compromised effectiveness of statins. Thus statins reduce cardiovascular events by about 30%, leaving a substantial residual event burden percentage of the events continuing to occur (Fig. 37.1). These findings underscore the complex nature of atherosclerosis and the need for additional novel interventions. These novel interventions basically operate on the following mechanisms: (1) lowering LDL cholesterol via non-HMG-COA reductase inhibition (2); augmenting HDL levels or HDL function (3); modulation of inflammatory or immune pathways.

LOWERING LDL CHOLESTEROL BEYOND HMG-COA REDUCTASE INHIBITION

Circulating cholesterol, VLDL and LDL are derived from two sources: endogenous synthesis via liver and exogenous absorption via alimentary tract. Numerous enzymes, transporters, and lipoprotein transfer pathways are involved, providing opportunities for pharmacological interventions beyond inhibition of HMG-COA reductase (Fig. 37.2).

Cholesterol Absorption Inhibitors

Plant stanols are intestinally active agents to prevent micellar cholesterol formation, thereby inhibiting intestinal absorption of cholesterol. They increase cholesterol efflux from intestinal cells into the intestinal lumen by activating intestinal activity of ABCA1 (ATP-binding cassette transporter) activity (7). Oil-based products enriched with plant stanol esters lowers LDL cholesterol concentrations by 10–14% (8).

Agents that inhibit the bile–acid transporter or the putative intestinal cholesterol permease on the intestinal brush border block intestinal transport of cholesterol. Ezetimibe is one such agent with Niemann-Pick C1-like 1 (NPC1L1), an intestinal cholesterol transporter, as its molecular target (9). Ezetimibe reduces total cholesterol levels by 15–20%, and its cholesterol-lowering effects are synergistic with those of statins (10). Ezetimibe produced a significant reduction in LDL cholesterol when combined with 80 mg simvastatin in patients with familial hypercholesterolemia compared with simvastatin alone (11). A combination of low-dose statin (10 mg of atorvastatin) and 10 mg of ezetimibe has been shown to produce the same magnitude of LDL lowering as monotherapy with high-dose atorvastatin (80 mg) (12), making ezetimibe a welcome addition to our armamentarium as monotherapy for patients who need modest LDL lowering or as combination therapy with statins (or fibrates) for patients who need greater LDL lowering but are unable to tolerate high doses of statin or respond poorly to statins alone. However, questions have been raised about its efficacy in reducing cardiovascular events (11) whether a combination of ezetimibe and statin provides an additional reduction of cardiovascular events compared with statin alone after an acute coronary syndrome. The currently ongoing clinical trial of ezetimibe (IMPROVE IT; ClinicalTrials.gov Identifier: NCT00202878; estimated completion date: June 2013) is likely to provide a clearer picture of whether ezetimibe-induced LDL-C lowering translates into clinical benefit (13). Although some studies suggested a potential increase in cancer-related deaths with ezetimibe, the totality of clinical trial data to date does not provide support for this hypothesis findings (14).

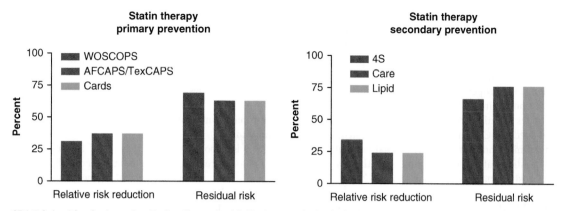

Figure 37.1 Relative risk reduction and residual cardiovascular risk (death or non-fatal MI) after statin therapy in primary and secondary prevention trials.

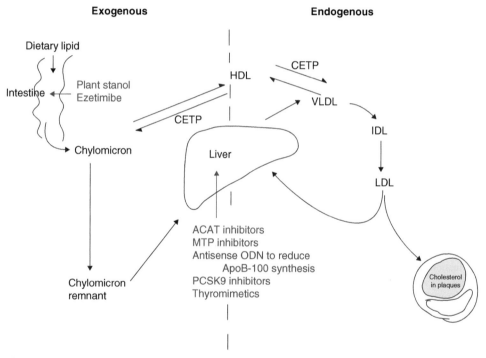

Figure 37.2 Schematic representation of LDL metabolism and potential steps that can be intervened by pharmacological therapies (in *red*).

Acyl-CoA Cholesterol Acyl Transferase Inhibitors

Acyl-CoA cholesterol acyltransferase (ACAT) is responsible for cholesterol esterification in the macrophages, liver, and intestines. Two forms of ACAT, ACAT-1, and ACAT-2, have been described. ACAT-1 in macrophages is responsible for cholesterol ester formation resulting in foam cell formation in atherosclerotic lesions. Therefore, ACAT-1 inhibition may theoretically provide anti-atherogenic effects. ACAT-2 inhibition in the intestine may reduce cholesterol absorption, resulting in a reduction in circulating cholesterol levels. However, preclinical studies utilizing strategies to completely eliminate ACAT-1

activity through gene targeting or transplantation of ACAT-1-null bone marrow did not reduce atherosclerosis in hypercholesterolemic mice but in fact increased lesion size and macrophage necrosis along with accumulation of cholesterol deposits in the skin and brain (15,16). These observations have raised concerns about selective and complete inhibition of ACAT-1.

Partial inhibition of ACAT activity by using nonselective inhibitors of both ACAT-1 and ACAT-2 has shown promising results in murine hypercholesterolemia atherosclerosis models (17). Similarly, inhibition of liver-specific ACAT-2

429

through gene targeting results in resistance to diet-induced hypercholesterolemia in mice (18), suggesting that selective ACAT-2 inhibition may be another approach to reduce dietary absorption of cholesterol. A selective partial ACAT-1 inhibitor, K-604, has demonstrated plaque stabilizing and anti-atherogenic properties in preclinical models (19) and is currently undergoing a Phase 2 clinical evaluation in the United States (ClinicalTrials.gov identifier: NCT00851500). Two non-specific ACAT inhibitors have been tested in clinical trials (avasimibe and pactimibe) with negative results raising further questions about the usefulness of these agents for atherosclerosis management in humans (20–22).

Microsomal Triglyceride Transfer Protein Inhibitors

Microsomal triglyceride transfer protein (MTP) is a heterodimeric lipid transfer protein present in the endoplasmic reticulum of hepatocytes and intestinal cells and its function is to transfer neutral lipids (triglyceride, phospholipids, cholesterol esters) to apoB in VLDL and chylomicron synthesis. In human, a defect in the MTP gene (producing a severe deficiency in MTP) causes marked reductions in plasma triglycerides, LDL, and VLDL cholesterol (abetalipoproteinemia) and also fat malabsorption, steatorrhea, and hepatic steatosis. Two small molecules of synthetic inhibitors of MTP have been tested and shown to produce marked reductions in atherogenic lipoproteins in hyperlipidemic Watanabe rabbits that lack a functional LDL receptor, a model of homozygous familial hypercholesterolemia in human (23).

Clinical testing of an MTP inhibitor, BMS-201038 (now known as lomitapide), in patients with homozygous familial hypercholesterolemia has demonstrated dose-dependent decrease in LDL and apoB levels but was associated with a high rate of gastrointestinal and hepatic adverse events (24). Recent additional studies with lomitapide showed that it lowered LDL-cholesterol in patients with moderate hypercholesterolemia either as a single agent or in combination with ezetimibe with elevation of transaminase as a major adverse effect (25). Lomitapide may offer a treatment option for patients who cannot tolerate statin therapy or who experience insufficient LDL-cholesterol reduction with available therapies. However, the use of lomitapide raised certain safety concerns due to GI adverse effects such as diarrhea, nausea, abdominal discomfort, vomiting, elevation of transaminase, and an increase in hepatic fatty content. These safety issues must be fully addressed before clinical use of this class of drugs can be recommended.

Antisense Oligonucleotide to Reduce ApoB-100 Production

Mipomersen is a second-generation antisense oligonucleotide developed to reduce the hepatic synthesis of apoB-100, a protein component of all atherogenic lipoproteins that is required for hepatic VLDL assembly and secretion. When given subcutaneously as an injection, mipomersen lowers LDL-C and apoB-100 levels by inhibiting the synthesis of apoB-100 when used as a single agent or in combination with other lipid-lowering drugs (26). In phase 3 human trials mipomersan lowered LDL-C in patients with homozygous FH or heterozygous

FH on maximally tolerated lipid-lowering therapy (27). Common adverse effects include local injection site reactions, flu-like symptoms, and elevation of hepatic enzymes. Mipomersan may also increase hepatic triglyceride content and since hepatic steatosis is a potentially serious adverse effect, additional long-term safety studies are needed for this novel agent (28).

Poprotein Convertase Subtilisin Kexin Type 9 (PCSK-9) Inhibitors

PCSK9 is responsible for degradation of LDL receptors and its inhibition increases LDL receptor number on cell surface (29,30). Loss-of-function mutation in PCSK-9 gene is associated with low LDL-C levels from birth and striking protection from CHD (31). Thus inhibition of PCSK-9 would be a potential strategy for LDL-C reduction and CHD prevention.

Antibody directed toward inhibition of PCSK9 to reduce LDL has been demonstrated in mice and cynomolgus monkeys (32) suggesting the feasibility and efficacy of this approach. AMG 145, developed by Amgen Inc., is a fully human monoclonal antibody to PCSK9 and being investigated for the treatment of hypercholesterolemia as an add-on to stable statin therapy. AMG 145 is currently undergoing Phase I clinical trial (ClinicalTrials.gov identifier: NCT01133522; estimated completion date: March 2012). Other PCSK 9 inhibiting antibodies such as REGN727 IgG (developed by Sanofi-Aventis; Clinicaltrials.gov identifier: NCT01288469) and RN316 IgG (developed by Pfizer; Clinicaltrilas.gov identifier: NCT01163851) are being tested in clinical trials as well.

Thyromimetics

Increased thyroid hormone levels reduce LDL-C levels but also adversely affect heart and bone. Thyroid hormone receptors consist of two major types (TRα and TRβ) along with several isoforms created by alternative splicing. TRα plays a major regulatory role in the heart whereas TRβ regulates cholesterol levels by mediating the activation of CYP7A in response to T3 in liver. Selective activation of TRβ, preferentially expressed in liver, by an experimental agonist KB2115, reduced LDL-C levels in humans without cardiac side effects in a short-term study (33). Another hepatic selective thyromimetic, T-0681, was shown to reduce cholesterol levels and atherosclerosis in hyperlipidemic animals (34,35). More data are needed to confirm long-term efficacy and safety of such agents in humans.

AUGMENTATION OF HDL LEVELS OR FUNCTION
HDL Metabolism

Lipid poor apoA-1 discoid particles receive cholesterol from peripheral tissues such as macrophages in the arterial wall via ABCA1 transporters. Subsequently, the cholesterol in these particles becomes esterified by lecithin-cholesterol acyltransferase (LCAT) leading to remodeling of HDL particles into spherical HDL2 and HDL3 particles. HDL then delivers cholesterol ester to the liver via SRB1 receptors or exchanges cholesterol ester for triglycerides from VLDL and LDL particles, an exchange facilitated by cholesteryl ester transfer protein

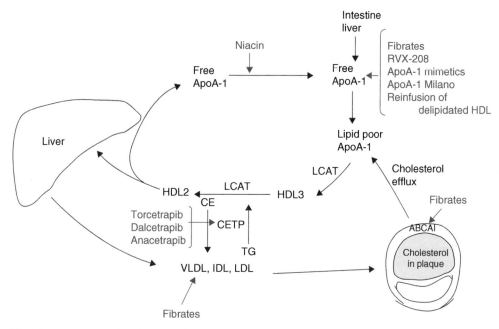

Figure 37.3 Schematic representation of HDL metabolism and potential steps that can be intervened by pharmacological therapies (in *red*).

(CETP). The cholesterol ester transferred to LDL and VLDL is then targeted for hepatic uptake via the LDL receptor pathway or accumulates in the arterial wall via subendothelial retention. Similar to LDL cholesterol metabolism, multiple steps, and transfer machineries are involved in this complicated pathway and provide opportunities for pharmacological intervention to enhance HDL levels or function (Fig. 37.3).

BIOLOGICAL BASIS FOR BENEFICIAL EFFECTS OF HDL ON ATHERO-THROMBOSIS

Stimulation of Reverse Cholesterol Transport

Since accumulation of cholesterol in the arterial wall is a major contributor to atherogenesis, one of the principal actions of HDL is to stimulate reverse cholesterol transport to mobilize free cholesterol from the peripheral tissues, including lipid laden macrophages, for hepatic uptake and elimination in feces through biliary sterols. Thus mobilization of free cholesterol from plaque macrophages by apoA-1 and HDL contributes to an anti-atherogenic effect (36).

Anti-inflammatory and Immuno modulatory Effects of ApoA-1 and HDL

The anti-inflammatory effects of HDL have been attributed to specific effects of apoA-1, inhibition of LDL oxidation, scavenging of pro-inflammatory lipids from oxidized LDL, sphingosine pathway activation, and activation of ABCA1-dependent JAK/STAT3 pathway attenuating TLR/MyD88-mediated pro-inflammatory responses (36–39). HDL may also promote migration of dendritic cells out of vascular lesions into regional lymph nodes (40), possibly by neutralizing the dendritic cell-immobilizing effects of

phospholipids generated during LDL oxidation. HDL also attenuates the inhibitory effects of inflammation on reverse cholesterol transport. Recent experimental observations have shown that ABCA1 and ABCG1, critical players in the initial steps of reverse cholesterol transport from macrophages and critical regulators of HDL particle formation, play an important role in suppressing atherosclerosis associated leukocytosis by inhibiting bone-marrow-derived progenitor cells (39).

Anti-oxidant Effects of ApoA-1 and HDL

LDL oxidation in the vessel wall likely plays a key role in atherogenesis. HDL inhibits LDL oxidation, scavenges toxic phospholipids from oxidized LDL, and protects vascular smooth muscle cells and endothelial cells from damaging effects of oxidized LDL. The anti-oxidant effects of HDL have been attributed to paraoxonase (PON), platelet-activating factor acetylhydrolase (PAF-AH) carried by HDL (36,37).

Endothelial Protective Effects of HDL

Endothelial dysfunction and endothelial denudation are important contributors and consequences of atherosclerosis. HDL has been shown to attenuate endothelial dysfunction induced by dyslipidemia and atherosclerosis by SRB-1-dependent induction of eNOS, attenuate endothelial cell apoptosis and stimulating endothelial reparative capacity (41–44).

Antithrombotic Effects of ApoA-1 and HDL

HDL inhibits platelet aggregation, activates protein c and inhibits assembly of the prothrombinase complex on anionic phospholipid surfaces (45).

Pancreatic β Cell Protective Effects of HDL

Insulin resistance and type II diabetes are often associated with reduced levels of HDL-C. HDL infusion was shown to improve pancreatic beta cell function in type 2 diabetic patients. Furthermore HDL may protect against diabetes by reducing stress-induced pancreatic beta cell apoptosis. Furthermore, ABCA1 and ABACG1 mediated anti-inflammatory effects of HDL may attenuate islet cell inflammation that is implicated in development of type 2 diabetes (46–48).

HDL FUNCTIONALITY AND THE CONCEPT OF DYSFUNCTIONAL HDL

High plasma HDL-cholesterol levels do not assure protection. Recent studies have shown that the reverse cholesterol-stimulating effects of HDL bear an inconsistent relationship to plasma HDL-cholesterol levels suggesting that HDL-cholesterol levels may not always be a reliable marker of HDL's anti-atherogenic effects. HDL may lose its beneficial effects by becoming pro-inflammatory and dysfunctional (49). Conversely, certain low HDL-cholesterol states, may not promote atherosclerosis because HDL function is intact or enhanced (50,51). Dysfunctional HDL occurs in inflammatory states or when HDL is exposed to to oxidants such as malondialdehyde and inflammatory mediators such as myeloperoxidase or serum amyloid A (49). Collectively, these observations have led to the notion that HDL functionality, rather than HDL cholesterol level alone, may be an additional determinant of its athero-protective effects and that HDL composition may influence its athero-protective effects. Such an assay for HDL functionality is not available for clinical application yet, but its development would help in understanding the role of HDL functionality in atherosclerotic cardiovascular disease and in monitoring the efficacy of HDL-raising therapies.

EMERGING NEW THERAPIES TARGETING HDL AND ITS APOPROTEINS

Niacin-Laropiprant Combination

Niacin is a B vitamin that is known to increase HDL cholesterol levels and reduce LDL cholesterol, Lp(a) levels, and triglyceride levels. Niacin decreases the hepatic production and release of VLDL, resulting in reduced levels of subsequent lipoproteins, such as VLDL remnants and LDL, in the endogenous cholesterol pathway. Niacin also reduces the catabolic rate of apoA-1, hence increases HDL level (52,53). A putative receptor for Niacin (GPR109A) has recently been identified that may mediate some of the biological actions of Niacin. In a phase 1 and 2 clinical trial, a partial agonist of niacin receptor, MK-0354, did not affect HDL, LDL, or triglyceride levels after 4 weeks of treatment (54). A recent pre-clinical study suggested that the anti-atherosclerotic activity of niacin is mediated through activation of GPR109A on immune cells leading to anti-inflammatory effects independent of the lipid-modulating activity of niacin (55). These observations raised more questions regarding the mechanisms of action of niacin.

Several small clinical trials have suggested that adding niacin to other lipid-lowering drugs reduces atherosclerosis progression, promotes regression, and has an overall favorable effect on clinical outcomes (56,57). However, widespread use of niacin has been difficult due to high rates of intolerance and adverse effects. The flushing-itching side effect of niacin has been attributed to its interaction with niacin receptor GPR109A on dermal Langerhans cells and keratinocytes that activate prostaglandin D_2 and E_2 pathways leading to vasodilatation through activation of prostaglandin DP1 receptors on vascular smooth muscle cells. Laropiprant is a selective DP1 receptor inhibitor that attenuates niacin-induced flushing (58). A combination of extened-release niacin and laropiprant has been approved in Europe for treatment of dyslipidemia. Laropiprant is currently being tested in combination with niacin in the Heart Protection-2—THRIVE clinical trial (Clinicaltrials.gov identifier: NCT00461630) for the efficacy in reducing cardiovascular events. This trial along with the ongoing AIM-high trial of niacin (Clinicaltrials.gov identifier: NCT00120289) could provide definitive data regarding the clinical benefits and tolerability/safety of niacin or niacin-laropiprant combination. However, NIH recently stopped the AIM-HIGH trial prematurely because during 32 months of follow-up, the combination treatment of extended-release niacin and simvastatin did not reduce fatal or non-fatal MI, strokes, hospitalizations for acute coronary syndrome, or revascularization procedures when compared with statin treatment alone (http://www.nih.gov/news/health/may2011/nhlbi-26.htm).

Fibrates

Fibrates are ligands of the nuclear receptor peroxisome proliferator-activated receptor α (PPARα) that regulates the expression of several genes involved in fatty acid and lipoprotein metabolism. Fibrates modestly increase HDL-C, reduce triglycerides, and have various effects on LDL-C levels. Studies have demonstrated the potential interaction of gemfibrozil but not fenofibrate with statin via competition for hepative glucoronidation, making fenofibrate safer to use with statins (59,60).

Pooled results from randomized trials showed that fibrates did not significantly reduce coronary mortality or all cause mortality despite a significant reduction in non-fatal cardiovascular events when compared to placebo (61). Given the HDL raising and triglyceride-reducing effect of fibrates, it seems logical to consider combination of fibrates and statins to maximize the benefit of lipid therapy. A recent clinical trial (ACCORD lipid trial) comparing fenofibrate plus simvastatin to simvastatin alone in patients with type 2 diabetes showed that combination therapy did not reduce cardiovascular events (62). Fibrates produce a high incidence of gastrointestinal side effects and less frequently cutaneous and musculoskeletal effects especially when used in combination with other lipid-modifying drugs. Thus the overall efficacy of fibrates in reducing cardiovascular events remains questionable at best.

CETP Inhibitors

CETP redistributes cholesterol ester from HDL to apoB-containing lipoprotein in exchange for triglycerides from ILD and LDL, leading to uptake by the LDL receptor in liver. Genetic studies showing low activity genetic variants of CETP were associated with elevated circulating levels of HDL cholesterol stimulated studies of inhibition of CETP to increase circulating levels of HDL cholesterol in the hope that this strategy would reduce cardiovascular events. The first major clinical trial using an oral CETP inhibitor, torcetrapib, demonstrated that patients enrolled in the torcetrapib plus atorvastatin group experienced a significant excess in cardiovascular and non-cardiovascular mortality despite a marked increase in HDL cholesterol and a significant LDL cholesterol lowering compared to recipients of atorvastatin alone (63). Similarly, torcetrapib added to atorvastatin had no significant effect on the progression of atherosclerosis in carotid or coronary arteries compared to atorvastatin alone (64,65). Although the failure of torcetrapib has been attributed to its molecule specific and CETP-independent angiotensin-aldosterone activation and hypertensive effects, it has also been argued that CETP inhibition may disrupt the reverse cholesterol transport pathway and generate large HDL cholesterol ester and apoE-enriched particles that are dysfunctional. Thus, at present, the role of CETP inhibition in the management of atherosclerosis remains controversial.

Two additional CETP inhibitors (dalcetrapib and anacetrapib) without angiotensin-aldosterone stimulating and hypertensive effects are currently in clinical trials (66,67). In a phase II 76-week human trial, anacetrapib at a dose of 100 mg daily resulted in a 39.8% reduction of LDL and 138% increase of HDL after treatment for 24 weeks without evidence for adverse effects on blood pressure, electrolytes, or aldosterone levels or a composite of clinical events; however, all cause mortality trended against anacetrapib and hs-CRP showed an increase instead of a decrease raising some concerns (68). A phase 3 morbidity and mortality trial with anectrapib is being planned (69). Another CETP inhibitor, dalcetrapib (originally developed by Japanese tobacco corporation and known as JTT-705) has been also shown not to activate the renin-angiotensin aldosterone pathway, has no effects on blood pressure, and modestly increases HDL-cholesterol levels (70). Recent studies have suggested that unlike anectrapib and torectrapib, dalcetrapib does not inhibit the transfer of cholesterol ester between HDL particles and only selectively inhibits cholesterol ester transfer between HDL and LDL/VLDL particles; hence it is being labeled as a CETP modulator (71). The precise biological advantages of this modulating effect of dalcetrapib remain unclear and the results of the recently completed morbidity and mortality phase 3 human trial (Dal-Outcomes Trial) should provide much needed outcomes data by 2013 (Clinicaltrials.gov identifier: NCT01323153). The results of these trials could provide definitive evidence in favor or against CETP inhibition and consequent increase in HDL cholesterol as a strategy for cardiovascular protection.

Small Molecule Stimulator Of apoa-1 Gene Transcription

RVX –208 is an oral small molecule that increases endogenous production of apoA-1 by stimulating its gene transcription (72). Experimental studies showed that RVX-208 increases HDL cholesterol and apoA-1 levels in monkeys and humans, specifically increasing pre-beta HDL particles believed to be highly effective stimulators of reverse cholesterol transport (73). A recent trial reported that administration of RVX-208 for 12 weeks was associated with a modest increase in apoA-I, HDL-C, and concentration of large HDL particles; however, a high incidence of liver enzyme elevations associated with its use have raised some concerns warranting additional studies (74).

Re Infusion of Autologous Delipidated HDL

Based on the hypothesis that lipid poor apoA-1 particles are effective in stimulating ABCA1-mediated reverse cholesterol transport, the idea of re-infusing ex-vivo delipidated autologous plasma HDL was tested in a small phase 1/2 human trial following favorable results in non-human primates (75). After 7 weekly sessions of delipidation apheresis and reinfusion, patients receiving autologous selective HDL-delipidated plasma showed a non-statistically significant coronary plaque regression as measured by intravascular ultrasound compared to patients receiving control plasma apheresis/reinfusions (76). Larger studies are needed to validate this interesting but logistically complicated and potentially expensive approach.

apoA-1 Mimetic Peptides

Several small peptides that simulate the lipid transport effects of apoA-1 have been synthesized and tested in experimental models of atherosclerosis with promising results. One such peptide, D-4F (18 mer peptide with 4 phenylalanine residues, made from dextro-isomers of amino acids to improve oral bioavailability, Novartis APP018) was shown to be highly athero-protective in murine models (77). One small human trial demonstrated modest anti-inflammatory activity of HDL isolated from subjects receiving a single dose of oral D-4F (78). Another peptide (ATI 5261, Artery Therapeutics) is on its way to clinical development after it was shown to increase fecal sterol excretion and reduce atherosclerosis on intraperitoneal delivery in mice (79). Human studies of these peptides have thus far been limited and their utility remains uncertain.

Intravenous Infusion of apoA-1Milano or Wild-Type apoA-1 (Synthetic HDL)

apoA-1$_{Milano}$ is a naturally occurring mutant (A173C) of apoA-1, carried by a small number of inhabitants of Limone sul Garda who, despite high triglycerides and very low HDL cholesterol and apoA-1 levels, have low incidence of cardiovascular disease, suggesting that apoA-I$_{Milano}$ may be a gain of function mutation (50). Several experimental studies have shown that infusion of recombinant apoA-1$_{Milano}$–phospholipid complex (synthetic HDL) rapidly and favorably remodels atherosclerotic plaques with reduced plaque lipid and inflammation, inhibits progression of lesions, reverses endothelial dysfunction, and promotes rapid regression in various experimental models (80–83). These observations were subsequently confirmed in a small phase 2 clinical trial in which sequential intravascular ultrasound studies done before and after 5 weekly is ambiguous of r-apoA-I$_{Milano}$ phospholipid complex (ETC216) showed rapid coronary plaque regression (84). Obstacles in developing this therapy further include the need for intravenous infusion, the expensive production process for large-scale manufacturing and challenges involved in preventing bacterial host derived protein contamination in the recombinant product produced by *Escherichia coli*. An alternative approach using plant biotechnology by SemBiosys genetics wherein apoA-I$_{Milano}$ can be expressed in safflower seed has given renewed interest to developing this therapy. This plant engineered protein appears to be functionally similar to *E. coli* derived recombinant protein despite lacking two amino acids (Des1,2 apoA-I$_{Milano}$), can be produced at low cost, is scalable and free of bacterial host derived protein.

Intravenous Infusion of Human Plasma Derived Wild-Type apoA-1

Human plasma derived wild type apoA-1 linked unclear soybean phospholipid (CSL111) was infused at 40 mg/kg/infusion in humans in a small proof-of-concept trial. Five weekly infusions did not show a significant benefit on coronary plaque in comparison to placebo (primary end point); however, when compared to pretreatment baseline, apo A-1 recipients showed regression in contradistinction to the placebo arm (85). The 80 mg/kg/infusion regimen was abandoned because of hepatic toxicity even though a single infusion of 80 mg/kg, in an unrelated study, was shown to favorably change femoral artery plaque composition (86).

Endothelial Lipase Inhibition to Raise HDL Levels

Endothelial lipase is a phospholipase, together with lipoprotein lipase and hepatic lipase, belongs to the lipoprotein lipase family. It is synthesized mainly by vascular endothelial cells and to lesser extent by macrophages and smooth muscle cells. These cells secrete endothelial lipase, which binds to proteoglycans at cell surface to exert its action. Over-expression of endothelial lipase in animals reduces plasma HDL-C levels whereas endothelial lipase gene knockout (87) or inhibition by an antibody increases plasma HDL-C levels (88). Increased endothelial lipase level has been associated with metabolic syndrome and coronary atherosclerosis (89), suggesting its inhibition may be a viable strategy for increasing HDL in humans.

Gene Transfer of HDL-associated Proteins (apo A-1, Paraoxonase, and PAF-AH)

Pre-clinical studies have demonstrated that effective transfer of genes encoding apoA-1 or apoA-1 mutants and other protective proteins associated with HDL, using viral vectors produce significant reduction and/or promote regression of atherosclerosis (90,91), however, clinical translation of such studies has

not been reported to date. There are many challenges that must be overcome before clinical translation of gene transfer for atherosclerosis can become a reality: these have largely to do with the development of high efficiency, safe, non-immunogenic, scalable vectors that can lead to stable and long-term transgene expression in the host without provoking adverse immunologic or non-immunologic complications. Various isoforms of adeno associated viral (AAV) vectors hold considerable promise for human gene transfer and are under active investigation (90).

MODULATION OF INFLAMMATORY OR IMMUNE PATHWAYS

Lipoprotein Associated Phospholipase (Lp-PLA-2) Inhibitor (Darapladib)

Lipoprotein associated phospholipase 2 is a circulating lipid-associated phospholipase that has been shown to be a marker for increased cardiovascular risk and has also been implicated as a pro-inflammatory risk factor that might contribute to plaque formation and plaque inflammation (92). A synthetic inhibitor, darapladib, has been shown to have athero-protective effects in preclinical models (93). In a phase 2 human clinical trial (IBIS-2), involving sequential coronary plaque assessment using intravascular ultrasound and palpography, darapladib-treated subjects showed no increase in necrotic lipid core whereas placebo-treated subjects showed a significant increase in necrotic lipid core size on secondary analysis but darapladib failed to reduce atherosclerosis progression, hs-CRP levels, or arterial stiffness (94). Two phase III clinical trials (STABILITY and SOLID TIMI 52 trial) will investigate the efficacy and safety of darapladib in nearly 13,000 individuals with coronary heart disease. When completed, these trials could provide important insights into the utility of darapladib to reduce myocardial infarction, stroke and cardiovascular death.

Inhibitors of Soluble Phospholipase A-2 (sPLA2, Varespladib)

Several circulating secretory phospholipases have been implicated in atherogenesis and inflammation and inhibitors of these secretory phospholipases have been developed as potential therapy for inflammatory disorders including atherosclerosis (95). In a Phase 2 trial of varespladib substantial dose-dependent reductions in plasma sPLA2-IIA concentration were observed, along with reduction in LDL-C levels, using four doses over 8 weeks (96). Another study of varespladib in ACS patients (FRANCIS-ACS trial; NCT00743925) reported similar LDL-lowering effect but without reducing adverse cardiovascular events (97).

Liver X Receptors (LXR) Agonists

Liver X receptors (LXRs) are nuclear receptors that are activated by endogenous oxysterols derived from oxidized lipids. LXRs act as cholesterol sensors: when cellular oxysterols accumulate as a result of increasing concentrations of cholesterol, LXR induces the transcription of genes that protect cells from cholesterol overload. The two isoforms of LXRs (α and β) function as sterol sensors with important roles in regulating lipid

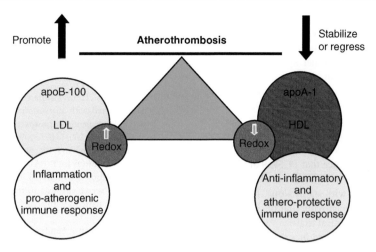

Figure 37.4 Key modulators such as atherogenic lipoproteins, oxidative stress, inflammatory activity, and immune activation play pivotal roles in atherosclerosis and its thrombotic complication.

homeostasis and inflammation, prompting interest in the development of synthetic LXR ligands as therapeutic agents for atherosclerotic cardiovascular disease (98).

Synthetic LXR ligands have been tested in animal models for the treatment of atherosclerosis. Two LXR agonists, GW3965 and T0901317, have been shown to reduce plaques in murine model of atherosclerosis, providing direct evidence for an atheroprotective effect of LXR agonists (99,100). These results suggest that LXR ligands may be useful therapeutic agents for the treatment of atherosclerosis. However, these therapeutic benefits have to be balanced by the adverse effects of LXR agonists wherein LXR activation is associated with stimulation of lipogenesis resulting in increased plasma triglyceride levels and hepatic fat accumulation (101–103). Recently, another potent synthetic steroidal LXR activator, N,N-dimethyl-3b-hydroxycholenamide (DMHCA), has been shown to reduce atherosclerosis in apoE-deficient mice, without elevating hepatic and plasma TG levels. Based on these observations, DMHCA could be a candidate for further development as a therapeutic agent for atherosclerosis (104).

Immune Modulation of Atherosclerosis with a Peptide-based Vaccine (CVX-210) or a Monoclonal Anti-LDL Epitope Antibody (BI-204)

Atherosclerosis is currently viewed as an immune-mediated chronic inflammatory disease of arterial walls. Many antigenic molecules such as LDL, heat shock protein have been demonstrated to elicit immune responses involved in atherogenesis. Active immunization of hyperlipidemic rabbits or mice using native or oxidized LDL as an immunogen reduces atherosclerosis without a significant change in circulating cholesterol levels (105–107). Using human apoB-100 as a target, several peptides with antigenicity have been identified within this molecule and synthetic mimics of these sequences consisting of 20 amino

acid peptide, have been tested as vaccines in mice (108–110). Several of these apoB100 related peptide vaccines have been shown to reduce atherosclerosis and plaque inflammation in hyperlipidemic mice (108–110).

In addition to active immunotherapy with a vaccine, passive immunization with a monoclonal antibody (BI-204) against one of the apoB100 related antigenic peptides can induce rapid plaque regression and anti-inflammatory response in hyperlipidemic mice (111,112). Such a strategy is now being tested in clinical trials.

PERSONAL PERSPECTIVE

Atherosclerosis and its thrombotic complication continue to be a major cause of morbidity and mortality. Numerous factors, some in favor promoting and some reducing or stabilizing atherosclerosis, are involved in the process (Fig. 37.4). As discussed above, many new potential therapeutic strategies including (*i*) non-statin drugs to reduce LDL cholesterol; (*ii*) various regimens to augment HDL levels and HDL function, and (*iii*) inflammation- or immune-modulation therapies are now being developed and tested in different phases of pre-clinical or clinical studies. Some of these novel therapies target patients for secondary prevention of future events (LDL-lowering or HDL-raising) whereas some aim at primary prevention (active immunization against atherosclerosis). Given that atherosclerosis is a chronic disease starting in youth with clinical disease generally becoming manifest at a much later stage, it is likely that various approaches ranging from prevention of atherosclerosis formation in at youth to further reduction of residual risk, after an initial event, are needed. The therapies discussed in this chapter will be valuable additions to our current pharmacological armamentarium to prevent and treat atherosclerotic vascular disease and its associated complications once they are proven effective and safe in humans.

Since this Chapter was written, new information regarding the efficacy of a PCSK9 antibody and dalcetrapib became available.

The first trial is a phase 2 study to evaluate the efficacy of 12-week treatment with a monoclonal antibody to PCSK 9, SAR236553/REGN727, in reducing LDL versus placebo in patients with LDL > 100 mg/dl on stable atorvastatin therapy (NCT 01288443; McKenney JM et al. JACC 2012;59:2344-2353). At the end of 12 weeks, SAR236553/REGN727 treatment resulted in a significant dose-related and dose-regimen dependent LDL-C reduction compared to placebo. This study provided proof-of-concept of evidence that PCSK 9 antibody can further reduce LDL-C in patients who are unable to achieve LDL-C goal on monotherapy with statin alone. If this can be translated into clinically beneficial reduction of cardiovascular hard en-points awaits further clinical trials.

Since torcetrapib treatment resulted in a significant excess in mortality despite a favorable increase in HDL-C and a reduction in LDL-C compared to recipients of atorvastatin alone (63), focus has been on a different CETP inhibitor, dalcetrapib, due to its lack of off-target effects on renin-angiotensin aldosterone pathway. Dalcetrapib has been tested in a global development program, The dal-HEART, by Roche. The dal-HEART consists of six clinical trials -- dal-PLAQUE, dal-VESSEL, dal-OUTCOMES, dal-OUTCOMES 2, dal-PLAQUE 2 and dal-ACUTE. In May 2012, Roche decided to terminate all the studies in the dal-HEART program after a second interim analysis of the dal-OUTCOMES Phase III trial demonstrated no clinically meaningful efficacy of dalcetrapib when added to existing standard of care in patients with stable coronary heart disease following an acute coronary syndrome (http://www.roche.com/media/media_releases/med-cor-2012-05-07.htm).

REFERENCES

1. Shah PK. Molecular mechanisms of plaque instability. Curr Opin Lipidol 2007; 18: 492–9.
2. Chyu KY, Shah PK. The role of inflammation in plaque disruption and thrombosis. Rev Cardiovasc Med 2001; 2: 82–91.
3. Andersson J, Libby P, Hansson GK. Adaptive immunity and atherosclerosis. Clin Immunol 2010; 134: 33–46.
4. Hansson GK. Inflammatory mechanisms in atherosclerosis. J Thromb Haemost 2009; 7(Suppl 1): 328–31.
5. Grundy SM, Becker D, Clark LT, et al. Third Report of the National Cholesterol Education Program (NCEP) Expert Panel on Detection, Evaluation, and treatment of high blood cholesterol in adults (Adult Treatment Panel III) final report. Circulation 2002; 106: 3143–421
6. Grundy SM, Cleeman JI, Merz CN, et al. Implications of recent clinical trials for the National Cholesterol Education Program Adult Treatment Panel III Guidelines. J Am Coll Cardiol 2004; 44: 720–32.
7. Plat J, Mensink RP. Increased intestinal ABCA1 expression contributes to the decrease in cholesterol absorption after plant stanol consumption. FASEB J 2002; 16: 1248–53.
8. Plat J, Mensink RP. Plant stanol and sterol esters in the control of blood cholesterol levels: mechanism and safety aspects. Am J Cardiol 2005; 96: 15D–22D.
9. Garcia-Calvo M, Lisnock J, Bull HG, et al. The target of ezetimibe is Niemann-Pick C1-Like 1 (NPC1L1). Proc Natl Acad Sci USA 2005; 102: 8132–7.
10. Kerzner B, Corbelli J, Sharp S, et al. Efficacy and safety of ezetimibe coadministered with lovastatin in primary hypercholesterolemia. Am J Cardiol 2003; 91: 418–24.
11. Kastelein JJ, Akdim F, Stroes ES, et al. Simvastatin with or without ezetimibe in familial hypercholesterolemia. N Engl J Med 2008; 358: 1431–43.
12. Ballantyne CM, Houri J, Notarbartolo A, et al. Effect of ezetimibe coadministered with atorvastatin in 628 patients with primary hypercholesterolemia: a prospective, randomized, double-blind trial. Circulation 2003; 107: 2409–15.
13. Cannon CP, Giugliano RP, Blazing MA, et al. Rationale and design of IMPROVE-IT (IMProved Reduction of Outcomes: Vytorin Efficacy International Trial): comparison of ezetimbe/simvastatin versus simvastatin monotherapy on cardiovascular outcomes in patients with acute coronary syndromes. Am Heart J 2008; 156: 826–32.
14. Peto R, Emberson J, Landray M, et al. Analyses of cancer data from three ezetimibe trials. N Engl J Med 2008; 359: 1357–66.
15. Accad M, Smith SJ, Newland DL, et al. Massive xanthomatosis and altered composition of atherosclerotic lesions in hyperlipidemic mice lacking acyl CoA: cholesterol acyltransferase 1. J Clin Invest 2000; 105: 711–9.
16. Fazio S, Major AS, Swift LL, et al. Increased atherosclerosis in LDL receptor-null mice lacking ACAT1 in macrophages. J Clin Invest 2001; 107: 163–71.
17. Kusunoki J, Hansoty DK, Aragane K, et al. Acyl-CoA: cholesterol acyltransferase inhibition reduces atherosclerosis in apolipoprotein E-deficient mice. Circulation 2001; 103: 2604–9.
18. Bell TA III, Brown JM, Graham MJ, et al. Liver-specific inhibition of acyl-coenzyme a: cholesterol acyltransferase 2 with antisense oligonucleotides limits atherosclerosis development in apolipoprotein B100-only low-density lipoprotein receptor-/- mice. Arterioscler Thromb Vasc Biol 2006; 26: 1814–20.
19. Ikenoya M, Yoshinaka Y, Kobayashi H, et al. A selective ACAT-1 inhibitor, K-604, suppresses fatty streak lesions in fat-fed hamsters without affecting plasma cholesterol levels. Atherosclerosis 2007; 191: 290–7.
20. Tardif JC, Gregoire J, L'Allier PL, et al. Effects of the acyl coenzyme A: cholesterol acyltransferase inhibitor avasimibe on human atherosclerotic lesions. Circulation 2004; 110: 3372–7.
21. Nissen SE, Tuzcu EM, Brewer HB, et al. Effect of ACAT inhibition on the progression of coronary atherosclerosis. N Engl J Med 2006; 354: 1253–63.
22. Meuwese MC, de GE, Duivenvoorden R, et al. ACAT inhibition and progression of carotid atherosclerosis in patients with familial hypercholesterolemia: the CAPTIVATE randomized trial. JAMA 2009; 301: 1131–9.
23. Wetterau JR, Gregg RE, Harrity TW, et al. An MTP inhibitor that normalizes atherogenic lipoprotein levels in WHHL rabbits. Science 1998; 282: 751–4.
24. Cuchel M, Bloedon LT, Szapary PO, et al. Inhibition of microsomal triglyceride transfer protein in familial hypercholesterolemia. N Engl J Med 2007; 356: 148–56.
25. Samaha FF, McKenney J, Bloedon LT, et al. Inhibition of microsomal triglyceride transfer protein alone or with ezetimibe in patients with moderate hypercholesterolemia. Nat Clin Pract Cardiovasc Med 2008; 5: 497–505.
26. Visser ME, Kastelein JJ, Stroes ES. Apolipoprotein B synthesis inhibition: results from clinical trials. Curr Opin Lipidol 2010; 21: 319–23.

27. Raal FJ, Santos RD, Blom DJ, et al. Mipomersen, an apolipoprotein B synthesis inhibitor, for lowering of LDL cholesterol concentrations in patients with homozygous familial hypercholesterolaemia: a randomised, double-blind, placebo-controlled trial. Lancet 2010; 375: 998–1006.

28. Kling J. Safety signal dampens reception for mipomersen antisense. Nat Biotechnol 2010; 28: 295–7.

29. Soutar AK, Naoumova RP. Mechanisms of disease: genetic causes of familial hypercholesterolemia. Nat Clin Pract Cardiovasc Med 2007; 4: 214–25.

30. Lambert G, Charlton F, Rye KA, Piper DE. Molecular basis of PCSK9 function. Atherosclerosis 2009; 203: 1–7.

31. Cohen JC, Boerwinkle E, Mosley TH Jr, et al. Sequence variations in PCSK9, low LDL, and protection against coronary heart disease. N Engl J Med 2006; 354: 1264–72.

32. Chan JC, Piper DE, Cao Q, et al. A proprotein convertase subtilisin/kexin type 9 neutralizing antibody reduces serum cholesterol in mice and nonhuman primates. Proc Natl Acad Sci USA 2009; 106: 9820–5.

33. Berkenstam A, Kristensen J, Mellstrom K, et al. The thyroid hormone mimetic compound KB2115 lowers plasma LDL cholesterol and stimulates bile acid synthesis without cardiac effects in humans. Proc Natl Acad Sci USA 2008; 105: 663–7.

34. Tancevski I, Wehinger A, Demetz E, et al. The thyromimetic T-0681 protects from atherosclerosis. J Lipid Res 2009; 50: 938–44.

35. Tancevski I, Demetz E, Eller P, et al. The liver-selective thyromimetic T-0681 influences reverse cholesterol transport and atherosclerosis development in mice. PLoS One 2010; 5: e8722.

36. Shah PK, Kaul S, Nilsson J, et al. Exploiting the vascular protective effects of high-density lipoprotein and its apolipoproteins: an idea whose time for testing is coming, part I. Circulation 2001; 104: 2376–83.

37. Shah PK, Kaul S, Nilsson J, et al. Exploiting the vascular protective effects of high-density lipoprotein and its apolipoproteins: an idea whose time for testing is coming, part II. Circulation 2001; 104: 2498–502.

38. Yin K, Liao DF, Tang CK. ATP-binding membrane cassette transporter A1 (ABCA1): a possible link between inflammation and reverse cholesterol transport. Mol Med 2010; 16: 438–49.

39. Yvan-Charvet L, Wang N, Tall AR. Role of HDL, ABCA1, and ABCG1 transporters in cholesterol efflux and immune responses. Arterioscler Thromb Vasc Biol 2010; 30: 139–43.

40. Angeli V, Llodra J, Rong JX, et al. Dyslipidemia associated with atherosclerotic disease systemically alters dendritic cell mobilization. Immunity 2004; 21: 561–74.

41. Pu DR, Liu L. HDL slowing down endothelial progenitor cells senescence: a novel anti-atherogenic property of HDL. Med Hypotheses 2008; 70: 338–42.

42. Mineo C, Shaul PW. Role of high-density lipoprotein and scavenger receptor B type I in the promotion of endothelial repair. Trends Cardiovasc Med 2007; 17: 156–61.

43. Kimura T, Tomura H, Mogi C, et al. Role of scavenger receptor class B type I and sphingosine 1-phosphate receptors in high density lipoprotein-induced inhibition of adhesion molecule expression in endothelial cells. J Biol Chem 2006; 281: 37457–67.

44. Seetharam D, Mineo C, Gormley AK, et al. High-density lipoprotein promotes endothelial cell migration and reendothelialization via scavenger receptor-B type I. Circ Res 2006; 98: 63–72.

45. Oslakovic C, Krisinger MJ, Andersson A, et al. Anionic phospholipids lose their procoagulant properties when incorporated into high density lipoproteins. J Biol Chem 2009; 284: 5896–904.

46. Fryirs M, Barter PJ, Rye KA. Cholesterol metabolism and pancreatic beta-cell function. Curr Opin Lipidol 2009; 20: 159–64.

47. Fryirs MA, Barter PJ, Appavoo M, et al. Effects of high-density lipoproteins on pancreatic beta-cell insulin secretion. Arterioscler Thromb Vasc Biol 2010; 30: 1642–8.

48. Kruit JK, Brunham LR, Verchere CB, et al. HDL and LDL cholesterol significantly influence beta-cell function in type 2 diabetes mellitus. Curr Opin Lipidol 2010; 21: 178–85.

49. Smith JD. Dysfunctional HDL as a diagnostic and therapeutic target. Arterioscler Thromb Vasc Biol 2010; 30: 151–5.

50. Sirtori CR, Calabresi L, Franceschini G, et al. Cardiovascular status of carriers of the apolipoprotein A-I(Milano) mutant: the Limone sul Garda study. Circulation 2001; 103: 1949–54.

51. Franceschini G, Calabresi L, Chiesa G, et al. Increased cholesterol efflux potential of sera from ApoA-IMilano carriers and transgenic mice. Arterioscler Thromb Vasc Biol 1999; 19: 1257–62.

52. Shepherd J, Packard CJ, Patsch JR, et al. Effects of nicotinic acid therapy on plasma high density lipoprotein subfraction distribution and composition and on apolipoprotein A metabolism. J Clin Invest 1979; 63: 858–67.

53. Lamon-Fava S, Diffenderfer MR, Barrett PH, et al. Extended-release niacin alters the metabolism of plasma apolipoprotein (Apo) A-I and ApoB-containing lipoproteins. Arterioscler Thromb Vasc Biol 2008; 28: 1672–8.

54. Lai E, Waters MG, Tata JR, et al. Effects of a niacin receptor partial agonist, MK-0354, on plasma free fatty acids, lipids, and cutaneous flushing in humans. J Clin Lipidol 2008; 2: 375–83.

55. Lukasova M, Malaval C, Gille A, et al. Nicotinic acid inhibits progression of atherosclerosis in mice through its receptor GPR109A expressed by immune cells. J Clin Invest 2011; 121: 1163–73.

56. Brown BG, Zhao XQ, Chait A, et al. Simvastatin and niacin, antioxidant vitamins, or the combination for the prevention of coronary disease. N Engl J Med 2001; 345: 1583–92.

57. Taylor AJ, Sullenberger LE, Lee HJ, et al. Arterial Biology for the Investigation of the Treatment Effects of Reducing Cholesterol (ARBITER) 2: a double-blind, placebo-controlled study of extended-release niacin on atherosclerosis progression in secondary prevention patients treated with statins. Circulation 2004; 110: 3512–7.

58. Sanyal S, Kuvin JT, Karas RH. Niacin and laropiprant. Drugs Today (Barc) 2010; 46: 371–8.

59. Prueksaritanont T, Tang C, Qiu Y, et al. Effects of fibrates on metabolism of statins in human hepatocytes. Drug Metab Dispos 2002; 30: 1280–7.

60. Prueksaritanont T, Zhao JJ, Ma B, et al. Mechanistic studies on metabolic interactions between gemfibrozil and statins. J Pharmacol Exp Ther 2002; 301: 1042–51.

61. Jun M, Foote C, Lv J, et al. Effects of fibrates on cardiovascular outcomes: a systematic review and meta-analysis. Lancet 2010; 375: 1875–84.

62. Ginsberg HN, Elam MB, Lovato LC, et al. Effects of combination lipid therapy in type 2 diabetes mellitus. N Engl J Med 2010; 362: 1563–74.

63. Barter PJ, Caulfield M, Eriksson M, et al. Effects of torcetrapib in patients at high risk for coronary events. N Engl J Med 2007; 357: 2109–22.

64. Nicholls SJ, Tuzcu EM, Brennan DM, et al. Cholesteryl ester transfer protein inhibition, high-density lipoprotein raising,

and progression of coronary atherosclerosis: insights from ILLUSTRATE (Investigation of Lipid Level Management Using Coronary Ultrasound to Assess Reduction of Atherosclerosis by CETP Inhibition and HDL Elevation). Circulation 2008; 118: 2506–14.

65. Bots ML, Visseren FL, Evans GW, et al. Torcetrapib and carotid intima-media thickness in mixed dyslipidaemia (RADIANCE 2 study): a randomised, double-blind trial. Lancet 2007; 370: 153–60.

66. Schwartz GG, Olsson AG, Ballantyne CM, et al. Rationale and design of the dal-OUTCOMES trial: efficacy and safety of dalcetrapib in patients with recent acute coronary syndrome. Am Heart J 2009; 158: 896–901.

67. Cannon CP, Dansky HM, Davidson M, et al. Design of the DEFINE trial: determining the EFficacy and tolerability of CETP INhibition with AnacEtrapib. Am Heart J 2009; 158: 513–9.

68. Bloomfield D, Carlson GL, Sapre A, et al. Efficacy and safety of the cholesteryl ester transfer protein inhibitor anacetrapib as monotherapy and coadministered with atorvastatin in dyslipidemic patients. Am Heart J 2009; 157: 352–60.

69. Cannon CP, Shah S, Dansky HM, et al. Safety of anacetrapib in patients with or at high risk for coronary heart disease. N Engl J Med 2010; 363: 2406–15.

70. Stein EA, Roth EM, Rhyne JM, et al. Safety and tolerability of dalcetrapib (RO4607381/JTT-705): results from a 48-week trial. Eur Heart J 2010; 31: 480–8.

71. Niesor EJ, Magg C, Ogawa N, et al. Modulating cholesteryl ester transfer protein activity maintains efficient pre-beta-HDL formation and increases reverse cholesterol transport. J Lipid Res 2010; 51: 3443–54.

72. McNeill E. RVX-208, a stimulator of apolipoprotein AI gene expression for the treatment of cardiovascular diseases. Curr Opin Investig Drugs 2010; 11: 357–64.

73. Bailey D, Jahagirdar R, Gordon A, et al. RVX-208: a small molecule that increases apolipoprotein A-I and high-density lipoprotein cholesterol in vitro and in vivo. J Am Coll Cardiol 2010; 55: 2580–9.

74. Nicholls SJ, Gordon A, Johansson J, et al. Efficacy and safety of a novel oral inducer of apolipoprotein a-I synthesis in statin-treated patients with stable coronary artery disease a randomized controlled trial. J Am Coll Cardiol 2011; 57: 1111–9.

75. Sacks FM, Rudel LL, Conner A, et al. Selective delipidation of plasma HDL enhances reverse cholesterol transport in vivo. J Lipid Res 2009; 50: 894–907.

76. Waksman R, Torguson R, Kent KM, et al. A first-in-man, randomized, placebo-controlled study to evaluate the safety and feasibility of autologous delipidated high-density lipoprotein plasma infusions in patients with acute coronary syndrome. J Am Coll Cardiol 2010; 55: 2727–35.

77. Sherman CB, Peterson SJ, Frishman WH. Apolipoprotein A-I mimetic peptides: a potential new therapy for the prevention of atherosclerosis. Cardiol Rev 2010; 18: 141–7.

78. Bloedon LT, Dunbar R, Duffy D, et al. Safety, pharmacokinetics, and pharmacodynamics of oral apoA-I mimetic peptide D-4F in high-risk cardiovascular patients. J Lipid Res 2008; 49: 1344–52.

79. Bielicki JK, Zhang H, Cortez Y, et al. A new HDL mimetic peptide that stimulates cellular cholesterol efflux with high efficiency greatly reduces atherosclerosis in mice. J Lipid Res 2010; 51: 1496–503.

80. Kaul S, Coin B, Hedayiti A, et al. Rapid reversal of endothelial dysfunction in hypercholesterolemic apolipoprotein E-null mice by recombinant apolipoprotein A-I(Milano)-phospholipid complex. J Am Coll Cardiol 2004; 44: 1311–9.

81. Kaul S, Rukshin V, Santos R, et al. Intramural delivery of recombinant apolipoprotein A-IMilano/phospholipid complex (ETC-216) inhibits in-stent stenosis in porcine coronary arteries. Circulation 2003; 107: 2551–4.

82. Shah PK, Yano J, Reyes O, et al. High-dose recombinant apolipoprotein A-I(milano) mobilizes tissue cholesterol and rapidly reduces plaque lipid and macrophage content in apolipoprotein e-deficient mice. Potential implications for acute plaque stabilization. Circulation 2001; 103: 3047–50.

83. Shah PK, Nilsson J, Kaul S, et al. Effects of recombinant apolipoprotein A-I(Milano) on aortic atherosclerosis in apolipoprotein E-deficient mice. Circulation 1998; 97: 780–5.

84. Nissen SE, Tsunoda T, Tuzcu EM, et al. Effect of recombinant ApoA-I Milano on coronary atherosclerosis in patients with acute coronary syndromes: a randomized controlled trial. JAMA 2003; 290: 2292–300.

85. Tardif JC, Gregoire J, L'Allier PL, et al. Effects of reconstituted high-density lipoprotein infusions on coronary atherosclerosis: a randomized controlled trial. JAMA 2007; 297: 1675–82.

86. Shaw JA, Bobik A, Murphy A, et al. Infusion of reconstituted high-density lipoprotein leads to acute changes in human atherosclerotic plaque. Circ Res 2008; 103: 1084–91.

87. Santamarina-Fojo S, Haudenschild C. Role of hepatic and lipoprotein lipase in lipoprotein metabolism and atherosclerosis: studies in transgenic and knockout animal models and somatic gene transfer. Int J Tissue React 2000; 22: 39–47.

88. Badellino KO, Rader DJ. The role of endothelial lipase in high-density lipoprotein metabolism. Curr Opin Cardiol 2004; 19: 392–5.

89. Badellino KO, Wolfe ML, Reilly MP, et al. Endothelial lipase concentrations are increased in metabolic syndrome and associated with coronary atherosclerosis. PLoS Med 2006; 3: e22.

90. Sharifi BG, Wu K, Wang L, et al. AAV serotype-dependent apolipoprotein A-I(Milano) gene expression. Atherosclerosis 2005; 181: 261–9.

91. Wang L, Sharifi BG, Pan T, et al. Bone marrow transplantation shows superior atheroprotective effects of gene therapy with apolipoprotein A-I Milano compared with wild-type apolipoprotein A-I in hyperlipidemic mice. J Am Coll Cardiol 2006; 48: 1459–68.

92. Corson MA. Emerging inflammatory markers for assessing coronary heart disease risk. Curr Cardiol Rep 2009; 11: 452–9.

93. Wilensky RL, Shi Y, Mohler ER III, et al. Inhibition of lipoprotein-associated phospholipase A2 reduces complex coronary atherosclerotic plaque development. Nat Med 2008; 14: 1059–66.

94. Serruys PW, Garcia-Garcia HM, Buszman P, et al. Effects of the direct lipoprotein-associated phospholipase A(2) inhibitor darapladib on human coronary atherosclerotic plaque. Circulation 2008; 118: 1172–82.

95. Suckling K. Phospholipase A2s: developing drug targets for atherosclerosis. Atherosclerosis 2010; 212: 357–66.

96. Rosenson RS, Hislop C, McConnell D, et al. Effects of 1-H-indole-3-glyoxamide (A-002) on concentration of secretory phospholipase A2 (PLASMA study): a phase II double-blind, randomised, placebo-controlled trial. Lancet 2009; 373: 649–58.

97. Rosenson RS, Hislop C, Elliott M, et al. Effects of varespladib methyl on biomarkers and major cardiovascular events in acute coronary syndrome patients. J Am Coll Cardiol 2010; 56: 1079–88.

98. Zhao C, Hlman-Wright K. Liver X receptor in cholesterol metabolism. J Endocrinol 2010; 204: 233–40.

99. Joseph SB, McKilligin E, Pei L, et al. Synthetic LXR ligand inhibits the development of atherosclerosis in mice. Proc Natl Acad Sci USA 2002; 99: 7604–9.

100. Terasaka N, Hiroshima A, Koieyama T, et al. T-0901317, a synthetic liver X receptor ligand, inhibits development of atherosclerosis in LDL receptor-deficient mice. FEBS Lett 2003; 536: 6–11.

101. Repa JJ, Liang G, Ou J, et al. Regulation of mouse sterol regulatory element-binding protein-1c gene (SREBP-1c) by oxysterol receptors, LXRalpha and LXRbeta. Genes Dev 2000; 14: 2819–30.

102. Schultz JR, Tu H, Luk A, et al. Role of LXRs in control of lipogenesis. Genes Dev 2000; 14: 2831–8.

103. Grefhorst A, Elzinga BM, Voshol PJ, et al. Stimulation of lipogenesis by pharmacological activation of the liver X receptor leads to production of large, triglyceride-rich very low density lipoprotein particles. J Biol Chem 2002; 277: 34182–90.

104. Kratzer A, Buchebner M, Pfeifer T, et al. Synthetic LXR agonist attenuates plaque formation in apoE-/- mice without inducing liver steatosis and hypertriglyceridemia. J Lipid Res 2009; 50: 312–26.

105. Ameli S, Hultgardh-Nilsson A, Regnstrom J, et al. Effect of immunization with homologous LDL and oxidized LDL on early atherosclerosis in hypercholesterolemic rabbits. Arterioscler Thromb Vasc Biol 1996; 16: 1074–9.

106. Chyu KY, Reyes OS, Zhao X, et al. Timing affects the efficacy of LDL immunization on atherosclerotic lesions in apo E (-/-) mice. Atherosclerosis 2004; 176: 27–35.

107. Nilsson J, Calara F, Regnstrom J, et al. Immunization with homologous oxidized low density lipoprotein reduces neointimal formation after balloon injury in hypercholesterolemic rabbits. J Am Coll Cardiol 1997; 30: 1886–91.

108. Chyu KY, Zhao X, Reyes OS, et al. Immunization using an Apo B-100 related epitope reduces atherosclerosis and plaque inflammation in hypercholesterolemic apo E (-/-) mice. Biochem Biophys Res Commun 2005; 338: 1982–9.

109. Fredrikson GN, Soderberg I, Lindholm M, et al. Inhibition of atherosclerosis in ApoE-Null mice by immunization with ApoB-100 peptide sequences. Arterioscler Thromb Vasc Biol 2003; 23: 879–84.

110. Fredrikson GN, Hedblad B, Berglund G, et al. Identification of immune responses against aldehyde-modified peptide sequences in ApoB associated with cardiovascular disease. Arterioscler Thromb Vasc Biol 2003; 23: 872–8.

111. Schiopu A, Bengtsson J, Soderberg I, et al. Recombinant human antibodies against aldehyde-modified apolipoprotein B-100 peptide sequences inhibit atherosclerosis. Circulation 2004; 110: 2047–52.

112. Schiopu A, Frendeus B, Jansson B, et al. Recombinant antibodies to an oxidized low-density lipoprotein epitope induce rapid regression of atherosclerosis in apobec-1(-/-)/low-density lipoprotein receptor(-/-) mice. J Am Coll Cardiol 2007; 50: 2313–8.

Index

Printed and bound by CPI Group (UK) Ltd, Croydon, CR0 4YY

24/10/2024

01778288-0005